CORONAVIRUSES AND THEIR DISEASES

ADVANCES IN EXPERIMENTAL MEDICINE AND BIOLOGY

Recent Volumes in this Series

Volume 273
TOBACCO SMOKING AND ATHEROSCLEROSIS: Pathogenesis and Cellular
Mechanisms
Edited by John N. Diana

Volume 274
CIRCULATING REGULATORY FACTORS AND NEUROENDOCRINE FUNCTION
Edited by John C. Porter and Daniela Ježová

Volume 275
PHOSPHOLIPASE A₂: Role and Function in Inflammation
Edited by Patrick Y-K Wong and Edward A. Dennis

Volume 276
CORONAVIRUSES AND THEIR DISEASES
Edited by David Cavanagh and T. David K. Brown

Volume 277
OXYGEN TRANSPORT TO TISSUE XII
Edited by Johannes Piiper, Thomas K. Goldstick, and Michael Meyer

Volume 278
IMMUNOBIOLOGY AND PROPHYLAXIS OF HUMAN HERPESVIRUS
INFECTIONS
Edited by Carlos Lopez, Ryoichi Mori, Bernard Roizman, and Richard J. Whitley

Volume 279
BIOCHEMISTRY, MOLECULAR BIOLOGY, AND PHYSIOLOGY OF
PHOSPHOLIPASE A₂ AND ITS REGULATORY FACTORS
Edited by Anil B. Mukherjee

Volume 280
MYOBLAST TRANSFER THERAPY
Edited by Robert C. Griggs and George Karpati

Volume 281
FIBRINOGEN, THROMBOSIS, COAGULATION, AND FIBRINOLYSIS
Edited by Chung-Yuan Liu and Shu Chien

A Continuation Order Plan is available for this series. A continuation order will bring delivery of each new volume immediately upon publication. Volumes are billed only upon actual shipment. For further information please contact the publisher.

CORONAVIRUSES AND THEIR DISEASES

Edited by

David Cavanagh

AFRC Institute for Animal Health
Huntingdon, United Kingdom

and

T. David K. Brown

University of Cambridge
Cambridge, United Kingdom

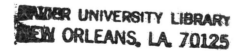
PLENUM PRESS • NEW YORK AND LONDON

Library of Congress Cataloging-in-Publication Data

International Symposium on Coronaviruses (4th : 1989 : Cambridge,
  England)
    Coronaviruses and their diseases / edited by David Cavanagh and T.
  David K. Brown.
       p.   cm. -- (Advances in experimental medicine and biology ; v.
  276)
    "Proceedings of the Fourth International Symposium on
  Coronaviruses, held July 16-21, 1989, in Cambridge, United Kingdom"-
  -T.p. verso.
    Includes bibliographical references and index.
    ISBN 0-306-43664-7
    1. Coronaviruses--Congresses. 2. Coronavirus infections-
  -Pathogenesis--Congresses.   I. Cavanagh, David, Ph. D. II. Brown,
  T. David K. III. Title. IV. Series.
  QR399.I595 1989
  616'.0194--dc20   90-14242
                                                            CIP

Proceedings of the Fourth International Symposium on Coronaviruses,
held July 16–21, 1989, in King's College, Cambridge, United Kingdom

ISBN 0-306-43664-7

© 1990 Plenum Press, New York
A Division of Plenum Publishing Corporation
233 Spring Street, New York, N.Y. 10013

Printed in the United States of America

PREFACE

Interest in the coronaviruses has never been greater. Their economic impact is considerable as they infect humans, livestock, poultry and companion animals. Murine hepatitis virus (MHV) infection of the mouse and rat central nervous systems are the subject of intense study ; these investigations are providing insights into the potential role of viruses in human neurological diseases and, more generally, into mechanisms causing neurological damage.

The single-stranded, positive-sense RNA genomes of two species of these enveloped viruses (IBV and MHV) have been cloned completely and one of them (IBV) sequenced in its entirety, revealing a genome size of some 27000 nucleotides. This has made possible more incisive investigations into the nature of those polypeptides, encoded by more than half of the genome, which are likely to contribute, in the main, to RNA polymerase/replicase activity. Intriguingly, ribosomal frameshifting is exhibited within the mRNA coding for these polypeptides.

The cloning/sequencing phase of coronavirology for which the 1980's will be partly remembered, has provided a sound framework for further studies of the virus structural proteins and also some provocative insights relevant to these studies. The large spike glycoprotein(s), responsible for membrane fusion and bearing important antigenic sites, varies amazingly in length and composition both within as well as between coronavirus species. Receptors on host cells have been identified. The integral membrane glycoprotein (M) has been shown to use internal hydrophobic sequences to direct translocation within membranes. For a long time virtually ignored, the phosphorylated nucleocapsid protein (N) is attracting renewed interest as a regulatory protein. Finally, and perhaps most surprisingly, the "extra" glycoprotein possessed by a sub-set of the genus has been shown not only to have acetyl-esterase receptor-destroying activity (in addition to haemagglutination), but also to have sequence homology with the HEF1, subunit of the influenza C virus glycoprotein. Consequently, this protein has been named the haemagglutinin-esterase glycoprotein (HE).

A high-point of the meeting was the presentation of data which demonstrate that, at least in the case of porcine transmissible gastroenteritis virus (TGEV), synthesis of subgenomic mRNAs occurs, in part, from subgenomic negative strand templates; this represents a novel amplification mechanism for viral mRNA synthesis. It may well turn out to be a general feature of coronavirus replication with interesting implications for the control of mRNA abundance.

An exciting observation with great relevance to coronavirus evolution has been the experimental demonstration of high frequency recombination, *in vivo* as well as *in vitro*. Circumstantial evidence for evolution of IBV in the field is now available. A new disease of pigs has been shown to be closely related to TGEV, but with a tropism for the respiratory tract as opposed to the gut, hence its name of porcine respiratory coronavirus (PRCV). Turkey enteric coronavirus (TCV) has at last attracted detailed analysis, results showing that it has much more in common with the HE-containing mammalian viruses than with avian infectious bronchitis virus (IBV) of chickens. The epizootiology of IBV, which exhibits remarkable antigenic diversity, is now being clarified by sequencing and monoclonal antibody analysis, as are antigenic sites of TGEV and bovine coronavirus (BCV).

Elegant studies, using rats and mice, have revealed much about the pathogenesis of MHV infection within the central nervous system e.g. the relative susceptibility of different cells such as oligodendrocytes and astrocytes, and the immunopathogenesis of demyelination. It is with MHV, and most recently PRCV, that molecular analysis is beginning to illuminate the basis for tissue-tropisms and other features of pathogenesis.

The great interest in the coronaviruses was reflected by the attendance of some 120 participants at the Fourth International Symposium on Coronaviruses, held in July 1989 at King's College, Cambridge, UK. Molecular and pathogenicity-based sessions were interspersed to encourage full participation, but in this volume the molecular and pathogenesis chapters have been presented separately for convenience. As during the Symposium, where they were well received, several chapters commence with an invited "Background Paper" to help put new data into context.

We take this opportunity to thank again those companies who supported the Symposium financially: Intervet International BV; Norden Laboratories; The Wellcome Foundation; Roche Products Limited and Ross Breeders Limited.

The Symposium was a great success and it was agreed that a Fifth International Symposium on Coronaviruses will be held in France in 1992, organised by Dr. Hubert Laude and colleagues.

David Cavanagh, Ph.D.
Agricultural & Food Research Council
Institute for Animal Health
UK

T. David K. Brown, Ph.D.
Department of Pathology
University of Cambridge
UK

CONTENTS

Revised Nomenclature for Coronavirus Structural Proteins, mRNAs
and Genes 1
    D. Cavanagh, D. Brian, L. Enjuanes, K. Holmes, M. Lai,
    H. Laude, S. Siddell, W. Spaan, F. Taguchi and P. Talbo

CHAPTER 1. THE SPIKE (S) GLYCOPROTEIN

Background Paper: Functions of Coronavirus Glycoproteins 5
    K.V. Holmes and R.K. Williams

Biosynthesis and Function of the Coronavirus Spike Protein 9
    H. Vennema, P.J.M. Rottier, L. Heijnen, G.J. Godeke,
    M.C. Horzinek and W.J.M. Spaan

Functional Analysis of the Coronavirus MHV-JHM Surface
Glycoproteins in Vaccinia Virus Recombinants 21
    M. Pfleiderer, E. Routledge and S.G. Siddell

Role of pH in Syncytium Induction and Genome Uncoating of
Avian Infectious Bronchitis Coronavirus (IBV) 33
    D. Li and D. Cavanagh

Is the 110K Glycoprotein the Only Receptor for MHV and Does Its
Expression Determine Species Specificity? 37
    K.V. Holmes, R.K. Williams, C.B. Cardellichio, S.R. Compton,
    C.B. Stephensen, S.W. Snyder, M.F. Frana, Gui-Seng Jiang,
    A. Smith and R.L. Knobler

MHV-Resistant SJL/J Mice Express a Non-Functional Homolog
to the MHV Receptor Glycoprotein 45
    R.K. Williams, S.W. Snyder and K.V. Holmes

Fc Receptor-like Activity of Mouse Hepatitis Virus E2
Glycoprotein 51
    E.L. Oleszak and J.L. Leibowitz

Mouse Fibroblast Mutants Selected for Survival Against
Mouse Hepatitis Virus Infection Show Increased
Resistance to Infection and Virus-induced Cell
Fusion 59
    M. Daya, F. Wong, M. Cervin, G. Evans, H. Vennema,
    W.J.M. Spaan and R. Anderson

On the Membrane Cytopathology of Mouse Hepatitis Virus
    Infection as Probed by a Semi-permeable
    Translation-inhibiting Drug 67
    G. Macintyre, C. Kooi, F. Wong and R. Anderson

Molecular Characterization of the 229E Strain of
    Human Coronavirus 73
    N. Arpin and P.J. Talbot

Sequence Analysis of the 3' End (8740 Nucleotides) of BECV Genome;
    Comparison with Homologous MHV Nucleotide Sequence 81
    P. Boireau, N. Woloszyn, C. Crucière, E. Savoysky and
    J. Laporte

CHAPTER 2. THE HAEMAGGLUTININ-ESTERASE (HE) AND MEMBRANE (M) GLYCOPROTEINS

Background Paper: Coronavirus M and HE: Two Peculiar
    Glycoproteins 91
    P.J.M. Rottier

Structure and Expression of the Bovine Coronavirus
    Hemagglutinin Protein 95
    T.E. Kienzle, S. Abraham, B.G. Hogue and D.A. Brian

The Haemagglutinin of Bovine Coronavirus Exhibits Significant
    Similarity to the Haemagglutinin of Type C
    Influenza Virus 103
    M.D. Parker, G.J. Cox, D. Yoo, D.R. Fitzpatrick and
    L.A. Babiuk

Isolation and Characterization of the Acetylesterase of
    Haemagglutinating Encephalomyelitis Virus (HEV) 109
    B. Schultze, R. Günter Heß, R. Rott, H-D. Klenk and
    G. Herrler

Differential Reactivity of Bovine Coronavirus (BCV) and
    Influenza C Virus with N-Acetyl-9-0-Acetylneuraminic
    Acid (NEU5,9AC$_2$)-Containing Receptors 115
    B. Schultze, H.J. Groß, H.D. Klenk, R. Brossmer and
    G. Herrler

Expression of the Porcine Transmissible Gastroenteritis
    Coronavirus M Protein 121
    B.G. Hogue and D.P. Nayak

Expression of MHV-A59. M Glycoprotein: Effects of Deletions on
    Membrane Integration and Intracellular Transport 127
    P.J.M. Rottier, J.K. Locker, M.C. Horzinek and W.J.M. Spaan

CHAPTER 3. B- AND T-CELL EPITOPES OF THE STRUCTURAL PROTEINS

Background Paper: Mapping Epitopes on Coronavirus Glycoproteins . . . 139
    H. Laude

Binding of Antibodies that Strongly Neutralise Infectious Bronchitis
  Virus is Dependent on the Glycosylation of the Viral
  Peplomer Protein 143
  G. Koch and A. Kant

Enteric Coronavirus TGEV: Mapping of Four Major Antigenic Determinants
  in the Amino Half of Peplomer Protein E2 151
  B. Delmas, M. Godet, J. Gelfi, D. Rasschaert, H. Laude

Location of Antigenic Sites of the S-Glycoprotein of Transmissible
  Gastroenteritis Virus and their Conservation in
  Coronaviruses 159
  L. Enjuanes, F. Gebauer, I. Correa, M.J. Bullido, C. Suñé,
  C. Smerdou, C. Sánchez, J.A. Lenstra, W.P.A. Posthumus
  and R.H. Meloen

Topological and Functional Analysis of Epitopes on the S(E2)
  and HE(E3) Glycoproteins of Bovine Enteric Coronavirus . . . 173
  J.F. Vautherot, M.F. Madelaine and J. Laporte

Linear Neutralizing Epitopes on the Peplomer Protein of
  Coronaviruses 181
  W.P.A. Posthumus, R.H. Meloen, L.Enjuanes, I.Correa, A.P. van
  Nieuwstadt, G.Koch, R.J. de Groot, J.G.Kusters, W.Luytjes,
  W.J.Spaan, B.A.M. van der Zeijst and J.A.Lenstra

The Nucleocapsid Protein of IBV Comprises Immunodominant
  Determinants Recognized by T-Cells 189
  A.M.H. Boots, J.G. Kusters, B.A.M. van der Zeijst
  and E.J. Hensen

CHAPTER 4:   EXPRESSION AND IMMUNOGENICITY OF THE STRUCTURAL PROTEINS

Background Paper: Progress Towards a Coronavirus Recombinant
  DNA Vaccine 201
  W.J.M. Spaan

Protection of Mice from Lethal Coronavirus
  MHV-A59 Infection by Monoclonal Affinity-Purified
  Spike Glycoprotein 205
  C.Daniel and P.J. Talbot

Expression of the Spike Protein of Murine Coronavirus JHM Using a
  Baculovirus Vector 211
  F.Taguchi, S. Yoden, S. Siddell and T. Kikuchi

Immunogenicity of Recombinant Feline Infectious Peritonitis
  Virus Spike Protein in Mice and Kittens 217
  H. Vennema, R.J. de Groot, D.A. Harbour, M. Dalderup,
  T. Gruffydd-Jones, M.C. Horzinek and W.J.M. Spaan

Expression of TGEV Structural Genes in Virus Vectors 223
  D.J. Pulford, P. Britton, K.W. Page and D.J. Garwes

CHAPTER 5: THE NUCLEOCAPSID (N) PROTEIN

Background Paper: Functions of the Coronavirus Nucleocapsid
    Protein 235
    P.S. Masters and L.S. Sturman

Structure and Function Studies of the Nucleocapsid Protein of
    Mouse Hepatitis Virus 239
    P.S. Masters, M.M. Parker, C.S. Ricard, C.Duchala,
    M.F. Frana, K.V. Holmes and L.S. Sturman

MHV Leader RNA Secondary Structure Affects Binding to
    the Nucleocapsid Protein 247
    L.M. Welter, S.A. Stohlman and R.J. Deans

In Vivo and In Vitro Models of Demyelinating Disease:
    A Phosphoprotein Phosphatase in Host Cell Endosomes
    Dephosphorylating the Nucleocapsid Protein of
    Coronavirus JHM 255
    D.V. Mohandas and S. Dales

In Vivo and In Vitro Models of Demyelinating Disease: Possible
    Relationship Between Induction of Regulatory Subunit
    from cAMP Dependent Protein Kinase and Inhibition of
    JHMV Replication in Cultured Oligodendrocytes 261
    G.A.R. Wilson, D.V. Mohandas and S. Dales

CHAPTER 6: THE POLYMERASE AND OTHER NON-STRUCTURAL PROTEINS

A Ribosomal Frameshift Signal in the Polymerase-Encoding Region
    of the IBV Genome 269
    S.C. Inglis, N. Rolley and I. Brierley

Products of the Polymerase-Encoding Region of the Coronavirus IBV . . 275
    I. Brierley, M.E.G. Boursnell, M.M. Binns, B. Bilimoria,
    N.J. Rolley, T.D.K. Brown and S.C. Inglis

Murine Coronavirus Gene 1 Polyprotein Contains an Autoproteolytic
    Activity 283
    S.C. Baker, N. La Monica, C.K. Shieh and M.M.C. Lai

Detection of Mouse Hepatitis Virus Nonstructural Proteins
    Using Antisera Directed Against Bacterial Viral
    Fusion Proteins 291
    P.W. Zoltick, J.L. Leibowitz, J. DeVries, C.J. Pachuk
    and S.R. Weiss

Nucleotide Sequence of the E2-Peplomer Protein Gene and Partial
    Nucleotide Sequence of the Upstream Polymerase Gene
    of Transmissible Gastroenteritis Virus (Miller Strain) . . . 301
    R.D. Wesley

The Polymerase Gene of Corona- and Toroviruses: Evidence for an
    Evolutionary Relationship 307
    P.J. Bredenbeek, E.J. Snijder, A.F.H. Noten, J.A. den Boon,
    W.M.M. Schaaper, M.C. Horzinek and W.J.M. Spaan

Characterization of the MHV-JHM Non-Structural Protein
Encoded by mRNA 2 317
B. Schwarz, E. Routledge and S. Siddell

CHAPTER 7: TRANSCRIPTION AND REPLICATION

Background Paper: Transcription and Replication of
Coronavirus RNA: a 1989 Update 327
M.M.C. Lai

Coronavirus Subgenomic Replicons as a Mechanism for mRNA
Amplification 335
P.B. Sethna, S.L. Hung and D.A. Brian

Studies of Coronavirus DI RNA Replication Using In Vitro
Constructed DI cDNA Clones 341
S. Makino and M.M.C. Lai

Murine Coronavirus Temperature Sensitive Mutants 349
R.S. Baric, M.C. Schaad, T.Wei, K. Fu, K. Lum, C. Shieh
and S.A. Stohlman

Genomic Organisation of a Virulent Isolate of Porcine
Transmissible Gastroenteritis Virus 357
P. Britton, K.W. Page, D.J. Pulford, D.J. Garwes,
K. Mawditt, F. Stewart, F. Parra, C.L. Otin,
J.M. Alonso and R.S. Carmenes

CHAPTER 8: ASPECTS OF CORONAVIRUS VARIATION AND EVOLUTION

Background Paper: Aspects of Coronavirus Evolution 367
D. Cavanagh and T.D.K. Brown

Molecular Basis of the Variation Exhibited by Avian Infectious
Bronchitis Coronavirus (IBV) 369
D. Cavanagh, P. Davis, J. Cook and D. Li

Sequence Comparisons of the 3' End of the Genomes of Five
Strains of Avian Infectious Bronchitis Virus 373
E.W. Collisson, A.K. Williams, R.V. Haar, W. Li
and L.W. Sneed

Selection of Variants of Avian Infectious Bronchitis Virus
Showing Tropism for Different Organs 379
K. Otsuki, K. Matsuo, N. Maeda, T. Sanekata, and M. Tsubokura

Monoclonal Antibody-Selected Variants of MHV-4 Contain
Substitutions and Deletions in the E2 Spike
Glycoprotein 385
T.M. Gallagher and M.J. Buchmeier

RNA Sequence Analysis of the E2 Genes of Wildtype and
Neuroattenuated Mutants of MHV-4 Reveals a
Hypervariable Domain 395
S.E. Parker and M.J. Buchmeier

Characterization of Attenuated Mutants of MHV3: Importance
    of the E2 Protein in Organ Tropism and Infection
    of Isolated Liver Cells 403
    J.P. Martin, W. Chen, G. Obert, and

Murine Hepatitis Virus JHM Variants Isolated from Wistar
    Furth Rats with Viral-Induced Neurological Disease 411
    V.L. Morris, G.A.R. Wilson, C.E. McKenzie, C. Tieszer,
    N. La Monica, L. Banner, D. Percy, M.M.C. Lai, and
    S. Dales

CHAPTER 9: PORCINE RESPIRATORY CORONAVIRUS

Background Paper: The Appearance of the Porcine Respiratory
    Coronavirus has Created New Problems and Perspectives 419
    M. Pensaert

Induction of Milk IgA Antibodies by Porcine Respiratory
    Coronavirus Infection 421
    P. Callebaut, E. Cox, M. Pensaert and K. van Deun

Sites of Replication of a Porcine Respiratory Coronavirus in
    5-Week-Old Pigs with or Without Maternal Antibodies 429
    E.Cox, M. Pensaert, J. Hooyberghs and K. van Deun

Infection with a New Porcine Respiratory Coronavirus in
    Denmark: Serologic Differentiation from Transmissible
    Gastroenteritis Virus Using Monoclonal Antibodies 435
    P. Have

Molecular Aspects of the Relationship of Transmissible
    Gastroenteritis Virus (TGEV) with Porcine Respiratory
    Coronavirus (PRCV) 441
    P. Britton, D.J. Garwes, K. Page and F. Stewart

CHAPTER 10: TURKEY AND BOVINE CORONAVIRUSES

Characterization and Location of the Structural Polypeptides
    of Turkey Enteric Coronavirus Using Monoclonal Antibodies
    and Enzymatic Treatments 449
    S. Dea, S. Garzon and P. Tijssen

Evidence of Close Relatedness Between Turkey and Bovine
    Coronaviruses 457
    P. Tijssen, A.J. Verbeek and S. Dea

A Comparison of Bovine Coronavirus Strains Using Monoclonal
    Antibodies 461
    M.A. Clark, I. Campbell, A.A. El-Ghorr, D.R. Snodgrass and
    F.M.M. Scott

Analysis of Different Probe-Labeling Systems for Detection
    by Hybridization of Bovine Coronavirus 467
    J.A. Verbeek, S. Dea and P. Tijssen

CHAPTER 11: NON-NEUROLOGICAL DISEASES

Canine Coronavirus Infection in Cats; a Possible Role in Feline
 Infectious Peritonitis 475
 F. McArdle, M. Bennett, R.M. Gaskell, B. Tennant,
 D.F. Kelly and C.J. Gaskell

Characterization of an Attenuated Temperature Sensitive
 Feline Infectious Peritonitis Vaccine Virus 481
 J.D. Gerber, N.E. Pfeiffer, J.D. Ingersoll,
 K.K. Christianson, R.M. Landon, N.L. Selzer and
 W.H. Beckenhauer.

Investigations into Resistance of Chicken Lines to Infection
 with Infectious Bronchitis Virus 491
 J.Cook, K. Otsuki, M. Huggins and N. Bumstead

Comparison of the Replication of Distinct Strains of Human
 Coronavirus OC43 in Organotypic Human Colon Cells
 (Caco-2) and Mouse Intestine 497
 A.R. Collins

Detection of Coronavirus RNA in CNS Tissue of Multiple
 Sclerosis and Control Patients 505
 R.S. Murray, B. MacMillan, G. Cabirac and J.S. Burks

Rabbit Dilated Cardiomyopathy 511
 R.S. Baric, S. Edwards and J.D. Small

Retinopathy Following Intravitreal Injection of Mice with
 MHV Strain JHM 519
 S.G. Robbins, B. Detrick and J.J. Hooks

Reproductive Disorders in Female SHR Rats Infected with
 Sialodacryoadenitis Virus 525
 K. Utsumi, Y. Yokota, T. Ishikawa, K. Ohnishi and K. Fujiwara

Mechanism of Protective Effect of Prostaglandin E in Murine
 Hepatitis Virus Strain 3 Infection: Effects on
 Macrophage Production of Tumour Necrosis Factor,
 Procoagulant Activity and Leukotriene B4 533
 S. Sinclair, M. Abecassis, P.Y. Wong, A. Romaschin,
 L.S. Fung and G. Levy

Mouse Hepatitis Virus 3 Pathogenicity and B and T
 Lymphotropisms 543
 P. Jolicoeur and L. Lamontagne

CHAPTER 12: NEUROLOGICAL CONSEQUENCES OF MURINE HEPATITIS
VIRUS INFECTION OF MICE

Background Paper: Advances in the Study of MHV Infection
 of Mice 555
 S. Kyuwa and S. Stohlman

T Cell-Mediated Clearance of JHMV from the Central Nervous
   System 557
   J. Williamson, S. Kyuwa, F.-I. Wang and S. Stohlman

Immunopathogenesis of Demyelination Induced by MHV-4 565
   J.O. Fleming, F.I. Wang, M.D. Trousdale, D.R. Hinton
   and S.A. Stohlman

Localization of Virus and Antibody Response in Mice Infected
   Persistently with MHV-JHM 573
   G. Jacobsen and S. Perlman

Regulation of MHC Class I and II Antigens of Cerebral
   Endothelial Cells and Astrocytes Following MHV-4
   Infection 579
   J. Joseph, R.L. Knobler, F.D. Lublin and M.N. Hart

Mouse Hepatitis Virus A59 Increases Steady-State Levels of
   mRNAs Encoding Major Histocompatibility Complex
   Antigens 593
   J.L. Gombold and S.R. Weiss

Vacuolar Degeneration Induced by JHM-CC Virus in the CNS of
   Cyclophosphamide-Treated Mice 601
   Y. Iwasaki, N. Hirano, T. Tsukamoto and S. Haga

Vacuolar Encephalomyelopathy in Mice Induced by Intracerebral
   Inoculation with a Coronavirus JHM-CC Strain 609
   T. Tsukamoto, Y. Iwasaki, N. Hirano and S. Haga

Difference in Response of Susceptible Mouse Strains to a
   Small Plaque Mutant (JHM-CC) of Mouse Coronavirus 617
   N. Hirano, T. Tsukamoto, S. Haga and Y. Iwasaki

CHAPTER 13: NEUROLOGICAL CONSEQUENCES OF MURINE HEPATITIS VIRUS INFECTION OF RATS

Background Paper: On the Role of the Immune Response in the Course
   of Coronavirus JHM-Induced Encephalomyelitides in Mice
   and Rats 623
   R. Dörries

Quantitation, Phenotypic Characterization and In Situ Localization
   of Lymphoid Cells in the Brain Parenchyma of Rats with
   Differing Susceptibility to Coronavirus JHM-Induced
   Encephalomyelitis 629
   R. Dörries, S. Schwender, H. Imrich, H. Harms and V. ter Meulen

Coronavirus Induced Demyelinating Encephalomyelitis in Rats:
   Immunopathological Aspects of Viral Persistency 637
   H. Wege, Jörn Winter, H. Körner, Egbert Flory, F. Zimprich and
   H. Lassman

Astrocytes as Antigen Presenting Cells for Primary and
   Secondary T Cell Responses: Effect of Astrocyte
   Infection by Murine Hepatitis Virus 647
   R. Mößner, J. Sedgwick, E. Flory, H. Körner, H. Wege
   and V. ter Meulen

Epigenetic Factors Influencing the Morphogenesis of Primary
    Neural Cell Cultures and the Concomitant Effects
    on Establishing JHMV Infections 655
  J.M.M. Pasick and S. Dales

Index   673

REVISED NOMENCLATURE FOR CORONAVIRUS STRUCTURAL

PROTEINS, mRNAs AND GENES

D. Cavanagh, D. Brian, L. Enjuanes, K. Holmes, M. Lai,
H. Laude, S. Siddell, W. Spaan, F. Taguchi and P. Talbot

At the Fourth International Symposium on Coronaviruses, July 1989, Cambridge, the Coronavirus Study Group (Vertebrate Virus Subcommittee, International Committee on Taxonomy of Viruses) recommended a simplified nomenclature for coronavirus proteins, mRNAs and genes. This was considered necessary because of the confusion being caused by the use of different terms, acronyms and numbering system. Some papers in this book already contain the new nomenclature while others do not. We present here the "old" and the "new" systems to aid the reader. The Study Group believed that, because of a lack of information, it was inappropriate to make recommendations regarding non-structural proteins. For an introduction to the proteins, mRNAs and genes of coronaviruses, the reader is referred to the review by Spaan et al. (1988) and to Background Papers in this volume by Holmes; Rottier; Masters and Sturman and Lai.

Acronyms for the Structural Proteins

Protein	Former acronym	Recommended acronym
Spike glycoprotein ⎤ ⎥ Peplomer glycoprotein ⎦	S,E2	S
N-terminal S cleavage product	S1,E2B	S1
C-terminal S cleavage product	S2,E2A	S2
Haemagglutinin- esterase glycoprotein	E3,H,HA	HE
Integral membrane glycoprotein	IMP,M,E1	M
Nucleocapsid protein	N, NC	N

mRNAs

mRNAs are to be referred to by NUMBERS 1,2,3...., starting with the

Coronaviruses and Their Diseases
Edited by D. Cavanagh and T.D.K. Brown
Plenum Press, New York, 1990

genome-sized mRNA. Consequently, the mRNAs of infectious bronchitis virus (IBV), previously denoted as F,E,D,C,B and A should be referred to as 1,2,3,4,5 and 6, respectively. When a protein has a name and an acronym e.g. S, HE, N, M, the corresponding mRNA may be referred to by number, by acronym or both e.g for the IBV mRNA encoding the spike glycoprotein one can use mRNA2, S mRNA or mRNA2 (S), as appropriate.

When "new" mRNAs are discovered, the use of numbers continues. For example, mRNA2 of murine hepatitis virus (MHV) JHM strain encodes a 30K protein. The more recently discovered mRNA which encodes HE should be referred to as "mRNA2-1", since mRNA3 has previously been used to denote the mRNA encoding S of MHV.

Genes/Open-reading-frames (ORFs)

Genes/ORFs are to be referred to by LETTERS. When the corresponding protein has a name, the acronym (UPPER CASE) should be used e.g. S,HE. Otherwise the gene/ORF should be referred to by the number of the corresponding mRNA plus a letter (lower case) when there is more than one ORF. For example, mRNA3 of IBV has three ORFs, 3a, 3b and 3c. Some strains of MHV-A59 do not have a separate message for the HE protein, indeed they do not make HE. Instead mRNA2 encodes, at its 5' end, a 30K protein (ORF 2a) and also has an untranslated ORF (ORF2b) encoding part of the HE protein.

Reference

1. W. Spaan, D. Cavanagh and M.C. Horzinek. Coronaviruses: Structure and Genome Expression. J.gen.Virol. 69: 2939 (1988).

Chapter 1

The Spike (S) Glycoprotein

BACKGROUND PAPER:

FUNCTIONS OF CORONAVIRUS GLYCOPROTEINS

Kathryn V. Holmes and Richard K. Williams

Department of Pathology
Uniformed Services University of the Health Sciences
Bethesda
Maryland 20814
USA

For coronaviruses, the glycoproteins have both historical and biological significance (1,2). Because some coronaviruses were difficult to isolate and propagate, their characteristic large, petal-shaped spikes first allowed coronaviruses to be identified as related agents in a common family. Viral glycoproteins play important roles throughout the life cycle of coronaviruses. Viral glycoproteins interact with receptors on the host cell membrane and are required for penetration of the viral genome into cells by fusion of the viral envelope with the plasma membrane or endosomal membranes. In virus-infected cells, coronavirus glycoproteins may be glycosylated, acylated, oligomerized, cleaved into subunits by proteases, and transported to specific membrane compartments. The viral glycoproteins participate in assembly of virions, and the intracellular location of viral glycoproteins may determine the location of coronavirus budding. Viral glycoproteins on the surface of infected cells may permit fusion with adjacent cells, and may make the cell susceptible to immune cytolysis or cell-mediated cytotoxicity, or permit hemadsorption. Epitopes of viral glycoproteins may be recognized by neutralizing, non-neutralizing or hemagglutination-inhibiting antibodies. Thus, elucidation of the structure and functions of coronavirus glycoproteins is of central importance in understanding the replicative cycle and pathogenesis of coronaviruses.

A model of a coronavirus virion is shown in Figure 1. All coronaviruses contain the membrane glycoprotein, (M), and the large spike glycoprotein, (S). Virions of serologic groups II and IV may also contain the third glycoprotein, the hemagglutinin esterase (HE), which forms a smaller spike in the viral envelope. These include bovine coronavirus (BCV), human coronavirus OC43 (HCV-OC43), some strains of mouse hepatitis virus (MHV), hemagglutinating encephalomyelitis virus of swine (HEV), and turkey coronavirus (TCV). The amount of HE relative to S in virions may vary considerably.

BIOCHEMICAL CHARACTERISTICS OF CORONAVIRUS ENVELOPE GLYCOPROTEINS

The membrane glycoprotein, (M), has a molecular weight in different coronaviruses which ranges from 20 to 30K. A small portion of the amino terminus extends from the outer surface of the lipid bilayer. On some coronaviruses, eg. MHV, this domain is glycosylated by addition in the Golgi apparatus of short oligosaccharides to serine or threonine residues. In IBV and some other coronaviruses, the oligosaccharides of M are N-linked. The membrane glycoprotein spans the membrane 3 times, and has a large domain beneath the lipid bilayer.

The glycoprotein which makes up the large spike, S, has an apparent molecular weight of 150 to 200K and appears to be a dimer held together by non-covalent bonds. A small carboxy-

Coronaviruses and Their Diseases
Edited by D. Cavanagh and T.D.K. Brown
Plenum Press, New York, 1990

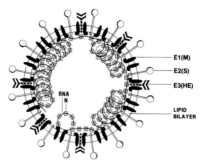

Figure 1. Model of coronavirus virions. The envelopes of all coronaviruses contain membrane glycoprotein, (M) and the spike, (S) glycoprotein. Hemagglutinating coronaviruses contain, in addition, a third glycoprotein hemagglutinin esterase (HE) which forms a short spike on their envelopes. A helical nucleocapsid composed of the nucleocapsid protein N and the plus-strand, genomic RNA is enclosed within the viral envelope. (Reproduced with permission from Academic Press.)

terminal domain rich in cysteine residues is located beneath the lipid bilayer, and the protein traverses the lipid bilayer only once. During maturation and intracellular transport, some molecules of S are cleaved by host cell proteases probably located in the Golgi apparatus to yield two large subunits called S1 and S2. The cleavage is host-cell dependent. Palmitic acid is covalently linked to the carboxy-terminal subunit of S2 which is anchored in the lipid bilayer. Numerous N-linked oligosaccharides are found on both of the subunits of this glycoprotein. Aggregation may occur at alkaline pH.

The 65K HE glycoprotein forms dimers linked together by disulfide bonds which have an apparent molecular weight of 140K. Each of the glycoproteins of several coronaviruses has been cloned, sequenced and expressed in eukaryotic cells.

FUNCTIONS OF CORONAVIRUS ENVELOPE GLYCOPROTEINS

Table 1 summarizes our current understanding of the functions of the three coronavirus glycoproteins. The membrane glycoprotein M of MHV interacts with the nucleocapsid *in vitro* and may aid in virus budding within infected cells by interaction of the cytoplasmic domain with the viral nucleocapsid. Because budding commences in the Golgi apparatus where this glycoprotein accumulates, it is possible that the intracellular location of M determines the site of virus maturation.

The large spike glycoprotein S has two functions which are essential for coronavirus infectivity. For MHV-A59, S interacts with a 110K glycoprotein receptor on the surface of susceptible murine cells, leading to infection. Blocking of the virus-binding domain of this receptor by monoclonal antireceptor antibody prevents infection of the cells. Comparable glycoprotein receptors for other coronaviruses have not yet been identified . S glycoproteins of many coronaviruses cause virus-induced cell fusion. For MHV, protease cleavage may occur either intracellularly, during glycoprotein synthesis and transport through the Golgi apparatus, or extracellularly, using trypsin. The S glycoproteins in IBV, MHV and BCV virions have protease-susceptible sites, but there is no protease susceptible site in the S glycoprotein of FIPV, although this virus can cause cell fusion. Different host cells vary in their susceptibility to fusion with coronaviruses. It is likely but not proven that the cell fusing activity of coronaviruses is caused by the same glycoprotein that fuses the viral envelope with host cell membranes during virus penetration. For IBV and TGEV, S is responsible for hemagglutination. The biological significance of this activity and the characteristics of the receptor for S on erythrocytes are not yet understood. The S glycoprotein stimulates both neutralizing and fusion-inhibiting antibodies. Neutralizing monoclonal antibodies directed against S have been used to select virus variants which show altered pathogenicity *in vivo*. The domains of S which are responsible for its biological activities are now being analyzed.

Table 1. <u>Functions of coronavirus envelope glycoproteins</u>

M	Interaction with nucleocapsid Virion assembly Determination of site virus budding
S	Binding to 110K receptor glycoprotein (MHV) Cell fusion (protease activated for MHV and BCV, not FIPV) Stimulation of neutralizing antibody Stimulation of fusion-inhibiting antibody Hemagglutination (TGEV, IBV)
HE	Hemagglutination (BCV, OC43, HEV, TCV) Binding to 9-O-acetylated neuraminic acid (BCV, OC43) Acetylesterase (BCV, OC43)

Hemagglutination by BCV, OC43, HEV, TCV and some strains of MHV is apparently due to interaction of the HE glycoprotein with a carbohydrate moiety on the surface of erythrocytes. The HE of BCV and HCV-OC43 recognize 9-O-acetylated sialic acid, the same binding moiety used by the influenza C glycoprotein. In addition, these glycoproteins have an acetylesterase activity which can cleave off the 9-O-acetyl group, thereby preventing hemagglutination. A central question is whether infection of cells *in vitro* or *in vivo* can result from the recognition of 9-O-acetylated sialic acid by the HE glycoprotein. If HE can function as a viral attachment protein leading to infection, then it will be important to determine whether S or HE is responsible for fusion of the viral envelope with cellular membranes. The effects upon infection of monoclonal antibodies directed against HE may help to elucidate the role of this glycoprotein in coronavirus infection. For MHV-JHM, there is a suggestion that the HE glycoprotein of this murine virus may be important for infection of the central nervous system of rats. A virus which expresses the mRNA which should encode the HE glycoprotein was selected by passage of MHV-JHM through rat brain. If the HE activity is not required for growth of the virus in cell culture, then virus which has lost the capacity to make HE could outgrow virus which expresses HE.

It is fascinating to consider how serogroups II and IV of the coronavirus family acquired the gene encoding the HE glycoprotein, which resembles in part the glycoprotein of influenza C. This additional glycoprotein may provide these coronaviruses with a broader host range and/or altered pathogenicity in comparison with coronaviruses which encode only the M and S glycoproteins. A careful study of the receptor recognition mechanisms of many coronaviruses may provide new insight into the evolution of the coronavirus family.

ACKNOWLEDGEMENTS

The authors are grateful for discussions with Dr. Lawrence S. Sturman and Dr. Mark F. Frana. This research was supported by NIH grant #18997. Dr. Williams is supported by NRSA #F32AI07810. The opinions or assertion contained herein are the private views of the authors and should not be construed as official or necessarily reflecting the views of the Uniformed Services University of the Health Sciences or the Department of Defense.

REFERENCES

1. Holmes, K.V. Replication of Coronaviruses, in Virology, 2nd Edition, B.N. Fields *et al..*, (eds) Raven Press, New York, in press, 1989.
2. Spaan, W., Cavanagh, D., Horzinek, M.C., Coronaviruses: Structure and genome expression. <u>J. Gen. Virol.</u> 69: 2939-2952, 1988.

BIOSYNTHESIS AND FUNCTION OF THE CORONAVIRUS SPIKE PROTEIN

H. Vennema, P.J.M. Rottier, L. Heijnen, G.J. Godeke,
M.C. Horzinek and W.J.M. Spaan

Department of Virology, Faculty of Veterinary Medicine
State University of Utrecht, Yalelaan 1, P.O. Box 80.165
3508 TD Utrecht, The Netherlands

INTRODUCTION

One of the most interesting aspects of coronavirus replication is their intracellular assembly. Budding is localized in the ER-pre Golgi region (8, 26). Both coronavirus glycoproteins are synthesized in the RER on membrane bound ribosomes (16). The integral membrane protein (M) accumulates in the perinuclear region and is believed to determine the site of budding. The spike protein (S) mediates binding of virions to the host cell receptor, possesses a fusogenic activity and is the major target for virus neutralizing antibodies (22). The primary nucleotide sequence and the predicted amino acid sequence of a number of spike protein genes revealed features characteristic of type I membrane proteins (22).

The S protein of all coronaviruses studied so far is cotranslationally glycosylated. The transport and maturation of S has been studied in coronavirus infected cells (22, 24). Due to the fact that virus budding takes place intracellularly, S protein can be transported in association with cellular or viral membranes. These two transport processes cannot be studied separately. In the present study we have used vaccinia virus recombinants expressing the S gene of three different coronaviruses to study the intracellular transport and maturation of the S protein in the absence of virus budding.

During its synthesis and transport in coronavirus infected cells the S protein is folded and assembled into the structure which finally constitutes the viral spike. From experimental data (1) combined with theoretical analyses (4) a model was deduced picturing the spike as a dimer of the S protein. In order to study this aspect of the maturation of S we have begun to analyze its oligomerization process.

MATERIALS AND METHODS

<u>Cloning of full-length spike protein genes; construction of recombinant vaccinia viruses.</u> The S genes of FIPV strain 79-1146, MHV-A59 and IBV M41 have been cloned and sequenced in our laboratory. The coding sequence of the FIPV S gene was recloned from cDNA clone B1 (5) as described (3). The coding region of the S gene of MHV was reconstructed from two overlapping cDNA clones, B24 and 1F11, (13). The S gene coding

sequence of IBV was isolated from cDNA clone 39 (18). The VSV G coding
region was isolated from plasmid pSVGL11, a derivative of pSVGL (19).
Isolated gene fragments were recloned in transfer vectors pGS20 (15), or
pSC11 (2). Recombinant vaccinia viruses were constructed using established
procedures described previously (2, 15).

Cell culture and protein labelling. FIPV infection was carried out on
NLFK cells at a multiplicity of infection (m.o.i.) of 10 $TCID_{50}$ per cell.
Subconfluent monolayers of NLFK or HeLa cells were infected with different
vaccinia virus recombinants at a m.o.i. of 10 PFU per cell. Protein
labelling was carried out at the times indicated in the legends in
methionine free medium supplemented with ^{35}S-methionine at a concentration
of 0.1mCi/ml. In some cases a pulse labelling period was followed by a
chase with medium containing 4 mM methionine and 10% fetal calf serum.
Cells were lysed in 20mM Tris-HCl pH7.5, 1mM EDTA, 100mM NaCl (TESV),
containing 1% Triton X-100 and 2mM phenyl-methyl-sulphonyl fluoride (PMSF).

Radio immunoprecipitation and endo H analysis. Immunoprecipitations
were carried out overnight at 4°C in TESV, 0.4% Triton X-100, at a 600-
fold antiserum dilution for lysates of recombinant vaccinia virus infected
cells and at a 100-fold dilution for lysates of FIPV and mock infected
cells. After the addition of KCl to 0.5M, immunecomplexes were bound to
Staph A (Pansorbin Cells, Calbiochem) for 2.5h at 4°C and pelleted by
centrifugation. Pellets were washed three times in TESV, 0.1% Triton X-100.
The final pellet was suspended in 50mM Tris-HCl pH 6.8, 0.25% SDS and
heated for 2 min at 95°C to dissolve immune complexes. Immunoprecipitated
proteins were treated with endo H (Boerhinger Mannheim) by adding 15μl
150mM Na-Citrate pH 5.3 and 1mU endo H to 10μl supernatant of dissolved
immunecomplexes and overnight incubation at 37°C or mock treated by
incubation without enzyme and analyzed in 10% SDS polyacrylamide gels.

Oligomerization assay. ^{35}S-labelled MHV-A59 was prepared from the
medium of infected Sac$^-$ cells (25cm^2) incubated from 6-9h p.i. in cysteine-
free MEM containing 2% foetal calf serum (FCS) to which was added 150μCi
^{35}S-cysteine at 6h and at 7.5h p.i. Virus was collected by precipitation
with 8% PEG in the presence of 2.3% NaCl and dissolved in MNT (20mM MES,
30mM Tris-HCl, 100mM NaCl, 1.25mM EDTA, 1mM EGTA, pH 5.8) containing 1%
Triton X-100. The cells were lysed in the same buffer, cleared by
centrifugation and the supernatant was used for gradient analysis. For the
pulse-chase experiment MHV-A59 infected Sac$^-$ cells (75cm^2) were trypsinized
and labelled in suspension in 200μl of the above labelling medium to which
now was added 400μCi ^{35}S-cysteine. After the 3 min pulse one 30μl sample of
the cells was lysed immediately in 220μl ice-cold MNT containing 1% Triton
X-100. Five similar samples were suspended in preincubated chase medium
(DMEM containing 5% FCS and 2mM cysteine), incubated for various times,
harvested and lysed in the same buffer.

For sedimentation analysis samples were loaded onto 5-20% (w/w)
continuous sucrose gradients in MNT buffer containing 0.1% Triton X-100 and
centrifuged in a SW50.1 rotor (Beckman Instruments) for 10h at 45,000rpm
and 4°C. Fractions were collected from the bottom. Viral proteins were
precipitated using 1μl rabbit polyclonal antiserum against MHV-A59 and 15μl
Staph A and prepared for SDS-PAGE. To analyze possible complexes pelleted
through the gradient, material at the bottom of the tube was dissolved and
immuneprecipitated as well. All samples were heated for 5 min at 95°C prior
to PAGE. As sedimentation markers the following proteins were used:
thyroglobulin, β-glucuronidase, catalase, lactate dehydrogenase and BSA,
which have molecular weights of 669, 280, 232, 140, and 67kD. Their
positions in the gradients were determined by Coomassie blue staining of
gels run with material from each fraction.

RESULTS

Expression of recombinant S proteins. Recombinant vaccinia viruses encoding S proteins of FIPV, MHV and IBV under control of the vaccinia 7.5kD promoter were constructed as described in materials and methods and designated vFS, vMS and vIS, respectively. Recombinant S proteins were labelled with ^{35}S-methionine and compared to their respective coronavirus counterparts after immunoprecipitation and SDS-PAGE analysis. Figure 1 shows the results for the FIPV spike protein. Endoglycosidase H (Endo H) was used to deglycosylate glycoproteins. Both the untreated as well as the deglycosylated recombinant and FIPV spike proteins comigrated in SDS-PAGE (FIG. 1). Similar results were obtained for IBV and MHV spike proteins (data not shown).

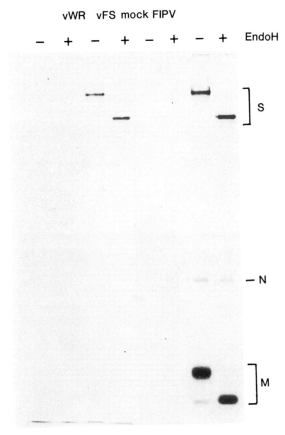

FIG. 1. Radio immunoprecipitation (RIP) and SDS-PAGE analysis of recombinant FIPV S protein. Recombinant (vFS) and wild type (vWR) vaccinia virus infected cells were labelled for 30 min at 16h p.i.. FIPV and mock infected cells were labelled at 8h p.i.. RIP was carried out. FIPV structural proteins (S, N and M) are indicated. Immunoprecipitates were split in two samples; one half was mock treated and the other was treated with endo H (indicated with - and +, respectively).

Biological activity of recombinant S proteins. Cell surface expression
was demonstrated by immunofluorescence staining of unfixed cells
(manuscript submitted). S protein expressed on the surface of infected
cells is thought to induce cell-cell fusion (24). This phenomenon was
evident from the appearance of large syncytia in vFS infected NLFK cells
and vMS infected Sac⁻ cells (FIG. 2). No syncytia formation was observed in
NLFK or Sac⁻ cells infected with wild type vaccinia virus or with vIS.
Induction of cell fusion by recombinant vFS was restricted to cells of
feline origin, whereas vMS induced fusion was observed only in murine
cells. These results suggest a relation between susceptibility of cells for
a certain coronavirus and the ability of the respective S protein to induce
fusion.

Intracellular transport of recombinant S proteins. During the transfer
from the RER to the trans-Golgi compartment, the oligosaccharide side
chains of N-glycosylated glycoproteins are processed and modified. The co-
translationally added high mannose side chains which are endo H sensitive
become endo H resistant in the medial-Golgi compartment (9). Therefore, the
rate of acquisition of endo H resistance can be used to study intracellular
transport kinetics. To analyze the rate of acquisition of resistance to
digestion by endo H we performed pulse chase experiments, followed by RIP
and endo H digestions, with vFS, vMS and vIS infected NLFK cells. In
addition a recombinant vaccinia virus, designated vVG, expressing the VSV G

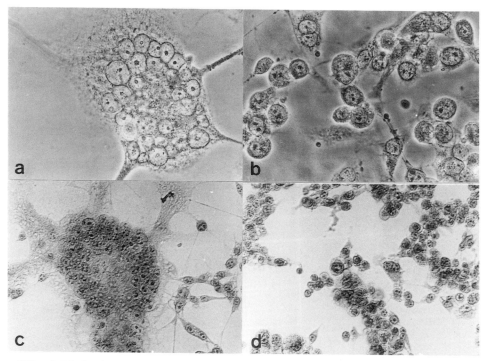

FIG. 2.Biological activity of recombinant S proteins. NLFK cells were
    infected with vFS (a) or vWR (b). Infected NLFK cells were
    photographed using dark field microscopy, x400. Sac⁻ cells were
    infected with vMS (c) or vWR (d). Infected Sac⁻ cells were
    stained for nuclei using hematoxylin and photographed under light
    microscopy, x100.

protein was included in this study. Figure 3 shows the results of a 30 min pulse labelling and a 60 min chase period. It can be seen that none of the three coronavirus S proteins acquired any detectable resistance to endo H during the 1h chase period. In the lanes of the vMS lysates two background bands can be seen besides the S protein band. The upper band appears to be a glycoprotein. At the end of the pulse labelling period this protein was already partially resistant to endo H and completely so after the 1h chase period.

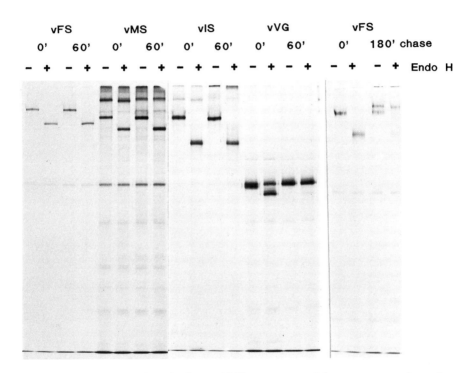

FIG. 3. Endo H analysis of three different recombinant coronavirus S
proteins and of recombinant VSV G protein. Infected NLFK cells
were pulse-labelled at 12h p.i for 30 min and lysed immediately
or after a chase of 1h or 3h (vFS). Recombinant vaccinia viruses
are indicated above each panel of 4 lanes.

In contrast to the S proteins, the VSV G-protein has become partially resistant to digestion by endo H during the 30 min pulse labelling period. After the 60 min chase period all of the VSV G-protein was resistant to endo H. During longer chase periods a higher molecular weight form of the recombinant FIPV S protein appeared which was resistant to digestion by endo H, albeit not completely. After a 3h chase period about half of the recombinant S protein was still sensitive to digestion by endo H (FIG. 3). The half time of acquisition of endo H resistance of the recombinant S proteins of MHV and IBV was also estimated to be approximately 3h (data not shown).

<u>Biosynthesis of the S protein in FIPV infected cells.</u> To study the biosynthesis of S in FIPV infected cells we analyzed the structural proteins in cell lysates and of virions released into the extracellular medium. Endo H analysis of intracellular and virion protein showed that the virion S protein was endo H resistant. The amount of intracellular S protein decreased during chases due to release into the medium. Intracellular S protein was endo H sensitive even after prolonged incubation (manuscript submitted).

The rate of acquisition of resistance to endo H digestion was determined using combined lysates, which were prepared by adding concentrated lysis buffer and protease inhibitor to a culture dish without removing the medium. FIPV infected NLFK cells were pulse labelled for 20 min at 9h p.i. and chased for different periods. The results of this experiment are shown in Figure 4. Approximately half of the labelled spike protein has become resistant to digestion by endo H after a chase period of 1h. After 2h the amount of endo H sensitive material has further decreased. A small amount of endo H sensitive material remains after a 4h chase period.

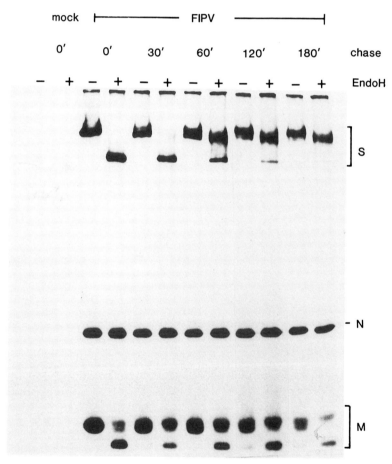

FIG. 4. Kinetics of endo H resistance acquisition of the S protein in FIPV infected NLFK cells. Metabolic labelling was carried out at 9h p.i. for 30 min. Lysates were prepared immediately or after the indicated chase times. Intracellular and virion proteins were analyzed together in combined lysates. More than half of the labelled S protein is endo H resistant after 1h.

Oligomeric structure and kinetics of oligomerization of the S protein in MHV infected cells. The analysis of the oligomeric state of the S protein in cells as well as in virions was performed in sucrose density gradients. Under the conditions described, the S protein of purified MHV-A59, dissolved in 1% Triton X-100 sedimented deep into the gradient peaking in fractions 2 and 3 (Fig. 5). It occurred there both in its 180kD uncleaved form and as the 90kD cleavage products. The same species were also found at the same position in gradients loaded with a lysate of MHV-A59 infected cells after a 3h labelling period. In addition, the S protein precursor gp150 was found in this gradient peaking at two positions namely around fractions 3 and 8 (Fig. 5). In order to determine the complexity of these S species their sedimentation rates were compared with those of a number of marker proteins. These analyses were perfomed both in the SW50.1 rotor and using the SW40 (data not shown). From this it followed that gp150 occurs as a momomer and as a dimer (peaks around fraction 8 and 3, respectively) and that the gp180 and gp90 species are present as the homodimer (gp180)$_2$ and the cleaved form thereof, the heterotetramer (90A/90B)$_2$.

The order and time-course of appearance of the various S structures in MHV-A59 infected cells were determined by gradient analysis of samples from a pulse-chase experiment. As illustrated in Fig. 6, S is synthesized as its precursor gp150 in the form of a monomer that dimerizes slowly. Then (gp150)$_2$ is converted to the (gp180)$_2$ form which subsequently undergoes cleavage giving rise to the (90A/90B)$_2$ structure.

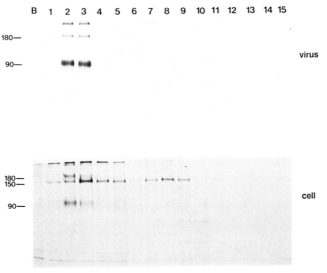

FIG. 5. Sedimentation analysis of MHV-A59 S protein from purified virus and from infected cells. Viral and cellular material was prepared by a 3h labelling with ^{35}S-cysteine and analyzed after sucrose gradient centrifugation. Numbers on top refer to the fractions obtained, 1 and 15 representing bottom and top of the gradient, respectively. In lane B the material was analyzed that pelleted through the gradient to the bottom of the tube. Arrows indicate the positions of the markers β-glucuronidase (280kD) and catalase (232kD) run in a parallel gradient.

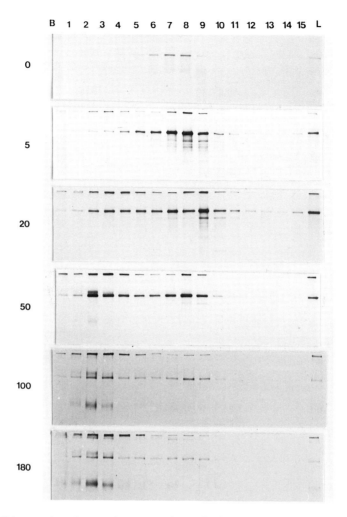

FIG. 6. Oligomerization and maturation of the S protein. The fate of S synthesized as its precursor gp150 during a 3 min pulse labelling was followed by analysis of cells chased for 5, 20, 50, 100. and 180 min. In the lanes marked L an unfractionated sample of each lysate was analyzed after immuneprecipitation. The precursor is seen to dimerize, to be subsequently converted to (gp180)$_2$ and to finally be cleaved.

DISCUSSION

In this paper we showed that several coronavirus S proteins expressed from cloned cDNA are transported slowly to the medial-Golgi where endo H resistance is acquired. Comparison of the transport rates of the recombinant S protein to the S protein in FIPV infected cells showed that the retention of the S protein only occurs in the absence of budding. This specific retention can be interpreted as transient accumulation between RER and medial-Golgi, possibly to allow efficient incorporation in budding virions. A second possible interpretation of this retention may be that the S protein localizes the budding event itself. The fact that the M protein of MHV accumulates in the perinuclear region in infected cells has led to the assumption that the M protein determines the site of budding (12). This view was supported by the observation that the M protein accumulates in the Golgi apparatus in cDNA expressing cells (14, 20). However, the rate of O-glycosylation and terminal sialylation of the MHV-A59 M protein in transfected COS cells (20) was the same as in MHV-A59 infected Sac⁻ cells. This means that the M protein is not specifically retained in the region where budding takes place, since sialylation occurs in trans-Golgi.

It has been shown that in the presence of tunicamycine spikeless non-infectious virus particles are assembled (12, 17, 21, 23). On the basis of these data it was assumed that the S protein is not necessary for virus budding. As was already pointed out, the unglycosylated S protein is probably degraded and this may occur after incorporation in virions (21, 23).

Control experiments with VSV G-protein expressed in the same way as the coronavirus S proteins showed that the observed phenomenon of slow intracellular transport is coronavirus specific and not due to the expression system we used.

In contrast to the M protein S is transported to the plasma membrane. This intrinsic property of the S protein may be responsible for transport of virus particles. Cell surface expression of recombinant S proteins was demonstrated among others by the induction of cell-to-cell fusion. The cell fusion data suggest a relationship between cell susceptibility for a coronavirus and the ability of the respective S protein to induce cell-to-cell fusion. Recombinant vaccinia viruses now offer the possibility to test factors influencing cell fusion, independent of coronavirus replication.

Our studies of the complexity of S in viral particles confirmed the models put forward earlier (1, 4). They demonstrated that the peplomers are indeed composed of 2 S molecules which in cases like MHV-A59 and IBV are cleaved. The biogenesis of the spikes involves the dimerization of the primary translation product of the S-mRNA. This is a slow process when compared to the trimerization of G and HA from VSV (6) and influenza virus (10), respectively, but occurs faster than trimerization of the Rous sarcoma virus env glycoprotein (11). Exactly where dimerization of gp150 occurs is still unclear. It is likely, however, to take place before its passage through the trans-Golgi compartment since it preceeds the appearance of gp180, the charactistic product resulting from the processing of the oligosaccharides in the Golgi apparatus. Assuming that the S protein is incorporated into the virion at the time of budding, the gp150-dimer constitutes the initial spike structure. Interestingly, no monomer forms of gp180 were detected in the gradients. This indicates that dimerization is a very efficient process or that it is a prerequisite for transport through the Golgi system. The latter has been shown for some viral glycoproteins destined for the plasma membrane (6, 7, 10). It may also indicate that dimerization is a precondition as well for incorporation into viral particles.

Cleavage of viral membrane glycoproteins is known to occur with many viruses. It generally constitutes one of the last steps in the maturation of the proteins and is required to activate viral infectivity. Though cleavage is not essential for all coronaviruses, the same principles seem to hold true for MHV-A59 (26). Our gradient analyses show that the first 90kD cleavage products are detectable as soon as gp180-dimers have appeared. This implies that cleavage of S occurs either while still in the trans-Golgi compartment or shortly after its exit to the cell surface.

LITERATURE

1. Cavanagh, D. 1983. Coronavirus IBV: Structural characterization of the spike protein. J. Gen. Virol. 64:2577-2583.

2. Chakrabarti, S., K. Brechling, and B. Moss. 1985. Vaccinia virus expression vector: Coexpression of β-galactosidase provides visual screening of recombinant virus plaques. Mol. Cell Biol. 5:3403-3409.

3. de Groot, R.J., R.W. van Leen, M.J.M Dalderup, H. Vennema, M.C. Horzinek, and W.J.M. Spaan. 1989. Stably expressed FIPV peplomer protein induces cell fusion and elecits neutralizing antibodies in mice. Virology 171:493-502

4. de Groot, R.J., W. Luytjes, M.C. Horzinek, B.A.M. van der Zeijst, W.J.M. Spaan, and J.A. Lenstra. 1987. Evidence for a coiled-coil structure in the spike proteins of coronaviruses. J. Mol. Biol. 196:963-966.

5. de Groot, R.J., J. Maduro, J.A. Lenstra, M.C. Horzinek, B.A.M. van der Zeijst, and W.J. Spaan. 1987. cDNA cloning and sequence analysis of the gene encoding the peplomer protein of feline infectious peritonitis virus. J. Gen. Virol. 68:2639-2646.

6. Doms, R.W., D.S. Keller, A. Helenius, and W.E. Balch. 1987. Role for adenosine triphosphate in regulating the assembly and transport of vesicular stomatits virus G protein. J. Cell Biol. 105:1957-1969.

7. Doms, R.W., A. Ruusala, C. Machammer, J. Helenius, A. Helenius, and J.K. Rose. 1988. Differential effects of mutations in three domains on folding, quarternary structure, and intracellular transport of vesicular stomatist virus G protein. J. Cell Biol. 107:89-99.

8. Dubois-Dalcq, M.E., E.W. Doller, M.V. Haspel, and K.V. Holmes. 1982. Cell tropism and expression of mouse hepatitis viruses (MHV) in mouse spinal cord cultures. Virology 119:317-331.

9. Dunphy, W.G., and J.E. Rothman. 1985. Compartmental organization of the golgi stack. Cell 42:13-21.

10. Gething, M.-J., K. McCammon, and J. Sambrook. 1986. Expression of wild-type and mutant forms of influenza hemagglutinin: The role of folding in intracellular transport. Cell 46:939-950.

11. Einfeld, D., and E. Hunter. 1988. Oligomeric structure of a prototype retrovirus glycoprotein. Proc. Natl. Acad. Sci. 85:8688-8692.

12. Holmes, K.V., E.W. Doller, and L.S. Sturman. 1981. Tunicamycin resistant glycosylation of a coronavirus glycoprotein: Demonstration of a novel type of viral glycoprotein. Virology 115:334-344.

13. Luytjes, W., L.S. Sturman, P.J. Bredenbeek, J. Charite, B.A.M. van der Zeijst, M.C. Horzinek, and W.J. Spaan. 1987. Primary structure of the glycoprotein E2 of coronavirus MHV-A59 and identification of the trypsin cleavage site. Virology 161:479-487.

14. Machamer, C.E., and J.K. Rose. 1987. A specific transmembrane domain of a coronavirus E1 glycoprotein is required for its retention in the Golgi region. J. Cell Biol. 105:1205-1214.

15. Mackett, M., G.L. Smith, and B. Moss. 1984. General method for production and selection of infectious vaccinia virus recombinants expressing foreign genes. J. Virol. 49:857-864.

16. Niemann, H., B. Boschek, D. Evans, M. Rosing, T. Tamura, and H.D. Klenk. 1982. Post-translational glycosylation of coronavirus glycoprotein E1: inhibition by monensin. EMBO. J. 1:1499-1504.

17. Niemann, H., and H.-D. Klenk. 1981. Coronavirus glycoprotein E1, a new type of viral glycoprotein. J. Mol. Biol. 153:993-1010.

18. Niesters, H.G., J.A. Lenstra, W.J. Spaan, A.J. Zijderveld, N.M. Bleumink-Pluym, F. Hong, G.J. van Scharrenburg, M.C. Horzinek, and B.A.M. van der Zeijst. 1986. The peplomer protein sequence of the M41 strain of coronavirus IBV and its comparison with Beaudette strains. Virus. Res. 5:253-263.

19. Rose, J.K., and J.E. Bergmann. 1982. Expression from cloned cDNA of cell-surface secreted forms of the glycoprotein of vesicular stomatitis virus in eucaryotic cells. Cell 30:753-762.

20. Rottier, P.J., and J.K. Rose. 1987. Coronavirus E1 glycoprotein expressed from cloned cDNA localizes in the Golgi region. J. Virol. 61:2042-2045.

21. Rottier, P.J.M., M.C. Horzinek, and Zeijst B.A.M. van der. 1981. Viral protein synthesis in mouse hepatitis virus strain A59-infected cells: effect of tunicamycin. J. Virol. 40:350-357.

22. Spaan, W., D. Cavanagh, and M.C. Horzinek. 1988. Coronaviruses: Structure and genome expression. J. Gen. Virol. 69:2939-2952.

23. Stern, D.F., and B.M. Sefton. 1982. Coronavirus proteins: structure and function of the oligosaccharides of the avian infectious bronchitis virus glycoproteins. J. Virol. 44:804-812.

24. Sturman, L., and K. Holmes. 1985. The novel glycoproteins of coronaviruses. TIBS 10:17-20.

25. Sturman, L.S., C.S. Ricard, and K.V. Holmes. 1985. Proteolytic cleavage of the E2 glycoprotein of murine coronavirus: Activation of cell-fusing activity of virions by trypsin and separation of two different 90K cleavage fragments. J. Virol. 56:904-911.

26. Tooze, S.A., J. Tooze, and G. Warren. 1988. Site of addition of N-acetyl-galactosamine to the E1 glycoprotein of mouse hepatitis virus-A59. J. Cell Biol. 106:1475-1487.

FUNCTIONAL ANALYSIS OF THE CORONAVIRUS MHV-JHM SURFACE

GLYCOPROTEINS IN VACCINIA VIRUS RECOMBINANTS

M. Pfleiderer, E. Routledge and S.G. Siddell

Institute of Virology
Versbacher Str. 7
8700 Würzburg

INTRODUCTION

Coronavirus MHV-JHM has two surface glycoproteins. The S protein is a heterodimer comprised of two non-covalently bound,
subunits of about 90,000 molecular weight (mol.wt.) (S_1 and S_2)
which are derived by proteolytic processing of the 180,000
mol.wt. precursor S. Multimers of the heterodimer assemble
together to produce the characteristic peplomer structures at
the surface of the virion. The second surface projection is
smaller and is comprised of disulphide-linked homodimer(s) of
the HE protein. The reduced HE monomer has a mol.wt. of 65,000
(Siddell et al., 1981).

In spite of an increasing amount of structural data regarding
these proteins there is still relatively little known about
their functions. Indirect evidence using S protein specific
monoclonal antibodies (Collins et al., 1982; Wege et al., 1984)
suggests that the MHV S protein mediates binding of the virus to
a cellular receptor and the fusion of viral and cellular membranes. A function for the MHV-JHM HE protein has not been
shown. Earlier results from King et al. (1985) correlated the
haemagglutinating activity of bovine coronavirus (BCV) with the
HE protein and recently Vlasak et al. (1988a) have demonstrated
that BCV and the human coronavirus HCV OC43 can recognize and
destroy a receptor on the cell surface which is similar or identical to the influenza C virus receptor. Moreover, Vlasak et al.
(1988b) could demonstrate that in the case of BCV the receptor
destroying activity associated with the HE protein had the
specificity of an acetylesterase.

Luytjes et al. (1988) have recently cloned and sequenced the
unique region of the MHV-A59 mRNA 2. They found two large open
reading frames (ORFs) of which the downstream ORF lacks an
amino-terminal initiation codon. These authors interpreted this
ORF as a pseudogene but noted a striking similarity with the
HEF_1 subunit of the Influenza C surface glycoprotein (Nakada et
al., 1984).

The aim of the experiments described in this paper were

1) to determine directly whether the MHV-JHM S protein was able to mediate cell fusion
2) to determine the primary sequence of the MHV-JHM HE protein and
3) to determine whether the MHV-JHM HE protein has receptor binding and receptor destroying activities.

RESULTS

I <u>Analysis of the fusion activity of the MHV-JHM S protein</u>

In order to demonstrate that the MHV-JHM S protein is responsible for the fusogenic activity of the virus, we have cloned complete copies of the S gene ORF into the unique Bam HI site of the Vaccinia virus cloning vector pTF7.5 (Fuerst et al., 1987). The isolation and characterization of the S gene cDNA clones will be described in detail elsewhere. The construct, pTF7.5/S+ was then used to transfect DBT cells which had been infected with Vaccinia virus recombinant vTF7.3, which expresses the T7 RNA polymerase gene. Fig. 1 shows the cytopathic effect (c.p.e.) 10 hours after infection and transfection with the Vaccinia virus recombinant vTF7.3 and the recombinant construct pTF7.5/S+. It is evident that the infected/transfected DBT cells display extensive syncytia formation, the characteristic cytopathic result of the MHV-JHM fusogenic activity. This result shows that the MHV-JHM S protein alone is sufficient to mediate the membrane fusion of infected cells. No further component on the surface of the virion is required for this effect.

II <u>Cloning and sequencing of the MHV-JHM HE gene</u>

A cDNA encompassing the unique region of the MHV-JHM mRNA 2-1 was made using a specific oligonucleotide primer, essentially according to the method of Gubler and Hoffman (1983). Within this region, which is 5' proximal to the S gene, is a large ORF of 428 aminoacids with the potential to encode a polypeptide of 47,000 mol.wt. (Fig. 2). Within the sequence are 8 potential N-glycosylation sites which would increase the apparent molecular weight of the protein to approximately 65,000 (the size of the HE protein). At the amino and carboxy-termini of the polypeptide are stretches of hydrophobic aminoacids which could represent a signal recognition sequence and a membrane anchor region respectively, both typical features for membrane bound proteins.

In order to identify the protein product of the MHV-JHM mRNA 2-1 ORF and to analyse its biological functions we have expressed this ORF using a Vaccinia virus expression system. The construction of the clone BSPMHV2-1/1 which contained the mRNA 2-1 ORF and 7 additional nucleotides upstream of the ATG start codon will be described in detail elsewhere. This cDNA was cloned into the unique BamHI site of the pTF7-5 vector with the ATG start codon next to the T7 RNA polymerase promoter. This construct, pTF7-5/MHV2-1, was used to transfect DBT cells which

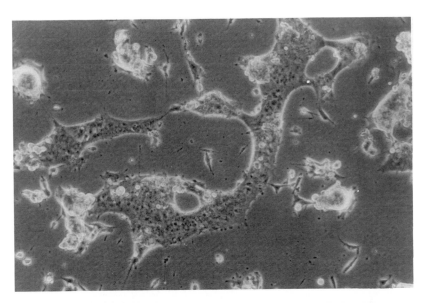

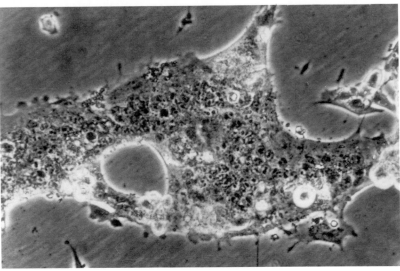

Fig. 1. Fusion activity of the MHV-JHM S protein
    2×10^6 DBT cells in a 6 cm petri dish were infected
    with the recombinant Vaccinia Virus vTF7-3 with a moi
    of 30 pfu/cell. Two hours p.i. the virus was removed
    and replaced by calciumphosphate coprecipitated pTF7-
    5/S+ plasmid DNA (20 μg). After 30 min at room
    temperature medium was added and incubation was
    continued at 37°C. The monolayers were photographed
    10 hours post transfection.

```
  1 MFFSLLLVLGLTEAEKIKICLQKQVNSSFSLHNGFGGNLYATEEKRMFEL 50
                 || ||   |   ||| |   |   ||||
  1 ......................MGSTCIAMAPRTLLLLIGCQLVFGF 25

 51 VKPKAGASVLNQSTWIGFGDSRTD......KSNSAFPRSADVSAK.TADK 92
    |   | |||  || |||||| |      || | |        ||
 26 NEPLNIVSHLND.DWFLFGDSRSDCTYVENNGHPKLDWLDLDPKLCNSGK 74

 93 FRFLSGGSLMLSMFGPPGKVDYLYQGCGKHKVFYEGVNWSPHAAINCY.. 140
    |   || ||| ||      |  | | | ||||||||||||| || |
 75 ISAKSGNSLFRSFHFTDF...YNYTGEGDQIVFYEGVNFSPNHGFKCLAY 121

141 ..RKNWTDIKLNFQKNIYELASQSHCMSLVNALDKTIPLQVTAGTAGNCN 188
      |||| |   |||   |  |||||||          || |
122 GDNKRWMGNKARFYARVYEKMAQYRSLSFVNVPYAYGGKAKPTSICKH.K 170

189 NSFLKNPALYTQEVKPSENKCGKENLAFFTLPTQFGTYESKLHLVASCYF 238
    | ||| |   |   || |||  |         |    || ||| |
171 TLTLNNPTFISKESNYVDYYESE........ANFTLAGCDEFIVPLCVF 212

239 IYDSKEVYNKRGCDNYF..QVIYDSFGKVVGGLDNRVSPYTGNSGDTPTM 286
    |||  |   |  | |     | | |  |  | || ||  |
213 NGHSKGSSSDPANKYYMDSQSYYNMDTGVLYGFNSTLDVGNTAKDPGLDL 262

287 QCDMLQLKPGRYSVRSSPRFLLMPERSYCFDMKEK.GPVTAVQSIWGKGR 335
    | |  | ||| |   |  ||  ||  | |   || ||| |  ||| | |
263 TCRYLALTPGNYKAVSLEYLLSLPSKAICLRKPKRFMPVQVVDSRWNSTR 312

336 ESDYAVDQACLSTPGCMLIQKQKPYIGEADDHHGDQEMRELLSGLDYEAR 385
    ||     ||        |   |  | ||| |||||||| |
313 QSDNMTAVACQLPYCFFRNTSADYSGGTHDVHHGDFHFRQLLSGLLLNVS 362

386 CISQSG..WVNETSPFTEKYLLPPKFGRCPLAAKEESIPKIPDGLLIPTS 433
    || | |     | |   |     || || | | |   ||
363 CIAQQGAFLYNNVSSSWPAY....GYGQCPTAANIGYMAPVCIYDPLPVV 408

434 GTDTTVTKPKSR 446              ( INFLUENZA C )
    |  | | |
409 LLGVLLGIAVLIIVFLILYFMTDSGVRLHEA 439 ( MHV-JHM )
```

Fig. 2. Nucleotide sequence of the unique region of the MHV-JHM mRNA 2-1.
The figure shows the nucleotide sequence and the deduced amino acid sequence of the MHV-JHM mRNA 2-1 unique region in comparison to the HEF$_1$ subunit of the Influenza C virus HEF protein (Pfeifer and Compans, 1984). The putative signal recognition sequence and the membrane anchor region of the MHV-JHM polypeptide are underlined. The potential glycosylation sites are marked.

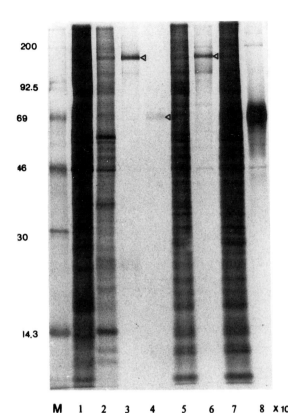

Fig. 3. Expression of the MHV-JHM HE protein using a Vaccinia
virus expression system
   2×10^6 DBT cells in a 6 cm petri dish were infected
with the recombinant Vaccinia virus vTF7-3 with a moi
of 30 pfu/cell and transfected with either a pTF7-5/S
gene plasmid DNA, or pTF7-5/MHV2-1 plasmid DNA. Six
hours after transfection the cells were metabolically
labelled with ^{35}S methionine for 60 minutes and then
lysed with 200 μl of lysis buffer (Siddell et al.,
1981). Alternatively 2×10^6 DBT cells were infected
with MHV-JHM with a moi of 5 and lysed 12 hours p.i.
5 μl of lysate were directly loaded on a 15 % SDS polyacrylamide gel, or 50 μl were used for the immunoprecipitation with either HE or S specific monoclonal
antibodies (Wege et al., 1984). M: MW marker; lane 1:
lysate from uninfected DBT cells; lane 2: lysate from
MHV-JHM infected DBT cells; lanes 3 and 4: immunoprecipitation of the lysate from lane 2 with S specific
or HE specific monoclonal antibodies; lane 5: lysate
from vTF7-3 infected/pTF7-5/S transfected DBT cells;
lane 6: immunoprecipitation of the lysate from lane 5
with S specific monoclonal antibodies; lane 7: lysate
from vTF7-3 infected/pTF7-5/MHV2-1 transfected DBT
cells; lane 8: immunoprecipitation of the lysate from
lane 7 with a HE specific monoclonal antibody.

had been infected previously with the recombinant Vaccinia virus vTF7-3. Lysates were made from the infected/transfected cells and immunoprecipitated with an MHV-JHM HE specific mono-clonal antibody (kindly provided by Dr. H. Wege). Figure 3, lane 8, shows the immunoprecipitate from vTF7-3 infected cells transfected with the pTF7-5/MHV2-1 plasmid DNA. Comparison with the immunoprecipitate from MHV-JHM infected DBT cells demonstrates that the protein product of the MHV-JHM mRNA 2-1 unique region, expressed via a Vaccinia virus expression system, has the same electrophoretic and antigenic properties as the HE protein from MHV-JHM infected cells.

This result shows that the mRNA 2-1 ORF is the gene for the MHV-JHM HE protein. In addition, the Vaccinia virus system pro-duces far more HE protein than MHV-JHM infected cells. This overexpression allowed the analysis of the biological functions of the protein.

III Analysis of the biological function of the MHV-JHM HE protein

The HEF$_1$ subunit of the Influenza C HEF protein has an acetylesterase activity which specifically cleaves off the acetate moiety on position 9 from the substrate N-acetyl-9-0-acetyl-neuraminic acid (Herrler et al., 1985). This activity can be analysed using the organic substrate p-nitrophenylace-tate (pNPA). Esterases specifically cleave off the acetate moiety from this substrate leaving the product p-nitrophenol. In order to demonstrate the esterase activity of the MHV-JHM HE protein we immunoprecipitated the HE expressed in the Vaccinia virus system with a specific monoclonal antibody and analysed the activity of the purified immunocomplexes. Figure 4 shows that the HE, but not the S protein, has an esterase activity. HE protein immunocomplexes from MHV-JHM infected cells also show esterase activity which is consistent with the low level of expression shown in Figure 3, lane 4.

Since we could demonstrate an HE specific acetylesterase activity, the next question was whether the protein can also recognize and bind to sialic acid containing receptors on the cell surface. Thus we investigated the ability of the HE pro-tein to bind rat erythrocytes, which are known to contain the receptor of the Influenza C virus in large amounts on their surface (G. Herrler, personal communication). DBT cells were infected with the recombinant Vaccinia virus vTF7-3, trans-fected with either pTF7-5/S plasmid DNA or pTF7-5/MHV2-1 plas-mid DNA and assayed for hemadsorption activity.

Fig. 5 clearly demonstrates that only DBT cells which express the MHV-JHM HE protein (2), specifically bind erythro-cytes. Uninfected DBT cells (3), or DBT cells which express the MHV-JHM S protein (1) do not have such an activity. This result shows that MHV-JHM has a second glycoprotein on its surface which binds to a specific receptor on the host cell. This second receptor is very similar or identical to that used by the Influenza C virus.

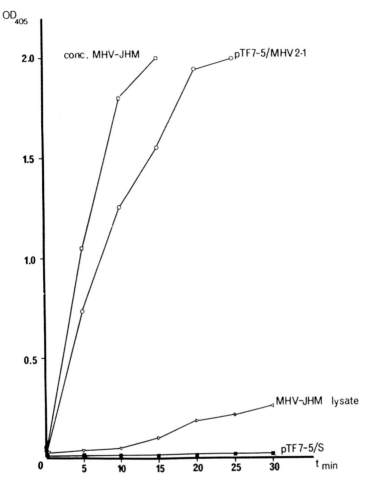

Fig. 4. Esterase activity of the MHV-JHM HE protein
2 x 10[6] DBT cells were infected with the Vaccinia virus
recombinant vTF7-3 with a moi of 30 pfu/cell and transfected with either pTF7-5/S plasmid DNA or pTF7-5/MHV2-
1 plasmid DNA. 24 hours post transfection cells were
lysed with 200 µl of lysis buffer (Siddell et al.,
1981). The lysate was immunoprecipitated with a specific monoclonal antibody and 1/10 of the purified
immunecomplexes was tested for esterase activity. 10 mg
of p-nitrophenylacetate (pNPA) was dissolved in 500 µl
ethanol and 100 µl of this solution was mixed with 10
ml PBS (final concentration 200 µg/ml). 20 µl purified
MHV-JHM (Siddell et al., 1980) or 20 µl purified HE
protein - antibody - protein A Sepharose were mixed
with the diluted pNPA solution (1 ml) and the increase
of the adsorption at OD_{405} was measured over a period
of 30 minutes.

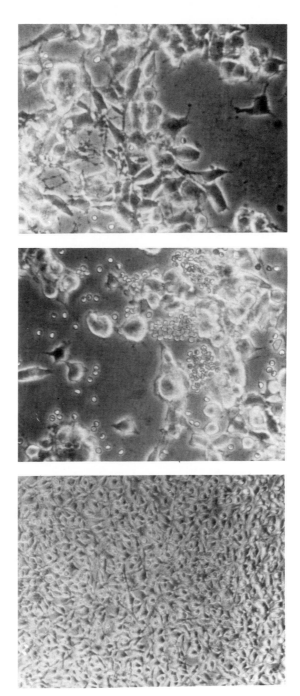

Fig. 5 Hemadsorption activity of the MHV-JHM HE protein
2 x 10^6 DBT cells were infected with the Vaccinia virus
recombinant vTF-3 with an moi of 30 pfu/cell and transfected with either pTF7-5/S plasmid DNA or pTF7-5/MHV2-1
plasmid DNA. Monolayers were chilled to 4°C on ice for
30 minutes 6 hours post transfection and incubated at
4°C with 1 ml of a 2 % solution of rat erythrocytes in
PBS. Unspecifically bound erythrocytes were washed away
with PBS at 4°C

DISCUSSION

Coronavirus MHV-JHM has two surface glycoproteins, the S protein and the HE protein. The experiments reported here, and earlier studies (Wege et al., 1984) suggest that both proteins have the ability to bind to cellular receptor(s). In addition, both proteins have a further biological function which is the fusion activity of the S protein and the esterase activity of the HE protein.

So far three paradigms of fusion have been described. The HA_2 subunit of the Influenza A virus HA protein mediates an acidic pH dependent fusion of viral and cellular membranes. This event is normally restricted to endosomal particles with their acidic pH environment (Wilson et al., 1981). In contrast, a pH independent membrane fusion is mediated by the F_1 subunit of the paramyxoviral F protein (Richardson et al., 1983). Both fusion mechanisms share one common feature, the highly hydrophobic N-terminus of the fusion active subunit.

Some members of the alphavirus group (Sindbis virus and Semliki Forest virus) seem to use a third fusion paradigm. In this case, the fusion event is pH dependent, but the fusion active E1 protein has no hydrophobic N-terminus. A stretch of hydrophobic amino acids, which is found 80 residues away from the N-terminus, implicates an internal rather than an external domain in membrane fusion (Garoff et al., 1980a and b).

It has been shown in this paper, that the MHV-JHM S protein is the fusion active component of the virus. This protein does not require acidic pH conditions to develop its activity (Sturman et al., 1985) and it has no terminal hydrophobic amino acid sequences in its S_2 subunit (Schmidt et al., 1987). Since it has not yet been directly shown that cleavage of the S protein is necessary for MHV-JHM fusion and since some members of the coronavirus family (TGEV and FIPV) (deGroot et al., 1987, 1989) have an uncleaved but fusion active S protein, one can argue that the MHV-JHM S protein mediated fusion activity, like the E1 protein of the alphaviruses, uses one or more internal domains. This idea seems to be supported by recent results obtained by Luytjes et al. (1989) for the closely related MHV-A59.

The second surface glycoprotein of MHV-JHM, the HE protein, has been shown in this paper to have an receptor binding and a receptor destroying (esterase) activity similar to that of the Influenza C virus. The exact role of these two activities for infectivity and pathogenesis of the virus is not yet clear.

ACKNOWLEDGMENTS

We would like to thank Dr. B. Moss for supplying the Vaccinia virus expression systems used in these studies. We also thank B. Schelle-Prinz for technical assistance and Helga Kriesinger for typing the manuscript. This work was supported by the DFG (SFB165/B1).

REFERENCES

Collins, A.R., Knobler, R.L., Powell, H., and Buchmeier, M.J., 1982, Monoclonal antibodies to Murine Hepatitis Virus-4 (strain JHM) define the viral glycoprotein responsible for attachment and cell-cell fusion. Virology 119:358.

de Groot, R.J., Maduro, J., Lenstra, J.A., Horzinek, M.C., and van der Zeijst, B.A., 1987, cDNA cloning and sequence analysis of the gene encoding the peplomer protein of Feline Infectious Peritonitits virus. J. gen. Virol. 68:2639.

de Groot, R.J., van Leen, R.W., Dalderup, M.J.H., Vennema, H., Horzinek, M.C., and Spaan, W., 1989, Stabley expressed FIPV peplomer protein induces cell fusion and elicits neutralizing antibodies in mice. Virology, 171:493.

Fuerst, T.R., Niles, E.G., Studier, F.W., and Moss, B., 1986, Eukaryotic transient expression system based on recombinant Vaccinia virus that synthesizes bacteriophage T7 RNA polymerase. Proc. Natl. Acad. Sci. USA 83:8122.

Garoff, H., Frischauf, A.-M., Simons, K., Lehrach, H., and Delius, H. (1980a). Nucleotide sequence of cDNA coding for Semliki Forest Virus membrane gylcoproteins. Nature 288:236.

Garoff, H., Frischauf, A.-M., Simons, K., Lehrach, H., and Delius, H. (1980b). The capsid protein of Semliki Forest Virus has clusters of basic amino acids and prolines in its amino terminal region. Proc. Natl. Acad. Sci. USA 77:6376.

Gubler, U., and Hoffman, B.J., 1983, A simple and very efficient method for generating cDNA libraries, Gene 25:263.

Herrler, G., Rott, R., Klenk, H.-D., Müller, H.-P., Shukla, A.-K., Schauer, R., 1985, The receptor destroying enzyme of Influenza C virus is a neuraminate-O-acetlyesterase, EMBO J 4:1503.

King, B., Potts, B.J., and Brian, D., 1985, Bovine Coronavirus hemagglutinin protein, Virus Research 2:53.

Luytjes, W., Bredenbeek, P.J., Noten, A.F.H., Horzinek, M.C., and Spaan, W., 1988, Sequence of the Mouse Hepatitis Virus A59 mRNA 2: indications for RNA recombination between Coronaviruses and Influenza C virus. Virology 166:415.

Luytjes, W., Geerts, D., Posthumus, W., Moloen, R., and Spaan, W., 1989, Amino acid sequence of a conserved neutralizing epitope of murine coronaviruses. J. Virol. 63:1408.

Nakada, S., Craeger, R., Krystal, R., Aaronson, R.P., and Palese, P., 1984, Influenza C virus hemagglutinin: comparison with Influenza A and B virus hemagglutinin. J. Virol. 50:118.

Pfeifer, J.B., and Compans, R.W., 1984, Structure of the Influenza C glycoprotein gene as determined from cloned cDNA. Virus Res. 1:281.

Richardson, C.D., and Choppin, P.W., 1983, Oligopeptides that specifically inhibit membrane fusion by paramyxoviruses: studies on the site of action. Virology 131:518.

Schmidt, I., Skinner, M.A., and Siddell, S.G., 1987, Nucleotide sequence of the gene encoding the surface projection glycoprotein of the Coronavirus MHV-JHM. J. gen. Virol. 68: 47.

Siddell, S.G., Wege, H., Barthel, A., and ter Meulen, V., 1980, Coronavirus JHM: cell free synthesis of structural protein p60. J. Virol. 33:10.

Siddell, S.G., Wege, H., Barthel, A., and ter Meulen, V., 1981, Coronavirus JHM: intracellular protein synthesis. J. gen. Virol. 53:145.

Sturman, L.S., Ricard, C., and Holmes, K.V., 1985, Proteolytic cleavage of the E2 glycoprotein of murine coronavirus: Activation of cell-fusing activity of virions by trypsin treatment and separation of two different 90K cleavage fragments. J. Virol 56:904.

Vlasak, R., Luytjes, W., Spaan, W., and Palese, P., 1988a, Human and bovine Coronaviruses recognize sialic acid-containing receptors similar those of Influenza C virus. Proc. Natl. Acad. Sci. USA 85:4526.

Vlasak, R., Juytjes, W., Leider, J., Spaan, W., and Palese, P., 1988b, The E3 protein of bovine Coronavirus is a receptor-destroying enzyme with acetylesterase activity. J. Virol. 62:4686.

Wege, H., Dörries, R., and Wege, H., 1984, Hybridoma antibodies to the murine Coronavirus JHM: characterization of epitopes on the peplomer protein (E2). J. gen. Virol. 65:1931.

Wilson, I.A., Skehel, J.J., and Wiley, D.C., 1981, Structure of the hemagglutinating membrane glycoprotein of Influenza C virus at 3 Å resolution. Nature 289:366.

ROLE OF pH IN SYNCYTIUM INDUCTION AND GENOME UNCOATING OF AVIAN

INFECTIOUS BRONCHITIS CORONAVIRUS (IBV)

D. Li and D. Cavanagh

AFRC Institute for Animal Health, Houghton Laboratory
Houghton, Huntingdon Cambridgeshire, PE17 2DA, UK

SUMMARY

Syncytium formation induced in Vero cells by IBV-Beaudette was optimal at pH 6.7 and absent at pH 7.5. Reduction of IBV-Beaudette replication by ammonium chloride, which raises the pH in endosomes, further
indicated that uncoating of the virus genome probably occurred within the
acidic environment of endosomes. However, this would not appear to apply
to all IBV strains, since one was unaffected by the drug. It would
appear that some strains of IBV have the capacity to fuse with the plasma
membrane at neutral pH, thereby leading to genome uncoating at that site.
Other strains of IBV might also uncoat at the plasma membrane when the
extracellular environment is slightly less than pH7.

INTRODUCTION

The large spike (S) glycoprotein of coronaviruses is involved in
several processes[1]: attachment of the virus to cells; fusion of the
virus envelope with cell membranes resulting in uncoating of the genome;
and fusion of the cell surface membrane of infected cells with that of
neighbouring cells to form syncytia. The latter process is caused by the
presence of S, synthesised following infection, at the cell surface and
is referred to as fusion-from-within (FFWI). Whether genome uncoating of
IBV occurs following fusion with the cell surface (plasma) membrane or
with internal membranes eg. within the acidic environment of endosomes or
lysosomes, is unknown. We have addressed this question.

MATERIALS AND METHODS

IBV strains. Beaudette-US (adapted to Vero cells)[2]; H120; D1466;
D274; UK/123/82.

Cells. Vero and chick kidney (CK) cells were used. Maintenance
medium for experiments was Eagle's minimal essential medium buffered with
20mM BES (N,N-bis[2-hydroxyethyl]-2-Aminoethane sulfonic acid) and
various concentrations of sodium bicarbonate to achieve the desired pH.

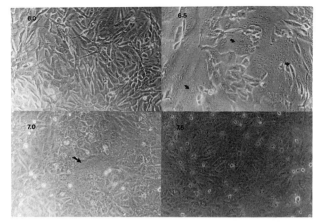

Fig.1. pH dependence of syncytium induction in Vero cells by IBV-Beaudette-US. Cells were infected at an MOI of 0.02 pfu/cell and incubated at the indicated pH for 36h at 38°C. Syncytia are indicated by arrows.

RESULTS

pH Requirement for IBV-induced cell-cell fusion. Vero cells inoculated with IBV-Beaudette-US (multiplicity of infection (MOI) 0.02 pfu/cell) were subsequently incubated at different pH. After 36h at 38°C there was extensive syncytium formation, resulting from FFWI, at pH 6.5 and 7.0 but none at pH 6.0 and 7.5 (Fig.1).

Analysis of infectious virus production and viral RNA synthesis (not shown), revealed that IBV replication was very low at pH 6.0 and 7.5. pH 6.0 itself was not inhibitory for membrane fusion. Thus cells inoculated at an MOI of 0.2pfu/cell and incubated at pH 7.5 did form syncytia when the infected cells were exposed to pH 6.0 for 30 min at 36h post inoculation (p.i.). Maximum fusion was obtained when cells were incubated at pH 6.7 (data not shown).

Table 1. Titre* of IBV-Beaudette-US grown in Vero cells in the presence of ammonium chloride

Multiplicity (pfu/cell)	hours p.i.	concentration of ammonium chloride (mM)				
		0	5	10	20	30
	12	2.4	1.5	0	0	0
0.3	24	4.7	3.3	2.0	2.0	0
	36	5.8	4.8	2.7	0	0

* Virus was titrated by plaque assay in Vero cells and is expressed as $\log_{10}$ pfu/ml.

Table 2. Effect of ammonium chloride on the early infection of
IBV-Beaudette-US in Vero cells[*]

Groups	NH$_4$Cl 0-2 hours p.i.	2-4	No of infected cells at 14 hours p.i.	No of infectious foci at 14 hours p.i.
1	+	-	10.5	2
2	-	-	138.5	38
3	-	+	180.0	31
4	-	-	171.5	35

[*] Vero cells were infected at a multiplicity of 0.3 pfu per cell.
Infected cells and infectious foci were detected by immunofluorescence.

Location of genome uncoating. Ammonium chloride raises the pH in endosomes and would be expected to inhibit genome uncoating of a virus which required an acidic endosomal environment for uncoating. Vero cells were incubated for 30 min with ammonium chloride and then inoculated, in the presence of the drug, with Beaudette-US at 0.3 pfu/cell. After washing incubation was continued in the presence of ammonium chloride. Table 1 shows that infectious virus production was reduced by 10 to 1000-fold, depending on the concentration of the drug. Preliminary work had established that the Vero cells remained viable under the conditions used.

Reduction of virus production also resulted when ammonium chloride was present only for the first 2h after infection but not when the drug was added after 2h of incubation (Table 2). Several experiments showed that ammonium chloride had not (a) had a direct virucidal effect, (b) reduced virus attachment to cells or (c) greatly inhibited cell RNA synthesis. The inhibitory effect of ammonium chloride also occurred with 3 other strains of IBV, as assessed by immunofluorescence of infected CK cells. However, strain UK/123/82 was reproducibly not affected by ammonium chloride, suggesting that the drug did not have general effects on IBV translation, transcription, protein processing and transportation and virus maturation. Thus, the replication of IBV-Beaudette and some but not all other IBV strains, was inhibited at a stage following attachment to cells but before RNA translation and transcription. The affected stage was most likely that of genome uncoating and indicates that some IBV strains enter cells by endocytosis followed by transfer to endosomes where a slightly acidic environment is required for optimum fusion of the virus and endosome membranes.

DISCUSSION

Our results show that FFWI of IBV-Beaudette was optimal at slightly acidic pH. This is in contrast to murine hepatitis virus, where the optimum pH was above 7.0 and when pH of about 6.8 was inhibitory to FFWI although not to replication[3-5]. The FFWI results obtained with IBV-Beaudette correlate with our studies using the lysosomotropic agent ammonium chloride which indicated that an acidic environment was optimal for genome uncoating, probably within endosomes. The finding that UK/-123/82 was not inhibited by this drug and that some cells were successfully infected (as shown by fluorescence) by Beaudette even in the presence of ammonium chloride indicates that as a group IBV strains require, at most, only a mildly acidic pH for genome uncoating. In this respect they resemble some flaviviruses (Ref [6]) rather than influenza A virus (ref [7]). IBV strains unaffected by ammonium chloride would appear to have the potential for uncoating by fusion of the virus envelope with the plasma membrane. Alternatively, or in addition, uncoating may occur in endocytic vesicles but without a requirement for acidic pH. With such strains the site of uncoating probably depends on the speed of fusion with the plasma membrane relative to the rate of entry by endocytosis. When the extracellular environment is below pH7, those strains which fuse optimally at a slightly acidic pH may also be able to fuse directly with the plasma membrane.

REFERENCES

1. Spaan, W., Cavanagh, D. and Horzinek, M.C. Coronaviruses: structure and genome expression. J. gen. Virol. 69: 2939 (1988).
2. Alonso-Caplen, F.V., Matsuoka, Y., Wilcox, G.E. and Compans, R.W. Replication and morphogenesis of avian coronavirus in Vero cells and their inhibition by monensin. Virus Research, 1: 153 (1984).
3. Sturman, L.S., Ricard, C.S. and Holmes, K.V. Proteolytic cleavage of the E2 glycoprotein of murine coronavirus: activation of cell-fusing activity of virions by trypsin and separation of two different 90K cleavage fragments. J. Virol. 56: 904 (1985).
4. Frana, M.F., Behnke, J.N., Sturman, L.S. and Holmes, K.V. Proteolytic cleavage of the E2 glycoprotein of murine coronavirus: host-dependent differences in proteolytic cleavage and cell fusion. J. Virol. 56: 912 (1985).
5. Sawicki, S.G. and Sawicki, D.L. Coronavirus Minus-strand RNA synthesis and effect of cycloheximide on coronavirus RNA synthesis. J. Virol. 57: 328 (1986).
6. Kimura, T and Ohyama A. Association between the pH-dependent conformational change of West Nile flavivirus E protein and virus-mediated membrane fusion. J. gen. Virol. 69: 1247 (1988).
7. Lenard, J. and Miller, D.K. pH-dependent hemolysis by influenza, Semliki Forest virus and Sendai virus. Virology 110: 479 (1981).

IS THE 110K GLYCOPROTEIN THE ONLY RECEPTOR FOR MHV AND DOES ITS EXPRESSION DETERMINE SPECIES SPECIFICITY?

Kathryn V. Holmes[1], Richard K. Williams[1], Christine B. Cardellichio[1], Susan R. Compton[1], Charles B. Stephensen[1], Stuart W. Snyder[1], Mark F. Frana[1], Gui-Sen Jiang[1], Abigail Smith[2], and Robert L. Knobler[3]

[1]Uniformed Services University of the Health Sciences, Bethesda, MD 20814, [2]Yale University School of Medicine, New Haven, CT 06510, and [3]Thomas Jefferson Medical College, Philadelphia PA 19107

INTRODUCTION

Coronaviruses exhibit strong tissue tropisms and species specificities, and the molecular mechanisms for these tropisms are of considerable interest. For mouse hepatitis virus, strain A59 (MHV-A59), a solid phase assay was developed to detect binding of virions to plasma membranes from normal target tissues of susceptible mice (1). Using a virus overlay protein blot assay, MHV-A59 was shown to bind specifically to a 100 to 110K protein from liver or intestine membranes of MHV-susceptible BALB/c mice. The specificity of virus binding was demonstrated by the observations that other enterotropic murine viruses did not bind to the same membrane protein and that MHV-A59 did not bind to any proteins from intestine or hepatocyte membranes from SJL/J mice, which are highly resistant to infection with MHV-A59 (2,3). Thus, SJL/J mice may be resistant to infection with MHV-A59 because the virus fails to bind to its normal target tissues, possibly because the virus-binding moiety is absent from the SJL/J plasma membranes.

The present study was undertaken to determine whether the tissue tropism and species specificity of MHV are determined by the expression of the 110K protein which serves as the receptor for MHV-A59.

Coronaviruses and Their Diseases
Edited by D. Cavanagh and T.D.K. Brown
Plenum Press, New York, 1990

METHODS AND RESULTS

Brush border membranes were purified from MHV-susceptible BALB/c mice as previously described (1), and membrane proteins were solubilized by treatment with NP40 and deoxycholate. Glycoproteins were adsorbed to lectin-coated beads, solubilized with SDS, separated by SDS-PAGE and blotted to nitrocellulose. Binding of MHV-A59 virus to membrane glycoproteins was detected using the virus-overlay protein blot assay (1). Essentially all of the virus-binding activity of the 110K protein was recovered in the lectin-selected glycoprotein fraction (4). This experiment showed that the 110K receptor from BALB/c intestine was a glycoprotein.

Removal of carbohydrates from membrane glycoproteins of either BALB/c membranes or affinity purified, radioiodinated receptor, with neuraminidase, endoglycosidase F, or endoglycosidase H reduced the apparent molecular weight of the receptor but failed to decrease its virus-binding activity. Treatment of BALB/c brush border membranes or purified receptor glycoprotein with protease, however, did reduce and, finally, eliminate virus-binding activity (R. K. Williams, et al., in preparation). These observations suggest that the virus-binding moiety of the 110K MHV receptor glycoprotein is a polypeptide and not a carbohydrate or oligosaccharide.

Antibody directed against the 110K glycoprotein was developed by immunizing SJL/J mice with intestinal brush border membranes from BALB/c mice (K. V. Holmes, in preparation). Hybridomas producing monoclonal antibodies (MAbs) specific for the 110K glycoprotein were prepared. Several receptor-specific MAbs reacted in immunoblots with the 110K glycoprotein from BALB/c brush border membranes and with a 58K fragment isolated from these membranes (5). One blocking MAb, called CC1, reacted specifically by immunofluorescence with the intestinal brush border of BALB/c mice but failed to bind to brush borders of MHV-resistant SJL/J mice. Thus, the specificity of binding of the anti-receptor MAb CC1 to intestine membranes from different strains of mice was similar to binding of MHV-A59 virions to these membranes.

Pre-treatment of L2 or 17 Cl 1 mouse fibroblast cultures with MAb CC1 prior to incubation with infectious virus prevented binding of MHV-A59 virions to the cells and prevented infection of the cultures. This MAb blocked infection of murine cell cultures with the following strains of MHV: MHV-A59, MHV-1, MHV-3, MHV-S and MHV-JHM. Immunoblot assays showed that MAb CC1 recognized the MHV-A59 receptor glycoprotein from purified intestinal brush border membranes and hepatocyte plasma membranes from mouse strains which are fully or partially susceptible to infection with MHV, including BALB/c, C3H, C57Bl/6, and A/J (6).

The evidence supporting the hypothesis that the 100 to 110K glycoprotein is a receptor for MHV-A59 is

TABLE 1

Evidence that the 110K Glycoprotein is a Receptor

for Mouse Hepatitis Virus

1. Virus binds specifically to the 110K
   glycoprotein in liver and intestine membranes
   of MHV-susceptible and semi-susceptible
   strains of mice.

2. Virus-binding activity is not detectable in
   membrane glycoproteins of liver or intestine
   of SJL/J mice, which are highly resistant to
   infection with MHV-A59.

3. Monoclonal anti-receptor antibody CC1
   recognizes the glycoprotein in liver and
   intestinal brush border membranes of MHV-
   susceptible and semi-susceptible mouse
   strains.

4. MAb CC1 fails to bind to liver or intestinal
   brush border membranes of MHV-resistant SJL/J
   mice.

5. MAb CC1 binds to membranes of MHV-susceptible
   murine cell lines and blocks infection with
   several strains of MHV.

summarized in Table 1. The blocking anti-receptor Mab CC1
was used for affinity purification of the receptor
glycoprotein (5). Studies on the characteristics of the
receptor are in progress.

In order to determine whether the 100 to 110K
glycoprotein serves as the only receptor for MHV-A59 on
cells from different tissues of susceptible BALB/c mice,
the binding of MAb CC1 to membranes from different tissues
was studied. Radioiodinated CC1 bound best to membranes
of large and small intestine and liver, and this binding
was blocked by excess unlabelled CC1 but not by an excess
of an irrelevant MAb of the same isotype. Binding of CC1
to membranes from other susceptible tissues of BALB/c
mice, such as lung, spleen and brain, could not be
detected by this method. Immunofluorescence of frozen
sections proved to be a more sensitive way to detect
binding of MAb CC1 to membranes of different tissues,
detecting the receptor in endothelial cells in tissues,
such as brain, which had appeared negative by binding of
radioiodinated CC1. However, even immunofluorescence did
not detect the presence of the receptor antigen on glial
or neuronal cells in the brain of BALB/c mice, a tissue
which is known to be susceptible to infection with MHV (7;

Table 2

Species Specificity of MHV-A59 Binding to

Intestinal Brush Border Membranes

Species of BBM	MHV-A59 Binding	MAb CC1 Binding
Mouse (BALB/c)	+	+
Mouse (C57Bl/6)	+	+
Mouse (C3H)	+	+
Mouse (SJL/J)	-	-
Rat (Wistar Furth)	-	-
Dog	-	-
Cat	-	-
Pig	-	-
Human	-	-

C. Gottfraind, in preparation). Therefore, experiments were done to evaluate whether CC1 could protect glial cell cultures from infection with MHV. Primary cultures of glial cells prepared from MHV-susceptible BALB/c mice or MHV-resistant SJL/J mice were pre-treated with anti-receptor MAb CC1 and then inoculated with MHV-A59. SJL/J glial cultures were resistant to infection with MHV-A59 even in the absence of CC1, as judged by failure of viral antigens to develop in cultures inoculated with virus. BALB/c glial cells pre-treated with an irrelevant MAb supported the replication of MHV-A59, but virus infection was completely blocked by pre-treatment with anti-receptor MAb CC1. These results suggest that all of the tissues of the BALB/c mouse which are susceptible to infection with MHV-A59 express the 100 to 110K glycoprotein, and that this may be the only receptor for MHV-A59 on the membranes of these tissues.

Many coronaviruses exhibit strong species specificity. For example, MHV naturally infects only mice, although experimental infection of some strains of rats at a young age has been demonstrated with MHV-JHM (8,9). The availability of the MHV-A59 binding determinant on intestinal brush border membranes isolated from different species was evaluated using the solid phase virus binding assay (6). The species selected for study were all natural hosts for either enteric or respiratory coronaviruses, and appropriate solid phase virus binding assays showed that coronaviruses native to each species did bind to the brush border membranes or other target

cell membranes of that species. Table 2 shows that
binding of MHV-A59 to intestinal brush border membranes
was detectable only on membranes from MHV-susceptible or
semi-susceptible strains of mice, and not from other
species. The specificity of virus binding correlated well
with the specificity of binding of the blocking anti-
receptor monoclonal antibody CC1 (Table 2).

DISCUSSION

     Early studies on virus receptors were predicated upon
the hypothesis that a single receptor moiety would be
responsible for binding of one virus to a variety of host
cells. More recently, it has become apparent that one
virus may bind to either of several different molecules on
the surfaces of different cell types in order to initiate
infection (10,11,12). As new and sensitive assays for
virus receptors are developed, increasing complexity of
virus-cell interactions may become apparent. Our initial
analysis of coronavirus receptors identified a 100 to 110K
glycoprotein which permitted binding of MHV-A59 to
membranes of enterocytes and hepatocytes from susceptible
strains of mice (1). The isolation of an anti-receptor
monoclonal antibody which can block virus infection led to
more sensitive assays for the expression of the MHV-
binding moiety on cell membranes. The data summarized in
Table 1 strongly support the hypothesis that the 100 to
110K glycoprotein is a biologically significant receptor
for MHV-A59, both on cultured murine cells and in tissues
of MHV-susceptible mice. Several different strains of MHV
apparently share the same receptor determinant, since the
same anti-receptor MAb can block infection of murine
fibroblasts with each virus strain. Expression of the
glycoprotein receptor on membranes from different murine
tissues correlates with the tissue tropism of MHV-A59.
The most sensitive assay for expression of the
glycoprotein and its role in infection with MHV-A59
appears to be blocking of virus infection by anti-receptor
MAb CC1, which demonstrated that the glycoprotein was a
functional receptor in cultured glial cells as well as
fibroblasts. The data summarized in Table 2 suggest that
the species specificity of MHV-A59 may be due to absence
of the virus-binding moiety recognized by MAb CC1 from
intestinal brush border membranes of other species.
Whether the MHV-A59 receptor moiety is expressed on other
tissues in these other species has not yet been
determined.

     Two additional observations add to the complexity of
the MHV receptor story. The first is the observation,
presented in the accompanying paper (5), that SJL/J mice
express on their intestinal brush border membranes a
shorter, homologous glycoprotein which cross-reacts with
antigens at the amino terminus of the MHV-A59 receptor
glycoprotein from BALB/c mice, but which lacks the moiety
or epitope(s) that permit attachment of virus or binding

a deletion or mutation in the glycoprotein which serves as an MHV-A59 receptor in BALB/c mice, rather than lacking the entire glycoprotein. The cellular function(s) of these murine membrane glycoproteins has not yet been determined.

The second complicating factor arises from the discovery that some hemagglutinating coronaviruses including bovine coronavirus (BCV), human coronavirus HCV-OC43, and several strains of MHV express a membrane glycoprotein, E3 or HE, which has hemagglutinin and acetyl esterase activities (13,14,15). This permits virions to bind to cell membrane molecules containing 9 O-acetylated sialic acid, and to elute from these molecules, destroying their virus-binding activity. It is possible that the interaction of the viral HE glycoprotein with a carbohydrate on the cell surface can serve as an alternate way for coronaviruses to infect cells in vitro or in vivo. The strains of MHV which were used for our studies did not express the HE glycoprotein, so our results indicate that the 100 to 110K glycoprotein alone is sufficient to initiate infection of susceptible cultured cells or animals with these virus strains. When strains of MHV which express the HE glycoprotein are tested by the methods described here, it will be possible to evaluate the roles of the two alternative modes of virus-cell interactions in the initiation of MHV infection. Coronaviruses in serogroups I and III do not have the gene for the HE glycoprotein, and further analysis will be required to determine the nature of their host cell receptors.

ACKNOWLEDGEMENTS

The authors gratefully acknowledge the excellent technical assistance of S. Wetherell and P. Elia. This research was supported by NIH grants AI 18997, AI 25231, and NS 22145 and grant number RG 1722 from the Multiple Sclerosis Society. Dr. Williams is the recipient of NIH NRSA # AI 07810. The opinions or assertions contained herein are the private ones of the authors and are not to be construed as official or reflecting the views of the Department of Defense or the Uniformed Services University of the Health Sciences.

REFERENCES

1. Boyle, J.F., D.G. Weismiller, and K.V. Holmes. 1987. Genetic resistance to mouse hepatitis virus correlates with absence of virus-binding activity on target tissues. J. Virol. 61:185-189.

2. S.W. Barthold, and Smith, A.L. 1984. Mouse hepatitis virus strain-related patterns of tissue tropism in suckling mice. Arch. Virol. 81:103-112.

3. Smith, M.S., R.E. Click, and P.G. Plagemann. 1984. Control of mouse hepatitis virus replication in macrophages by a recessive gene on chromosome 7. J. Immunol. **133**:428-432.

4. Holmes, K.V., Boyle, J.F., Weismiller, D.G., Compton, S.R., Williams, R.K., Stephensen, C.B., and Frana, M.F. 1987. Identification of a receptor for mouse hepatitis virus. Adv. Exp. Med. Biol. **218**:197-202.

5. Williams, R.K., S.W. Snyder, and K.V. Holmes. 1989. MHV-Resistant SJL/J mice express a non-functional homolog to the MHV receptor glycoprotein. This volume.

6. Compton, S.R. 1988. PhD Thesis. Uniformed Services University of the Health Sciences, Bethesda, MD.

7. Knobler, R.L., Dubois-Dalcq, M., Haspel, M.V., Claysmith, A.P., Lampert, P.W., and Oldstone, M.B. 1981. Selective localization of wild type and mutant mouse hepatitis virus (JHM strain) antigens in CNS tissue by fluorescence, light and electron microscopy. J. Neuroimmunol. **1**:81-92.

8. Sorensen, O., and S. Dales. 1985. In vivo and in vitro models of demyelinating disease: JHM virus in the rat central nervous system localized by in situ cDNA hybridization and immunofluorescent microscopy. J. Virol **56**:434-438.

9. Wege, H., M. Koga, R. Watanabe, K. Nagashima, and V. ter Meulen. 1983. Neurovirulence of murine coronavirus JHM temperature-sensitive mutants in rats. Infect. Immun. **39**:1316-1324.

10. Paulson, J.C., G.N. Rogers, J. Murayama, G. Sze, and E. Martin. 1986. Biological implications of influenza virus receptor specificity. Virus Attachment and Entry into Cells 144-151.

11. Weis, W., Brown, J.H., Cusack, S., Paulson, J.C., Skehel, J.J., and Wiley, D.C. 1988. Structure of the influenza virus hemagglutinin complexed with its receptor, sialic acid. Nature Jun 2,333(6172):426-31.

12. Reagan, K.J., B. Goldberg, and R.L. Crowell. 1984. Altered receptor specificity of coxsackievirus B3 after growth in rhabdomyosarcoma cells. J. Virol. **49**:635-640.

13. Luytjes, W., P.J. Bredenbeek, A.F. Noten, M.C. Horzinek, and W.J. Spaan. 1988. Sequence of mouse hepatitis virus A59 mRNA 2: Indications for RNA recombination between coronaviruses and influenza C virus. Virology 166:415-422.

14. Vlasak, R., W. Luytjes, J. Leider, W. Spaan, and P. Palese. 1988. The E3 protein of bovine coronavirus is a receptor-destroying enzyme with acetylesterase activity. J. Virol. **62**:4686-4690.

15. Vlasak, R., W. Luytjes, W. Spaan, and P. Palese. 1988. Human and bovine coronaviruses recognize sialic acid-containing receptors similar to those of influenza C viruses. Proc. Natl. Acad. Sci. U. S. A. 85:4526-4529.

MHV-RESISTANT SJL/J MICE EXPRESS A NON-FUNCTIONAL HOMOLOG TO THE MHV

RECEPTOR GLYCOPROTEIN

Richard K. Williams, Stuart W. Snyder and Kathryn V. Holmes

Department of Pathology, Uniformed Services University of the
Health Sciences, Bethesda, Maryland, USA, 20814

ABSTRACT

MHV-A59 recognizes a 100-110 K glycoprotein receptor on intestinal and liver
plasma membranes. The receptor protein was affinity purified using an anti-
receptor monoclonal antibody. Purified receptor was sequenced from the 1st to
the 15th amino acids. Antiserum raised against a synthetic peptide having this
sequence bound to the 110 K receptor from BALB/c intestine and a 58 K
fragment of the receptor. SJL/J mice are resistant to MHV-A59 and their plasma
membranes were previously shown to lack binding to MHV. However, anti-
peptide antibody bound to a 105 K protein and a 53 K protein fragment from
SJL/J plasma membranes. These SJL/J proteins did not bind MHV or to the
blocking monoclonal anti-receptor antibody. Genetic resistance of SJL/J mice to
MHV-A59 appears to be due to mutation of the receptor glycoprotein resulting
in a molecule that does not bind MHV.

INTRODUCTION

Infection of a host animal with a coronavirus requires specific host
functions. Susceptibility to mouse hepatitis virus (MHV) is under host genetic
control. Different outcomes of inoculation with MHV are seen in different
genetically pure strains of mice[1-7]. Of 12 mouse strains tested only SJL/J mice
were resistant to CNS infection with JHM strain of MHV[5]. This resistance is due
to a recessive locus, hv-2, that is independent of H2 haplotype and Ir
genotype[5,6]. Resistance of SJL/J macrophages to MHV strain A59 is also due to a
recessive gene that is independent of the H2 complex[7]. Resistance to MHV-A59 is
found at early ages and macrophages isolated from SJL/J mice as young as one
week old are resistant. The resistance locus for MHV-A59 in SJL/J mice maps
near the centromere on chromosome 7.

Coronavirus MHV binds to a glycoprotein receptor found in plasma
membrane fractions from susceptible tissues[8,9]. This MHV receptor is 100 K in
liver and 110 K in intestine. Polyclonal and monoclonal antibodies directed
against the receptor block infection of cultured cells by MHV-A59 indicating
that this is the biological receptor for MHV-A59 on these cells[10].

Genetic control of susceptibility to MHV-A59 is strongly correlated with presence or absence of this receptor. Plasma membranes isolated from susceptible mouse strains have the 100-110 K receptor glycoprotein[8]. SJL/J mouse tissues have no detectable MHV receptor activity. SJL/J mice immunized with crude preparations of receptor developed strong immune responses against the receptor glycoprotein. Polyclonal antibodies and monoclonal antibodies from these immunized mice react with the receptor glycoprotein from susceptible mice such as BALB/c but not with any proteins in the SJL/J mice[10]. The SJL/J immune system therefore sees the receptor protein as foreign. It was not known whether SJL/J mice entirely lack the protein that serves as the receptor for MHV or if they express a variant protein that does not have the ability to bind virus. If a variant of the receptor protein is present in the SJL/J mouse, this protein must lack the binding sites for virus and for the polyclonal and monoclonal anti-receptor antibodies.

In order to characterize the MHV receptor we affinity purified the protein and began sequencing. We used a partial sequence to produce a synthetic peptide derived from the amino terminal region (NTR) of the receptor. Antibody raised against this synthetic peptide (anti-NTR) was used to look for an SJL/J protein homologous to the MHV receptor from BALB/c mice.

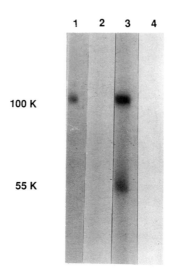

Figure 1.   Immunoblot of affinity purified MHV receptor protein with antibody directed against the amino terminal peptide of the MHV receptor. Affinity purified receptor was treated with 2-mercaptoethanol, run on an SDS gel and blotted to nitrocellulose. Blot strips were reacted with polyclonal anti-receptor antibody (lane 1), rabbit pre-immune serum (lane 2), anti-NTR antibody (lane 3) or with anti-NTR antibody which had been pre-absorbed with excess NTR peptide before applying to the blot (lane 4). Molecular weight of the receptor in daltons calculated from standard proteins is shown to the left.

METHODS and RESULTS

Monoclonal antibody CC1 (MAb) directed against the receptor protein was produced by immunizing SJL/J mice with BALB/c intestinal brush border membrane as described[10]. MAb CC1 recognizes receptor protein on Western blots and live cells and blocks virus binding to receptor. Affinity purification of the receptor was accomplished using this monoclonal antibody. A crude membrane fraction from susceptible mouse liver was produced by homogenization and differential centrifugation. Receptor was solubilized from the membranes using nonionic detergent in the presence of protease inhibitors. Solubilized receptor was then allowed to bind to the monoclonal antibody and eluted with 6 M sodium thiocyanate.

Purity of the receptor protein increased 3,000 to 10,000 fold in this single affinity purification step. Final purification of receptor was achieved by preparative SDS-gel electrophoresis followed by electroblotting the receptor to PVDF membrane (Immobilon P, Millipore Corp.). Receptor on PVDF was then stained for protein and the receptor band was cut out and used directly for amino sequencing using the method of Matsudaira[11]. The preliminary sequence for the amino terminus of the intact receptor was determined for amino acids 1 through 15 of the receptor. A single first amino acid was found indicating complete purity of the receptor.

Solid phase synthesis was used to produce a synthetic peptide designated NTR representing the first 15 amino acids of the receptor protein. Antibodies directed against this peptide were produced in rabbits by coupling the peptide to keyhole limpet hemocyanin. The antiserum produced was tested for reactivity with the receptor purified from susceptible mouse liver. Anti-NTR antibody reacted with the affinity purified receptor at 100 K and with a 55 K protein fragment of the receptor (Fig. 1). The specificity of this reaction is shown by

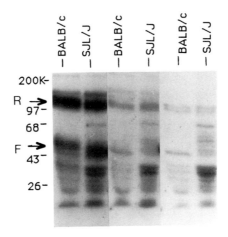

Anti-NTR   Anti-NTR   Preimm.
+Peptide

Figure 2. Immunoblot of intestinal brush border membranes from susceptible BALB/c mice and resistant SJL/J mice. Proteins blots were reacted with the anti-NTR antibody or pre-immune serum as indicated. Anti-NTR + peptide indicates that this blot was reacted with Anti-NTR antibody that had been pre-absorbed with excess NTR peptide. R and F mark the position of the BALB/c receptor and the fragment of the receptor respectively.

the ability of the NTR peptide to block the reaction of the anti-NTR antibody with the receptor. The 100 K receptor protein and the 55 K protein therefore share a common amino terminal region. These data confirm the sequence for the amino terminal region of the receptor and suggest that the 55 K protein is a fragment of the receptor generated by the loss of approximately half of the molecule from the middle to the carboxy terminal end.

To determine if the intestinal receptor, like the hepatocyte receptor, would react with the anti-NTR antibody, intestinal brush border membranes from BALB/c mice were immunoblotted with anti-NTR antibody or pre-immune rabbit serum. The anti-NTR antibody specifically bound to the intact receptor (R in Fig. 2) which is 110 K in BALB/c intestine and a 58 K fragment of the receptor (F in Fig. 2). Pre-absorption of the anti-NTR antibody with excess NTR peptide eliminated the binding to both the 110 K and 58 K bands. Binding of the antibody to several background bands was non-specific and occurred with the pre-immune rabbit serum and with the anti-NTR serum that had been pre-absorbed with the NTR peptide.

The anti-NTR antibody was used to test if the SJL/J membranes have a protein that shares the NTR sequence. In SJL/J intestinal brush border membranes (Fig 2) an upper band of about 105 K and a fragment at about 53 K reacted specifically with the anti-NTR antibody. As was found in the BALB/c proteins the binding of anti-NTR with these two specific SJL/J bands could be blocked by pre-absorption of the serum with the NTR peptide. These data show that polypeptides antigenically related to the MHV receptor of BALB/c mice are found in the SJL/J mouse intestine membranes.

We can begin to map the functional and antigenic domains of MHV receptor protein using anti-NTR, MAb CC1 and virus binding as probes to compare the BALB/c MHV receptor with the homologous inactive SJL/J protein. These data, summarized in Figure 3, suggest that the BALB/c receptor, its fragment, the

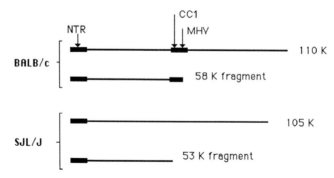

Figure 3.   Model for the BALB/c intestine receptor for MHV and its inactive homolog from SJL/J mice and their naturally occurring protein fragments. The location of the NTR peptide and the proposed binding sites for the CC1 monoclonal antibody and for MHV are indicated.

SJL/J variant protein and the SJL/J fragment are all co-terminal at the amino end. The blocking monoclonal antibody CC1 binds to the BALB/c receptor and its 58 K fragment but not to the SJL/J variant proteins. MHV binds to the large 110 K receptor from BALB/c and to the BALB/c receptor fragment. Blocking of virus binding to the receptor by MAb CC1 suggests that the MAb binding site and the virus binding site are near each other in the receptor molecule. Immunoblots containing approximately equal amounts of the 58 K fragment and the intact 110 K receptor, as determined by binding of anti-NTR and MAb CC1 show much more binding of MHV to the 110 K receptor than to the 58 K fragment (data not shown). This result suggests that the MHV binding site overlaps the end of the 55 K fragment in BALB/c intestine.

DISCUSSION

We have found that the intestinal brush border membranes from SJL/J mouse which lacks a functional receptor for MHV expresses a variant protein that shares its amino terminal region with the receptor found in BALB/c mice This variant SJL/J protein is approximately 5 K smaller on than the BALB/c receptor. We have also found that the SJL/J mouse has a similar lower band at about 53 K in intestine which appears to be a naturally occurring fragment. This reduction in molecular weight from 110 K in the BALB/c receptor protein to 105 in the SJL/J variant protein appears to be located within the first half of the variant molecule between the NTR sequence and the middle of the molecule since the fragment of the variant protein is also reduced 5K. We have not ruled out the formal possibility, however, that the lower receptor band is made from a smaller mRNA. The smaller size seen in the SJL/J bands may be due to deletion of part of the coding region of the receptor gene or to splicing out of an exon in the SJL/J mRNA. Alternatively, the smaller size could be due to a mutation that removes a site for glycosylation of the receptor core protein. We will now be able to examine these possibilities by directly comparing the MHV receptor and the non-binding variant protein.

The cellular function of the MHV receptor protein is not yet known. Presumably this protein has an important function in the host animal. The finding that the SJL/J mouse does not entirely lack this protein but expresses a variant molecule suggests that the variant protein serves the same cellular function as the related BALB/c protein. Further information on the structure of the MHV receptor protein and the variant SJL/J protein, including the complete amino acid sequence will depend on the analysis of cDNA clones for the receptor gene. Comparison of the complete amino acid sequence of the BALB/c and its SJL/J homolog should permit identification of the domain of the receptor protein that binds to MHV.

ACKNOWLEDGEMENTS

The authors are grateful for the excellent technical assistance of P. Elia, C. Cardellichio and S. Wetherell and for helpful discussions with Drs. John Hay, C. Dieffenbach, M. Pensiero, M. Frana and G. S. Jiang. This research was supported by NIH grants; AI18997 and AI25234. Dr. Williams is an NIH NRSA recipient; AI07810. The opinions or assertions contained herein are the private ones of the authors and are not to be construed as official or reflecting the views of the Department of Defense or the Uniformed Services University of the Health Sciences. Dr. Snyders current address is Laboratory for Molecular Virology and Carcinogenesis, National Cancer Institute, Fredrick Cancer Research Facility, Fredrick, MD, USA, 21701.

REFERENCES

1. Bang, F. B., and A. Warwick. 1960 Mouse macrophages as host cells for the hepatitis virus and the genetic basis of their susceptibility. Proc. Natl. Acad Sci. USA 46: 1065.

2. Kantock, M., A. Warwick, and F. B. Bang. 1963. The cellular nature of genetic susceptibility to a virus. J. Exp. Med. 117:781.

3. Weiser, W., I. Vellisto, and F. B. Bang. 1976 Congenic strains of mice susceptible and resistant to mouse hepatitis virus. Proc. Soc. Exp. Biol. Med. 152:499.

4. Levy-Leblond, E., D. Oth, and J. M. Dupuy. 1979. Genetic study of mouse sensitivity to MHV-3 infection: influence of the H2 complex. J. Immunol. 122: 1359.

5. Stohlman, S. A. and J. A. Frelinger. 1978. Resistance to fatal central nervous system disease by mouse hepatitis virus, strain JHM. I. Genetic analysis. Immunogenetics 6: 277.

6. Knobler, R. L., M. V. Haspel, and M. B. A. Oldstone. 1981. Mouse hepatitis virus type 4 (JHM strain)-induced fatal central nervous system disease. I. Genetic control and the murine neuron as the susceptible site of disease. J. Exp. Med. 153:832.

7. Smith, M. S., R. E. Click, and P. G. W. Plagemann. 1984. Control of mouse hepatitis virus replication in macrophages by a recessive gene on chromosome 7. J. Immunol. 428.

8. Boyle, J. F., D. G. Weismiller, and K. V. Holmes. 1987. Genetic resistance to mouse hepatitis virus correlates with absence of virus binding activity on target tissues. J. Virol. 61:185.

9. Holmes, K. V., J. F. Boyle, D. G. Weismiller, S. R. Compton, R. K. Williams, C. B. Stephensen, and M. F. Frana. 1987. Adv. Exp. Med. Biol. 181:197.

10. Holmes, K. V., R. K. Williams, and C. B. Stephensen. 1989. Coronavirus receptors. In Concepts in viral pathogenesis, A. Notkins and M. B. A. Oldstone (Eds). Springer Verlag, New York.

11. Matsudaira, P.1987. Sequence from picomole quantities of proteins electroblotted onto polyvinylidene difluoride membranes. J. Biol. Chem. 10035.

Fc RECEPTOR-LIKE ACTIVITY OF MOUSE HEPATITIS VIRUS E2 GLYCOPROTEIN

Emilia L. Oleszak and Julian L. Leibowitz

Department of Pathology and Laboratory Medicine
University of Texas Health Science Center at Houston
Houston, TX 77030

INTRODUCTION

The JHM strain of mouse hepatitis virus (MHV-JHM) is a member of
the coronavirus family, which experimentally induces encephalomyelitis
in susceptible mice and rats. In surviving animals a chronic white
matter disease ensues.[1] The development of demyelinating lesions is
thought to be a primary effect of infection of oligodendrocytes.[2,3]
MHV-JHM virus has been shown to persist in the infected brain as long as
1 year after infection. Persistent infections of mice with other
strains of MHV such as MHV-A59 and MHV-3 have also been reported.[4,5,6]
Murine coronaviruses have four structural proteins: a matrix like
transmembrane glycoprotein (E1), a nucleocapsid protein (N), a peplomer
protein (E2), and for some laboratory strains of MHV-JHM a 65,000 Da
glycoprotein. [7,8] The E2 glycoprotein (180,000 Da) is responsible for
the attachment of MHV to the host cell plasma membrane, induction of
cell-to-cell fusion and eliciting of the production of neutralizing
antibody.[9,10] In the course of immunological staining of MHV-infected
cells with rabbit antisera we observed at moderate dilution (1:50 –
1:100) normal and preimmune serum stained MHV-JHM infected, but not
uninfected, cells. This staining could not be removed by absorption of
rabbit antiserum with uninfected cells. This observation suggested that
infection of cells with MHV may result in the expression of receptors
for the Fc region of immunoglobulin G (IgG). It has been reported, that
herpesviruses induce FcR on the surface of infected cells. The IgG Fc-
binding receptors induced by HSV-1 are composed of a complex of two
virally encoded glyproteins, gE and gI, and both of them are required
for Fc receptor activity.[11,12] We report here that MHV-JHM infected
cells express Fc binding ability. We have demonstrated that the E2
protein is responsible for Fc binding on infected cells.

MATERIALS AND METHODS

Viruses and Cells: The L-2 and WEHI-3 cell lines have been
described previously.[13,14] The origin and growth of MHV-JHM, MHV-A59 and
MHV-3 have been described.[8,15]

Antibodies: The 1.38.1 mab specific for the MHV E2 glycoprotein[16]
and a hyperimmune rabbit serum which recognizes N and E2 were develop in
this laboratory. Goat antiserum against purified MHV-A59 glycoprotein

E2 was a generous gift from Dr. K. Holmes. Rat anti-surfactant monoclonal antibodies were generously supplied by Dr. D. Strayer. The rat anti-mouse FcγR monoclonal antibody 2.4G2 was originally described by Unkeless.[17] Purified whole rabbit IgG specific for Micrococcus lysodeikticus as well as F(ab')$_2$ fragments were a generous gift of Dr. D. Rodkey. Affinity purified rabbit anti-goat IgG, goat anti-rabbit IgG, rabbit anti-mouse IgG and goat anti-rat IgG, and their FITC conjugates, were purchased from Jackson Immunoresearch Laboratories (West Grove, PA).

Metabolic labeling of cells and immunoprecipitation. Cytoplasmic lysates of MHV infected cultures which had been labeled with ^{35}S-methionine were prepared as described previously.[8] Secondary antibody coated Staphylococcus aureus Cowan strain (SAC) were washed with PBS and incubated with the desired primary antibody for one hour on ice. Unbound antibodies were washed away from the SAC cells with PBS and the SAC-antibody complexes were resuspended in 10 mM phosphate, pH 7.4, 500 mM NaCl, 0.25% NP-40, 0.2 TIU/ml of aprotinin, 1 mM PMSF. ^{35}S-labeled cell lysate was added to antibody coated SAC and incubated on ice for 1 hour. The precipitated material was extensively washed with the buffer described above. Bound antigens were dissociated by heating at 70°C in SDS-PAGE sample buffer and subsequently analyzed by SDS-polyacrylamide gel electrophoresis.[18]

Indirect immunofluorescence microscopy was carried out by standard techniques.

Partial proteolysis mapping: V-8 protease mapping was carried out by the technique described by Cleveland.[19]

RESULTS

In the course of immunofluorescence staining MHV-infected cells with rabbit antisera raised against MHV nonstructural proteins we observed that normal rabbit serum (NRS) at dilutions of 1:50 to 1:100 stained MHV-JHM infected L-2 cells (Fig. 1, Panel B) but not uninfected cells (Fig. 1, Panel E). Similar staining was observed with purified rabbit IgG specific for M. lysodeikticus (Panel C), but not with F(ab')$_2$ fragments of rabbit IgG (Panel F). Neither rabbit IgG specific for M. lysodeikticus nor its F(ab')$_2$ fragments stained uninfected cells (not shown). These data suggested, that the staining of MHV-JHM infected cells requires the Fc portion of immunoglobulin. NRS, rabbit IgG, and rabbit anti-MHV serum (Panel A) stained syncytia but not uninfected cells. The immune reaction was diffuse and restricted to the cytoplasm and the cell membrane.

Molecular mimicry of MHV E2 glycoprotein and mouse FcγR.

To examine the hypothesis that FcR-like structures are responsible for the immunostaining of MHV-JHM infected cells we carried out immunoprecipitation experiments using purified rabbit IgG specific for M. lysodeikticus and its purified F(ab')$_2$ fragments. This IgG immunoprecipitated a polypeptide of 180,000 Da from extracts of ^{35}S-labeled MHV-JHM infected cells (Figure 2, lane j) but not from uninfected cells. However F(ab')$_2$ fragments did not immunoprecipitate any polypeptides from MHV-JHM infected cells (lane i). This 180,000 Da polypeptide corresponded to 180,000 Da polypeptide precipitated by the neutralizing anti-E2 monoclonal antibody 1.38.1 (Figure 2, lane c and k). Furthermore, rat mab 2.4G2 specific for FcγR also

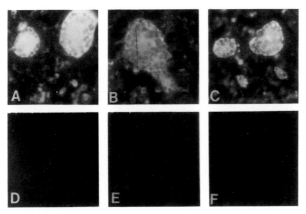

Fig. 1.   Indirect immunofluorescence staining of MHV-JHM infected cells.
          MHV-JHM infected L-2 cells were stained with rabbit anti-MHV
          serum (A) (1:100); NRS (B) (1:100); purified rabbit IgG 50μg,
          (C); rabbit F(ab')2 fragments 50μg, (F). Rabbit IgG (E) and
          rabbit anti-MHV serum (D) were used to stain mock infected cells.

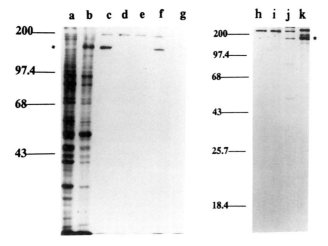

Fig. 2.   Immunoprecipitation of MHV-E2 glycoprotein by rabbit anti-M.
          lysodeikticus IgG. [^{35}S]-methionine labeled MHV-JHM infected
          and mock-infected cytoplasmic extracts were prepared as described
          in Materials and Methods. Lanes a and b display 0.5μl of mock-
          infected and MHV-JHM infected lysate respectively. MHV-JHM in-
          fected cell lysates were immunoprecipitated with the anti-E2
          mab 1.38.1 (lane c and k), with goat anti-mouse IgG (lane d), goat
          anti-rat IgG (lane e), rat anti-FcγR mab 2.4G2 (lane f), goat
          anti-rabbit IgG (lane h), 50μg rabbit anti-M.lysodeikticus
          F(ab')$_2$ fragments (lane i), 50μg of purified rabbit anti-
          M.lysodeikticus IgG (lane j). Mock-infected cell lysate was
          immunoprecipitated with the 2.4G2 mab (lane g). Immunoprecipitates
          were resolved by SDS-PAGE on a 8% gel (lanes a-g) or 10% gel (lanes
          h-k). The position of the 180,000 Da polypeptide is indicated
          (asterisk).

immunoprecipitated a 180,000 Da polypeptide from MHV-JHM-infected (Figure 2, lane f), but not from uninfected cells (Figure 2, lane g). Secondary goat anti-mouse IgG, goat anti-rat IgG and goat anti-rabbit IgG did not immunoprecipitate this 180,000 Da band.

Since MHV infects both mice and rats we investigated the ability of several irrelevant rat and mouse monoclonal antibodies to immunoprecipitate the E2 protein. Rat mabs specific for lung surfactant (IgG1 and IgG2b) immunoprecipitated a 180,000 Da polypeptide which coelectrophoresed with the protein immunoprecipitated with the 2.4G2 mab (Fig. 3). These rat mabs immunoprecipitated the 180,000 Da polypeptide from cells infected with additional strains of MHV, namely MHV-A59 and MHV-3 (Fig. 3).

Irrelevant mouse mab of the IgG2a subclass (OKT3, OKT8, MKD6) and IgG2b subclass (OKT4) but not IgG1 (anti-Leu 4 and mab specific for the T cell receptor gamma chain) also immunoprecipitated a 180,000 Da polypeptide from MHV-JHM infected cells but not from uninfected cells (data not shown). Therefore, we concluded that rat, mouse and rabbit IgG immunoprecipitated from MHV-JHM infected L-2 cells 180,000 Da polypeptide, which has identical molecular size to the MHV-E2 protein.

MHV-E2 glycoprotein and mouse FcγR are structurally identical

To determine if the 180,000 Da polypetide immunoprecipitated by the anti-E2 mab 1.38.1 and the anti-Fc γR mab 2.4G2 are structurally related we employed V-8 protease peptide map analysis.[19] V-8 protease digestion of the polypeptides immunoprecipitated by anti-E2 mab yielded an identical peptide map to that obtained by V-8 digestion of the polypeptide immunoprecipitated by the anti-FcγR mab (Fig. 4).

Since rabbit, rat and mouse IgG immunoprecipitated E2 glycoprotein from MHV-JHM infected L-2 cells we tested the ability of goat anti-E2 antibodies to bind to FcγR on the representative FcR bearing cell line, WEHI-3. The 2.4G2 mab, a rat anti-surfactant mab (IgG1), mouse mab MKD6 specific for I A^d and goat anti-E2 serum immunoprecipitated a 75,000 – 77,000 Da polypeptide typical of FcγR from ^{35}S-methionine labeled WEHI-3 cells (Fig. 5). Nonimmune goat serum did not precipitate any labeled proteins from WEHI-3 cells, suggesting, that the goat anti-E2 antibody immunoprecipitated the FcγR via its Fab region.

DISCUSSION

Molecular mimicry is defined as the presence of common antigenic sites, either linear or conformational, between microorganisms and normal host cell components.[20] The immune response initiated against foreign viral material, which is homologous to "self" host protein may lead to autoimmune disease.[21] In this work we report the antigenic mimicry between FcγR and the MHV-JHM E2 glycoprotein. Purified rabbit IgG, but not F(ab')$_2$ fragments, irrelevant rat mabs (IgG1 and IgG2b); irrelevant mouse mabs (IgG2a and IgG2b) immunoprecipitated a 180,000 Da polypeptide from MHV-JHM infected L-2 cells. Furthermore a rat 2.4G2 mab specific for FcγRII also immunoprecipitated also a 180,000 Da polypeptide from MHV-JHM infected cells which coelectrophoresed with the 180,000 Da molecule immunoprecipitated by a mab specific for MHV-E2 glycoprotein. The 180,000 Da polypeptide recognized by the 2.4G2 anti-FcγR mab and the 1.38.1 anti-E2 mab yield identical V-8 protease peptide maps (Fig. 4) and therefore, are almost assuredly the same molecular species. Furthermore, actinomycin D did not inhibit the expression of the 180,000 Da polypeptide that was immunoprecipitated by the anti-FcγR

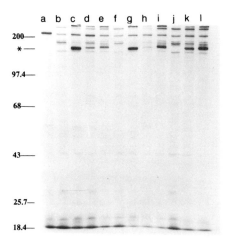

Fig. 3. Immunoprecipitation of MHV-E$_2$ by 2.4G2 anti-FcγR mab and anti-
         surfactant antibodies (IgG1 and IgG2b). MHV-JHM infected cells
         were immunoprecipitated with 2.4G2 mab (lane c), rat anti-surfactant
         mab (IgG1) (lane g) and rat anti-surfactant mab (IgG2b) (lane k).
         MHV-A-59 infected cells reacted with 2.4G2 mab (lane d); rat anti-
         surfactant mab (IgG1) (lane h) and rat anti-surfactant mab (IgG2b)
         (lane l). MHV-3 infected cells reacted with 2.4G2 mab (lane e);
         rat anti-surfactant mab (IgG1) (lane i). Goat anti-rat IgG were
         reacted with MHV-JHM infected cells (lane a). Mock-infected cells
         were reacted with 2.4G2 mab (lane b); rat anti-surfactant (IgG1)
         (lane f) and rat anti-surfactant (IgG2b) (lane j).

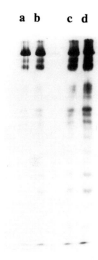

Fig. 4. Comparison of the Cleveland partial proteolytic fragments derived
         from 180,000 Da polypeptide immunoprecipitated by 2.4G2 anti-
         FcγR mab (lanes a,b) and by 1.38.1 anti-E$_2$ mab (lanes c,d).
         Lanes b and d contained approximately twice as much material
         as lanes a and c.

55

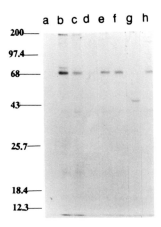

Fig. 5. Radioimmunoprecipitation of FcγR by goat anti-E2 antibodies.
^{35}S-methionine labeled WEHI-3 cell lysates were immunoprecipitated with goat anti-rat IgG (lane a); mab 2.4G2 (lane b);
rat anti-surfactant mab (lane c); goat anti-mouse IgG (lane d);
mab MKD6 (lane e); anti E2 mab (lane f); normal goat serum
(lane g); goat anti-E2 (lane h).

mab, indicating that this protein is of viral origin (data not shown).
Rabbit IgG, the 2.4G2 anti-FcγR mab and polyclonal goat anti-E2 specific
serum immunoprecipitated a typical FcγR molecule of 75,000-77,000 Da
from the myelomonocytic WEHI-3 cell line (Fig. 5). Nonimmune goat
serum, goat anti-mouse IgG and goat anti-rat IgG did not precipitate any
band from ^{35}S-labeled lysates of WEHI-3 cells. The binding of goat
anti-E2 to the FcγR suggests that this molecule shares an antigenic
determinant with the MHVE2 protein as well as an Fc binding activity.

Fc receptors for all immunoglobulin classes are found on B
lymphocytes, some T cells, macrophages, NK cells and polymorphonuclear
leukocytes.[22] The function of these Fc receptors is to bind Ig via the
Fc region of the Ig molecule. They provide a link between humoral and
cellular immune response by permitting antibody-dependent cell mediated
cytotoxicity (ADCC) to take place.[23,24,25] FcγRII recognized by the
2.4G2 mab is present on macrophages and lymphocytes[17]. The receptor is
a transmembrane glycoprotein with two extracellular domains that are
homologous to members of the Ig gene superfamily.[26]

Expression of receptors for the Fc regions of IgG are induced also
by members of Herpesviridae: HSV-1, HSV-2, cytomegalovirus and
varicella zoster[11,27,28,29,30] The FcγR- like molecules induced by HSV-1
are encoded in the virus genome and are comprised of a complex
containing gE and gI (g70) glycoproteins.[12,31] Both are required for Fc
receptor activity. No significant common structural basis for the Fc
binding activities of the MHV-E2, HSV-1 gE and gI and FcγR molecules
could be demonstrated on the basis of their primary sequences using the
Dayhoff Align program.[32]

The antigenic mimicry observed here between E2 viral antigen and
FcγR may have important biological implications. It has been postulated
that coating of infected cells with IgG molecules attached by their Fc
fragment may mask viral antigens from neutralizing anti-viral
antibody.[33] Such binding may allow the infected cells to escape
destruction by immunological mechanism, namely ADCC and complement
mediated lysis, and may contribute in maintenance of persistent
infection.

ACKNOWLEDGEMENTS

       We would like to thank Dr. K. Holmes, Dr. S. Rodkey, Dr. C.
Platsoucas and Dr. D. Strayer for generously providing several
antibodies used in this study. We gratefully acknowledge Dr. Ch.
Lawrance and the Molecular Biology Information Resource of the Baylor
College of Medicine for the use of their molecular biology software.
This work was supported by NIH grants NS-20834 and BRSG grant RR-05745.

REFERENCES

1.   O. Sorensen, R. Dugre, D. Percy, and S. Dales, In vivo and in vitro
     models of demyelinating diseases: endogenous factors influencing
     demyelinating disease caused by murine hepatitis virus in rats
     and mice. Infect. Immun. 37: 1248 (1982).
2.   P. W. Lampert, J. K. Sims, and A. J. Kniazeff, Mechanism of
     demyelination in JHM virus encephalomyelitis. Electron microscope
     studies. Acta. Neuro. Pathol. 24:76 (1976).
3.   H. S. Wege, S. Sidell, and V. ter Meulen, The biology and
     pathogenesis of coronaviruses. Curr. Top. Microbiol. Immunobiol.
     99:165 (1982).
4.   C. LePrevost, J. L. Virelizier, and J. M. Dupuy, Immunopathology
     of mouse hepatitis virus type 3 infection. III. Clinical and
     virologic observation of persistent viral infection. J. Immunol.
     115:640 (1975).
5.   T. Tamura, F. Taguchi, K. Veda, K. Fujiwara, Persistent infection
     with mouse hepatitis virus of low virulence in nude mice.
     Microbiol. Immunol. 21:683 (1977).
6.   J. L. Virelizier, Pathogenicity and persistence of mouse hepatitis
     virus in inbred strains of mice. In: Biochemistry and Biology
     of Coronaviruses (Adv. Exp. Biol. and Med., Vol. 142), Ter Meulen,
     V., Siddell, S., Wege, H. (eds.), 349-358, Plenum Press, New
     York (1981).
7.   S. Siddell, H. Wege, A. Barthel, and V. ter Meulen, Coronavirus
     JHM: intracellular protein synthesis. J. Gen. Virol 53:145 (1981).
8.   C. W. Bond, K. Anderson, and J. L. Leibowitz, Protein synthesis in
     cells infected by murine hepatitis viruses JHM and A:59. Tryptic
     peptide analysis. Arch. Virol. 80:333 (1984).
9.   A. R. Collins, R. L. Knobler, H. Powell, and M. J. Buchmeier, Monoclonal
     antibodies to murine hepatitis virus 4 (strain JHM) define the viral
     glycoprotein responsible for attachment and cell-cell fusion.
     Virology 119:358 (1982).
10. L. S. Sturman, C. S. Ricard, and K. V. Holmes, Proteolytic cleavage
     of the E2 glycoprotein of murine coronavirus: activition of cell-
     fusing activity of virions by trypsin and separation of two
     different 90K cleavage fragments. J. Virol. 56:904 (1985).
11. J. F. Watkins, Adsorption of sensitized sheep erythrocytes to HeLa
     cells infected with Herpes simplex virus. Nature 202:1364 (1964).
12. D. C. Johnson, M. C. Frame, M. W. Ligas, A. M. Cross and N. D. Stew,
     Herpes simplex virus immunoglobulin G Fc receptor activity depends
     on a complex of two viral glycoproteins, gE and gI. J. Virol.
     62:1347 (1988).
13. K. H. Rothels, A. A. Axelrad, L. Siminovitch, F. A. McCulloch, and
     R. C. Parker, The origin of altered cell lines from mouse, monkey,
     and man as indicated by chromosome and transplantation studies. Can.
     Cancer Conf. 3:189 (1959).
14. P. M. Hogarth, M. L. Hibbs, L. Bonadonna, B. M. Scott, E. Witort,
     G. A. Pietersz, and I. F. C. McKenzie, The mouse Fc receptor for
     IgG (Ly-17): molecular cloning and specificity. Immunogenetics
     26:161 (1987).
15. G. A. Levy, J. L. Leibowitz, and T. S. Edgington, The induction of

monocyte procoagulant activity by murine hepatitis virus (MHV-3) parallels disease susceptibility in mice. J. Exp. Med. 154:1150 (1981).

16. J. L. Leibowitz, J. D. DeVries, and M. Rodriguez, Increased hepatotropism of mutants of MHV, strain JHM, selected with monoclonal antibodies. Adv. Exp. Med. Biol. 218, 321-331, M.M.C. Lai and S. A. Stohlman, eds. Plenum Press, New York, NY. (1986).

17. J. C. Unkeless, Characterization of a monoclonal antibody directed against mouse macrophage and lymphocyte Fc receptors. J. Exp. Med. 150:580 (1979).

18. U. K. Laemmli, and M. Favre, Maturation of the head of bacteriophage T4. I. DNA packaging events. J. Mol. Biol. 80:575 (1973).

19. D. W. Cleveland, S. G. Fischer, M. W. Kirschner, and U. K. Laemmli, Peptide mapping by limited proteolysis in sodium dodecyl sulfate and analysis by gel electrophoresis. J. Biol. Chem. 252:1102 (1977).

20. T. Dyrberg, and M. B. A. Oldstone, Peptides as probes to study molecular mimicry and virus-induced autoimmunity. Curr. Top. Microbiol. Immunobiol. 130:25 (1986).

21. M. B. A. Oldstone, Molecular mimicry and autoimmune disease. Cell 50:819 (1987).

22. A. Froese, and F. Paraskevas, Structure and function of Fc receptors, Dekker, New York (1983).

23. C. F. Nathan, H.W. Murray, and Z. A. Cohn, The macrophage as an effector cell. N. Engl. J. Med. 303:622 (1980).

24. I.S. Mellman, H. Plutner, R. Steinman, J. C. Unkelles, and Z.A. Cohn, Internalization and degradation of macrophage Fc receptors during receptor-mediated phagocytosis. J. Cell Biol. 96:887 (1983).

25. R. G. Q. Leslie, Complex aggregation: a critical event in macrophage handling of soluble immune complexes. Immun. Today 6:183 (1985).

26. A. F. Williams, and A. N. Barclay, The immunoglobulin superfamily-domains for cell surface recognition. Ann. Rev. Immunol 6:381 (1988).

27. M. Ogata, and S. Shigeta, Appearance of immunoglobulin G Fc receptor in cultured human cells infected with varicella-zoster virus. Infect. Immun. 26:770 (1979).

28. M. F. Para, L. Goldstein, and P. G. Spear, Similarities and differences in the Fc binding glycoprotein (gE) of Herpes simplex virus types 1 and 2 and tentative mapping of the viral gene for this glycoprotein. J. Virol. 41:137 (1982).

29. T. Murayama, S. Natsuume-Sakai, K. Shimokawa, and T. Furnakawa, Fc receptor(s) induced by human cytomegalovirus bind differentially with human immunoglobulin G subclasses. J. Gen. Virol. 67:1475 (1986).

30. Y. Eizuru, and Y. Minamishima, Induction of Fc (IgG) receptor(s) by simian cytomegaloviruses in human embryonic lung fibroblasts. Intervirol. 29:339 (1988).

31. D. C. Johnson, and V. Feenstra, Indentification of a novel Herpes simplex virus type 1 - induced glycoprotein which complexes with gE and binds immunoglobulin. J. Virol. 61:2208 (1987).

32. M. O. Dayhoff, W. C. Barker, and L. T. Hunt, Establishing homologies in protein sequences. Methods Enzymol. 91: 524 (1983).

33. R. Adler, J. C. Glorioso, J. Cossman, and M. Levine, Possible role of Fc receptors on cells infected and transformed by Herpes-viruses: Escape from immune cytolysis. Infect. Immun. 21:442 (1978).

MOUSE FIBROBLAST MUTANTS SELECTED FOR SURVIVAL AGAINST MOUSE HEPATITIS VIRUS INFECTION SHOW INCREASED RESISTANCE TO INFECTION AND VIRUS-INDUCED CELL FUSION

M. Daya[1], F. Wong[1], M. Cervin[1], G. Evans[1], H. Vennema[2], W.J.M. Spaan[2] and R. Anderson[1]

[1]Department of Microbiology & Infectious Diseases
University of Calgary, Alberta, T2N 4N1, Canada, and
[2]Institute of Virology, Department of Infectious Diseases &
Immunology, Veterinary Faculty, State University, Utrecht
The Netherlands

ABSTRACT

We describe here a genetic approach to the analysis of host cell functions involved in determining permissiveness to mouse hepatitis virus (MHV). Using the chemical mutagen, ethyl methane sulfonate (EMS), mouse fibroblast cell mutants were generated which were selected for resistance to cell-killing by MHV. These mutants were then screened for their susceptibility to MHV infection, ability to replicate MHV and relative sensitivity to MHV-induced cell fusion. In contrast to wild type L-2 cells which were acutely and terminally infected by MHV, all five mutants examined replicated MHV in a persistent manner. These mutants showed a reduced susceptibility to MHV infection and an increased resistance to MHV-induced cell fusion. Fusion resistance was specific to that mediated by the MHV E2 protein; mutant as well as wild type L-2 cells were equally sensitive to fusion by polyethylene glycol. The combined effect of reduced infectability and increased fusion resistance was to limit MHV infection to only a small percentage of the total cells in culture, thereby permitting survival of both virus and cells. The observed high rate of generation of the cell mutants suggests that the conversion of a fully MHV-susceptible cell to a semi-resistant one (capable of supporting a persistent infection) is a fairly common event, possibly involving a single mutation.

INTRODUCTION

Cell mutants which are resistant to virus infection have proven to be useful in the elucidation of host cell functions required for virus replication. Although most exploited in prokaryotic systems (1), the analysis of virus-resistant cell mutants has also yielded interesting results in eukarotic cell-virus interactions (2-5).

Genetic resistance to mouse hepatitis virus (MHV)-induced disease can be demonstrated, at least in part, at the level of the virus-cell interaction. Various cell types including macrophages, hepatocytes and fibroblasts show relative permissiveness to MHV infection which correlates with susceptibility of the murine host to MHV-induced disease (6-9). Results from these and other studies indicate that cellular resistance to MHV may occur at the initial stage of virus binding (10, 11) or at post-adsorption stages (12, 13).

In an effort to define host cell functions which might discriminate between acute, subacute and abortive infections of MHV, we have isolated and characterized

Coronaviruses and Their Diseases
Edited by D. Cavanagh and T.D.K. Brown
Plenum Press, New York, 1990

a number of L-2 fibroblast-derived cell mutants which were selected for their ability to survive a normally cytocidal MHV infection.

MATERIALS AND METHODS

Cells and Viruses. Monolayers of L-2 (14), LM-K (15) and mutant L-2 (described below) cells were cultured in minimal essential medium (MEM) supplemented with 5% fetal calf serum (FCS). The A59 strain of MHV (16) was obtained from the American Type Culture Collection. The vMS strain of vaccinia is a recombinant virus containing the E2 gene of MHV(A59) (Vennema et al., manuscript in preparation). Cells were inoculated with virus by adsorbing for 30 min at room temperature and subsequently incubated at 37° in MEM containing 5% FCS. Plaque assays were performed using standard techniques (eg. 17) employing L-2 cells for MHV and vero cells for vMS. Cytopathic effect was documented by phase contrast photomicrography of Giemsa-stained cultures.

Generation of MHV-semi-resistant L-2 cell mutants. Confluent monolayers of L-2 cells in three 75 cm^2 flasks (5 x 10^7 cells/flask) were incubated for 18 h at 37° in minimal essential medium (MEM) supplemented with 5% fetal calf serum (FCS) and containing ethyl methanesulfonate (EMS; 300 μg/ml). Cell monolayers were washed with citrate saline and incubated in medium (EMS-free) for 48 h. The cells were then trypsinized and incubated for a further five days. Cultures were inoculated with MHV at an approximate multiplicity of infection (moi) of 0.1 and incubated for 36 h. After this time, most of the monolayer was destroyed, although a few isolated cells remained attached to the plastic substrate. The medium was replaced and these cells allowed to grow for 10 days after which time they had formed individual colonies. An average of 8-10 colonies was observed per 5 x 10^7 of MHV-challenged cells. When unmutagenized L-2 cells were subjected to a similar regimen of MHV-challenge and subsequent regrowth, a smaller number (1-2 colonies) was observed. Thus the rate of generation of spontaneous MHV- resistant cell mutants is apparently increased by EMS treatment. Cultures were trypsinized and cloned by limit dilution in 96-well plates. Five independent clones were grown up and analyzed as described below.

Immunofluorescence. Immunofluorescence was used to determine cellular susceptibility to MHV or vMS infection. Cell cultures (2 x 10^6 cells) were inoculated with MHV or vMS (8 x 10^6 pfu, as titered on L-2 cells) for 30 min at room temperature, washed three times with medium containing 5% FCS, and incubated at 37°. In order to prevent cell fusion and secondary spread of infection, cultures were treated at 3h PI with fusion-inhibiting anti-E2 MAb (18). At 6h (MHV infection) or 9h (vMS infection) cultures were fixed with 5% acetic acid/95% ethanol for 3 min, washed, blocked with 30% goat serum, incubated overnight with polyclonal anti-MHV antiserum, washed and treated 1h with goat anti-mouse FITC. After washing and mounting, cells were examined by immunofluorescent microscopy.

Contact fusion assay (19, 20). Sparsely seeded coverslip cultures (3 x 10^5 cells) of L-2, LM-K or L-2 mutant cells were either mock-infected or infected with either MHV or vMS. At either 4 (MHV) or 8 (vMS) h PI, cultures were overlaid with a ten-fold excess of uninfected L-2 or L-2 mutant cells and incubated at 37° for 4 h. Cultures were stained with Giemsa and examined by phase contrast microscopy.

RESULTS

Generation of L-2 cell mutants selected for survival against MHV infection

As described in Materials and Methods, a number of mutant L-2 cell clones was obtained which survived a normally cytocidal infection by MHV. Following limiting dilution none of the five mutant L-2 cell clones tested were found to be producing virus indicating that they had escaped infection by MHV.

Several cell lines in which MHV infection is persistent show a restricted susceptibility to infection, as shown by infectious centre assay (13, 19, 21). One possible explanation, therefore, for the ability of L-2 cell mutants to survive MHV infection is a partial resistance to the establishment of the infectious process. In order to examine this possibility, cultures of wild type L-2, LM-K and mutant L-2 cells were inoculated with the same stock of pretitered MHV, and subsequently monitored for infection by immunofluorescence. The results, shown in Table I, demonstrate a diverse ability, among the five mutant cell lines, to permit MHV infection. When exposed to the same MHV inoculum, mutant L-2 cells showed reduced numbers of infected cells as indicated by immunofluorescence. Because of the risk of secondary infection arising from cell-cell fusion, cells were incubated in the presence of fusion-inhibiting. MAb (18). By this method we could assure that only cells infected by the initial inoculum would be scored as positive. The results thus suggest a relative resistance of the L-2 cell mutants (as compared to wild type L-2 cells) to become infected by MHV and consequently escape its cell-killing effects. This fact is likely of critical importance to the success of generating the mutant L-2 cells by the selection procedure employed. By comparison, infection of the mutant L-2 cells with vMS showed no such severe restriction of infection (Table 1).

Table 1

Susceptibility of mutant L-2 cells to infection by MHV and vMS*

Cell	% immunofluorescent positive	
	MHV	vMS
L-2	100	100
LM-K	0.5 ± 0.4	100
M2	11 ± 4	78
M10	10 ± 5	65
M12	3 ± 1	83
M22	11 ± 5	88
M26	3 ± 1	73

*Monolayer cultures were inoculated with MHV or vMS, incubated and stained for immunofluorescence using polyclonal anti-MHV antiserum. Results for MHV-infected cells are the means ± standard deviations for three experiments.

Immunofluorescence analysis of MHV-infected L-2 cell mutant cultures maintained for 14 days at 37° showed fluctuating numbers of MHV-infected cells which generally ranged from 0.5 - 5% of the total cells in each culture (data not shown).

Mutant L-2 cells replicate MHV in a persistent fashion

In order to study the longer-term behaviour of MHV infection in the mutant cells, cultures were inoculated with virus and maintained for a period of two weeks.

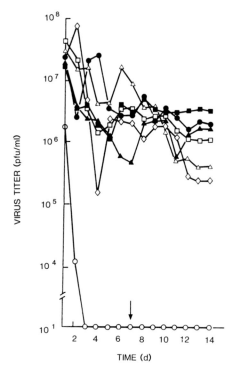

Figure 1

Persistent MHV infection of L-2 cell mutants. Confluent cultures (ca. 10^7 cells) of LM-K and L-2 (wild type and mutant) cells were inoculated with MHV and incubated at 37°. Media were changed daily and titrated for infectious virus by plaque assay. On day 7, surviving cultures were subpassaged by trypsinization (arrow). Symbols: L-2,○; M2,●; M10,□; M12,■; M22,△; M26,▲; LM-K,◇.

All mutant cells tested showed a remarkably similar pattern of virus production, characterized by continued, fluctuating levels of MHV, over the experimental period of 14 days. Although the monolayers showed evidence of syncytial development, this was much reduced compared to the wild type L-2 cells which survived and produced virus for only two days (Fig. 1). For comparison, MHV production in LM-K cells, previously shown to support a persistent infection of MHV (19), was also monitored in parallel over the l4-day period and was found to follow a pattern similar to that observed with the mutant L-2 cells (Fig. 1).

Mutant L-2 cells express fusion-active E2 at the cell surface

Although, as suggested above, the L-2 cell mutants show resistance to MHV-mediated fusion, they are themselves not deficient in expressing fusogenic E2 protein at their cell surfaces. This was demonstrated by a contact fusion procedure in which sparsely seeded cultures of vMS-infected L-2, LM-K or L-2 cell mutant cells were overlaid with an excess of uninfected L-2 cells at 8h PI and incubated for 4h at 37°. As shown in Fig. 2, all cells which were infected with vMS induced fusion with the uninfected L-2 cell neighbours indicating that the former were expressing fusion-active E2 at their outer surfaces.

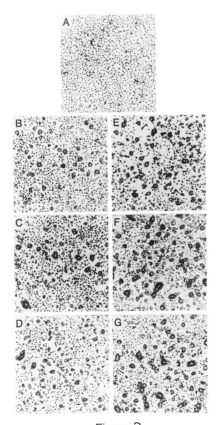

Figure 2

L-2 cell mutants express fusion-active E2 protein at the cell surface. Sparsely seeded L-2 (A, B) or L-2 mutant (M2, C; M10, D; M12, E; M22, F or M26, G) were mock-infected (A) or infected with vMS (B-G). At 8h PI cultures were overlaid with a ten-fold excess number of uninfected L-2 cells and examined for contact fusion.

Mutant L-2 cells show resistance to MHV-induced fusion

Since it was noted that the progression of MHV-induced cell fusion appeared more slowly in the mutant cell lines as compared to wild type L-2 cells, it seemed likely that the cell mutants might be relatively more fusion-resistant and therefore able to restrict virus spread and accompanying cytopathology throughout the cultures. To test this idea directly a contact fusion assay was performed (19) in which sparsely seeded MHV-infected wild type L-2 cells were overlaid with a ten-fold excess number of cells (either mutant or wild type) and the resultant cell-cell fusion monitored after 4 h at 37°. As shown in Fig. 3 syncytial development was markedly reduced in the mutant cell lines, confirming the idea that they are relatively resistant to MHV-induced fusion.

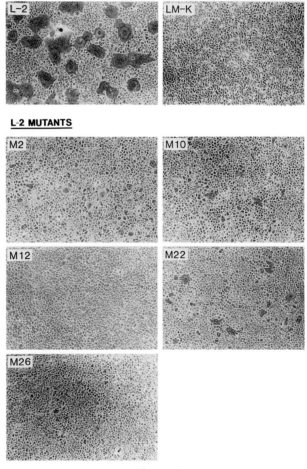

Figure 3

L-2 cell mutants are resistant to MHV-mediated cell fusion. Contact fusion was monitored between sparsely seeded MHV-infected L-2 cells and a ten-fold excess of uninfected L-2, LM-K, or L-2 mutant cells.

Although it is clear that the mutant L-2 cells are resistant to E2- mediated fusion, they do not show generalized resistance to fusogenic agents. This was tested by determining numbers of multinucleate cells formed by treatment of wild type L-2 and mutant L-2 (M2, M10, M12, M22 and M26) with polyethylene glycol (PEG); no difference was observed among the cells tested (data not shown). Taken together, the results are compatible with the hypothesis that the mutant L-2 cells are defective in a cell surface E2- specific recognition factor (possibly a receptor) which is required for efficient membrane fusion to occur.

DISCUSSION

The present results confirm an earlier hypothesis that host cell differences in susceptibility to MHV infection correlate with differences in susceptibility to MHV-mediated cell fusion (19, 20). All five mutants tested in the present study showed a similar phenotype of reduced infectability and reduced susceptibility to MHV E2-mediated fusion. The relatively high mutational frequency observed during the generation of these mutants suggests that the two factors (infectability and fusion susceptibility) are co-mutable. This conclusion may find rationalization in the likely involvement of membrane fusion in two steps of the virus replication cycle, i.e. internalization/uncoating and late cell-cell fusion. The mutagenesis studies thus point toward the alteration of a single cellular component which is required for efficient virus infection as well as for membrane fusion. A possible candidate may be a cell surface protein required for the facilitation of fusogenic activity of the E2 protein.

Indications that host resistance to MHV-mediated fusion plays an important role in permissiveness to MHV infection come also from other studies. Host restriction of MHV-JHM replication in peritoneal macrophages is coupled with reduced virus dissemination by a cell fusion-dependent mechanism (22). Genetic control of resistance to MHV-induced cell fusion has also been reported in hepatocytes (8) and in cells of the central nervous system (23).

It is apparent from the present study that a cell population's tolerance to long term MHV infection can arise by mechanisms other than those which drastically restrict virus replication. Resistance to MHV-induced fusion represents not only a protective mechanism against a severe cytopathic effect but also against an important mode of MHV dissemination. It is likely that these factors permit the development of a persistently infected state by limiting the numbers of infected cells and permitting a dynamically changing proportion of the total cell population to escape infection.

ACKNOWLEDGMENTS

The Medical Research Council of Canada is gratefully acknowledged for grant support. H.V. is supported by a grant from Duphar B.V. (Weesp, The Netherlands). We also thank Leo Heynem for technical assistance in the preparation of vMS.

REFERENCES

1. Friedman, D.I., Olson, E.R., Georgopoulos, C., Tilly, K., Herskowitz, I. and Banuett, F. (1984) Interactions of bacteriophage and host macromolecules in the growth of bacteriophage lambda. Microbiol. Rev. 48, 299-325.
2. Toyama, S., Toyama, S. and Uetake, H. (1977) Altered cell-fusion capacity in lines of KB cells resistant to Sendai virus-induced cytolysis. Virology 76, 503-515.
3. Tufaro, F., Snider, M.D. and McKnight, S.L. (1987) Identification and characterization of a mouse cell mutant defective in the intracellular transport of glycoproteins. J. Cell Biol. 105, 647-657.

4. Hara, T., Hattori, S. and Kawakita, M. (1989) Isolation and characterization of mouse FM3A cell mutants which are devoid of Newcastle Disease Virus receptors. J. Virol. 63, 182-188.
5. Kaplan, G., Levy, A. and Racaniello, V.R. (1989) Isolation and characterization of HeLa cell lines blocked at different steps in the poliovirus life cycle. J. Virol. 63, 43-51.
6. Virelizier, J.L. and Allison, A.C. (1976) Correlation of persistent mouse hepatitis virus (MHV-3) infection with its effects on mouse macrophage cultures. Arch. Virol. 50, 279-285.
7. MacNaughton, M.R. and Patterson, S. (1980) Mouse hepatitis virus strain 3 infection of C57, A/Sn and A/J strain mice and their macrophages. Arch. Virol. 66, 71-75.
8. Arnheiter, H., Baechi, T. and Haller, O. (1982) Adult mouse hepatocytes in primary monolayer culture express genetic resistance to mouse hepatitis virus type 3. J. Immunol. 129, 1275-1281.
9. Lamontagne, L.M. and Dupuy, J.M. (1984) Natural resistance of mice to mouse hepatitis virus type 3 infection is expressed in embryonic fibroblast cells. J. Gen. Virol. 65, 1165-1171.
10. Tardieu, M., Boespflug, O., Barbe, T. (1986) Selective tropism of a neurotropic coronavirus for ependymal cells, neurons and meningeal cells. J. Virol. 60, 574-582.
11. Boyle, J.F., Weismiller, D.G. and Holmes, K.V. (1987) Genetic resistance to mouse hepatitis virus correlates with absence of virus-binding activity on target tissues. J. Virol. 61, 185-189.
12. Van Dinter, S. and Flintoff, W.F. (1987) Rat glial C6 cells are defective in murine coronavirus internalization. J. Gen. Virol. 68, 1677-1685.
13. Kooi, C., Mizzen, L., Alderson, C., Daya, M. and Anderson, R. (1988) Early events of importance in determining host cell permissiveness to mouse hepatitis virus infection. J. Gen. Virol. 69, 1125-1135.
14. Rothfels, K.H., Axelrad, A.A., Siminovitch, L., McCulloch, E.A. and Parker, R.C. (1959) The origin of altered cell lines from mouse, monkey and man as indicated by chromosome and transplantation studies. Canad. Cancer Conf. 3, 189-214.
15. Kit, S., Dubbs, D.R., Piekarski, L.J., Hsu, T.C. (1963) Deletion of thymidine kinase activity from L cells resistant to bromodeoxyuridine. Exp. Cell Res. 31, 297-312.
16. Manaker, R.A., Piczak, C.V., Miller, A.A. and Stanton, M.F. (1961) A hepatitis virus complicating studies with mouse leukemia. J. Natl. Cancer Inst. 27, 29-44.
17. Lucas, A., Flintoff, W., Anderson, R., Percy, D., Coulter, M. and Dales, S. (1977) In vivo and in vitro models of demyelinating diseases: tropism of the JHM strain of murine hepatitis virus for cells of glial origin. Cell 12, 553-560.
18. Mizzen, L., Macintyre, G., Wong, F. and Anderson, R. (1987) Translational regulation in mouse hepatitis virus infection is not mediated by altered intracellular ion concentrations. J. Gen. Virol. 68, 2143-2151.
19. Mizzen, L., Cheley, S., Rao, M., Wolf, R. and Anderson, R. (1983) Fusion resistance and decreased infectability as major host cell determinants of coronavirus persistence. Virology 128, 407-417.
20. Mizzen, L., Daya, M. and Anderson, R. (1987) The role of protease-dependent cell membrane fusion in persistent and lytic infections of murine hepatitis virus. Adv. Exp. Med. Biol. 218, 175-186.
21. Lucas, A., Coulter, M., Anderson, R., Dales, S. and Flintoff, W. (1978) In vivo and in vitro models of demyelinating diseases. II. Persistence and host-regulated thermosensitivity in cells of neural derivation infected with mouse hepatitis and measles viruses. Virology 88, 325-337.
22. Knobler, R.L., Tunison, L.A. and Oldstone, M.B.A. (1984) Host genetic control of mouse hepatitis virus type 4 (JHM strain) replication. I. Restriction of virus amplification and spread in macrophages from resistant mice. J. Gen. Virol. 65, 1543-1548.
23. Wilson, G.A.R. and Dales, S. (1988) In vivo and in vitro models of demyelinating disease: efficiency of virus spread and formation of infectious centers among glial cells is genetically determined by the murine host. J. Virol. 62, 3371-3377.

ON THE MEMBRANE CYTOPATHOLOGY OF MOUSE HEPATITIS VIRUS INFECTION AS PROBED BY A SEMI-PERMEABLE TRANSLATION-INHIBITING DRUG

G. Macintyre, C. Kooi, F. Wong and R. Anderson

Department of Microbiology & Infectious Diseases
University of Calgary, Calgary, Alberta
T2N 4N1, Canada

ABSTRACT

Previous studies of the membrane fusion process have permitted the characterization of membrane permeability changes concomitant with MHV-induced cytopathology. One indication of membrane permeability in MHV-infected cells is their sensitivity to translational inhibition by the normally impermeable amino-glycoside, hygromycin B (Macintyre, G., Wong, F. and Anderson, R. (1989) J. Gen. Virol. 70, 763-768). In the present study, we examine the hygromycin B sensitivity of acutely infected mouse fibroblast L-2 cell and macrophage cultures as well as persistently infected mouse fibroblast LM-K cell cultures. The results suggest that membrane permeability alterations (as indicated by hygromycin B sensitivity) are a common feature of these MHV infections. Hygromycin B "cured" persistently infected LM-K cells as indicated by the absence of detectable virus antigen by immunofluorescence and by the absence of infectious virus even after removal of the drug or co-cultivation with untreated L-2 cells. The results argue against the maintenance of MHV infection by a mechanism involving latently or non-cytolytically infected cells. We conclude therefore that at least one mechanism for MHV persistence depends on virus propagation by cytolytic infection of a small, dynamically changing, fraction of the total cells present in culture.

INTRODUCTION

Murine coronaviruses, typified by murine hepatitis virus (MHV) are able to produce infections of either an acute or persistent nature. Some evidence from in vitro (1,2) and in vivo (3,4) studies suggests that virus variants are produced which may account for the persistence of infection, while other studies (5-7) showed that persistent infections of MHV could be established in the absence of detectable levels of virus variants.

Some strains of MHV can produce persistent infections of the nervous system, which are characterized by symptoms similar to those of certain slowly degenerative neurological conditions in humans. MHV infection may persist due to a state of co-existence between isolated pockets of virus infected cells and normal, uninfected tissue (8-12). However, other evidence (13) suggests that virus infection of certain areas of the brain can proceed in a virtually latent manner in the absence of overt cytopathic effect (c.p.e.).

We have previously noted membrane permeability changes during acute MHV infection of mouse L-2 fibroblasts (14). Mouse LM-K fibroblasts which

Coronaviruses and Their Diseases
Edited by D. Cavanagh and T.D.K. Brown
Plenum Press, New York, 1990

support persistent infection of MHV also show membrane permeability alterations, as determined by sensitivity to the normally impermeable translation-inhibiting drug, hygromycin B (15). MHV persistence of LM-K cells, which normally involves a steady state infection of 0.1 - 1% of the cells in culture, was found to be cured by hygromycin B treatment, as measured by the elimination of infectious virus from the supernatant media. Hygromycin B also resulted in the eradication of MHV-specific RNA from LM-K cells (15).

In the present paper, we investigate further the mechanism of MHV persistence in LM-K cells and extend our studies using hygromycin B to mouse macrophages, which are an important target of MHV infection in the animal.

MATERIALS AND METHODS

Cells and Virus. L-2 cells (16) and LM-K cells (17) were grown as monolayers in minimal essential medium (MEM) supplemented with 5% fetal calf serum (FCS). After inoculation with MHV-A59 (18), virus was allowed to absorb for 30 min at room temperature. The cells were then incubated at 37°C in MEM containing 5% FCS and the relevant concentration of hygromycin B. The amount of infectious virus present in culture medium after drug treatment was measured by titration on L-2 cells by plaque assay (5).

Co-cultivation rescue study. MHV-inoculated LM-K cells, maintained in various concentrations of hygromycin B for 108 h, were trypsinized, centrifuged and mixed with an equal number of untreated L-2 cells. Following plating and incubation at 37°C, aliquots were taken from the supernatant media for assay of infectious virus by plaque assay (5).

Isolation of Peritoneal Macrophages. Four month old Balb/c mice were injected (i.p.) with 1.5ml 2% starch in 0.9% NaCl two days prior to the harvesting of peritoneal macrophages. Mice were sacrificed by cervical dislocation and the peritoneal cavity was washed twice with MEM plus 20% FCS. The total peritoneal wash was centrifuged at 1000g for 1 min and the pellet washed with MEM plus 20% FCS. The final pellet was resuspended in MEM plus 10% FCS, plated out and incubated overnight to allow the macrophages to adhere to the wells. Erythrocytes were removed by gently rinsing the monolayers with MEM plus 10% FCS. The monolayers were then infected with MHV as described for L-2 cells.

Immunofluorescence. At 42h PI cultures incubated in the absence or presence of hygromycin B were fixed with 5% acetic acid/95% ethanol for 3 min and washed. After blocking with 30% goat serum, samples were incubated overnight with polyclonal anti-MHV antiserum, washed and treated for 1h with goat anti-mouse FITC. After washing and mounting, cells were examined by immunofluorescent microscopy and scored for the presence of viral antigen.

RESULTS

Curing of Persistent MHV Infection by Hygromycin B

As previously reported, treatment of persistently infected LM-K cells with hygromycin B (0.5mM or higher) reduced virus propagation, viral RNA and viral antigen to undetectable levels (15). As a further verification that complete curing of persistent MHV infection could be achieved by hygromycin B treatment, persistently infected LM-K cultures, maintained for 108 h in the presence of drug, were returned to drug-free medium (indicated by arrow in fig. 1) and monitored for a further 108 h for the appearance of infectious virus. As shown in Fig. 1, cultures which were treated with drug at concentrations of 0.5mM or higher were in fact cured, showing no subsequent release of virus after removal of the drug.

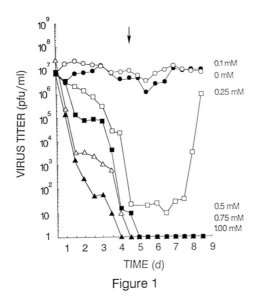

Figure 1

Curing of Persistent MHV Infection by Hygromycin B:
Removal of Drug Does Not Reactivate Infection

As a further check of the efficacy of hygromycin B in curing persistently infected LM-K cells, a co-cultivation rescue experiment was performed. This type of experiment is based on those used with occasional success in other virus systems in which release of infectious virus from a latently infected cell may be achieved by co-cultivation with a permissive cell type.

Accordingly, L-2 cells, known to be highly permissive to MHV (5-7), were added in a 1:1 ratio to persistently infected LM-K cells which had been treated for 108 h with various concentrations of hygromycin B. Following incubation in drug-free medium aliquots were removed from the supernatant media for infectious virus assay. As shown in Table 1, no virus was released by this co-cultivation rescue method from persistently infected LM-K cells which had been treated with hygromycin B at 0.5mM or higher.

In conjunction with our previous results using cDNA and antibody probes (15) the above studies strongly argue against the presence of even a small fraction of persistently infected LM-K cells in which the infection is resistant to hygromycin B and therefore free of virus-induced membrane cytopathology.

Susceptibility of MHV Infection of Macrophages to Hygromycin B

Peritoneal macrophages from Balb/c mice are susceptible to MHV infection and show a similar outcome to the infection as L-2 cells, including virus production and overt c.p.e. characterized by fusion of the cell monolayer (19). Monolayer cultures of L-2 cells and peritoneal macrophages were infected with MHV at an m.o.i. of 0.1. The cultures were incubated in the absence or presence of hygromycin B at various concentrations. At 42h PI the monolayers were examined by immunofluorescent microscopy and scored for the presence of viral antigen. The amount of viral antigen that could be detected in L-2 cells decreased with increasing concentrations of the drug. Hygromycin B had a similar but more severe effect on the MHV infection of peritoneal macrophages. At the lowest concentration of drug, 0.1mM, there was a marked decrease in the amount of viral antigen as compared to the infected, untreated macrophage culture. Treatment with hygromycin B at 0.25mM and above decreased viral antigen to undetectable levels in the peritoneal macrophages (Table 2). Thus, MHV infection of both L-2 cells and peritoneal macrophages can be cured by treatment with hygromycin B.

Table 1

Curing of Persistent MHV Infection by Hygromycin B:
Absence of "Rescuable" Virus by Co-cultivation

	Virus Titer (pfu/ml)	
	6h	24h
[Hygromycin B, mM]		
0	4.6×10^6	3.4×10^6
0.1	5.1×10^6	3.4×10^6
0.25	1.4×10^5	3.2×10^6
0.5	0	0
0.75	0	0
1.0	0	0

MHV-infected LM-K cells treated for 108h with the
relevant concentration of hygromycin B were harvested,
mixed with an equal number of L-2 cells and plated out.
The amount of virus present in media harvested at 6 and
24h post-mixing was quantitated by plaque assay.

Table 2

Susceptibility of MHV Infection of Macrophages to Hygromycin B

[Hygromycin B, mM]	Relative Immunofluorescence	
	L-2	Macrophages
0	+ + + +	+ + + +
0.1	+ + + +	+
0.25	+ + +	-
0.5	+ + +	-
0.75	+	-
1.00	-	-

MHV-infected L-2 cells and peritoneal macrophages were treated with various concentrations of hygromycin B for 42h PI. The monolayers were then stained for immunofluoresence as described in Materials and Methods.

DISCUSSION

The results from this and our previous study (15) suggest that hygromycin B sensitivity may be a common feature of MHV infections in various cell types. Hygromycin B sensitivity is also associated with infections of several other viruses (20). While the mechanism of action of hygromycin B in virus-infected cells remains uncertain, evidence has been presented by other groups, suggesting the involvement of virus-induced membrane changes, either at the level of the plasma membrane (20) or the endosome (21). From our results, it is evident that whatever these changes are, they occur in both acute and persistent infections of MHV. Persistent MHV infection of LM-K cells, for example, can be cured by hygromycin B treatment which selectively eliminates MHV-infected cells. The maintenance of MHV persistence, at least in LM-K cells, therefore involves the expression of this aspect of viral cytopathology which predisposes the host cell to hygromycin B sensitivity.

REFERENCES

1. Stohlman, S.A., Sakaguchi, A.Y. and Weiner, L.P. (1979) Characterization of the cold-sensitive murine hepatitis virus mutants rescued from latently infected cells by cell fusion. Virology 98:448-455.
2. Holmes, K.V. and Behnke, J.N. (1981) Evolution of a coronavirus during persistent infection in vitro. Adv. Exp. Med. Biol. 142:287-299.
3. Jackson, D., Percy, D. and Morris, V.L. (1984) Characterization of murine hepatitis virus (JHM) RNA from rats with experimental encephalomyelitis. Virology 137:297-304.

4. Taguchi, F., Siddell, S., Wege, H., Massa, P. and ter Meulen, V. (1987) Characterization of JHMV variants isolated from rat brain and cultured neural cells after wild type JHMV infection. Adv. Exp. Med. Biol. 218:343-349.
5. Lucas, A., Flintoff, W., Anderson, R., Percy, D., Coulter, M. and Dales, S. (1977) In vivo and in vitro models of demyelinating diseases: Tropism of the JHM strain of murine hepatitis virus for cells of glial origin. Cell 12:553-560.
6. Lucas, A., Coulter, M., Anderson, R., Dales, S. and Flintoff, W. (1978) In vivo and in vitro models of demyelinating diseases. II. Persistence and host-regulated thermosensitivity in cells of neural derivation infected with mouse hepatitis and measles viruses. Virology 88:325-337.
7. Mizzen, L., Cheley, S., Rao, M., Wolf, R. and Anderson, R. (1983) Fusion resistance and decreased infectability as major host cell determinants of coronavirus persistence. Virology 128:407-417.
8. Bailey, O.T., Pappenheimer, A.M. and Cheever, F.S. (1949) A murine virus (JHM) causing disseminated encephalomyelitis with extensive destruction of myelin. II. Pathology. J. Exptl. Med. 90:195-212.
9. Weiner, L.P., Johnson, R.T. and Herndon, R.M. (1973) Viral infections and demyelinating diseases. New Engl. J. Med. 288:1103-1110.
10. Haspel, M.V., Lampert, P.W. and Oldstone, M.B.A. (1978) Temperature-sensitive mutants of mouse hepatitis virus produce a high incidence of demyelination. Proc. Natl. Acad. Sci. U.S.A. 75:4033-4036.
11. Nagashima, K., Wege, H., Meyermann, R. and ter Meulen, V. (1978) Demyelinating encephalomyelitis induced by long-term coronavirus infection in rats. A preliminary report. Acta Neuropathol. 45:205-213.
12. Sorensen, O., Percy, D. and Dales, S. (1980) In vivo and in vitro models of demyelinating diseases. III. JHM virus infection of rats. Arch. Neurol. 37:478-484.
13. Sorensen, O., Beushausen, S., Puchalski, S., Cheley, S., Anderson, R., Coulter-Mackie, M. and Dales, S. (1984) In vitro and in vivo models of demyelinating diseases - VIII: genetic, immunologic and cellular influences on JHM virus infection of rats. Adv. Exp. Med. Biol. 173:279-298.
14. Mizzen, L., Macintyre, G., Wong, F. and Anderson, R. (1987) Translational regulation in mouse hepatitis virus infection is not mediated by altered intracellular ion concentrations. J. Gen. Virol. 68:2143-2151.
15. Macintyre, G., Wong, F. and Anderson, R. (1989) A model for persistent murine coronavirus infection involving maintenance via cytopathically infected cell centres. J. Gen. Virol. 70:763-768.
16. Rothfels, K.H., Axelrad, A.A., Siminovitch, L., McCulloch, E.A. and Parker, R.C. (1959) The origin of altered cell lines from mouse, monkey and man as indicated by chromosome and transplantation studies. Can. Cancer Conf. 3:189-214.
17. Kit, S., Dubbs, D.R., Piekarski, L.J. and Hsu, T.C. (1963) Deletion of thymidine kinase activity from L cells resistant to bromodeoxyuridine. Exp. Cell Res. 31:297-312.
18. Manaker, R.A., Piczak, C.V., Miller, A.A. and Stanton, M.F. (1961) A hepatitis virus complicating studies with mouse leukemia. J. Natl. Cancer Inst. 27:29-44.
19. Taguchi, F., Yamaguchi, R., Makino, S. and Fujiwara, K. (1981) Correlation between growth potential of mouse hepatitis viruses in macrophages and their virulence for mice. Infect. Immun. 34:1059-1061.
20. Benedetto, A., Rossi, G.B., Amici, C., Belardelli, F., Cioe, L., Carruba, G. and Carrasco, L. (1980) Inhibition of animal virus production by means of translation inhibitors unable to penetrate normal cells. Virology 106:123-132.
21. Cameron, J.M., Clemens, M.J., Gray, M.A., Menzies, D.E., Mills, B.J., Warren, A.P. and Pasternak, C.A. (1986) Increased sensitivity of virus-infected cells to inhibitors of protein synthesis does not correlate with changes in plasma membrane permeability. Virology 155:534-544.

MOLECULAR CHARACTERIZATION OF THE 229E STRAIN OF HUMAN

CORONAVIRUS

Nathalie Arpin and Pierre J. Talbot

Virology Research Center
Institut Armand-Frappier, Université du Québec
531, boulevard des Prairies
Laval, Québec, CANADA H7N 4Z3

ABSTRACT

Human coronaviruses (HCV) cause various respiratory, gastrointestinal and possibly neurological disorders. Very little is known of the molecular biology of these ubiquitous pathogens. We have undertaken the molecular characterization of the prototype 229E strain of HCV. The virus grew to the highest titers on a human embryonic lung cell line (L132) at 33°C and purification was optimal on Renografin-60® gradients. Metabolic labeling with [^{35}S]methionine or [^{3}H]glucosamine or galactose and analysis by SDS-PAGE revealed at least five structural proteins, which could be identified by analogy with murine coronaviruses as follows: the spike glycoprotein (E2/S), in both monomeric (88-97 kDa) and dimeric (190-200) forms, the nucleoprotein (N) at 52-53 kDa and the matrix protein (E1/M), in both glycosylated (25-26 kDa) and non-glycosylated (20-22 kDa) forms. Monomeric, dimeric and multimeric (>200 kDa) forms of E2/S incorporated glucosamine and galactose, whereas only galactose was incorporated into E1/M. Multimers of E1/M, with apparent molecular masses of 44, 74 and 140 kDa, were formed in the absence of a reducing agent.

INTRODUCTION

Human coronaviruses belong to either one of two antigenic groups, represented by the prototype strains 229E and OC43[1]. They are responsible for as much as 25% of common colds[2], and a possible involvement in neurological disorders was suggested by the observation of corona-like virus particles in the brain of one multiple sclerosis (MS) patient[3], the isolation of two coronaviruses from MS brain tissue passaged in mice[4] and the detection of intrathecal antibodies against coronaviruses in MS patients[5]. Nevertheless, our limited knowledge of the molecular structure and biology of human coronaviruses and the lack of molecular probes have not yet allowed a verification of their medical importance. We report here our initial studies on the molecular structure of the 229E strain of human coronavirus.

METHODS

Cells and virus

The L132 human embryonic lung cell line[6,7], the Vero african green monkey kidney cell line and the 229E strain of HCV (HCV-229E) were obtained from the American

Type Culture Collection (ATCC; Rockville, MD, U.S.A.). The RD151 human rhabdomyosarcoma[8,9] and the HRT18 human adenocarcinoma[10] cell lines were kindly provided by Dr. Arlene R. Collins (State University of New York, Buffalo, NY, U.S.A.) and Dr. David A. Brian (University of Tennessee, Knoxville, TN, U.S.A.), respectively. The IMHP human embryonic lung cell line was obtained fron the Tissue Culture Service of this Institute. Cells were grown as monolayers at 37 °C in Earle's minimum essential medium : Hank's M199 (1:1, v/v) containing 0.13 % (w/v) sodium bicarbonate, 50 µg/ml of gentamicin and 5% (v/v) fetal bovine serum (FBS). The virus was plaque-purified twice and a stock obtained by three serial passages at an MOI of 0.001. Infectious titers were determined by plaque assay as described[11], except that plaques were revealed after a 7-day incubation period of infected L132 cells at 33°C. Viral infections were performed on half-confluent cell monolayers in medium which had a FBS content reduced to 1% (v/v). For viral growth curves in L132 cells, infectious titers were obtained by plaque assay with both culture medium clarified at 1500 x g for 7 min (extracellular virus) and cell monolayers lysed by three cycles of freezing at -70°C and thawing at 37°C (intracellular virus).

Radiolabeling of viral polypeptides

The infectious titer of the HCV-229E stock was concentrated after a fourth passage at low MOI in L132 cells. The medium, harvested at 43 hrs p.i., was clarified by centrifugation at 10,000 x g for 20 min and virus pelleted at 100,000 x g for 90 min. Resuspension into a small volume of culture medium boosted the viral titer from 1.2 x 10^6 to 2.6 x 10^8 PFU/ml. This allowed infection of cells at a higher MOI, in order to optimize the incorporation of radiolabeled precursors into viral polypeptides. At 4 hrs after infection of cells with HCV-229E at an MOI of 1, either 0.33 mCi/ml of [^{35}S]methionine (^{35}S-E. coli hydrolysate containing 70 % methionine) or 70 µCi/ml of [^{3}H]glucosamine or [^{3}H]galactose (ICN, Ville St-Laurent, PQ, Canada) was added to the culture medium.

Virus purification

Infected fluids were harvested at 43 hrs p.i., clarified by centrifugation at 10,000 x g for 20 min, and virus precipitated with 10 % (w/v) polyethylene glycol in the presence of 0.5 M NaCl. After centrifugation at 10,000 x g for 30 min, the pellet was resuspended in TMEN buffer (50 mM Tris-acid-maleate, pH 6.2, 0.1 M NaCl, 1 mM EDTA) and applied to a discontinuous 10 and 50% (v/v) Renografin-60® (Squibb Canada, Montréal, PQ, Canada) gradient, which was centrifuged at 148,000 x g for 2 hrs. The viral band was further purified on a continuous gradient of the same material, centrifuged at the same speed for 18 hrs. In one experiment, the following gradient materials were compared to Renografin-60® for the optimization of viral purification: 10-50 % (w/w) sucrose or potassium tartrate or 10-50% (w/w) Nycodenz® (Accurate Chemicals, Westbury, NY, U.S.A.).

Polyacrylamide gel electrophoresis (SDS-PAGE)

Samples were resuspended in sample buffer [50 mM Tris-HCl, pH 6.8, 1% (w/v) sodium dodecyl sulfate (SDS), 1% (v/v) 2-mercaptoethanol (omitted in one experiement), 10% (v/v) glycerol, 0.003% (w/v) bromophenol blue] and treated at 100 °C for 2 min. Polypeptides were separated on 7 to 15% (w/v) polyacrylamide gels[12] and revealed by fluorography with Enlightning® (Dupont, Montréal, PQ, Canada). Radiolabeled molecular weight standards were used to estimate the size of viral polypeptides.

RESULTS

The initial step in our molecular characterization of HCV-229E consisted in optimizing virus growth and purification conditions. A viral growth curve was established in L132 cells at 37°C, as shown in Fig. 1. After infection at low MOI, infectious virus was detectable by 10 hrs p.i. and started to appear in the culture medium at 14 hrs p.i., before reaching a peak at 42-44 hrs p.i.. However, much higher infectious titers could be obtained

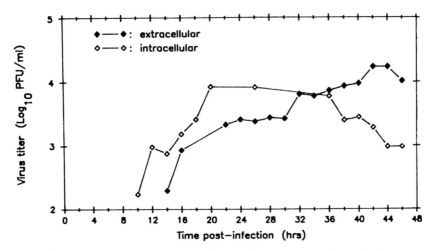

Fig. 1. Growth curve of HCV-229E on L132 cells at 37 °C (MOI = 0.001)

after infection at 33°C. Growth curves were obtained at this temperature for both intracellular (Fig. 2) and extracellular (Fig. 3) virus. Even though infectious titers were as much as 1000-fold higher at 33°C, the growth curves showed a similar time-dependence on the production of infectious virus particles. Moreover, there was no difference in the infectious virus titers obtained at 42-44 hrs after infection at MOIs of 0.01, 0.1 or 1, although extracellular virus titers were slightly reduced after infection at an MOI of 0.001. Thus, an MOI of 0.01 was chosen for virus passages, and a time of 43 hrs p.i. determined to be optimal for the obtention of extracellular virions. We then compared the infectious virus titers which could be obtained after infection of various cell lines. As shown in Table 1, given the fact that IMHP cells were more difficult to grow, L132 cells represented the best of the cell lines tested. Finally, of four gradient materials tested for virus purification, Renografin-60® allowed the best recovery of infectious virus and integrity of virions as seen in the electron microscope (data not shown)

Table 1. Growth of HCV-229E on various cell lines

Cell line	Temperature (°C)	Infectious virus titer (PFU/ml)	n[1]
L132	37	$1.3 \pm 0.7 \times 10^5$	7
IMHP	37	$2.8 \pm 0.2 \times 10^5$	2
RD151	37	1.2×10^4	2
Vero	37	<20	2
HRT18	37	<20	2
L132	33	$1.2 \pm 0.9 \times 10^6$	9

[1] number of experiments

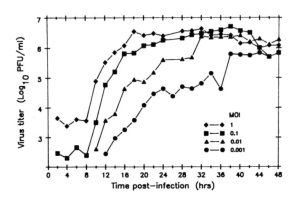

Fig. 2. Growth curves of HCV-229E on L132 cells at 33°C and various MOIs
(intracellular virus)

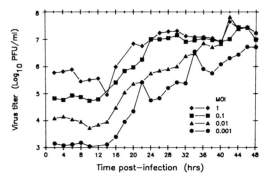

Fig. 3. Growth curves of HCV-229E on L132 cells at 33°C and various MOIs
(extracellular virus)

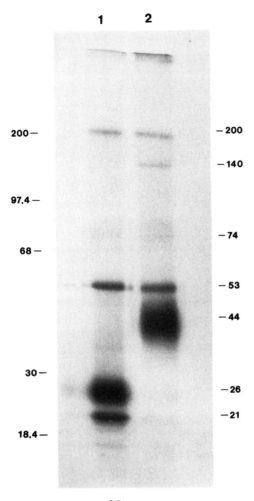

Fig. 4. Effect of reducing agent on [^{35}S]methionine-labeled HCV-229E
polypeptides. Sample buffer for SDS-PAGE contained (lane 1) or was free
of (lane 2) 2-mercaptoethanol. The migration of radiolabeled molecular
weight standards is shown on the left and the calculated molecular weights
of observed viral polypeptides is shown on the right.

Having optimized virus growth and purification conditions, we undertook the molecular characterization of the viral proteins. Labeling of HCV-229E with [^{35}S]methionine
and analysis of purified virions by SDS-PAGE showed four major viral polypeptides
which migrated with apparent molecular masses of 200, 53, 26 and 21 kDa. These masses
varied slightly between experiments and the following ranges were observed: 190-200, 52-
53, 25-26 and 20-22 kDa. An additionnal polypeptide of 88-97 kDa was occasionnally observed. Omission of the reducing agent caused a disappearance of the 26 and 21 kDa molecules and the appearance of 44, 74 and 140 kDa polypeptides.

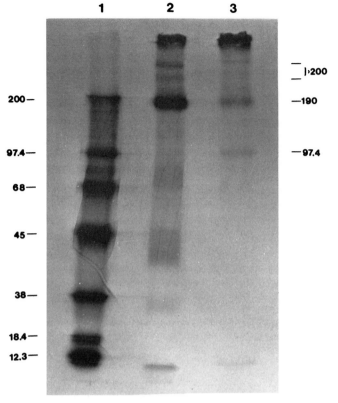

Fig.5. Labeling of HCV-229E glycoproteins with [^{3}H]glucosamine.The migration of radiolabeled molecular weight standards is shown on the left and the calculated molecular weights of observed viral polypeptides is shown on the right.

Finally, the incorporation of radiolabeled sugars was used to identify viral glycoproteins. As shown in Fig. 5, polypeptides of 97 and 190, as well as two large species which migrated above the 200 kDa marker, incorporated [^{3}H]glucosamine. On the other hand, [^{3}H]galactose was also incorporated into a 26 kDa viral polypeptide (data not shown).

DISCUSSION

We have shown that the growth of HCV-229E in the human embryonic lung cell line L132 at 33°C after infection at an MOI of at least 0.01, followed by purification on Renografin-60® gradients, represented the optimal experimental conditions tested for the most efficient recovery of infectious viral particles needed for molecular studies. Growth curves allowed the determination of optimal harvesting times for the analysis of viral structural proteins and will prove invaluable for the study of non-structural proteins. After metabolic radiolabeling with [^{35}S]methionine, four to five structural viral proteins could be identified. By analogy with murine coronaviruses, they could be identified as the spike glycoprotein (E2/S), in both monomeric (88-97 kDa) and dimeric (190-200) forms, the nucleoprotein (N) at 52-53 kDa and the matrix protein (E1/M), in both glycosylated (25-26 kDa) and non-glycosylated (20-22 kDa) forms.

Other authors have identified putative E2/S glycoprotein dimers at 160-196 kDa[13,14,15] and monomers at 105 kDa[13,14], which is consistent with our observation of

190-200 and 88-97 kDa. However, the putative E2/S multimers which migrated at >200 kDa after labeling with [^{3}H]glucosamine have not been previously observed, although their significance is unclear since they could not be detected after labeling with [^{35}S]methionine. The inconsistent appearance of the putative E2/S monomer of 88-97 kDa may relate to variations in the presumed proteolytic cleavage of the dimeric form of the molecule.

On the other hand, we have observed an apparently larger nucleoprotein than the previously reported 47-50 kDa molecule[13,14,15], as well as larger E1/M polypeptides when compared to the previously reported 17-24 kDa molecules[13,14,15]. The only study which reported on the glycosylation of the E1/M protein showed incorporation of [^{14}C]glucosamine into a 17 kDa molecule[13]. We have been unable to detect incorporation of glucosamine into the 25-26 kDa putatively glycosylated form of E1/M, although we could confirm glycosylation by the incorporation of [^{3}H]galactose. Moreover, we could not observe the 165 and 31 kDa glycoproteins that were previously reported[13], which is consistent with other studies[14,15].

The apparent multimerization of the E1/M matrix protein in the absence of a reducing agent has not to our knowledge been observed to date with any coronaviruses. The apparent molecular masses of the observed putative multimers suggest dimers (44 kDa), trimers (74 kDa) and hexamers (140 kDa). Putative dimers were most prominent and their absence in the presence of 2-mercaptoethanol is contrary to the reducing agent - enhanced appearance of a 38 kDa polypeptide of MHV-A59[16]. Moreover, the predicted primary sequence of the E1/M protein of HCV-229E, deduced from the nucleotide sequence of the cloned gene reveals, unlike other coronaviruses, the presence of only one cysteine residue (P. Jouvenne *et al.*, submitted for publication), which may be available to the formation of intermolecular disulfide bridges. Previous studies with MHV-A59 and HCV-OC43 have estimated the molar ratios of E1/M to E2/S to be 16:1[17] or 33:4[18], respectively. Presumably, several E1/M molecules could be joined by intermolecular disulfide bridges and other molecular links and interact with E2/S glycoproteins to stabilize viral peplomers. Thus, it would be conceivable that mutations in the E1/M gene could alter the stability of peplomers, which could alter virus pathogenesis. This would further emphasize the important role of this protein in virus biology, as was recently exemplified by the observation of passive anti- E1/M monoclonal antibody protection from MHV-JHM - induced encephalitis[19], and which would be consistent with the extensive antigenic conservation of E1/M already observed among various strains of murine coronaviruses[20].

Further molecular studies of human coronaviruses are important to gain a better understanding of their biology and involvement in human disease. Such studies are now in progress.

ACKNOWLEDGMENTS

This work was supported by grant MT-9203 to P.J. Talbot from the Medical Research Council of Canada. A studentship support to N. Arpin from Institut Armand-Frappier is gratefully acknowledged, as well as a scholarship to P.J. Talbot from the Natural Sciences and Engineering Research Council of Canada. The authors thank the excellent technical assistance of Francine Lambert and Francine Allard.

REFERENCES

1. M.R. Macnaughton, M.H. Madge, and S.E. Reed, Two antigenic groups of human coronaviruses detected by using enzyme-linked immunosorbent assay, Infect. Immun. 33: 734 (1981).
2. K. McIntosh. Coronaviruses. A comparative review, Curr. Top. Microbiol. Immunol. 63: 85 (1974).
3. R. Tanaka, Y. Iwasaki, and H. Koprowski, Intracisternal virus-like particles in brain of a multiple sclerosis patient, J. Neurol. Sci. 28: 121 (1976).

4. J.S. Burks, B.L. DeVals, L.D. Jankovsky, and J.C. Gerdes, Two coronaviruses isolated from central nervous system of two multiple sclerosis patients, Science 209: 933 (1980).

5. A. Salmi, B. Ziola, T. Hovi, and M. Reunanen, Antibodies to coronaviruses OC43 and 229E in multiple sclerosis patients, Neurology 32: 292 (1982).

6. E.V. Davis, and V.S. Bolin, Continuous cultivation of isogenous cell lines from the human embryo, Fed. Proc. 19: 386 (1960).

7. G. Chaloner-Larsson, and M. Johnson-Lussenburg, Establishment and maintenance of a persistent infection of L132 cells by human coronavirus strain 229E, Arch. Virol. 69: 117 (1981).

8. R.M. MacAllister, J. Melnyk, J.Z. Finklestein, E.C. Adams, and M.B. Gardner, Cultivation in vitro of cells derived from a human rhabdomyosarcoma, Cancer 24: 520 (1969).

9. O.W. Schmidt, M.K. Cooney, and G.E. Kenny, Plaque assay and improved yield of human coronaviruses in a human rhabdomyosarcoma cell line, J. Clin. Microbiol. 9: 722 (1979).

10. W.A.F. Tompkins, A.M. Watrach, J.D. Schmale, R.M. Schulze, and J.A. Harris, Culture and antigenic properties of newly established cell strains derived from adenocarcinomas of the human colon and rectum, J. Natl. Cancer Inst. 52: 101 (1974).

11. C. Daniel, and P.J. Talbot, Physico-chemical properties of murine hepatitis virus, strain A59, Arch. Virol. 96: 241 (1987).

12. U.K. Laemmli, Cleavage of structural proteins during the assembly of the head of bacteriophage T4, Nature (Lond.) 227: 680 (1970).

13. J.C. Hierholzer, Purification and biophysical properties of human coronavirus 229E, Virology 75: 155 (1976).

14. M.R. Macnaughton, The polypeptides of human and mouse coronaviruses, Arch. Virol. 63: 75 (1980).

15. O.W. Schmidt, and G.E. Kenny, Polypeptides and functions of antigens from human coronaviruses 229E and OC43, Infect. Immun. 35: 515 (1982).

16. L.S. Sturman, Characterization of a coronavirus. I. Structural proteins: Effects of preparative conditions on the migration of protein in polyacrylamide gels, Virology 77: 637 (1977).

17. L.S. Sturman, K.V. Holmes, and J. Behnke, Isolation of coronavirus envelope glycoproteins and interaction with the viral nucleocapsid, J. Virol. 33: 449 (1980).

18. B.G. Hogue, and D.A. Brian, Structural proteins of human respiratory coronavirus OC43, Virus Res. 5: 131 (1986).

19. J.O. Fleming, R.A. Shubin, M.A. Sussman, N. Casteel, and S.A. Stohlman, Monoclonal antibodies to the matrix (E1) glycoprotein of mouse hepatitis virus protect mice from encephalitis, Virology 168: 162 (1989).

20. P.J. Talbot, and M.J. Buchmeier. Antigenic variation among murine coronaviruses: Evidence for polymorphism on the peplomer glycoprotein, E2, Virus Res. 2: 317 (1985).

SEQUENCE ANALYSIS OF THE 3' END (8740 NUCLEOTIDES) OF BECV GENOME ; COMPARISON WITH HOMOLOGOUS MHV NUCLEOTIDE SEQUENCE

Pascal Boireau[2], Nathalie Woloszyn[1], Catherine Crucière[2], Ericka Savoysky[3] and Jacques Laporte[1]

[1]Station de Virologie et d'Immunologie Moléculaires I.N.R.A.,C.R.J.J. Domaine de Vilvert, 78350 Jouy en Josas, France
[2]Laboratoire de Virologie Moléculaire, L.C.R.V. C.N.E.V.A., 22 rue Pierre Curie, BP 67, 94703 Maisons-Alfort Cedex, France
[3]Laboratoire de Microbiologie Appliquée et Industrielle, Faculté des Sciences Pharmaceutiques et Biologiques, 5 rue A. Lebrun 5400 Nancy, France

INTRODUCTION

Bovine enteritic coronavirus (BECV) is one of the major pathogen of neonatal calves. The viral genome is a unique 20 Kb large RNA molecule which is polyadenylated at its 3' end. Studies of viral mRNAs suggest that eight genes are translated (Crucière & Laporte, personnal communication) and as established for MHV[1] the possibility of functional bicistronic genes cannot be excluded. BECV is made of 4 major structural proteins[2,3,4], a 50 kD phosphorylated nucleocapsid N, a 180 kD peplomer glycoprotein S (present on the virions as 105 and 95 kD glycosylated subunits), a 125 kD haemagglutinin HE (made up of two disulfide bridge-linked glycosylated subunits of 65 kD) and a 28 kD transmembrane glycoprotein M. The complete amino-acid sequences of these proteins have recently been deduced from nucleotide sequences of the viral genome[5,6,7,8,9].

In this paper we present the complete nucleotide sequence of the first eight Kb of BECV strain F15 genome and discuss the number and the location of the genes and the possible role of the encoded proteins ; we also compare our results with the already published data concerning MHV-A59 or JHM.

RESULTS

1- BECV specific intracellular RNAs

In a one-step growth experiment, the analysis of the poly(A+) RNAs extracted from BECV infected HRT18 cells 7 hours after virus penetration showed, after electrophoresis in denaturing agarose gel, 8 different molecular mass species (Fig. 1, Table 1). Northern blot analysis of these RNAs by cDNA probes corresponding to the viral N gene established their viral origin.

Coronaviruses and Their Diseases
Edited by D. Cavanagh and T.D.K. Brown
Plenum Press, New York, 1990

81

Table 1. Sizes of BECV mRNAs.

BECV mRNA	MOLECULAR WEIGHT OF BECV mRNA[1]	PREDICTED SIZE OF THE mRNA (IN BASES)		PREDICTED SIZE OF THE POLYPEPTIDE ENCODED BY mRNA[4]
		EXPERIMENTAL DATA[2]	NUCLEOTIDE SEQUENCE DATA[3]	
1	5,75			
2	2,70	8120		
3	2,45	7420	8700	47 730 (HE)
4	2,10	6360	7400	150 740 (S)
5	0,87	2630	3005	12 800 (NS2)
6	0,80	2400	2735	9 585 (NS3)
7	0,71	2160	2345	26 370 (M)
8	0,56	1690	1650	49 370 (N)

(1) in kD
(2) size of BECV mRNA obtained in denaturing agarose gel .
(3) size of BECV mRNA predicted from the location of the consensus nucleotide sequence CNAAAC (N=C or T)
(4) size of polypeptide deduced from the ORF immediatly downstream the conserved sequence (in D).

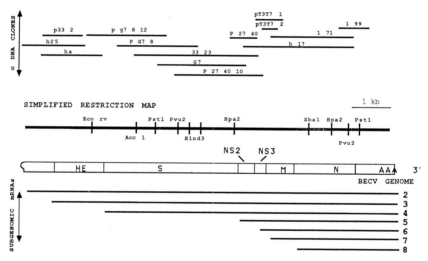

Figure 1. Organization of BECV Genome and Location of cDNA Clones Used in Sequence Determination.

Furthermore hybridization with a panel of viral probes showed that each mRNA had a common 3' end with the next smaller mRNA.

2- cDNA cloning and sequencing

From 14 overlapping cDNA clones (Fig. 1) we have sequenced the first 8.8 Kb of the 3' end of the viral genome. CDNA libraries were obtained by using synthetic oligonuleotide priming. CDNA inserts amplified by the polymerase chain reaction (PCR) were cloned into PT3T7 18U vector to obtain the whole length of some genes (NS2, NS3, HE). Location of cDNA clones was performed by restriction mapping, Southern and northern blot hybridizations. Nucleotide sequence of both cDNA strands was obtained from cDNA clones shown in Fig.1. From a database of nucleotide sequences containing about 60 000 nucleotides, a large unique 8740 nucleotide sequence was established. It contains six large non-overlapping open reading frames (ORF). Starting from the 3' end of the genome, the two first ORF encode, as previously reported[5,6], for the viral N and M structural proteins. Downstream two smaller ORFs NS3 and NS2 have coding capacities for 84 and 110 amino-acids respectivelly. After an intergenic sequence of 377 nucleotides, the next large ORF is 4092 nucleotides long. It belongs to the S gene encoding the major viral glycoprotein ; the predicted polypeptide (1364 amino-acids) has a relative molecular mass of about 150,5 kD[8]. The last ORF we have sequenced encodes for a polypeptide of 424 amino-acids with a relative molecular mass of 47729 D corresponding to the unglycosylated subunit of the gP 125 protein of BECV.

DISCUSSION

1- Genome organization of BECV

As determined by electrophoresis in denaturing gel the size of BECV poly(A$^+$) genomic RNA comprises between 18 Kb and 23 Kb. Seven subgenomic RNA species are evidenced in the infected cells and northern blot hybridization confirms that they form a 3'end coterminal nested set. These results are in good agreement with those of Keck et al.[9] concerning BECV RNA synthesis and lead us to conclude that at leat 8 non overlapping genes constitute the viral genome..
Sequencing of the first 8740 nucleotides of the 3' end of the genome demonstrate 6 different genes coding respectively for the N, M, NS3, NS2, S, and HE viral proteins. The rest of the genome should comprise the 2 missing genes (NS1 and Pol) if we compare with the MHV genome. Among the 6 sequenced genes N and HE present respectively 2 and 3 overlapping ORFs (Fig. 2). The already published sequences of IBV[10], MHV[1], or TGEV[11] demonstrate large overlapping ORFs only for genes encoding non structural proteins. Nevertheless the consensus nucleotide sequence surrounding the putative initiation codon of the secondary ORF of the BECV N gene is one of the optimal environments for initiation of mRNA translation[12]. This observation is not true for ORF2 of the HE gene which exhibits a U in +4 but the situation is the same for the initiation

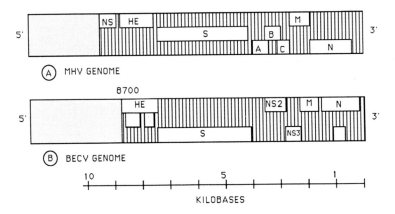

Figure 2. Location of ORFs (Larger than 200 Bases) in BECV and MHV Genomes.

codon of N, S and HE BECV genes. We cannot exclude a biological role for the secondary ORFs, but their expression in infected cells remains to be proved.

Immediatelly upstream from the initiation codon of the four structural genes we found a conserved nucleotide sequence : (A/T)C(C/T)AAAC. This sequence is very similar to the intergenic transcription initiation sites of some MHV mRNAs[13] which have the common TC(C/T)AAAC sequence. For the BECV NS2 and NS3 genes the sequence TCCAAAC is located far upstream of the putative initiation codon (80 and 130 nucleotides respectivelly). The location of the -CTAAAC- sequences that we observed for the different genes is in good agreement with the experimentally determined size of the BECV mRNAs (Table 1.) ; nevertheless because of the molecular mass markers we used, the experimental size given for the larger mRNAs appeared to be underestimated.

2- Properties of the BECV proteins predicted from the main ORFs

N and M proteins. The properties of these structural proteins and their comparison with the MHV homologous protein have been already described elsewhere[5,6].

S protein. The S gene[8] encodes the larger BECV glycoprotein (gp180) which shares some properties with other coronavirus S proteins i.e. : their amino-acid sequences revealed two main hydrophobic domains and a putative protease cleavage site. The 19 first N terminal amino-acids constitute the first hydrophobic domain consistent with a role as a signal sequence[14]. The second (amino-acids 1309 to 1335) is predicted as a transmembrane α helix and could be involved in the anchorage of the spikes in the viral membrane.

Because of the 19 putative glycosylation sites of this protein its relative molecular mass is estimated at about 185 kD. This glycoprotein has a putative protease cleavage site -Lys-Arg-Arg-Ser-Val-Arg- (amino-acids 763 to 769) colinear with the experimentally established cleavage site of MHV-A59 S protein[15]. The resulting framents S1 and S2 have a relative molecular mass (102,592 D and 85,175 D respectively) very similar to the molecular mass of the gp105 and gp 95 BECV structural proteins previously described[3,16].

HE protein. The amino-acid sequence deduced from the HE gene of BECV F15 isolated in France is very similar to the HE amino-acid sequence established for BECV Quebec strain[7] (5 amino-acids difference).

Luytjes et al.[17] have shown a fairly good similarity between the amino-acid sequence of the HA glycoprotein of Influenza C virus[18] and the MHV-A59 pseudogene product homologous to the BECV HE gene product. When comparing these 3 proteins by Dayhoff optimal alignment (Multalin program[19] Fig. 3) three highly conserved domains are evidenced : 1) from amino-acids 57 to 70, 2) from 124 to 134, 3) from 370 to 382. The esterase site of influenza C virus HA is identified as the -Gly-Phe-Gly-Asp-Ser-Arg-Thr- amino-acid sequence[20]. This sequence is the highly conserved sequence 1) except for a serine to threonine change in BECV and MHV-A59. Experiments have shown that purified BECV particles possess such an esterase activity[21].

Non structural proteins NS3 and NS2. The protein predicted from the ORF of the gene NS3 has a relative molecular mass of 9585 D,

```
                  1        10        20        30        40        50
         PHA59    MKGCMCUFVFTLLVUJAYYFVEKGRMCI...AMAPRTLLLLIUCQL......VFGFNEP
                       :*  **  : :*    **               *       *  * **
         PHAF15         MF.LLP..RFILVS....CI...IGS..........L.....GFD.NFP
                               *  *   *: : *              *        *: *
         PHANC    MFFSLLLMLGLTEAEKIKICLQKQVISSFSLHNGFGGNLYATEEKRMFELVKP

                        60        70        80        90        100
         PHA59    LNIVSHLNDD.WFLFGDSRSDCTYVENNGHPKLDWLDLDPKLCNSGKISAKSGNSLFRSF
                  *:*****  ** **********  **  **:* ** ** : ** *  *** :****
         PHAF15   TNVVSHLNGD.WFLFGDSRSDCNHVVNTNPRNYSYMDLNPALCDSGKISSKAGNSIFRSF
                   * ***  * * ****** *   :     **          :     *:*
         PHANC    KAGASVLNQSTWIGFGDSRTD..QSNSAFPRSLMSAKTADKF..RSLSGGSLMLSMFGPP

                     120       130       140       150       160
         PHA59    HFTDFYNYTGEGDQIVFYEGVNFSPSHGFKCLAHGDNKRWMGNKARFYARVYEKMAQYRS
                  ***********:**:*******  *** ****  **     ** * ** **  ***
         PHAF15   HFTDFYNYTGEGQQIIFYEGVNFTPYHAFKCTTSGSNDIWMQNKGLFYTQVYKNMAVYRS
                  * * ***  :*****  * *   *     * *       *  :* * *
         PHANC    GKVD.YLYQGCGHKVFYEGVNWSPHAAIDCY....RKNWTDIKLNFQKSIYELASQSHC

                        180       190       200       210       220
         PHA59    LSFVNV...SYAYGGNAKPASICKDNTL...TLNNPTFISKESNYVD...YYYESEANFT
                  * ****    **     :**   :**     ****  :** *: *   *** **:*
         PHAF15   LTFVNV...PYVYNGSAQSTALCKSGSL...VLNNPAYIAREANFGD...YYYKVEADFY
                  : :**     **       *    *       *   *   * *:    :: : :*
         PHANC    MSLVNALDKTIPLQVTKGVAKNCNNSFLKNPALYTQEVKPLEQICGEENLAFFTLPTQFG

                     230       240       250       260       270
         PHA59    LEGCDEFIVPLCGFNGHSKGS.SSDAANKYYTDSQSYYNMDIGVLYGFNSTLDVGNTAKD
                  * ****:***** **       *** **:*:* **:**:***  :
         PHAF15   LSGCDEYIVPLCIFNGKFLSN.T.....KYYDDSQYYFNKDTGVIYGLNSTETITT....
                  * :* **      **       *:   * :: *: **:
         PHANC    TYECKLHLVASCYFIYDSKEVYNKRGCGNYF...QVIYDSSGKVVGGLDNRVSPYTGNSG

                        290       300       310       320       330
         PHA59    PGLDLTCRYLALTPGNYKAVSLEYLLSLPSKAICLHKTKRFMPVQVVVDSRWSSIRQSDNM
                  *:*: **  *** ***:*  **:* :* * :** :* * :** *  * *:*  ******
         PHAF15   .GFDFNCHYLVLPSGNYLAISNELLLTVPTKAICLNKRRKDFTPVQVVHSRWNNARQSDNM
                  *   **   *    *:*  : :      * :** :*   : *:* ** * ** * *
         PHANC    DTPTMQCDMLQLKPGRYSVRSSSRFLLMPERSYCFDMKEK.GPVTAVQSIWGKGRKSDYA

                     350       360       370       380       390
         PHA59    TAAAC.QLPYCFFRNTCANYSGGTHDAHHGDFHFRQLLSGLLYNVSCIAQQG.AFLYNNV
                  ** ** ** ***:***  ** *  :*** *:*:****** ; *** *****
         PHAF15   TAVAC.QPPYCYFRNSTTNYVG.VYDINHGDAGFTSILSGLLYDSPCFSQQG.VFRYNNV
                  ** * *  ***:***     ::*:**** * :****:  *  * ** **
         PHANC    VDQACLSTPGCMLIQKQKPYIG.EADDHHGDQEMRELLSGLDYEARCISQSGWVNETSPF

                  400       410       420       430
         PHA59    SSSWPAYG.YGHCP............TAANIGYMA.PVCIYDPLPVILL..
                  ** ** * **:**              ***:*  *:*:*****:***
         PHAF15   SSVWPLYP.YGRCP............TAADINTPDVPICVYDPLPLILL..
                   * *  ****                *  *   * *  * * :**
         PHANC    TEEYLLPPKFGRCPLAAKQESIPKIPDGLLIPTSGTDTTVTKPKSRIFGIDDLIIGLLFV

                                                               440
         PHA59    .......GVLLG.................IAVL.......
                         *:***                  :**:
         PHAF15   .......GILLG.................VAVI.......
                         * ***                  : ::
         PHANC    AIVEAGIGGYLLGSRKESGGGVTKESAEKGFEKIGNDIQILRSSTNIAIEKLNDRISHDE

         PHA59    ..................IIVFLNVL...
                                   *** * :*
         PHAF15   ..................IIVVL.LL...
                                   : ::   **
         PHANC    QAIRDLTLEIENARSEALLGELGIIRALLVGNISIGLQESLWELASEITNRAGDLAVEVS

                                                                 450
         PHA59    ..............................FY...........
                                                 ::
         PHAF15   ..............................YF...........
                                                 ::
         PHANC    PGCWIIDNNICDQSCQNFIFKFNETAPVPTIPPLDTKIDLQSDPFYWGSSLGLAITAANL

                  456
         PHA59    ......DGURC
                        :* *
         PHAF15   ...MVDNGTRL
                  :* *  :
         PHANC    MAALVISGIAICRTK
                  650 654
```

Figure 3. Comparison by Dayhoff Alignment of Amino Acid Sequences Deduced from BECV HE Gene (PHAF 15), Homologous MHV A59 Pseudogene (PHA59) and Influenza C HA Gene (PHANC). Highly Conserved Esterase Site is Boxed.
(*) Exact Homology.
(:) Conservative Change.

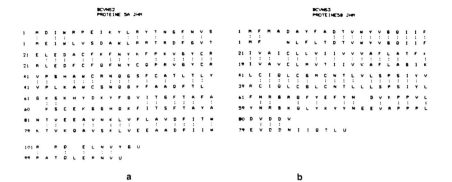

Figure 4. Alignments and Comparisons of Amino Acid Sequences of MHV JHM, 5A.5B Polypeptides and BECV NS2.NS3 Putative Polypeptides.

is highly hydrophobic and has 62% homology with the non structural MHV-JHM 10.2 kD protein[1]. There are 2 in-frame ATG at the beginning of this ORF (Fig. 4b). The second ATG seems, as a translation initiation codon, in a better environment[12] (G in +4 and T in -3). This observation is strengthened by comparison with the amino-acid sequence of the homologous MHV-JHM NS protein encoded by mRNA 4[13].

The 12.8 kD polypeptide deduced from NS2 gene (Fig 4a) has 53% homology with the 12.4 kD protein of MHV-JHM[1]. It has one potential glycosylation site and a C terminal hydrophobic α-helix structure looking like a transmembrane domain. The 12.4 kD non-structural polypeptides of IBV[10] and of MHV have a similar structure ; these 3 molecules should have a similar, but as yet unknown biological function.

This part of the BECV genome comprises only two genes (NS2 and NS3) but the homologous part of the MHV-JHM genome contains three genes A, B and C (Fig. 2). In fact between the NS and S BECV genes there is a small ORF (but no methionine as initiation codon) from which we can deduce a polypeptide having 52% homology with the C terminal end of the 15.2 kD polypeptide of MHV-JHM deduced from mRNA4[13]. A second small putative BECV polypeptide, deduced from another ORF located in the same part of the genome, has a similar homology with the N terminal end of the 15.2 kD MHV-JHM protein. Moreover, upstream of these two short hypothetical ORFs, in both cases we found a -GTAAAC-nucleotide sequence very similar to the consensus sequence - CTAAAC- putative transcription initiation site. These pseudogenes could be the memory of an ancestor gene unnecessary for virus replication at least in cell culture.

REFERENCES

1. M. A. Skinner, D. Ebner and S. G. Siddell, Coronavirus MHV-JHM mRNA 5 has a sequence arrangement which potentially allows translation of a second, downstream open reading frame. J. gen. Virol. 66:581 (1985).

2. J. Laporte and P. Bobulesco, Polypeptide structure of bovine enteritic coronavirus: comparison between a wild strain purified from feces and a HRT18 cell adapted strain, in: "Biochemistry and Biology of Coronaviruses," pp. 181-184. Edited by V. ter Meulen, S. Siddell and H. Wege, ed., Plenum Press, New York (1981).

3. J.F. Vautherot, J. Laporte, M.F. Madelaine, P. Bobulesco and A. Roseto, Antigenic and polypeptide structure of bovine enteritic coronavirus as defined by monoclonal antibodies, in "Molecular Biology and Pathogenesis of Coronaviruses" pp. 117-132. Edited by P.J.M. Rottier, B.A.M. van der Zeijst, W.J.M. Spaan and M.C. Horzinek, ed., Plenum Press, New York (1984).

4. B. King and D.A. Brian, Bovine coronavirus structural proteins. J. Virol., 42:700 (1982).

5. W. Lapps, B.G. Hogue and D.A. Brian, Sequence analysis of the bovine coronavirus nucleocapsid and matrix protein genes, Virology 157:47 (1987).

6. C. Crucière and J. Laporte, Sequence and analysis of bovine enteritic coronavirus (F15) genome I.- Sequence of the gene coding for the nucleocapsid protein; analysis of the predicted protein. An. Inst. Pasteur/Virology 139: 123 (1988).

7. M.D.Parker, G.J. Cox, D.R. Deregt, D.R. Fitzpatrick and L.A. Babiuk, Cloning and in vitro expression of the E3 haemagglutinin glycoprotein of Bovine Coronavirus. J. Gen. Virol. 70:155 (1989).

8. P. Boireau, C. Crucière and J. Laporte, Nucleotide sequence of the glycoprotein S (E2) gene of the bovine enteric coronavirus ; comparison with mouse hepatitis virus. J. gen. Virol. in the press (1990).

9. J.G. Keck, B.G. Hogue, D.A. Brian and M.M.C. Lai, Temporal regulation of bovine coronavirus RNA synthesis. Virus Res. 9:343 (1988).

10. M.E.G. Boursnell, M.M. Binns and T.D.K. Browm, Sequencing of coronavirus IBV genomic RNA : three open reading frames in the 5' "unique" region of mRNA D. J. gen. Virol. 66:2253 (1985).

11. D. Rasschaert, J. Gelfi and H. Laude, Enteric coronavirus TGEV : partial sequence of the genomic RNA, its organization and expression. Biochimie 69:591 (1987).

12. M. Kozak, At least six nucleotides preceding the AUG initiator codon enhance translation in mammalian cells, J. Mol. Biol. 196:947 (1987).

13. M.A. Skinner and S.G. Siddell, Coding sequence of coronavirus MHV-JHM mRNA 4. J. gen. Virol. 66:593 (1985).

14. M.E.E. Watson, Compilation of published signal sequences. Nucl. Acids Res. 12:5145 (1984).

15. W. Luytjes, L.S. Sturman, P.J. Bredenbeek, J. Charite, B.A.M. van der Zeijst, M.C. Horzinek and W.J.M. Spaan (1987), Primary structure of the glycoprotein E2 of coronavirus MHV-A59 and identification of the trypsin cleavage site, Virology 161:179 (1987).

16. D.Deregt and L.A. Babiuk. Monoclonal antibodies to bovine coronavirus: characteritics and topographical mapping of neutralizing epitopes on the E2 and E3 glycoproteins. Virology 161:410 (1987).

17. W. Luytjes, P.J. Bredenbeek, A.F.H. Noten, M.C. Horzinek and W.J.M. Spaan (1988), Sequence of mouse hepatitis virus A59 mRNA2 : Indication for RNA recombination between

coronaviruses and influenza C virus, <u>Virology</u> 166:415 (1988).

18. S. Nakada, R.S. Creager, M. Krystal, R.P. Aaronson and P. Palese, Influenza C virus hemagglutinin : comparison with influenza A and B virus hemagglutinins. <u>J. Virol.</u> 50:118 (1984).

19. F. Corpet, Multiple sequence aligment with hierarchical clustering. <u>Nucl. Acids Res.</u> 16:10881 (1988).

20. R. Vlasak, T. Muster, A.M. Lauro, J.C. Powers and P. Palese, Influenza C virus esterase : analysis of catalytic site, inhibition, and possible function. <u>J. Virol.</u> 63:2056 (1989).

21. R. Vlasak, W. Luytjes, J. Leider, W. Spaan and P. Palese, The E3 protein of bovine coronavirus is a receptor-destroying enzyme with acetylesterase activity. <u>J. Virol.</u> 62:4686 (1988).

Chapter 2

The Haemagglutinin-Esterase (HE) and Membrane (M) Glycoproteins

BACKGROUND PAPER

CORONAVIRUS M AND HE: TWO PECULIAR GLYCOPROTEINS

Peter J.M.Rottier

Institute of Infectious Diseases and Immunology
Department of Virology
Veterinary Faculty
State University of Utrecht
The Netherlands

Enveloped viruses carry in their membranes one or more surface glycoproteins. In coronaviruses three such proteins have been identified: a small integral membrane protein (M), a large glycoprotein constituting the characteristic viral spikes (S), and an intermediate-sized glycoprotein (HE). This paper will summarize published knowledge on the properties and function of the small and the intermediate-sized membrane proteins. They will be referred to as M and HE, respectively.

THE HE GLYCOPROTEIN

With only a few exceptions (e.g. MHV-A59 and FIPV), coronaviruses possess haem-agglutinating activity. For IBV and TGEV, whose virions lack a HE protein, this activity resides in the S protein. All other coronaviruses have a HE glycoprotein that has been shown or is supposed to represent the haemagglutinin. Interestingly, a second type of surface projection has been observed in coronaviruses possessing HE: a fringe of small granular projections situated at the base of the characteristic bulbous spikes. These short projections do indeed account for the haemagglutinating activity. Treatment of purified BCV with bromelain did not affect it. The enzyme degraded both the S and M protein while leaving HE intact; treated virions appeared to have lost the peplomers, whereas the fringe of short projections was still in place. Similar results were obtained with the human coronavirus OC43. Additional confirmation of the identity of HE as the haemagglutinin was recently obtained from experiments showing that monoclonal antibodies specific to the HE protein of BCV inhibited haemagglutination by this virus.

HE of coronaviruses is a glycoprotein of M_r approximately 60-65K with an apoprotein of about 45K. It is a typical class I membrane protein having a N-terminal signal sequence and a membrane anchor domain close to its C terminus. The protein is glycosylated only through N-linked oligosaccharides. The BCV HE sequence, which is the only HE sequence available so far, contains 9 potential N-glycosylation sites,the majority of which seems to be actually used. It is not known whether the protein is acylated or carries other modifications.

In infected cells HE is synthesized as a precursor glycoprotein that dimerizes rapidly by disulphide bond formation. The resulting homodimeric units are assembled into virions and transported out of the cell. En route to the plasma membrane part of the N-linked high-mannose oligosaccharides on the HE protein are processed to the complex type. Exactly how many homodimeric units make up one small projection has still to be determined.

The gene encoding the HE protein is located immediately upstream of the S gene and has probably been acquired by heterologous recombination. Interestingly, the indications for these features originally came from work with one of the few coronaviruses devoid of haemagglutinating activity, MHVA59. When the unique region of mRNA 2 of this virus was sequenced a second open reading frame was found downstream of the sequence encoding the 30K non-structural protein. This reading frame appeared to lack a translation initiation codon and is probably a pseudogene in MHV-A59. Most surprisingly, the sequence showed considerable homology to the HE haemagglutinin sequence of influenza C virus; at the amino acid level some 30% identity exists. It is believed that these influenza-like sequences were acquired during evolution by non-homologous recombination of some coronavirus with an influenza virus.

These observations prompted experiments to compare the biological properties of coronavirus HE to those of the influenza C HE protein. The latter is known to have both receptor binding and receptor-destroying activity, the receptor being characterized by the presence of a 9-O-acetylneuraminic acid modification. Indeed, the haemagglutinating coronaviruses HCV OC43 and BCV were found to recognize and bind to similarly sialylated receptors. In addition, receptor inactivation was demonstrated using BCV and shown to be of a type similar to that of influenza C, but distinct from that of influenza A. It is interesting to note that a similar observation was reported years ago for a mouse enteric coronavirus namely diarrhoea virus of infant mice (DVIM).

Further characterization of the receptor destroying activity showed that:

1. the activity is associated with the HE glycoprotein,
2. it is an acetylesterase activity that removes acetyl groups from O-acetylated sialic acids,
3. it is a serine esterase type of enzyme,
4. inactivation of the esterase activity strongly reduces the infectivity of the virus suggesting a role in one of the earliest stages of infection.

IBV and MHV-A59 being prototypes in the study of coronaviruses, interest in the HE glycoprotein has long lagged behind that for the other structural proteins. One realizes now that the presence of this protein in virions is the rule rather than the exception. Given the important features of the protein as they now emerge, focus on HE is expected to increase considerably. The central issues that will need to be addressed include:

1. the receptor binding activity: its function and, in relation to this, the function of the S glycoprotein in binding to the target cell; the further characterization of the receptor(s),
2. the receptor destroying activity: its mechanism and the precise role in coronavirus infection,
3. the biogenesis and structure of the small surface projections.

THE M GLYCOPROTEIN

Together with the nucleocapsid protein the small integral membrane protein M is the most abundant polypeptide constituent of coronavirions. M is a glycoprotein of M_r 25-30K that may either be N-glycosylated or carry only O-linked oligosaccharides as is the case with BCV, MHV and DVIM. The biological relevance of these differential glycosylations is obscure.

The gene encoding the M protein is located in the 3'-terminal region of the genome upstream from the N gene and is consequently expressed through one of the smaller subgenomic mRNAs. The M gene of several coronaviruses has been cloned and sequenced. The deduced amino acid sequences reveal common features but also some differences. The general structure of the mature protein is characterized by the presence of three successive stretches of hydrophobic amino acid residues in the N-terminal half of the molecule. This region is preceded by a hydrophilic N-terminus containing potential N- or O-glycosylation sites and followed by a more amphiphilic C-terminal half. Sequence homology among the various proteins is significant in some parts of the hydrophobic domains of the polypeptide, but is very high in the centre of the molecule where a stretch of 8 residues is identical among all viruses studied so far. A conspicuous feature in the sequences of the TGEV and FIPV M proteins is the presence of an N-terminal hydrophobic extension. As will be discussed below, this extension apparently functions as a membrane insertion signal.

Investigations of the organization of M in microsomal membranes and in the virion membrane using proteases have led to a model in which the protein is anchored in the lipid bilayer by its three hydrophobic domains. Protruding from one side of the membrane into the lumen of the microsomes is the N-terminus of the molecule. In virions this side corresponds to the external domain which carries the oligosaccharides. On the opposite side of the membrane most of the C-terminal half appears to be protected from protease attack and supposedly is tightly associated with the polar surface of the bilayer. Only the extreme C-terminal tail is accessible.

Several studies have focussed on the way this complex protein is assembled into membranes. As noted above, coronavirus M proteins generally lack an amino-terminal signal sequence. Yet they are targeted to the membane in a signal recognition particle-dependent manner and inserted cotranslationally. Both the first and the third transmembrane domain may function as targeting signals as either of them is able to direct insertion and anchoring of mutant M proteins from which the other two hydrophobic segments are deleted. Membrane integration of TGEV and FIPV M is mediated by a N-terminal signal sequence. Apparently this signal is cleaved off. It was suggested that cleavage may occur posttranslationally. Although *in vitro* the amino-terminal signal sequence appeared not to be an absolute requirement, its presence greatly enhanced the correct membrane assembly of the polypeptide.

An interesting biological feature of the M protein is its restriction to internal cell membranes. In contrast to most other viral membrane glycoproteins M accumulates in coronavirus infected cells in the perinuclear region. It is not transported to the plasma membrane except when in virions which are subsequently shed from the cell. As was shown by electron microscopy with MHV-A59 the protein is largely retained in the so-called budding compartment located between the endoplasmic reticulum and Golgi system. In addition, some M also reaches the Golgi membranes as an integral membrane protein.

Intracellular restriction is an intrinsic property of the M protein and is not dependent on other coronaviral factors. Expression of M proteins from different coronaviruses in various cells has revealed that M is transported efficiently to the Golgi apparatus. In the case of MHV-A59 M protein the majority of the O-linked sugars on the expression product acquire the sialic acid modification indicating that the protein has reached the trans cisternae of the organelle.

Its accumulation in the Golgi apparatus makes the M protein attractive in studies of the targeting of membrane proteins. Deletion mutagenesis has shown that removal of transmembrane domains can have diverse effects. A mutant M protein having only the first hydrophobic region appeared to accumulate intracellularly in a manner indistinguishable from the wild type protein. In contrast, a mutant with only the third transmembrane domain was not retained in the Golgi region but transported to the plasma membrane. These observations suggest that information for retention in the Golgi apparatus resides in the first transmembrane domain.

The domain structure and the biological features of the M protein presumably reflect its functions in the coronavirus life cycle:

1. The hydrophilic N-terminal virion ectodomain elicits antibodies. These antibodies can neutralize the virus but only in a complement-dependent manner. The role of the O-linked sugars carried by the ectodomain of some coronavirus M proteins is still unknown.
2. The cluster of transmembrane segments has been related to the intracellular budding of coronaviruses. The perinuclear region where M accumulates in infected cells coincides with the location of virion formation. In addition, this hydrophobic domain of M may be involved in the interaction with the S protein. Since no complexes between M and S have been observed in detergent-disrupted cells or virus, interaction probably occurs at the level of the membrane.
3. The C-terminal half of the protein most likely interacts with the nucleocapsid and is thus of key importance for the budding process. Association of the nucleocapsid of detergent-solubilized MHV-A59 with M but not with S has been demonstrated. Both the extreme C-

terminal tail and the highly conserved domain in the center of the M protein are candidate domains for binding to genomic RNA and/or nucleocapsid protein.

As more information is becoming available, the various functions of M will soon be understood in greater molecular detail. As a consequence, some functions may need to be redefined such as the exclusive role of M in determining the intracellular budding site. The recent finding that M, when expressed from cloned cDNA, is transported beyond the budding compartment, indicates that in the coronavirus-infected cell some factor is required to retain M in this compartment. It may well turn out that the S protein serves such a function and that the budding site is determined by the concerted action of both viral membrane proteins. Support for this assumption is provided by the finding that S accumulates in this very region of the cell and is transported to the cell surface only very slowly unless it is incorporated in virions.

The M protein has a number of interesting features both as a virion protein and as a model membrane glycoprotein. Future research will certainly concentrate on both of these aspects. The expected main issues will be:

    1. its role in viral budding, as part of the attempt to understand the process of virus assembly in molecular terms
    2. the significance of the N-terminal signal peptide in the TGEV and FIPV M sequence
    3. the function of O-linked vs. N-linked oligosaccharides
    4. the mechanism of membrane integration
    5. the identification of targeting information within the protein's structure.

Intracellular budding among positive strand RNA viruses is not restricted to coronaviruses; it has also been observed with toroviruses and arteriviruses. These viruses also share some replication characteristics and there are indications that they specify a membrane protein with features similar to M. It is an exciting idea, therefore, that these features may have more general relevance which makes the M protein all the more interesting.

STRUCTURE AND EXPRESSION OF THE BOVINE CORONAVIRUS HEMAGGLUTININ PROTEIN

Thomas E. Kienzle, Sushma Abraham, Brenda G. Hogue[1]
and David A. Brian

Department of Microbiology
The University of Tennessee
Knoxville, Tennessee 37996-0845

INTRODUCTION

cDNA clones prepared from genomic RNA of the Mebus strain of bovine coronavirus (BCV) were sequenced to reveal the hemagglutinin (H) gene of 1,272 bases that predicts a 47,700 mol. wt. apoprotein of 424 amino acids. The H gene mapped on the immediate 5' side of the peplomer gene. The H protein sequence revealed a putative N-terminal signal peptide of 18 amino acids, 9 potential glycosylation sites, 14 cysteine residues, and a potential C-terminal anchor region of 26 amino acids. When transcripts of the gene were translated *in vitro* in the presence of microsomes, signal cleavage, glycosylation, and membrane anchorage were observed, but not disulfide-linked dimerization. Translation of a truncated mRNA having no sequence for the C-terminal anchor resulted in a nonanchored, intraluminal (intramicrosomal) protein. When the H protein was expressed in cells in the absence of other coronaviral proteins, it became glycosylated, dimerized, and transported to the cell surface. The BCV hemagglutinin protein, therefore, is a type 1 glycoprotein that contains all the information it needs for signal cleavage, glycosylation, disulfide-linked dimerization, and transport to the cell surface.

MATERIALS AND METHODS

cDNA Cloning of BCV Genomic RNA

The Mebus strain of BCV was grown on human rectal tumor (HRT) cells and purified as previously described (Lapps *et. al.*, 1987). cDNA cloning was done essentially as described (Lapps *et. al.*, 1987), except that random 5-mer oligodeoxynucleotides (Pharmacia) were used as primers for first strand synthesis to generate several clones, one of which was I1 (Fig. 1A). A synthetically made primer (5' ATTATGACCGCACACC 3') was used to extend genomic sequence 5'-ward from clone I1, and this was used to generate several clones one of which was LA6 (Fig. 1A). Clones were selected by colony hybridization to randomly primed cDNA prepared from

---

[1]Current address: Department of Microbiology and Immunology, UCLA School of Medicine, Center for Health Sciences, Los Angeles, CA 90024

Coronaviruses and Their Diseases
Edited by D. Cavanagh and T.D.K. Brown
Plenum Press, New York, 1990

genomic RNA, and clones were mapped relative to one another and to the 3'
end of the genome using a matrix spot hybridization technique.

DNA Sequencing and Sequence Analysis

Dideoxy sequencing was used throughout. The ends of clones I1 and
LA6 were sequenced using universal primers for pUC vectors, and the clones
were ligated at the Hae 3 site (Fig. 1A) to form a continuous sequence
mapping in the region of the H gene. The reconstructed sequence was
subcloned into pGEM3Z (Promega) and a 3' and 5' nested set of subclones
was generated using exonuclease III and S1 nuclease (Henikoff, 1984).
Subclones were sequenced using universal primers for the pGEM vector, and
by synthetic primers that were made complementary to regions within the H
gene. Sequences were analyzed with the aid of the Microgenie program
(Beckman).

Expression Analyses

A construct of the H gene beginning 15 bases upstream (i.e.,
beginning with the CTAAAC intergenic sequence) from the putative ATG start
codon (an exonuclease III/S1-generated subclone of the LA6/I1 construct in
pGEM4Z) and under the control of the Sp6 polymerase promoter, was made and
named pHSp6 (Fig. 1B). The same insert was also subcloned into pGEM3Z
(using the Eco R1 and Hind III sites within the multiple cloning region)
such that the H gene was under the control of the T7 polymerase promoter.
This was named pHT7 (Fig. 1C).

For *in vitro* expression analyses, pHSp6 was linearized with Hind III
to yield full-length transcripts, or with Eco R5 to yield transcripts
lacking the coding region for the C-terminal anchor, and transcribed with

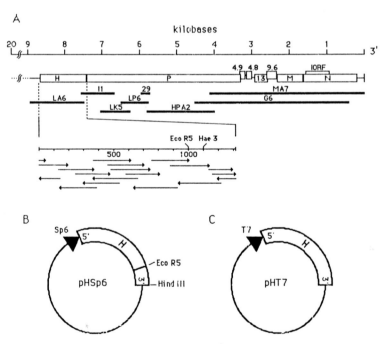

Fig 1. A. Gene map of the BCV genome, cDNA clone positions, and strategy
for sequencing the H gene. B. Plasmid construct for generating H
transcripts with Sp6 polymerase. C. Plasmid construct for generating H
transcripts with T7 polymerase.

SP6 polymerase (Promega protocol for yielding capped transcripts). Translation was done in wheat germ extract (Promega) in the presence or absence of canine pancreatic microsomes (Promega). Protein was labeled with ^{35}S-methionine (ICN). Immunoprecipitates were made using polyclonal rabbit anti gp65 (H subunit) (Hogue et. al., 1984) by the method of Anderson and Blobel (1983). Carbonate extractions at pH 11 were done by the method of Fujiki et. al., (1982). Competitive inhibition of N-Linked glycosylation was accomplished with 30μM octanoyl-asparagine-leucine-threonine (a gift from Dr. F. Naider, City University of New York), in the microsomal-containing translation mixture (Lau et. al., 1983). Polyacrylamide gel electrophoresis analyses were done as previously described (Hogue et. al., 1984).

For in vivo expression and analysis by immunofluorescence, HRT cells were infected with a vaccinia virus recombinant (vTF7-3, moi of 30) that expresses T7 polymerase (Fuerst et. al., 1987), transfected with pHT7 plasmid (1 μg per 1 cm^2) using Lipofectin Reagent (BRL) to mediate transfection, and prepared at 32h for internal or surface immunofluorescence using the method of Kaariainen et. al., (1983). For

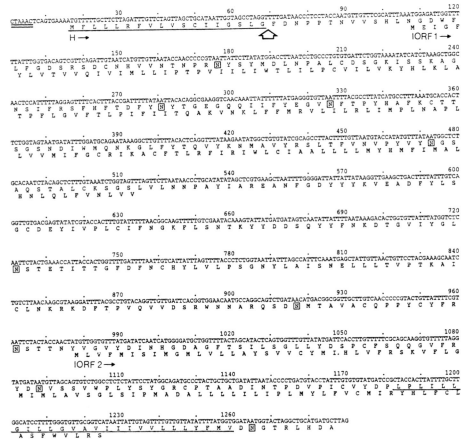

Fig. 2. Sequence of the H gene and deduced amino acid sequences of H, IORF1, and IORF2. The nucleotide sequence begins with the CTAAAC intergenic sequence 15 bases upstream from the presumed start condon of the H gene. The N-terminal signal peptide and presumed C-terminal anchor sequences are underlined. The signal cleavage site is indicated by an arrow. Potential N-linked glycosylation sites (NXS or NXT, where X $\neq$ P) are boxed.

analysis by immunoprecipitation, CV-1 cells were infected with vaccinia vTF7-3 (moi of 2), and transfected with pHT7 (0.2 μg per cm^2) using Lipofectin reagent, incubated 16 h at 37°, and labeled for 1 hr with 100 μCi each of ^{35}S-cysteine (Amersham) and ^{35}S-methionine (ICN). Immunoprecipitation was done on cell lysates as described above.

RESULTS

Based on the facts that (1) the hemagglutinating mammalian coronaviruses BCV and HCV OC43 have the H protein, while the antigenically related MHV A59 does not (Hogue et al., 1984), and, (2) BCV has an additional mRNA species (species 2a) that the nonhemagglutinating MHV does not have (Keck et. al., 1988), the H gene was predicted to be approximately 1.2 Kb in length and to lie on the 5' side of the peplomer protein gene (Hogue et. al., 1989; Keck et. al., 1988). The genome map position and sequences within clone I1 suggested that it contained the 5' end of the BCV peplomer (P) gene (because of sequence similarities with the MHV P gene), the intergenic CTAAAC sequence preceding the P gene, and part of an open reading frame immediately 5'-ward of the P gene. The open reading frame immediately 5' of the P gene was tentatively identified as the H gene. To find the 5' end of the putative H ORF, cDNA cloning was done with a primer sequence from the 5' end of clone I1 and a 1.6 Kb clone, LA6, was obtained (Fig. 1A). Partial sequencing suggested that it

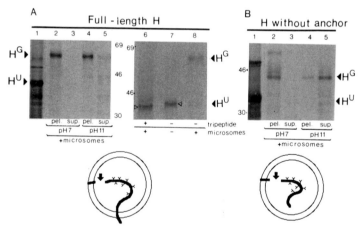

Fig. 3. Membrane anchorage and signal cleavage of the H protein. A. Full-length H subunit synthesized and glycosylated (H^G) in the presence of microsomes remains with the pelleted membrane after treatment at pH 11 (lane 4). Full-length H subunit undergoes signal cleavage, but not glycosylation, when translated in the presence of the tripeptide glycosylation inhibitor and microsomes (lane 6). This is schematically pictured in the lower left corner. B. The C-terminally truncated and glycosylated H subunit (H^G) is released from microsomes and is found mostly in the supernate when microsomes are treated at pH 11 (lane 5). This is schematically pictured in the lower right corner. All lanes represent translation products treated as indicated (lane 1 in parts A and B had no treatment) and electrophoresed in a 12% SDS polyacrylamide gel after reduction with 5% 2-mercaptoethanol.

probably contained the 5' end of the H gene and a LA6/I1 construct was made and completely sequenced (Fig. 1A). An open reading frame identifying the H gene was obtained (Fig. 2).

The following features were found from an analysis of the potential BCV H gene (Fig. 2). (1) The ORF is preceded 15 bases upstream by a CTAAAC intergenic consensus sequence of the type that precedes other BCV genes (Lapps *et. al.*, 1987). (2) The H ORF is 1,272 nucleotides long, encoding a potential apoprotein of 424 amino acids and having a predicted mol. wt. of 47,700. This is near the size expected from studies on H synthesis and processing (Deregt *et. al.*, 1987; Hogue *et. al.*, 1989). (3) There are two strongly hydrophobic regions, one covering a stretch of 18 aa at the N terminus and a second covering a stretch of 26 aa near the C terminus. An N-terminal sequence of NH_2-F-D-N-P-P-T-N-V-V- on the virion H protein (Hogue *et. al.*, 1989) that matches with amino acids 19 through 27 (Fig. 2) indicates first that the H gene sequence is authentic, and second that the N-terminal hydrophobic region functions as a signal peptide for membrane translocation and is cleaved between amino acids 18 and 19. The C-terminal hydrophobic region may function as a stop transfer signal and protein anchor. (4) There are 9 potential N glycosylation sites consistent with the high level of N-linked glycosylation for this protein which would suggest that nearly all of these must be used (Hogue *et. al.*, 1989). (5) There are 14 cysteine residues, some of which must be used for interchain disulfide bonding (King and Brian, 1982). (6) There are two large internal open reading frames, the significance of which is not yet known. The first (IORF1), from nucleotide 107 to 514, and the second (IORF2) from nucleotide 977 to 1,225, potentially encode proteins of 15,741 and 9,514 respectively.

To confirm by a second method that the H ORF does, in fact, encode the hemagglutinin, and to study the synthesis, orientation, processing and cellular localization of the hemagglutinin in the absence of other coronaviral proteins, H gene expression was studied *in vitro* and *in vivo*.

In vitro expression of H revealed the following: (1) Unglycosylated H subunit (H^u) migrated as a protein of 43Kd whereas glycosylated H subunit (H^G) migrated as a 65Kd glycoprotein, similar to the size of subunits obtained from infected cells or virions (Fig. 3A, lanes 1 and 2,

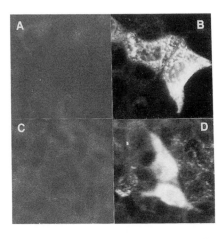

Fig. 4. Surface immunofluorescence of H protein. A. Uninfected HRT cells. B. BCV-infected cells. C. Vaccinia (vTF7-3)-infected cells. D. Cells infected with vaccinia vTF7-3 and transfected with pHT7 DNA.

and Hogue *et. al.*, 1989). (2) Both forms (H^u and H^G) were immunoprecipitable with H-specific rabbit antiserum (data not shown). (3) The H protein is almost entirely protected by protease when made in the presence of microsomes indicating that it is translocated into microsomes (data not shown). (4) H protein is not released from microsomes by carbonate (pH 11) extraction indicating that it is membrane anchored (Fig. 3A, lanes 2-5). (5) H protein made in the presence of microsomes and an inhibitor of glycosylation migrates as a protein approximately 2Kd smaller (Fig. 3A, lane 6) indicating that the signal peptide was cleaved. (6) H protein with its C-terminal hydrophobic sequence missing is not anchored in microsomal membranes but is secreted into the lumen of the microsomes (Fig. 3B, lanes 2-5), indicating that the C-terminal hydrophobic sequence serves as the membrane anchor. (7) No dimeric forms of H (either full-length or truncated) were found after *in vitro* translation.

In vivo expression of H revealed that it is found in the cytoplasm (data not shown) and on the external surface of the cell membrane (Fig. 4D). Immunoprecipitation of this product revealed a dimeric protein of 140 Kd reducible with 2-mercaptoethanol to subunits of 65 Kd (data not shown).

DISCUSSION

While this work was in progress, the sequence and *in vitro* expression of the H gene of the Quebec isolate of BCV was reported by Parker *et. al.* (1989). The Mebus gene sequence differs by only two bases from the Quebec sequence, and these are at base 322 where in our sequence it is G (rather than C) making amino acid 103 a valine (rather than leucine), and base 522 which is T (rather than A) resulting in no amino acid difference. The two large internal ORFs are present in both isolates.

Our results demonstrate for the first time that the BCV H protein is a type 1 glycoprotein and is not dependent upon other viral proteins for signal cleavage, dimer formation and transport to the cell surface. The scheme is summarized in Fig. 5.

A presumably incomplete form of the H gene is found in MHV A59 and maps on the 5' side of the peplomer protein gene (Luytjes *et. al.*, 1988). The MHV A59 protein (ORF2), although apparently not expressed during infection, possesses the putative active site (FGDS) for esterase activity (Luytjes *et. al.*, 1988). Remarkable sequence homology between the MHV A59 ORF2 and the hemagglutinin of influenza virus C, which also possesses esterase activity, has suggested an evolutionary relationship between these two proteins (Luytjes, 1988; Vlasak *et. al.*, 1987).

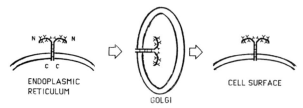

Fig. 5. Model illustrating the *in vivo* expression of BCV H protein in the absence of other coronaviral proteins. H is synthesized at the endoplasmic reticulum where it becomes translocated into the endoplasmic reticulum, becomes anchored at its C-terminus, loses the signal peptide from its N-terminus, becomes disulfide linked, and acquires sugars. It migrates through the Golgi and then to the plasma membrane.

Since BCV H protein shares 60% amino acid sequence homology with the potential product of MHV A59 ORF2, possesses the FGDS sequence of the esterase active site (beginning at base 124 in Fig. 2), and demonstrates esterase activity (Vlasak *et. al.*, 1988), it too may be evolutionarily related to the influenza C virus hemagglutinin. Interestingly, the influenza C hemagglutinin protein is derived by cleavage of a large precursor molecule (Herrler *et. al.*, 1988) and in this sense it is evolutionarily diverged from the BCV H protein.

ACKNOWLEDGEMENTS

This work was supported by NIAID Grant AI14367 and by USDA Grant 82-CRSR-2-1090.

REFERENCES

Anderson, D. J., and G. Blobel. 1983. Immunoprecipitation of protein from cell-free translations. Meth. Enzymol., 96:111-120.
Deregt, D., M. Sabara, and L. A. Babiuk, 1987. Structural proteins of bovine coronavirus and their intracellular processing. J. Gene Virol., 68:2863-2877.
Fuerst, T. R., P. L. Earl, and B. Moss. 1987. Use of a hybrid vaccinia virus-T7 RNA polymerase system for expression of target genes. Mol. Cell. Biol., 7:2538-2544.
Fujiki, Y., A. Hubbard, S. Fowler, and P. Lasarow. 1982. Isolation of intracellular membranes by means of sodium carbonate treatment: application to endoplasmic reticulum. J. Cell Biol., 93:97-102.
Henikoff, S. 1984. Unidirectional digestion with exonuclease III creates targeted breakpoints for DNA sequencing. Gene, 28:351-359.
Herrler, G., I. Durkop, H. Becht, and H. Klenk. 1988. The glycoprotein of influenza C virus is the hemagglutinin, esterase, and fusion factor. J. Gen. Virol., 69:839-846.
Hogue, B. G., T. E. Kienzle, and D. A. Brian. 1989. Synthesis and processing of the bovine enteric coronavirus hemagglutinin protein. J. Gen. Virol., 70:345-352.
Hogue, B. G., B. King, and D. A. Brian. 1984. Antigenic relationships among proteins of bovine coronavirus, human respiratory coronavirus, OC43, and mouse hepatitis coronavirus A59. J. Virol., 51:384-388.
Kaariainen, L., I. Virtanen, J. Saraste, and S. Keranen. 1983. Transport of virus membrane glycoproteins, use of temperature-sensitive mutants and organelle-specific lectins. Meth. Enzymol., 96:453-465.
Keck, J. G., B. G. Hogue, D. A. Brian and M. M. C. Lai. 1988. Temporal regulation of bovine coronavirus RNA Synthesis. Virus Res., 9:343-356.
King, B., and D. A. Brian. 1982. Bovine coronavirus structural proteins. J. Virol., 42:700-707
King, B., B. J. Potts, and D. A. Brian. 1985. Bovine coronavirus hemagglutinin protein. Virus Res., 2:53-59.
Lapps, W., B. G. Hogue, and D. A. Brian. 1987. Sequence analysis of the bovine coronavirus nucleocapsid and matrix protein genes. Virology, 157:47-57.
Lau, J. T. V., J. Welply, P. Shenbagamurthi, F. Naider, and W. J. Lennarz. 1988. Substrate recognition of oligosaccharyl transferase: Inhibition of cotranslational glycosylation by acceptor peptides. J. Biol. Chem., 258:15,255-15,250.
Luytjes, W., P. Bredenbeck, A. Noten, M. Horzinek, and W. Spaan., 1988. Sequence of mouse hepatitis virus A59 mRNA2: indications for RNA recombination between coronaviruses and influenza C virus. Virol., 166:415-422.

Parker, M. D., G. J. Cox, D. Deregt, D. R. Fitzpatrick, and L. A. Babunk. 1989. Cloning and *in vitro* expression of the gene for the E3 hemagglutinin glycoprotein of bovine coronavirus. J. Gen. Virol., 70:155-164.

Vlasak, R., M. Krystal, M. Nacht, and P. Palese. 1987. The influenza C virus glycoprotein (HE) exhibits receptor-binding (hemagglutinin) and receptor-destroying (esterase) activities. Virol., 160:419-425.

Vlasak, R., W. Luytjes, J. Leider, W. Spaan, and P. Palese. 1988. The E3 protein of bovine coronavirus is a receptor-destroying enzyme with acetyl esterase activity. J. Virol., 62:4686-4690.

THE HAEMAGGLUTININ OF BOVINE CORONAVIRUS EXHIBITS SIGNIFICANT

SIMILARITY TO THE HAEMAGGLUTININ OF TYPE C INFLUENZA VIRUS

Michael D. Parker, Graham J. Cox, Dongwan Yoo,
David R. Fitzpatrick and Lorne A. Babiuk

Veterinary Infectious Disease Organization
University of Saskatchewan
Saskatoon, Saskatchewan

INTRODUCTION

Coronaviruses are large enveloped RNA viruses containing a single-stranded genome complexed with a phosphorylated nucleocapsid protein which is surrounded by an envelope derived from intracellular membranes. The envelope contains two or three species of glycoproteins. The largest, E2 or S, is cleaved to S1 and S2 subunits and forms the large club-shaped peplomers on the surface of the virion which gives the virus its characteristic appearance. The E1 glycoprotein is believed to be responsible for determining the intracellular site of viral morphogenesis. A smaller group of coronaviruses contain a third membrane glycoprotein (Hogue and Brian, 1986, King et al., 1985, Pocock and Garwes, 1977), E3 or H, which, in the case of bovine coronavirus , exhibits haemagglutinating and acetylesterase activities.

Bovine coronavirus is one cause of severe scours in newborn cattle and is responsible for significant morbidity and mortality. Previous work has demonstrated that monoclonal antibodies against E2 or E3 are capable of neutralization and are protective in vivo (Deregt et al., 1989). In order to examine the biochemical and immunological properties of these glycoproteins in more detail, the gene for the E3 polypeptide has been molecularly cloned (Parker et al., 1989). Expression of the cloned E3 gene has shown that the polypeptide possesses receptor-destroying activity similar to that exhibited by the haemagglutinin/esterase (HE) of type C influenza virus. In addition, the sequence of the E3 polypeptide is very similar to the HE polypeptide of type C influenza virus.

RESULTS AND DISCUSSION

A series of cDNA clones representing the 3' 10kb of the bovine coronavirus genome have been mapped and sequenced and the resulting map is shown in Figure 1. The E2 and E3 genes are immediately adjacent on the genome. The open reading frame of the E2 gene is 4089 nucleotides in length and encodes a 145K polypeptide (Parker et al., submitted). Immediately upstream is the E3 gene which encodes a polypeptide of 47K (Parker et al., 1989). Immediately downstream of the E2 gene is a sequence of 946 nucleotides thought to encode two non-structural polypeptides (Leibowitz et al., 1982). As shown in the map in Figure 1,

Coronaviruses and Their Diseases
Edited by D. Cavanagh and T.D.K. Brown
Plenum Press, New York, 1990

103

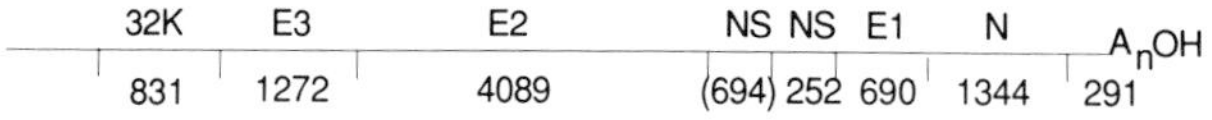

```
  32K      E3         E2        NS NS  E1    N    A_nOH
 |___|_____|_____|__|___|___|_____|_____
   831   1272        4089    (694) 252 690  1344   291
```

Figure 1. The 3' end of the genome of bovine coronavirus. The numbers below each designated gene indicate the length of the open reading frame exclusive of intergenic regions. The number in parentheses indicates the length of an uncharacterized sequence.

we have tentatively identified a 252 nucleotide open reading frame which would encode a 9.5K polypeptide (Cox and Parker, submitted). The remaining 694 nucleotides in this region adjacent to the E2 gene have consistently failed to generate and open reading frame capable of generating a polypeptide of greater than 7K. Further characterization of this region is underway. The E1 and N genes are adjacent and preceed a non-coding sequence of 291 nucleotides immediately upstream of the poly-A at the 3' terminus of the genomic RNA (Lapps et al., 1987). Therefore, the characteristic gene order reported for other coronaviruses is also found in BCV.

Characterization of the Esterase Activity of Bovine Coronavirus

Recently, Vlasak et al. (1989a, 1989b) reported that the bovine coronavirus exhibited receptor binding specificity and receptor-destroying activity similar to the type C influenza viruses. Indirect evidence that the BCV haemagglutinin was responsible for the observed enzymatic activity was obtained by radiolabeling the E3 polypeptide with ^{3}H-DFP which specifically inhibited the hydrolysis of p-nitrophenyl acetate. We previously reported that E3-specific monoclonal antibodies which inhibited haemagglutination also neutralized infectivity (Parker et al., 1989). In order to determine if the BCV E3 polypeptide was responsible for the virus-specific hydrolysis of acetate from O-acetylated sialic acids, we tested the ability of monoclonal antibodies specific for the E3-polypeptide to inhibit the release of acetate from bovine submaxillary mucin. When 2 ug of purified virus was incubated in phosphate buffered saline containing 25 mg/ml of BSM, an average of three determinations showed that 26 ug of acetate was released as determined with a commercially available kit. When the virus was incubated with a pool of E3-specific monoclonal antibodies (Deregt et al., 1988) prior to addition of substrate, background levels of free acetate were detected. Of the three monoclonals which bind three distinct epitopes, the monoclonal antibodies KD9-40 and HC10-5 completely inhibited esterase activity. The third antibody, BD9-8C, which shows minimal neutralizing and haemagglutination inhibiting (HI) activity, partially inhibited the esterase activity. The specificity of the inhibition was indicated by the lack of inhibition of non-immune sera or a pool of monoclonals

Table I

Antibody Inhibition of BCV Acetylesterase

Antibody	Specificity Antigenic Group	Neutralization	HI	Acetate Released (ug)
None	–	–	–	26
Pooled	E3	+++	+++	2
KD9-40	E3(A2)	+++	+++	2
HC10-5	E3(A1)	+++	+++	2
BD9-8C	E3(C)	+	–	15
Anti-BHV gIII	–	–	–	25

specific for the bovine herpesvirus gIII glycoprotein. Similar results were obtained with monoclonal antibodies specific for the BCV N, E1 and E2 polypeptides. Therefore, these data further support the notion that the acetylesterase activity of BCV is a property of the E3 polypeptide.

In order to determine if the acetylesterase activity of BCV is an intrinsic property of only the E3 polypeptide, a cDNA clone representing the E3 gene (Parker et al., 1989) was inserted into the genome of the baculovirus Autographa californica. Infection of insect cells (SF9) with the recombinant virus, BVLE3, results in the production of a 130K dimer which dissociates into 58K monomers under reducing conditions (Parker et al., submitted) Intact S. frugiperda cells infected with the recombinant virus were assay for acetylesterase activity. As shown in Table II, 6×10^6 BCV-infected MDBK cells were capable of hydrolyzing approximately 15 ug of acetate from submaxillary mucin. While uninfected insect cells failed to release acetate from BSM, BVLE3 infection of insect cells resulted in significant esterase activity. The esterase activity on BVLE3-infected insect cells was inhibited by the same antibody which inhibited the esterase in purified virus (data not shown). The ability of the E3 polypeptide produced in BVLE3-infected insect cells to hydrolyze the substrate in the absence of other viral components proves that the acetylesterase of bovine coronavirus is an intrinsic property of the E3 polypeptide.

Comparison of the BCV E3 Amino Acid Sequence with the HE of Type C Influenza Virus

In agreement with previous reports (Vlasak et al., 1988a, 1988b), the data above indicate that the receptor-destroying enzyme of BCV is similar in substrate specificity to that of the HE of type C influenza. A search of the protein sequence database of the National Biomedical Research Foundation indicated that extensive amino acid sequence homology existed between the E3 and HE of type C influenza.

Figure 2 shows a comparison of the sequence of the BCV E3 polypeptide and the HE of C/Cal/78 influenza virus (Nakada et al., 1984). A similar result was observed in a comparison between C/Cal/78 and an apparent pseudogene located in the MHV-A59 genome at a position analogous to the location of the BCV E3 gene (Luytjes et al., 1988).

The similarity becomes apparent beginning at amino acid 19 of BCV E3 and amino acid 47 of the C/Cal/78 HE. Amino acid 19 is the amino terminus of the mature E3 polypeptide as the preceeding 18 amino acids represent the signal sequence and are removed during maturation of the

Table II

Expression of BCV Acetylesterase in Virus-Infected Cells

Cells	ug Acetate Released
MDBK	
uninfected	4
BCV-infected	15
Spodoptera frugiperda	
uninfected	3
BVLE3-infected	
-cells	37
-medium[a]	6

[a] Immunoprecipitated from culture medium with Mab BD9-3C prior to assay

of the polypeptide (Hogue et al., 1989). The similarity extends to
position 384 of the E3 sequence which is six amino acids upstream of a
hydrophobic sequence thought to be the membrane anchor of the polypeptide
(Parker et al., 1989). The similar portion of the C/Cal/78 HE extends
to position 427 which is 20 amino acids upstream from the cleavage site
of the HE precursor. Within these boundaries, the similarity is 27%
when only identical residues are considered. However, optimization of
the alignment through the use of the Dayhoff scoring matrix increases
the similarity to 52% as indicated by the boxed positions shown in Figure
2.

Several aspects of the C/Cal/78 sequence emphasize the differences
between the polypeptides being compared. The HE is a disulfide-linked
heterodimer composed of subunits derived by proteolytic cleavage of a
common precurosr. As a result, the cysteine residues at positions 20
and 582, thought to be involved in the formation of the intermolecular
linkages (Nakada et al., 1984) are located in regions lacking similarity
to the E3 and are not shown in Figure 2. In addition, the HE is anchored
in the virion envelope by a hydrophobic domain near the carboxy-terminus
of the HA2 subunit which is also outside of the regions compared in
Figure 2.

Of the six cysteines in the HE thought to be involved in
intramolecular disulfide formation, only 3 are conserved in the BCV E3.
The cysteines at positions 347 and 371 are conserved in both viruses and
may be involved in intramolecular linkages in the HE of C/Cal/78.
However, at present the only disulfide known to exist in E3 is in the
linkage which is responsible for dimer formation.

With one exception at the asparagine at position 104 of E3, the
location of the potential N-glycosylation sites are not conserved between
the two polypeptides.

Although both polypeptides exhibit similar receptor specficities and
enzymatic activities, only the identity of the active site of the HE has
been investigated. After radiolabeling with DFP, Vlasak et al. (1989)
determined that the labeled tryptic peptide of the HE contained the
sequence TWIGFGDSR with the radiolabel attached to the serine residue.
Examination of the E3 sequence shows that the sequence is very highly
conserved from positions 33 to 41 which is analogous to the position of
the sequence in the C/Cal/78. Experiments are underway to determine
if this region comprises the active site of the BCV esterase.

Inspection of the sequence comparison in Figure 2 clearly indicates
that the two polypeptides are related. The lack of significant nucleotide
sequence similarity (data not shown) as well as the dissimilarity in the
locations of glycosylation sites, potential positions of disulfide
linkages and the different pathways leading to the formation of the
dimeric structures of the final gene products strongly suggests that
any proposed genetic interaction between these viruses undoubtedly
occurred between an ancient influenza-like virus and a coronavirus
progenitor. Reports that an E3-like molecule may be found in variants
of murine hepatitis virus (Taguchi et al., 1985, 1986) also suggests
that E3 may be a non-essential polypeptide in those viruses which
contain it. It may also be argued, based upon these same consideration
that the two polypeptides represent convergent evolution. However,
based upon the similarities of the binding and enzymatic properties of
the two polypeptides, it seems appropriate that the term HE indicating
haemagglutinin-acetylesterase be adopted as the designation for the
BCV haemagglutinin.

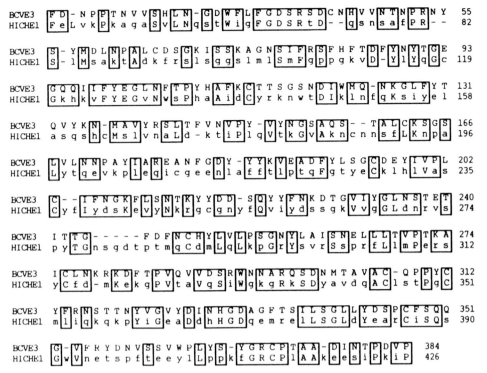

Figure 2. Amino acid sequence comparison of bovine coronavirus E3 glycoprotein and C/Cal/78 influenza virus HE. Similar amino acids determined by Dayhoff scoring matrix are boxed. "-" indicates a single residue gap introduced to maximize sequence alignment.

REFERENCES

Deregt, D., Gifford, G. A., Ijaz, M. K., Watts, T. C., Gilchrist, J. E., Haines, D. M., Babiuk, L. A., 1989, Monoclonal antibodies to bovine coronavirus glycoproteins E2 and E3: Demonstration of in vivo virus neutralizing activity, J. Gen. Virol., 70:993.

Hogue, B. G., Brian, D. A., 1986, Structural proteins of human respiratory coronavirus OC-43, Virus Res., 5:131.

Hogue, B. G., Green, T. E., Brian, D. A., 1989, Synthesis and processing of the bovine enteric coronavirus hemagglutinin protein, J. Gen. Virol., 70:345.

King, B., Potts, B. J., Brian, D. A., 1985, Bovine coronavirus hemagglutinin protein, Virus Res., 2:53.

Lapps, W., Hogue, B. G., Brian, D. A., 1987, Sequence analysis of the bovine coronavirus nucleocapsid and matrix protein genes, Virology, 157:47.

Leibowitz, J. L., Weiss, S. R., Paavola, E., Bond, C. W., 1982, Cell free translation of murine coronavirus RNA, J. Virol., 43:905.

Luytjes, W., Breenbeek, P. J., Noten, A. F. H., Horzinek, M. C., Spaan, W. J., 1988, Sequence of mouse hepatitis virus A59 mRNA 2: Indications for RNA recombination between coronaviruses and influenza C virus, Virology, 166:415.

Nakada, S., Creager, R. S., Krystal, M., Aaronson, R. P., Palese, P., 1984, Influenza C virus hemagglutinin: Comparison with influenza A and B virus hemagglutinins, J. Virol., 50:118.

Parker, M. D., Cox, G. J., Deregt, D., Fitzpatrick, D. R., Babiuk, L. A., 1989, Cloning and in vitro expression of the gene for the E3 hemagglutinin of bovine coronavirus, J. Gen. Virol., 70:155.

Pocock, D. H., Garwes, D. J., 1977, The polypeptides of haemagglutinating encephalomyelitis virus and isolated subviral particles, J. Gen. Virol., 37:487.

Taguchi, F., Siddell, S. G., Wege, H., Ter Meulen, V., 1985, Characterization of a variant virus selected in rat brains after infection by coronavirus mouse hepatitis virus JHM, J. Virol., 54:429.

Taguchi, F., Massa, P. T., Ter Meulen, V., 1986, Characterization of a variant virus isolated from neural cell culture after infection of mouse coronavirus JHMV, Virology, 155:267.

Vlasak, R., Luytjes, W., Leider, J., Spaan, W, Palese, P., 1988a, The E3 protein of bovine coronavirus is a receptor-destroying enzyme with acetylesterase activity, J. Virol., 62:468.

Vlasak, R., Luytjes, W., Spaan, W., Palese, P., 1988b, Human and bovine coronaviruses recognize sialic acid-containing receptors similar to those of influenza C viruses, Proc. Natl. Aca. Sci., 85:4526.

ISOLATION AND CHARACTERIZATION OF THE ACETYLESTERASE OF

HEMAGGLUTINATING ENCEPHALOMYELITIS VIRUS (HEV)

Beate Schultze[1], R. Günter Heß[2], Rudolf Rott[3],
Hans-Dieter Klenk[1] and Georg Herrler[1]

[1]Institut für Virologie, Philipps-Universität Marburg
[2]Landesveterinäruntersuchungsamt Koblenz
[3]Institut für Virologie, Justus-Liebig-Universität
Gießen

INTRODUCTION

Receptor-destroying enzymes have long been thought to be
present only on influenza viruses and paramyxoviruses but not on
other animal viruses. Paramyxoviruses as well as influenza A and B
viruses are able to inactivate their own receptors by virtue of a
neuraminidase which cleaves terminal sialic acid from glycoproteins or gangliosides (Drzeniek, 1972). The corresponding enzyme
of influenza C virus is a sialate 9-O-acetylesterase which releases acetyl residues from position C-9 of N-acetyl-9-O-acetyl-
neuraminic acid (Neu5,9Ac$_2$) (Herrler et al., 1985). Recently, sequencing of the genome of mouse hepatitis virus revealed an open
reading frame which surprisingly showed some similarity to the
glycoprotein HEF of influenza C virus (Luytjes et al., 1988). This
finding prompted a search which resulted in the discovery that bovine coronavirus (BCV) contains a sialate O-acetylesterase similar
to the receptor-destroying enzyme of influenza C virus (Vlasak et
al., 1988a). This enzyme is inhibited by diisopropylfluorophosphate (DFP), which binds covalently to serine in the active-site
of serine proteases and esterases. By using a radioactive form of
this inhibitor protein E3 of BCV was identified as esterase
(Vlasak et al., 1988b). The same glycoprotein has been shown previously to be involved in the hemagglutinating activity of BCV
(King et al., 1985). Therefore, E3 is designated HE.
   Here we report that an acetylesterase is also present on
hemagglutinating encephalomyelitis virus (HEV), a porcine coronavirus. The purification of this esterase is described.

RESULTS

HEV is related to BCV both serologically and in its
hemagglutinating properties. We analyzed whether HEV also has acetylesterase activity like BCV. Strain NT-9 of HEV, which has been
isolated by nasal swab from a pig (Heß and Bachmann, 1978), was
grown in MDCK I cells and purified by centrifugation through a
sucrose gradient. The purified virus was analyzed for its ability
to release acetate from p-nitrophenylacetate (PNPA). As shown in

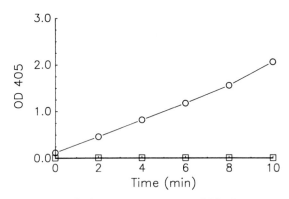

Fig. 1. Esterase activity of HEV. Purified HEV was incubated
for various times with p-nitrophenylacetate at room
temperature. Cleavage of the substrate was assayed
by determining the optical density at 405 nm.
Control virus (circles) and virus pretreated with
1 µM of diisopropylfluorophosphate for 30 min
at 4°C (squares) were compared.

Fig.1, HEV cleaved the substrate resulting in a time-dependent increase of the optical density. As the esterases of both BCV and
influenza C virus have been reported to be serine hydrolyses which
are inhibited by diisopropylfluorophosphate (DFP), it was of interest to find out whether the enzyme of HEV is also sensitive to
this inhibitor. As shown in Fig. 1, no enzyme activity was detectable after pretreatment of virus with 1 µM DFP for 30 min. This
result indicates that the esterase of HEV is a serine hydrolase.
In order to identify the viral protein responsible for the
acetylesterase activity of HEV, the same approach was chosen,
which had been used in the case of BCV (Vlasak et al., 1988b). Purified HEV was incubated with ^{3}H-DFP for 30 min at 4°C and then
analyzed by SDS-polyacrylamide gel electrophoresis. The result is
shown in Fig. 2. Following staining with Coomassie Brilliant Blue
the viral proteins N, M, S, and HE became visible. The radioactive
label was found to comigrate only with the latter glycoprotein.
The identity of the ^{3}H-DFP-labeled protein was confirmed by analyzing the sample in the absence and presence of reducing agents.
Under non-reducing conditions the labeled protein was detected in
a position expected for a protein with a molecular weight of
about 140 kDal. In the presence of dithiotreitol the apparent size
is reduced to about 65 kDal indicating that in the native protein
monomers are connected by disulfide bonds to form a dimeric
structure. This migration behavior is characteristic for the viral
protein involved in the hemagglutinating activity of HEV
(Callebaut and Pensaert, 1980) and therefore, in analogy to BCV,
is designated HE.
In order to isolate the esterase of HEV from the viral membrane,
purified virions were treated with 1% octylglucoside (OG). The
nucleocapsid as well as the M-protein were pelleted by centrifugation for 30 min at 25.000 x g (not shown). The glycoproteins
remaining in the supernatant (S and HE) were loaded onto a 10-30%

110

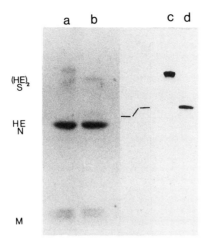

Fig. 2. Identification of the esterase protein of HEV. Purified virus was incubated in the presence of ^{3}H-DFP for 30 min on ice and then analyzed by SDS-polyacrylamide gel electrophoresis in the absence (lanes a and c) and presence (lanes b and d) of dithiotreitol. The gel was stained with Coomassie Brilliant Blue (lanes a and b) and processed for fluorography (lanes c and d)

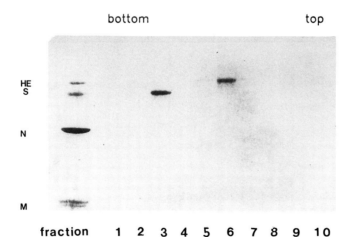

Fig. 3. Purification of the acetylesterase of HEV. The supernatant of octylglucoside-treated virions was centrifuged through a sucrose gradient (see text) and the fractions were analyzed by SDS-polyacrylamide gel electrophoresis under non-reducing conditions.

Table 1. Effect of the acetylesterase from HEV on the
receptors for HEV, BCV, influenza A (WSN) and
C (JHB/1/66) virus on chicken erythrocytes

treatment of erythrocytes	hemagglutination titer (HA-units/ml)			
	BCV	HEV	JHB/1/66	WSN
none	256	256	512	1024
acetylesterase	<2	<2	<2	1024

sucrose gradient in PBS containing 1% OG. Following centrifugation
at 42.000 rpm for 16 h in SW55 rotor, fractions were collected
from the bottom of the tube and analyzed by SDS-polyacrylamide gel
electrophoresis. As shown in Fig. 3, S-protein was detected in
fraction 3, while most of HE was recovered from fraction 6. Analysis of the fractions for acetylesterase activity revealed that
only fractions containing HE were able to release acetate from
PNPA. This result confirms that HE is responsible for the esterase
activity of HEV.

The purified acetylesterase of HEV was analyzed for its
ability to function as a receptor-destroying enzyme. Chicken red
blood cells suspended in PBS were incubated with purified acetylesterase (fraction 6, Fig. 3) for 60 min at 37°C. The treated
erythrocytes were used for a hemagglutination assay with two coronaviruses as well as with influenza A and C viruses. The result is
shown in Table 1. While high hemagglutination titers of all four
strains were obtained with control erythrocytes, only strain WSN
of influenza A virus agglutinated chicken red blood cells treated
with acetylesterase from BCV. Erythrocytes incubated in the presence of HE were completely resistant to agglutination not only by
HEV but also by BCV and strain JHB/1/66 of influenza C virus. This
result shows that the purified HE can function as receptor-destroying enzyme and that HEV uses the same type of receptors to
agglutinate erythrocytes as BCV and influenza C virus.

DISCUSSION

A sialate 9-O-acetylesterase has been reported to be present
on influenza C viruses (Herrler et al., 1985) and on bovine coronavirus (Vlasak et al., 1988a). We have shown here that this enzyme is also present on HEV. The acetylesterase inactivates the
erythrocyte receptors for BCV, HCV-OC43 (Vlasak et al., 1988a) and
HEV (this report) indicating that $Neu5,9Ac_2$ is a receptor determinant for attachment of these viruses to red blood cells. With the
acetylesterase available now in purified form, the question can be
adressed, whether $Neu5,9Ac_2$ is required on the surface of cultured
cells to initiate an infection. It will also be interesting to
find out whether the acetylesterase of HEV or BCV has an effect on
the receptors of other coronaviruses.

As in the case of BCV, the esterase activity of HEV was found to be a function of the HE-protein, which forms a dimer, the monomers of which are held together by disulfide bond(s). Such a protein has also been detected on human coronavirus strain OC43 as well as on several murine coronaviruses. All these strains are serologically more closely related to each other than to other coronaviruses such as TGEV, FIPV and IBV, respectively. The latter viruses are lacking an HE-protein and presumably also an esterase activity. An HE-protein is also missing in strain A59 of mouse hepatitis virus (MHV), which is serologically related to BCV and HEV. However, this virus contains genetic information for such a protein, but the corresponding open reading frame cannot be expressed (Luytjes et al., 1988). A protein of about 110 kDalton has been shown to function as a receptor for attachment of MHV-A59 to the cell surface (Boyle et al., 1987). The biological importance of the acetylesterase for coronaviruses is not known. Considering the different diseases caused by the members of this virus family, it will be interesting to find out whether the presence of an esterase affects the pathogenicity of coronaviruses

ACKNOWLEDGMENT

The technical assistance of Birgit Döll is gratefully acknowledged. This work was supported by Deutsche Forschungsgemeinschaft.

REFERENCES

Boyle, J. F., Weismiller, D. G., and Holmes, K. V., 1987, Genetic resistance to mouse hepatitis virus correlates with absence of virus-binding activity on target tissues, J. Virol., 61:185.
Callebaut, P. E. and Pensaert, M. B., 1980, Characterization and isolation of structural polypeptides in haemagglutinating encephalomyelitis virus, J. Gen. Virol., 48:193.
Drzeniek, R., 1972, Substrate specificities of neuraminidases, Histochem. J., 5:271.
Herrler, G., Rott, R., Klenk, H.-D., Müller, H.-P., Shukla, A. K., and Schauer, R., 1985, The receptor-destroying enzyme of influenza C virus is neuraminate-O-acetylesterase, EMBO J., 4:1503.
Heß, R. G. and Bachmann, P. A., 1978, Erbrechen und Kümmern der Ferkel: Vorkommen und Verbreitung in Süddeutschland, Tierärztliche Umschau, 33:571.
King, B., Potts, B. J., and Brian, D. A., 1985, Bovine coronavirus hemagglutinin protein, Virus Res., 2:53.
Luytjes, W., Bredenbeek, P. J., Noten, A. F. H., Horzinek, M. C., and Spaan, W. J. M., 1988, Sequence of mouse hepatitis virus A59 mRNA 2: Indications for RNA recombination between coronaviruses and influenza C virus, Virology, 166:415.
Vlasak, R., Luytjes, W., Spaan, W., and Palese, P., 1988a, Human and bovine coronaviruses recognize sialic acid containing receptors similar to those of influenza C viruses, Proc. Natl. Acad. Sci. USA, 85:4526.
Vlasak, R., Luytjes, W., Leider, J., Spaan, W., and Palese, P., 1988b, The E3 protein of coronavirus is a receptor-destroying enzyme with acetylesterase activity, J. Virol., 62:4686.

DIFFERENTIAL REACTIVITY OF BOVINE CORONAVIRUS (BCV) AND INFLUENZA

C VIRUS WITH N-ACETYL-9-O-ACETYLNEURAMINIC ACID (NEU5,9AC$_2$)-

CONTAINING RECEPTORS

Beate Schultze[1], Hans-Jürgen Groß[2], Hans-Dieter Klenk[1]
Reinhard Brossmer[2], and Georg Herrler[1]

[1]Institut für Virologie, Philipps-Universität Marburg
[2]Institut für Biochemie II, Universität Heidelberg

INTRODUCTION

Only little information is available about the initial
events in the infectious cycle of coronaviruses. Attachment of
strain A59 of mouse hepatitis virus to the cell surface has been
shown to be mediated by a protein of about 110 kDalton (Boyle et
al., 1988). Recently, bovine coronavirus (BCV) and human coronavirus OC43 (HCV-OC43) have been shown to recognize receptors on
erythrocytes similar to influenza C virus. The evidence is based
on the finding that both influenza C virus and BCV contain a
sialate O-acetylesterase, which functions as a receptor-destroying
enzyme (Vlasak et al, 1988). Incubation of chicken red blood cells
with the esterase of either virus renders the erythrocytes resistant to agglutination by both viruses as well as by HCV-OC43. This
result indicates that N-acetyl-9-O-acetylneuraminic acid
(Neu5,9Ac$_2$) is a receptor determinant for attachment of BCV and
HCV-OC43 to erythrocytes as has been shown previously for influenza C virus (Rogers et al., 1986). Here we confirm the importance
of Neu5,9Ac$_2$ for the binding of BCV to the cell surface by resialylation of erythrocytes. We present evidence that strain Johan-
nesburg/1/66 of influenza C virus is more efficient in recognizing
Neu5,9Ac$_2$-containing receptors than BCV.

RESULTS

There is a great variation among erythrocytes from different
species as far as the presence of 9-O-acetylated sialic acids on
the cell surface is concerned (Shukla and Schauer, 1982). While
red blood cells from mice and rats are very rich in Neu5,9Ac$_2$ (50%
and more of the total content of sialic acid), chemical analysis
has failed to detect any O-acetylated sialic acid on cells from
some other species such as human erythrocytes. In the case of
chicken red blood cells the presence of Neu5,9Ac$_2$ has been shown
to be a developmental marker (Herrler et al., 1987). Chemical analysis has revealed that this type of sialic acid is present on
erythrocytes from adult chicken, but not on cells from one-day-old
chicken. In order to obtain information about the hemagglutinating

Table 1. Agglutination of red blood cells by bovine coronavirus (BCV) and influenza A (FPV/Rostock/34(H7N1)) and C virus (JHB/1/66).

erythrocytes	hemagglutination titer (HA-units/ml)		
	BCV	JHB/1/66	FPV/Rostock
chicken, adult	64	512	512
chicken, 1-day-old	<2	<2	256
human	<2	<2	1024

activity of BCV, a hemagglutination assay was performed with erythrocytes from adult and one-day-old chicken as well as with human red blood cells. As shown in Table 1, only influenza A virus is able to agglutinate cells from all three sources. HA-titers of BCV and influenza C virus (strain JHB/1/66) were only obtained with erythrocytes from adult chicken, while cells from one-day-old chicken and human erythrocytes were resistant to agglutination. Considering the type of sialic acid present on the red blood cells (see above), the result from Table 1 is compatible with $Neu5,9Ac_2$ being a receptor determinant for attachment of BCV to erythrocytes.

With influenza C virus direct evidence for the importance of $Neu5,9Ac_2$ as an essential part of the receptors on red blood cells was obtained by resialylation of human erythrocytes (Rogers et al., 1986). The same approach was applied to BCV. Human red blood cells were incubated with neuraminidase from Vibrio cholerae to release most of the native sialic acids. The asialo-cells were resialylated using purified rat liver $Gal\beta1,4GlcNAc$ $\alpha2,6-$

Table 2. Generation of receptors for bovine coronavirus (BCV) and influenza C virus (JHB/1/66) by resialylation of human erythrocytes.

type of sialic acid attached to cells	hemagglutination titer (HA-units/ml)	
	BCV	JHB/1/66
none	<2	<2
Neu5Ac	<2	<2
$Neu5,9A_2$	128	128

Table 3. Comparison of the efficiency of bovine coronavirus (BCV) and influenza C virus (JHB/1/66) to utilize Neu5,9Ac$_2$ as a receptor determinant for agglutination of human red blood cells.

erythrocytes	hemagglutination titer (HA-units/ml)	
	BCV	JHB/1/66
chicken, untreated	256	256
human, untreated	<2	<2
human, resialylated with Neu5,9Ac$_2$		
4 μM	264	512
2 μM	16	512
1 μM	<2	512

sialyltransferase (specifically attaching sialic acid to galactose in an α-2,6-linkage) (Sticker et al., 1988) and activated sialic acids (CMP-Neu5Ac and CMP-Neu5,9Ac$_2$). As shown in Table 2, neither BCV nor influenza C virus is able to agglutinate cells resialylated to contain Neu5Ac on the surface. High hemagglutination titers were obtained, however, following attachment of 9-O-acetylated sialic acids to cell surface glycoproteins of asialocells. This result provides direct evidence that agglutination of red blood cells by BCV requires the presence of Neu5,9Ac$_2$ on the cell surface.

The efficiency of BCV and influenza C virus to recognize Neu5,9Ac$_2$-containing receptors was compared by determining the amount of 9-O-acetylated sialic acid required for generation of virus receptors on red blood cells. Following treatment with sialidase from Vibrio cholerae, human erythrocytes were incubated with sialyltransferase and different amounts of CMP-Neu5,9Ac$_2$ at 37°C. After 3 h cells were washed with PBS and used as a 1% suspension to determine the hemagglutination titer of BCV and influenza C virus. As shown in Table 3, optimal titers of influenza C virus were already obtained, when red blood cells were incubated in the presence of 1 μM CMP-Neu5,9Ac$_2$. Hemagglutination by BCV was only detectable with cells incubated in the presence of 2 μM of activated sialic acid, optimal titers requiring 1 μM CMP-Neu5,9Ac$_2$ during the resialylation reaction. This result indicates that strain JHB/1/66 of influenza C virus is more efficient in recognizing Neu5,9Ac$_2$-containing receptors on erythrocytes.

In order to get further information about the receptor-binding activity of BCV, an artificial sialic acid analogue was analyzed for its ability to function as a receptor determinant. 9-acetamido-9-deoxy-N-acetylneuraminic acid is very similar to Neu5,9Ac$_2$, the only difference being that the acetyl residue is

Table 4. Comparison of the ability of bovine coronavirus (BCV) and influenza C virus (JHB/1/66) to agglutinate human erythrocytes resialylated to contain the sialic acid analogue 9-N-acetyl-Neu5Ac.

type of sialic acid attached to cells	hemagglutination titer (HA-units/ml)	
	BCV	JHB/1/66
9-O-acetyl-Neu5Ac	128	128
9-N-acetyl-Neu5Ac (9-acetamido-Neu5Ac)	<2	256

attached to position C-9 via a nitrogen rather than an oxygen atom. The activated form of this sialic acid analogue has been shown previously to be a suitable donor substrate for Galβ1-4GlcNAc α2,6-sialyltransferase from rat liver (Groβ et al., 1987, 1989). Following transfer to the surface of human erythrocytes, this synthetic sialic acid functions as a receptor determinant for influenza C virus (J.C.Paulson, personal communication). As shown in Table 4, cells resialylated to contain 9-acetamido-Neu5Ac were agglutinated by influenza C virus, but not by BCV. This result provides further evidence that BCV and influenza C virus differ in their ability to recognize sialic acid-containing receptors.

DISCUSSION

The results presented above confirm that attachment of coronavirus to erythrocytes requires the presence of Neu5,9Ac$_2$-containing receptors on the cell surface. The resialylation method enabled us to compare two viruses with respect to their efficiency in recognizing Neu5,9Ac$_2$-containing receptors. Strain JHB/1/66 of influenza C virus requires less 9-0-acetylated sialic acid on the surface of erythrocytes to cause hemagglutination than BCV. This result does not implicate that influenza C viruses in general have a higher affinity for their receptors compared to coronaviruses. Analysis of more strains of the corresponding virus families will probably show that there is some variation in the number of receptors required for attachment of virus to the cell surface. In the case of strain JHB/1/66 a mutant was isolated which is more efficient in recognizing Neu5,9Ac$_2$-containing receptors than the wild type (Szepanski et al., 1989). This mutant has a broader cell tropism compared to the parent virus. It is very well possible, that there is also variation in the receptor-binding activity of different strains of BCV. Adaptation of BCV to growth in MDBK cells has been described. This cell line has a low amount of 9-0-acetylated sialic acid on the cell surface as judged by its resistance to infection by influenza C virus. We expect that MDBK-adapted BCV requires less Neu5,9Ac$_2$ on the surface of erythrocytes in order to cause hemagglutination than our strain of BCV, which has been grown in MDCK I cells. Another difference between strain JHB/1/66 of influenza C virus and bovine coronavirus was evident when 9-acetamido-Neu5Ac was analyzed for its ability to serve as a recep-

tor determinant. In contrast to influenza C virus BCV was unable
to agglutinate red blood cells sialylated with the synthetic sialic acid analogue. This result shows that the ester linkage between the acetyl residue and position C-9 of sialic acid is crucial
for binding of BCV. Sialic acid with an acetyl residue attached
via an amide-linkage is recognized as a receptor determinant only
by influenza C virus but not by BCV. The use of synthetic sialic
acid analogues should be very helpful in the future to characterize the interaction between coronaviruses and their receptors.
The resialylation method described here for analysis of erythrocyte receptors should be applicable also to cultured cells and
give an answer to the question whether $Neu5,9Ac_2$ is required for
BCV and other coronaviruses to initiate an infection.

ACKNOWLEDGMENT

     The technical assistance of Birgit Döll is gratefully
acknowledged. This work was supported by Deutsche Forschungs-
gemeinschaft (Forschergruppe Kl 238-1/1).

REFERENCES

Boyle, J. F., Weismiller, D. G., and Holmes, K. V., 1987, Genetic
     resistance to mouse hepatitis virus correlates with absence
     of virus-binding activity on target tissues, J. Virol.,
     61:185.
Groß, H. J., Bünsch, A., Paulson, J. C., and Brossmer, R., 1987,
     Activation and transfer of novel synthetic 9-substituted
     sialic acids, Eur. J. Biochem., 168:595.
Groß, H. J., Rose, U.,Krause, J. M., Paulson, J. C., Schmid, K.,
     Feeney, R. E., and Brossmer, R., 1989, Transfer of
     synthetic sialic acid analogues to N- and O- linked
     glycoprotein glycans using four different mammalian
     sialyltransferases, Biochemistry, in press.
Herrler, G., Reuter, G., Rott, R., Klenk, H.-D., and Schauer, R.,
     1987, N-acetyl-9-O-acetylneuraminic acid, the receptor
     determinant for influenza C virus, is a differentiation
     marker on chicken erythrocytes, Biol. Chem. Hoppe-Seyler,
     368:451.
Rogers, G. N., Herrler, G., Paulson, J. C., and Klenk, H.-D.,
     1986, Influenza C virus uses 9-O-acetyl-N-acetylneuraminic
     acid as a high affinity receptor determinant for attachment
     to cells, J. Biol. Chem., 261:5947.
Shukla, A. K. and Schauer, R., 1982, Fluorimetric determination of
     unsubstituted and 9(8)-O-acetylated sialic acids in
     erythrocyte membranes, Hoppe-Seyler's Z. Physiol. Chem.,
     363:255.
Sticker, U., Groß, H. J., and Brossmer, R., 1988, Purification of
     α2,6-sialyltransferase from rat liver by dye
     chromatography, Biochem. J., 253:577.
Szepanski, S., Klenk, H.-D., and Herrler, G., 1989, Analysis of a
     mutant of influenza C virus with a change in the receptor
     specificity, in: "Cell Biology of Virus Entry, Replication,
     and Pathogenesis", R. W. Compans, A. Helenius, and M. B. A.
     Oldstone, eds., Alan R. Liss, Inc., New York.
Vlasak, R., Luytjes, W., Spaan, W., and Palese, P., 1988, Human
     and bovine coronaviruses recognize sialic acid containing
     receptors similar to those of influenza C viruses,
     Proc. Natl. Acad. Sci. USA, 85:4526.

EXPRESSION OF THE PORCINE TRANSMISSIBLE

GASTROENTERITIS CORONAVIRUS M PROTEIN

Brenda G. Hogue and Debi P. Nayak

Department of Microbiology and Immunology
UCLA School of Medicine
Los Angeles, CA 90024

ABSTRACT

Cloned cDNA encoding the M protein of the porcine transmissible gastroenteritis coronavirus (TGEV) was introduced into a vaccinia virus to examine the function of the amino-terminal signal peptide. The M protein expressed by the recombinant virus was targeted to the Golgi region of infected cells, as is the M protein in cells infected with TGEV. The protein appeared not to undergo processing other than glycosylation. However, the vaccinia-expressed M protein was slightly larger than the protein found in TGEV-infected cells, suggesting that a difference in modification exists between the proteins.

INTRODUCTION

The TGEV M protein has been cloned and shown to be different from the M proteins of the mouse hepatitis virus (MHV), the bovine coronavirus (BCV), and the avian infectious bronchitis virus (IBV)[1,2]. Unlike the others, the TGEV M protein has a sixteen-amino-acid amino-terminal domain, which has the properties of a cleavable signal sequence. Otherwise, the TGEM M is like the others, in that it has three internal hydrophobic domains that presumably result in the protein being anchored in the lipid bilayer by three successive transmembrane helices[3]. Initial experiments suggested that there may be two forms of TGEV M, one that is virion-associated and has the signal peptide removed[2] and another intracellular uncleaved form[1]. It was hypothesized that interaction with other viral components is required for cleavage and that the additional hydrophobic sequence results in the intracellular transport of TGEV M being different from that of the other coronaviruses[1].

This paper reports the initiation of studies on the intracellular biogenesis of the M protein in the absence of other TGEV proteins. We have expressed the M protein using a vaccinia virus recombinant which includes a cDNA copy of the gene for the protein. The synthesis and processing of the protein has been studied and compared with the protein synthesized in TGEV-infected cells. The results indicate that the protein is localized to the Golgi. The vaccinia-expressed protein is slightly larger than the M from TGEV-infected cells, a result consistent with noncleavage of the signal. Other recent data suggest, however, that signal cleavage does occur, even in the absence of other viral components.

Coronaviruses and Their Diseases
Edited by D. Cavanagh and T.D.K. Brown
Plenum Press, New York, 1990

MATERIALS AND METHODS

Generation of a Vaccinia Recombinant Expressing the TGEV M Protein

A cDNA copy of the TGEV M protein gene was removed from the pGEM-M-1 construct[1] with Bam HI and Eco RI and was filled in with the Klenow fragment of DNA polymerase I. The gene was then subcloned into the pSC11 vector[4] in the unique Sma I site under the vaccinia promoter P7.5K. The plasmid containing the M gene in the correct orientation was transfected into CV-1 cells by calcium phosphate coprecipitation, after infection with wild-type vaccinia (WR strain) had been performed at a multiplicity of 0.05. Recombinant viruses were isolated by plaque assay on TK$^-$ cells in the presence of 5-bromodeoxyuridine and by including 5-bromo-4-chloro-3-indoyl-β-D-glactopyranoside (X-gal) in the plaquing overlay as previously described[4]. Recombinant viruses encoding the M protein (VVM) were plaque-purified three times on TK$^-$ cells prior to preparation of large stocks in HeLa cells.

Protein Expression Analyses

The Purdue strain of TGEV was grown on swine testicle cells (ST) as previously described[5]. Cells were infected at a multiplicity of infection (moi) of 5. At 8-9 hours postinfection (hpi) cells were labeled with 100 μCi of [^{35}S]methionine or 50 μCi each of [^{35}S]methionine and [^{35}S]cysteine. After labeling, cells were lysed on ice in 0.5 ml of buffer containing 50 mM pH 8.0 Tris, 1% TX-100, 0.5% deoxycholate, 150 mM NaCl, 20 mM EDTA, and 100 kallikrein units/ml Aprotinin. The M protein was immunoprecipitated using 1-2 μl of a monoclonal against the TGEV M (1A6)[6]. Antigen-antibody complexes were isolated with protein A sepharose CL-4B (Pharmacia) and washed in the buffer described above, to which was added 0.1% SDS. In some cases, cells were pretreated with 10 μg/ml tunicamycin for 2 h and then labeled in the presence of the same concentration of the drug. Endo H digestions were carried out as previously described[7], after elution of immunoprecipitated M from protein A sepharose by boiling in the presence of 1.0% SDS. Proteins were detected by immunofluorescence after cells were fixed with acetone:methanol (1:1) for 10 minutes at -20°C. M was detected by incubation with the 1A6 monoclonal (dilution 1:100) followed by incubation with affinity-purified fluorescein-conjugated goat anti-mouse IgG. Cells were visualized with a Nikon Optiphot microscope equipped with fluorescence epiillumination and a Nikon 40X objective. For vaccinia expression of the M protein, CV-1 or ST cells were infected with a moi of 1. Infected cells were harvested at 16 hpi. All procedures were carried out as described above.

RESULTS

Cellular Localization of Vaccinia Expressed M

To determine the cellular localization of M synthesized in the absence of other TGEV proteins, cells infected with the vaccinia recombinant were monitored by indirect immunofluorescence. Using monoclonal 1A6, specific M fluorescence was observed near the nuclei in the Golgi region of infected cells (Fig. 1, lower left). The fluorescence pattern was similar to that observed for the internal expression of M in TGEV-infected cells (Fig. 1, upper left).

Biosynthesis of Vaccinia Expressed M

The biosynthesis of M was followed by immunoprecipitation of infected cell lysates. Using monoclonal 1A6, a protein with a molecular weight of

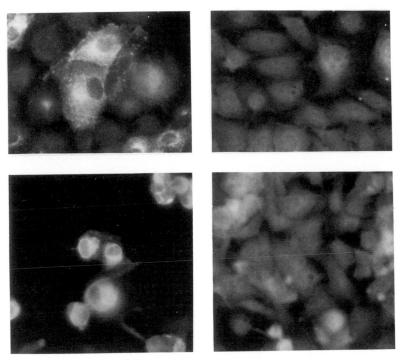

Fig. 1.   Internal immunofluorescence of M in ST cells infected with
          TGEV and VVM: Upper left, TGEV-infected cells; lower left,
          VVM-infected. Controls were either uninfected cells (upper
          right) or cells infected with a vaccinia recombinant
          expressing the influnenza neuraminidase (lower right).

30 kDa was immunoprecipitated from cell lysates infected with VVM (Fig. 2A,
lanes 8-12, and 2B, lanes 3-5). When electrophoresed in parallel with the M
protein immunoprecipitated from TGEV-infected cells (Fig. 2A, lanes 2-5 and
7, and 2B, lane 2), the VVM expressed protein was observed to migrate
slower. A molecular weight difference between the two protein species of
approximately 2 kDa was estimated. The molecular weight of TGEV M has been
estimated to be 28-30 kDa[8,9,10].

   To follow posttranslational processing of the proteins, infected cells
were pulsed for 5 minutes and chased. During a 3 hour chase, M synthesized
by VVM did not appear to undergo processing, as evidenced by no change in
molecular weight (Fig. 2A, lanes 8-12). The protein appeared to remain
stable during this time. The TGEV synthesized M appeared to undergo some
type of processing, since a heterogeneous smear began to appear above the
major protein species after only a 10 minute chase (Fig. 2A, lane 3) and
appeared to increase with time (Fig. 2A, lanes 4, 5, 7).

   Infected cells were maintained in the presence of tunicamycin, to
determine if the difference in mobility between VVM and TGEV M is due to an
N-linked glycosylation difference. Glycosylation of the TGEV M has been
shown to be of the N-linked type[11]. In the presence of tunicamycin, the M
synthesized by VVM (Fig. 2B, lanes 7 and 8) continued to run with a mobility
less than the M from TGEV-infected cells (Fig. 2B, lane 7), indicating that
the difference in molecular weight is not due to N-linked glycosylation. To
assess the extent of processing of the N-linked sugar chains, proteins
immunoprecipitated from both recombinant and TGEV-infected cells were

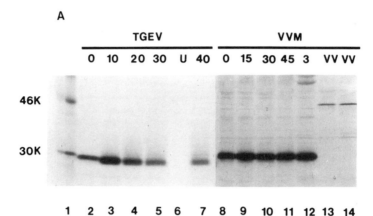

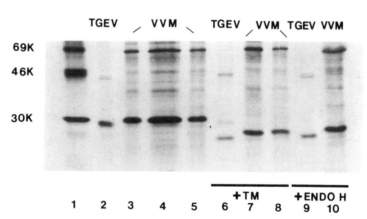

Fig. 2.   In vivo expression of M in TGEV- and VVM-infected cells.   (A)
Pulse-chase results: Lanes 2 through 5 and 7 are
immunoprecepitates from TGEV-infected cells harvested at 0,
10, 20, 30, and 40 minutes, respectively, after a 5 minute
pulse with [^{35}S]methionine.   Lanes 8-12 are immunoprecipates
from VVM-infected cells chased for 0, 15, 30, 45 minutes, and
3 hours, respectively.   Lane 6 is uninfected cells after a 40-
minute chase.   Lanes 13 and 14 are wild-type vaccinia-infected
cells chased for 0 and 3 hours, respectively.   Lane 1 contains
molecular weight markers.   (B) Tunicamycin-treatment and endo
H digestion results: Infected cells were pulsed for 30
minutes with [^{35}S]methionine and [^{35}S]cysteine then chased for
1.5 hours with excess cold amino acids.   Lanes 6-8 are
immunoprecipitations from cells maintained in the presence of
tunicamycin.   Lanes 9 and 10 are immunoprecipitations digested
with endo H.   Lanes 2-5 are untreated immunoprecipitates.
Lane 1 contains molecular weight markers.

digested with endo H. Both species were sensitive to endo H (Fig. 2B, lanes 9 and 10), indicating that neither protein was transported as far as the medial Golgi compartment, where endo H resistance is acquired[12].

Results identical to those described above were obtained using a transient vaccinia expression system. A recombinant vaccinia virus expressing bacteriophage T7 RNA polymerase[13] was used in conjunction with a transfected cDNA copy of the M gene under a T7 promoter (data not shown).

DISCUSSION

We describe here the results of in vivo expression of the TGEV M protein in the absence of other TGEV proteins. We have generated a vaccinia recombinant virus which includes a cDNA copy of the M gene. Even though we did not quantify expression by the recombinant, it was high; therefore, this expression system is a reasonable one to be used for transport and function studies of M. The VVM-expressed protein was specifically recognized by a monoclonal against the TGEV M; however, as judged by electrophoretic mobility, the VVM expressed protein was larger than the protein precipitated from TGEV-infected cells.

The results of previous work[1] suggested that M signal cleavage may depend on interaction with another viral protein or viral RNA. The results described in this paper are consistent with this hypothesis. However, we now have sequenced the amino terminus of the VVM M protein and find, surprisingly, that it is cleaved (Hogue and Nayak, unpublished data). In addition, the M gene which lacks the amino-terminal signal[1] has been expressed in vivo and found to comigrate with the VVM expressed M. (Hogue and Nayak, unpublished data). Taken together, these findings suggest that some other modification is responsible for the molecular weight difference. We are presently developing new hypotheses and performing further analyses to account for the observed molecular weight difference between the M proteins synthesized in TGEV- and VVM-infected cells.

The localization of M in the Golgi region of permeabilized cells is consistent with that observed by others for the expression of the M proteins of MHV[14] and IBV[15]. This site of localization also correlates with the site of intracellular budding for coronaviruses, consistent with the idea that M determines the budding site[16,17].

We did not detect definitive surface fluorescence of the VVM-expressed protein on nonpermeabilized cells (data not shown). No surface expression was seen in studies of MHV[14] and IBV[15], but we and others[18] have detected apparent surface fluorescence of M on TGEV-infected cells. The failure to observe surface fluorescence from VVM may be due to the extensive cytopathic effect (cpe) on cells infected with vaccinia. However, using a transient vaccinia expression system[13] which results in less cpe of infected cells, we are currently reexamining the surface fluoresence of cells expressing the M gene. We should be able to determine if the TGEV M protein is targeted to the cell surface in the absence of the other viral proteins or if the apparent surface expression on TGEV-infected cells represents transport of the protein to the surface by Golgi derived vessicles or mature virions remaining attached to the surface after release from the cell.

ACKNOWLEDGEMENTS

This work was supported by USPHS grant R01 AI16348 from the National Institutes of Health and by a PHS postdoctoral fellowship F32GM11788 (BGH) from the National Institute of General Medical Sciences. We thank David Brian for many helpful discussions.

REFERENCES

1. Kapke, P. A., Tung, F. Y. T., Hogue, B. G., Brian, D. A., Woods, R. D., and Wesley, R., The amino-terminal signal peptide on the porcine transmissible gastroenteritis coronavirus matrix protein is not an absolute requirement for membrane translocation and glycosylation, Virology 165:367-376 (1988).

2. Laude, H., Rasschaert, D., and Huet, J.-C., Sequence and N-terminal processing of the transmembrane protein E1 of the coronavirus transmissible gastroenteritis virus, J. Gen. Virol. 68:1687-1693 (1987).

3. Rottier, P. J. M., Brandenburg, D., Armstrong, J., and van der Zeijst, B. A. M., Assembly in vitro of a spanning membrane protein of the endoplasmic reticulum: the E1 glycoprotein of coronavirus mouse hepatitis virus A59, Proc. Natl. Acad. Sci. USA 81:1421-1425 (1984).

4. Chakrabarti, S., Brechling, K., and Moss, B., Vaccinia virus expression vector; coexpression of B-galactosidase provides visual screening of recombinant virus plaques, Mol. Cell. Biol. 5:3403-3409 (1985).

5. Kapke, P. A., and Brian, D. A., Sequence analysis of the procine transmissible gastroenteritis coronavirus nucleocapsid protein gene, Virology 151:41-49 (1986).

6. Woods, R. D., Wesley, R. D., and Kapke, P. A., Neutralization of transmissible gastroenteritis virus by complement-dependent monoclonal antibodies, Amer. J. Vet. Res. 49:300-304 (1987).

7. Hogue, B. G., Kienzle, T. E., Brian, Synthesis and processing of the bovine coronavirus hemagglutinin protein, J. Gen. Virol. 70:345-352 (1989).

8. Brian, D. A., Hogue, B. G., Lapps, W., Potts, B. J., and Kapke, P. A., Comparative structure of coronaviruses, in "Proceedings from the Fourth International Symposium of Neonatal Diarrhea," S. D. Acres, ed., University of Saskatoon, Saskatoon, Saskatchewan, Canada (1983).

9. Garwes, D. J., and Pocock, D. H., The polypeptide structure of transmissible gastroenteritis virus, J. Gen. Virol. 29:25-34.

10. Wesley, R. D., and Woods, R. D., Identification of a 17,000 molecular weight antigenic peptide in transmissible gastroenteritis virus, J. Gen. Virol. 67:1419-1425 (1986).

11. Jacobs, L., van der Zeijst, B. A. M., and Horzinek, M. C., Characterization and translation of transmissible gastroenteritis virus mRNAs, J. Virol. 57:1010-1015 (1986).

12. Dunphy, W. G., and Rothman, J. E., Compartmental organization of the Golgi stack, Cell 42:13-21 (1985).

13. Fuerst, T. R., Niles, E. G., Studier, F. W., and Moss, B., Eukaryotic transient-expression system based on recombinant vaccinia virus that systhesizes bacteriophage T7 RNA polymerase, Proc. Natl. Acad. Sci. USA, 83:8122-8126 (1986).

14. Rottier, P. J. M. and Rose, J. K., Coronavirus E1 glycoprotein expressed from cloned cDNA localizes in the Golgi region, J. Virol. 61:2042-2045 (1987).

15. Machamer, C. E., and Rose, J. K., A specific transmembrane domain of a coronavirus E1 glycoprotein is required for its retention in the Golgi region, J. Cell Biol. 105:1205-1214 (1987).

16. Holmes, K. V., Doller, E. W., and Sturman, L. S., Tunicamycin resistant glycosylation of coronavirus glycoprotein: Demonstration of a novel type of viral glycoprotien, Virology 115:334-344 (1981).

17. Tooze, J., Tooze, S. A., and Warren, G., Laminated cisternae of the rough endoplasmic reticulum induced by coronavirus MHV-A59, Eur. J. Cell Biol. 36:108-115 (1985).

18. Welch, S.-K. W., and Saif, L., Monoclonal antibodies to a virulent strain of TGEV, Arch. Virol. 101:221-235 (1988).

EXPRESSION OF MHV-A59 M GLYCOPROTEIN: EFFECTS OF DELETIONS ON

MEMBRANE INTEGRATION AND INTRACELLULAR TRANSPORT

P.J.M.Rottier, J.Krijnse Locker, M.C.Horzinek, and
W.J.M.Spaan

State University, Veterinary Faculty
Department of Infectious Diseases and Immunology
Institute of Virology
Yalelaan 1, 3584 CL Utrecht
The Netherlands

INTRODUCTION

The M protein of coronaviruses is an integral membrane protein, the general properties of which have been described elsewhere in this volume. The protein is ascribed a pivotal role in the budding process of these viruses. Its restriction to internal membranes suggests it to be a major factor in determining the intracellular site of virion assembly. In addition, M is thought to effect budding through the interaction of its cytoplasmic tail with the nucleocapsid.

Coronaviral M is a glycoprotein carrying oligosaccharides only at its amino-terminus. For most members of the family these are of the N-glycosidic type, but in the case of mouse hepatitis virus (MHV-A59) the sugars are added to serines and/or threonines through O-linkages (1). O-glycosylation is a post-translational event; the responsible enzymes do not reside in the endoplasmic reticulum (ER) but are encountered by the protein only en route to and through the Golgi apparatus.

M is a complex-type membrane protein. In most coronaviruses it has no cleavable signal sequence, yet needs signal recognition particle (SRP) for its integration in the ER (2). Three successive membrane-spanning segments anchor the protein in the ER membrane. They separate a hydrophilic N-terminus exposed to the lumen of the organelle from a C-terminal half of the molecule facing the cytoplasm (3,4,5). From the latter only the extreme terminal domain is accessible to proteases. Exactly how the protein acquires its topology is not known but the functioning as topogenic element of one or more of the hydrophobic segments seems clear. Deletion experiments with the M protein of infectious bronchitis virus (IBV) have shown both the first and the third segment to independently act as signal-anchor sequence (6). In contrast, no indication for a role in topogenesis of the N-terminal or C-terminal domain were obtained (7).

The M proteins of MHV-A59 and IBV have been expressed in cells from cloned cDNA (6,8) as well as by microinjection of mRNA (7,9). Both proteins were found by immunofluorescence to accumulate in the Golgi region. Little is known about the signals that target membrane proteins but it is clear that sorting information must somehow reside in the protein's structure. With respect to coronavirus M protein one interesting study has appeared supporting this view. IBV M proteins with deletions of either the first and second or the second and third transmembrane domain were assembled in cell membranes in the same orientation as the wild-type virus protein (6). It was found that deletion of the second and third domain did not alter the mutant protein's localization to the Golgi region. In contrast, the mutant protein possessing only the third domain was efficiently transported to the plasma membrane. These data suggested that the first transmembrane domain contains a Golgi specific retention signal (6).

We are interested in the M protein of MHV-A59 for its role in virus assembly and because it enables us to address fundamental questions concerning membrane assembly and protein sorting. Using in vitro mutagenesis we have prepared a number of mutant M proteins which we are now studying with respect to membrane integration and intracellular transport. Here we present the first results obtained with some of these mutants.

MATERIALS and METHODS

Plasmid constructions. The M gene was excised with HindIII and EcoRI from the vector pT3/T7-18 in which it had been cloned (8) and was ligated into the transcription vector pTZ19R (10; a kind gift from Dr.D.Mead). To generate the deletion mutants, oligonucleotide-directed mutagenesis was performed with single-stranded phagemid DNA by the method of Zoller and Smith (11). Template DNA was produced from the pTZ vector with the helper phage M13K07 (10). The following oligonucleotides, prepared by the DNA-synthesis service of Yale Medical School (New Haven) were used:
* mutant △N   : 5'-ATGAGTAGTACTACTCAGCTGAAGGAATGGAACTTC-3'
* mutant △C   : 5'-GGTGGAGCTTCAACCCCGGGGTTAGCGGTTTTGCTG-3'
* mutant △(a+b) : 5'-GTTCAATTCCTTAAGGAAGTGTATCTTGGATTTTCT-3'
* mutant △(b+c) : 5'-CCTTATGCTATTAACAAAACGGCTCGTGTAACCG-3'
* mutant △a△c   : 5'-GTTCAATTCCTTAAGGAAATGTTTATTTATGTTGTG-3' and
                   5'-GTATGCGCTAAATAATGTGAGCATAAGGTTGTTTATC-3'.
Primer-extended DNA was transfected onto competent E.Coli NM522. Mutants were identified by differential hybridization to the corresponding 5'-^{32}P-labeled oligonucleotide. Mutations were confirmed by DNA sequencing using the chain-terminator method (12). For the preparation of vaccinia virus recombinants the genes were transferred into the vector pSC11 (13). The wild-type M gene was cut out of the plasmid pJCE1 (8) with BamHI, blunted with the Klenow fragment of DNA polymerase I and ligated into SmaI-digested pSC11. For the transfer of the mutant genes a BglII-site was first introduced into the SmaI-site of pSC11 by linker ligation and the genes, taken out of the pTZ vectors using BamHI, were cloned into this new site.

Preparation of recombinant vaccinia viruses. M genes were recombined into the vaccinia virus genome by transfection of infected HeLa cells with the pSC11 plasmids and recombinants were identified as described by Machamer and Rose (6).

In vitro transcription and translation; alkaline extractions; protease digestions. Transcription reactions were carried out using T7-RNA polymerase (Bethesda Research Laboratories) according to the manufacturer's instructions in 50 or 100µl volumes containing 1 or 2 µg of EcoRI-linearized transcription plasmid, respectively. After a 1h incubation template DNA was degraded for 10 min at 37°C with RQ1 DNase (30U/ml; Promega). Then samples were put on ice and EDTA and yeast tRNA were added to a final concentration of 10mM and 20µg/ml, respectively. RNA was isolated by phenol extraction and ethanol precipitation. Dried pellets were dissolved in half the volume of the original transcription reaction of 10mM Tris-HCl (pH7.4) containing 0.1mM EDTA. Translations of the mRNAs (0.75µl

128

mRNA/10µl reaction) were done for 1h at 30°C in the Amersham reticulocyte lysate N.90Z in the presence of dog pancreas microsomes (a kind gift from Dr.D.I.Meyer). In one experiment (Fig.1) a reticulocyte lysate and microsomes purchased from New England Nuclear were used. To assay for membrane integration, translation reactions (10µl) were mixed on ice with an equal volume of 0.2M Na_2CO_3 (pH 11.5) and left on ice for at least 15 min. The samples were then layered over a sucrose step gradient (80µl 0.2M on top of 20µl 2M sucrose in 2mM $MgAc_2$ and 130mM KAc adjusted to pH 11.5 with NaOH) in tubes of the Beckman airfuge and spun for 10 min at 25 p.s.i. and 4°C. The upper 90µl of the supernatant (s) was separated from the rest (p) and the samples were diluted to 1ml with detergent solution (50mM Tris-HCl, 62.5mM EDTA, 0.4% DOC, 1% Nonidet P-40, pH8.0) containing 2mM PMSF and 100U kallikrein inhibitor. SDS was added to 0.2% followed by 2.5µl of rabbit antiserum to the carboxy-terminus of M. After an overnight incubation at 4°C immune complexes were collected using 20µl of a 10% suspension of Staph. aureus (Pansorbin; Sigma) and washed three times with RIPA buffer (10mM Tris-HCl, 150mM NaCl, 0.1% SDS, 1% DOC, 1% Nonidet P-40, pH7.4) before analysis in a 20% polyacrylamide gel.

Protease protection experiments were carried out essentially as described before (4). Briefly, samples of translation reactions were diluted with half a volume of proteinase K solution (1mg/ml) and incubated in the absence or in the presence of 0.05% saponin for 1h at room temperature. Samples were put on ice and reactions stopped by adding excess PMSF. Aliquots were then taken for direct analysis, for immunoprecipitation as described above or for extraction with Triton X-114 as described previously (4). Final analyses were done in 20% polyacrylamide gels.

In vivo labeling. COS cells were infected with recombinant vaccinia viruses at a m.o.i. of 20. Proteins were labeled from 4 to 7 hours p.i. with ^{35}S-methionine (30µCi/ml) in methionine-free medium. Cells were lysed and the M proteins were immunoprecipitated with 2 µl of a polyclonal MHV-A59 antiserum and 15µl Staph. aureus suspension. The samples were electrophoresed without heating in 15 % polyacrylamide gel.

Indirect immunofluorescence microscopy. Infected COS cells were fixed with 3 % paraformaldehyde at 6h p.i. and permeabilized with 1 % Triton X-100 in PBS. Cells were stained with polyclonal MHV-A59 antiserum (1:150) followed by affinity-purified fluorescein-conjugated goat anti-rabbit IgG (1:150, Kallestad) according to Rose and Bergman (14). For cell surface fluorescensce, infected COS cells were incubated at 10h p.i. with polyclonal MHV-A59 antiserum (1:150 in PBS + 5 % FCS) and then with fluorescein-conjugated anti-rabbit IgG (1:150), both for 30 min at room temperature. Cells were then fixed, washed and visualized with a Zeiss microscope.

Antisera. The preparation of polyclonal antiserum to purified MHV-A59 has been described (15). Antiserum to the carboxy-terminal tail of the MHV-A59 M protein was prepared in 2 rabbits with a synthetic peptide corresponding to the C-terminal 18 amino acids coupled to BSA. Both animals were immunized with 3mg of conjugate emulsified in complete Freund adjuvant, giving about 25 intradermal 50µl injections. Rabbits were boosted similarly 3 times over a period of 3.5 months with 2.5mg of conjugate now emulsified in incomplete Freund adjuvant. The animals were killed 3 weeks later; blood was collected and serum stored at -20°C. The N-terminus specific monoclonal antibody J.1.3 (16) was a kind gift from Drs.S.Stohlman and J.Fleming.

RESULTS

Generation of mutant proteins. As a first approach to test for a role of potentially relevant domains of the M molecule in membrane integration

129

and transport, precise deletions were made by in vitro mutagenesis of the M gene. The following mutants were constructed:

* ΔN: deletion of 16 of the 25 N-terminal amino acids, residues A(7) through F(22)
* ΔC: deletion of 75 amino acids from the cytoplasmic domain, residues E(121) through D(195)
* Δ(a+b): removal of the first two transmembrane domains, residues W(26) through N(81)
* Δ(b+c): removal of second and third transmembrane domain, residues S(49) through Y(101)
* ΔaΔc: deletion of first and third domain, residues W(26) through S(49) and Y(83) through N(104).

Being constructed in the transcription vector pTZ19R (10) the mutant genes could be expressed directly in vitro by translation of the T7-polymerase derived mRNAs. In addition, the genes were recombined into vaccinia virus for expression in eukaryotic cells.

In vitro membrane integration of mutant M proteins. The effect of the mutations on the protein's ability to be stably integrated into membranes was investigated by translation of in vitro transcribed M gene mRNAs in a reticulocyte lysate in the presence of rough microsomes. Integration was assayed by alkaline treatment of the reaction mixture followed by separation of integrated and unintegrated translation products by centrifugation of the membrane sheets. As shown in Fig. 1 (left lanes) both wild-type M and the mutant proteins are efficiently inserted: in each case the majority of the products cosedimented with the membranes. Deletion of most of the N-terminal residues or of a major part of the C-terminal domain was without effect. M proteins lacking two of the three hydrophobic segments also sedimented with the membranes. Apparently, each transmembrane domain can individually direct insertion into the lipid bilayer as well as anchor the protein.

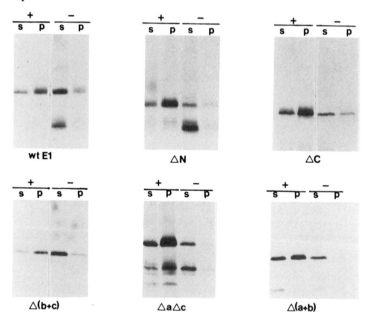

Fig.1. In vitro membrane integration. Wild-type and mutant M mRNAs were translated in a reticulocyte lysate. Microsomes were present during the translation (+) or added post-translationally (-). After treatment of the samples with alkali the membranes were sedimented through a sucrose gradient. Both the supernatant (s) and the membranes (p) were analyzed.

As we have shown earlier, wild-type M inserts into membranes co-translationally (2,4). Indeed, addition of microsomes to the translation mixture post-translationally, after having blocked further polypeptide synthesis with cycloheximide, showed only a background amount of sedimentable M (Fig.1, right lanes). When similar post-synthesis incubations with microsomes were applied to the mutant polypeptides, the same pictures were obtained. Thus, the insertion signals only function in a co-translational manner, post-translational insertion occurring to an insignificant extent, if at all.

Membrane topology of integrated proteins. Two approaches were taken to analyze the organization of the assembled proteins. In one assay we made use of antibodies specifically recognizing the extreme N-terminus and C-terminus, respectively, of M. The former was the monoclonal antibody J.1.3 developed by Fleming et al. (16) which neutralizes MHV in the presence of complement, the latter an antiserum raised in rabbits to a synthetic peptide corresponding to the 18 carboxy-terminal amino acids of M protein. As shown in Fig. 2 both antibodies precipitated the wild-type M protein synthesized in a reticulocyte lysate in the presence of rough microsomes. When treated with proteinase K, which is known to remove the C-terminus of the integrated protein (4,7), only the N-terminus specific antibodies brought down the M-fragment. Digestion from both sides of the membranes by including 0.05% saponin also abolished precipitation with this monoclonal antibody. When such analyses were done with mutant proteins, identical results were obtained with mutants ΔN and ΔC. Apparently, the deletions

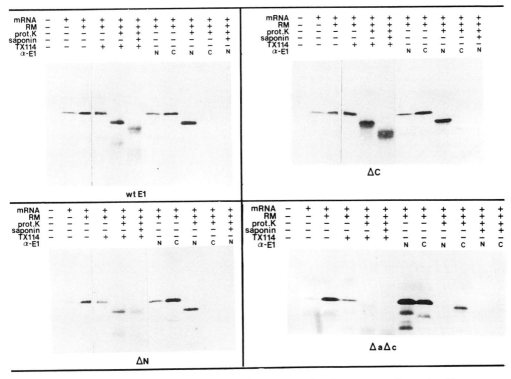

Fig.2. Topology of integrated proteins. Translations were done in the presence or absence of rough microsomes (RM). Aliquots were then taken for direct analysis and for proteinase K treatment in the presence or absence of saponin. Some samples were extracted with Triton X-114 and the detergent phase analyzed; others were immuno-precipitated with antibodies specific for the N- or C-terminus of M.

introduced into these proteins are not involved in the topogenesis of M. Of the single-spanning mutants, which lack two of the three hydrophobic domains, Δ(a+b) and Δ(b+c) did not yield unequivocal results. Mutant ΔaΔc, however, appeared to attain an orientation opposite to that of wild-type M. Protease treatment now showed that the C-terminus of the polypeptide was protected, but only when the membrane vesicles were intact.

In order to confirm and extend these findings, a second approach was taken; the mutant proteins were expressed in cells and glycosylation was used as a marker to assay for translocation of the protein's N-terminus across the membrane. It should be kept in mind, however, that O-glycosylation is a post-translational event, the first step of which is supposed to occur in the transitional "budding compartment" followed by additional glycosylation steps in the Golgi apparatus (17). In Fig. 3 immune precipitates of proteins expressed from a vaccinia virus vector in COS cells after a 3h labeling period are compared with the respective primary translation products obtained in a reticulocyte lysate in the absence of microsomes. Clearly, glycosylated products were obtained in the case of the wild-type protein and with mutants Δ(a+b) and ΔC. While this came as no surprise for ΔC, it indicates that the N-terminus of Δ(a+b) is translocated. As could also be expected, the mutants ΔaΔc and ΔN did not acquire oligosaccharides. In the former case this is in agreement with its reversed orientation, in the latter case the mutation in the N-terminal region apparently affected the functioning of this domain as a substrate for glycosyl transferases. Mutant Δ(b+c) protein comigrated with the in vitro synthesized product; however, a small amount of material migrating slightly slower was also observed. This band may well represent polypeptides to which only the initial N-acetylgalactosamine has been added as the protein seems not to be transported to the Golgi compartments (see below).

Intracellular transport. In order to extend the information obtained from the in vivo labeling experiments, immunofluorescence staining of COS cells infected with the different recombinant vaccinia viruses was performed to visualize the location of the respective proteins. Figure 4 shows the results of indirect staining of the cells at 6h p.i. with a polyclonal MHV-A59 antiserum followed by a fluorescein-conjugated second antibody. Wild-type M was localized in the same juxtanuclear region as we have observed earlier using a SV40-derived vector and which was shown to co-localize with a Golgi marker (8). This typical fluorescence distribution is not specific for COS cells; it was also seen in various other cell types such as HeLa, AtT20, CHO, Ratec, and Sac(-) (not shown). A similar staining pattern was observed with the mutants ΔN, ΔC and Δ(a+b). These proteins apparently

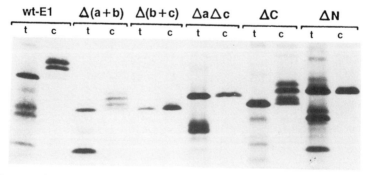

Fig.3. Expression of M proteins in culture cells. Wild-type and mutant proteins synthesized in recombinant vaccinia virus infected COS cells (c) during a 3h labeling period were compared by PAGE with the respective in vitro translation product (t).

reach the Golgi apparatus. Mutants △a△c and △(b+c) showed up clearly
differently. Staining now extended into the cell from all around the
nucleus. Though somewhat diffuse, the stained material was of a reticular
appearance.

Indirect immunofluorescence microscopy on non-permeabilized cells was
performed to analyze transport of M proteins to the plasma membrane. As
shown in Fig.4, surface staining was positive with mutant △(a+b). All other
mutants as well as wild-type M were negative (not shown).

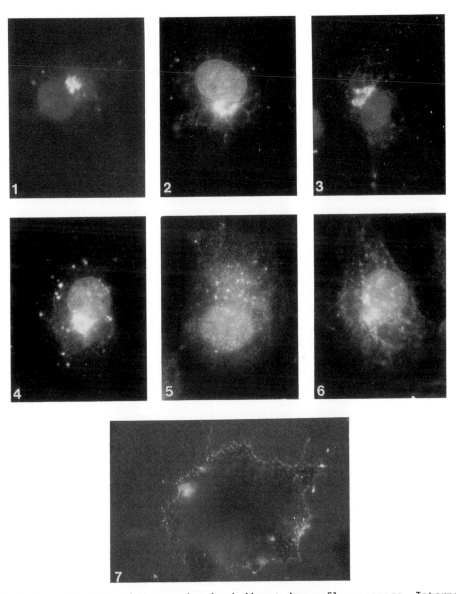

Fig.4. Localization of M proteins by indirect immunofluorescence. Internal
staining of COS cells infected with recombinant vaccinia viruses
expressing wild-type M (1) and the mutants △N (2), △C (3), △(a+b)
(4), △a△c (5) and △(b+c) (6). Cell surface staining of cells
expressing the mutant △(a+b) protein (7).

DISCUSSION

The general conclusion from the data reported here is that the region of the coronavirus M protein comprising the three membrane-spanning domains determine both its membrane topology and its intracellular location. Neither the amino-terminal domain nor the cytoplasmic part of the polypeptide seem to be involved in directing membrane assembly or intracellular transport. A role, however, for the regions immediately flanking the hydrophobic domains cannot be excluded yet.

The N-terminus of the MHV M protein is not cleaved (4,7). Its hydrophilic nature strongly argues against a role as a membrane insertion signal (3,5). The unchanged assembly of the protein lacking 16 out of the 25 N-terminal residues confirms this idea and is in agreement with conclusions drawn from similar work by Mayer et al. (7). Interestingly, the M proteins of porcine transmissible gastroenteritis virus (18,19) and feline infectious peritonitis virus (H. Vennema, pers. comm.) do have a cleaved signal peptide. This peptide precedes the hydrophilic domain and can thus be considered an extension of the N-terminus. It is not clear why these very proteins have an extra signal sequence, but it might be required to aid in translocating the hydrophilic region, which in these viruses has a higher positive charge.

Each of the possible single-spanning M mutants was found to stably integrate into the lipid bilayer. This indicates that each membrane-spanning domain can act as a signal-anchor sequence by itself. This is not so surprising, as the overall hydrophobicity seems to be the major requirement. Having identical amino-terminal and carboxy-terminal domains and thus differing only in the hydrophobic region, these mutant proteins are particularly interesting with respect to their orientation in the membrane. It appeared that the mutant possessing only the third membrane-spanning region has its N-terminus translocated to the lumen, as has been found with a comparable IBV M mutant (6). In contrast, when only the middle hydrophobic domain is present, the N-terminus is in the cytoplasm and the C-terminus exposed to the lumen. No clear conclusion could be drawn about mutant $\triangle$(b+c) but it is likely to also translocate its N-terminus across the membrane. Such an observation has been made with a similar IBV M mutant (6) as well as with a MHV-A59 M protein lacking residues 45-132 which includes the second and third transmembrane domain (7). This implies that the orientation of the hydrophobic domain in each mutant is identical to the orientation of this domain in the assembled wild-type M protein. In other words: each transmembrane domain has an intrinsic preferred orientation in the membrane. It remains to be assessed whether this preference is determined by the hydrophobic segments or by the sequences directly flanking them.

Targeting of the M protein in cells to the Golgi apparatus was affected neither by deleting most of the hydrophilic N-terminus nor by taking about one-third of the polypeptide out of the C-terminal half. Apparently, these domains do not contain sorting information. In contrast, deletions in the hydrophobic cluster generating single-spanning mutant proteins had drastic effects. Deletion of the first and second transmembrane domain generated a mutant protein that was no longer retained in the Golgi apparatus but was transported to the cell surface. A similar deletion in the IBV M protein had the same effect (6). Deletion either of the first and third domain or of the second and third domain both yielded polypeptides that appeared to be retained in the ER region. In the case of the mutant having only the second transmembrane domain this may be explained by its reversed orientation, possible targeting signals no longer being presented to the proper compartment. The location of the mutant with only the first domain is surprising since a similar mutation in IBV M did not change its Golgi accumulation (6). The latter result combined with the cell surface expression of the IBV mutant having only the third transmembrane domain suggested the presence of a Golgi retention signal in the first membrane-spanning segment. Our data do not support such a conclusion. We can only speculate about the reason why the mutants anchored by the first transmembrane region behave differently. The most plausible explanation is the difference in the mutations themselves: in the case of the IBV mutant the deletion comprised 59 residues which is 6 more than was the case with our MHV mutant. Clearly, more work will be required to straighten out this interesting discrepancy since this might give further clues about the signals involved in the targeting of this complex protein.

ACKNOWLEDGEMENTS

Part of this work was done in the laboratory of Dr.J.K.Rose (Yale University, New Haven). We thank Dr.Rose for his interest and support. We are also grateful to Dr.W.Balch for the use of the airfuge.

REFERENCES

1. Niemann, H., Geyer, R., Klenk, H.-D., Linder, D., Stirm, S., and Wirth, M. (1984). EMBO J. 3, 665-670.
2. Rottier, P., Armstrong, J., and Meyer, D.I. (1985). J.Biol.Chem. 260, 4648-4652.
3. Armstrong, J., Niemann, H., Smeekens, S., Rottier, P., and Warren, G. (1984). Nature 308, 751-752.
4. Rottier, P., Brandenburg, D., Armstrong, J., van der Zeijst, B., and Warren, G. (1984). Proc.Natl.Acad.Sci.USA 81, 1421-1425.
5. Rottier, P.J.M., Welling, G.W., Welling-Wester, S., Niesters, H.G.M., Lenstra, J.A., and van der Zeijst, B.A.M. (1986). Biochem. 25, 1335-1339.
6. Machamer, C.E., and Rose, J.K. (1987). J.Cell Biol. 105, 1205-1214.
7. Mayer, T., Tamura, T., Falk, M., and Niemann, H. (1988). J.Biol.Chem. 263, 14956-14963.
8. Rottier, P.J.M., and Rose, J.K. (1987). J.Virol. 61, 2042-2045.
9. Armstrong, J., McCrae, M., and Colman, A. (1987). J.Cell.Biochem. 35, 129-136.
10. Mead, D.A., Szczesna-Skorupa, E., and Kemper, B. (1986). Prot.Eng. 1, 67-74.
11. Zoller, M.J., and Smith, M. (1982). Nucleic Acids Res. 10, 6487-6500.
12. Sanger, F., Coulson, A.R., Barrell, B.J., Smith, A.J.H., and Roe, B.A. (1980). J.Mol.Biol. 143, 161-178.
13. Chakrabarti, S., Brechling, K., and Moss, B. (1985). Mol.Cell.Biol. 5, 3403-3409.
14. Rose, J.K., and Bergmann, J.E. (1982). Cell 30, 753-762.
15. Rottier, P.J.M., Spaan, W.J.M., Horzinek, M.C., and van der Zeijst, B.A.M. (1981). J.Virol. 38, 20-26.
16. Fleming, J.O., Shubin, R.A., Sussman, M.A., Casteel, N., and Stohlman, S.A. (1989). Virol. 168, 162-167.
17. Tooze, S.A., Tooze, J., and Warren, G. (1988). J.Cell Biol. 106, 1475-1487.
18. Laude, H., Rasschaert, D., and Huet, J.-C. (1987). J.gen.Virol. 68, 1687-1693.
19. Kapke, P.A., Tung, F.Y.T., Hogue, B.G., Brian, D.A., Woods, R.D., and Wesley, R. (1988). Virol. 165, 367-376.

Chapter 3

B- and T-Cell Epitopes of the Structural Proteins

BACKGROUND PAPER

MAPPING EPITOPES ON CORONAVIRUS GLYCOPROTEINS

Hubert Laude

Institut National de la Recherche Agronomique
Station de Recherches de Virologie et d'Immunologie Moléculaires
78350 Jouy-en-Josas
France

INTRODUCTION

The purpose of this paper is to summarise the state of coronavirus epitope research, with an emphasis laid on the most recent achievements, i.e. the correlation between antigenicity and polypeptide primary structure. The antigenic properties of coronaviruses reside mainly in their envelope glycoproteins: the S (spike) protein, a high molecular weight polypeptide which constitutes the petal-shaped peplomers and the M (membrane) protein, a smaller integral membrane polypeptide. Some coronaviruses possess an additional surface glycoprotein, the haemagglutinin-esterase (HE) protein.

PEPLOMER PROTEIN S

Analysis of the predicted amino acid sequences now established for 5 coronaviruses (IBV, MHV, TGEV, FIPV and BCV) has led to a model in which the protein is divided into 2 domains: the amino-terminal half, which is assumed to form the globular part of the peplomer, and the carboxy-terminal half, which is assumed to form an elongated structure, the stalk of the peplomer, and also contains a putative transmembrane anchoring region near the carboxy terminus. Both parts bear numerous asparagine-linked complex glycan sidechains, which may modulate their antigenicity. The sequences of the amino-terminal halves exhibit very little conservation, whereas homologies averaging 30% are observed in the carboxy-terminal halves. Several coronaviruses, including IBV, MHV and BCV have a S protein which is cleaved approximately in the middle, thus defining an amino-terminal subunit (S1) and a carboxy-terminal subunit (S2). Several major antigenic sites have been identified on the S proteins of MHV, TGEV and IBV by competitive binding experiments; a number of these sites could be oriented, if not precisely localised, on the primary structure of the molecule.

MHV S Protein

Recombinant viruses generated *in vivo* by RNA-RNA recombination which contain approximately the 5' two-thirds of the MHV-JHM peplomer gene and the 3' one-third of the MHV-A59 peplomer gene have lost their reactivity to monoclonal antibodies (MAbs) defining the sites designated A and B on the JHM S protein. It was inferred that both sites are probably contained within the carboxy-terminal one-third of the protein (Makino *et al.*, 1987). However the positions of the crossover sites have only been mapped by ologonucleotide finger-printing and require confirmation by nucleotide sequencing. Site A was defined by neutralising or non-neutralising MAbs and site B by neutralising MAbs; site A MAbs also inhibited cell fusion. Both sites contained epitopes which exhibited a natural variation from strain to strain and allowed the generation of escape mutants. In addition site B escape mutants showed markedly altered neurovirulence when inoculated into mice. Reactivity analysis of selected or spontaneous variants suggested that sites A and and B are topologically related (Fleming *et al.*, 1986; Taguchi and Fleming, 1989). Three antigenic sites delineated by other groups on the JHM S protein, designated B and C (Talbot *et al.*, 1984) and Ba (Wege *et al.*, 1984), apparently possess the same characteristics with respect to neutralisation, fusion inhibition, variation and generation of attenuated mutants (Dalziel *et al.*, 1986; Wege *et al.*, 1988). It is therefore tempting to speculate that sites B, B-C and Ba are topographically related to the above-mentioned site A. At least part of the latter sites might be conformation-dependent, as was the case for sites B and C (Talbot *et al.*, 1984); this would explain why they could not be mapped using a bacterial expression system.

Expression of fragments of a protein as a fusion polypeptide using a procaryotic vector such as pEX is a classical approach to the mapping of antigenic determinants. Most probably, however, this method mainly detects epitopes that are conformation-independent. Fine mapping of a linear epitope on JHM S protein has been achieved by combining pEX expression and peptide scanning (Lutyes *et al.*, 1989). This epitope belongs to the site designated A (Talbot *et al.*, 1984); this site is: i) recognised by strongly neutralising and fusion-inhibiting MAbs, ii) resistant to denaturation, iii) highly conserved among MHV strains, and iv)possibly crucial for virus infectivity (failure to select escape mutants). The antibody binding site stretched from residue 848 to 856, i.e. about 130 residues from the N-terminus of subunit S2. This 9 amino acid sequence is markedly hydrophobic and located immediately upstream of a region largely conserved in the coronavirus peplomer protein.

Finally, a synthetic decapeptide corresponding to the sequence 993-1002 of the JHM S protein , which was delineated using a surface probability algorithm, elicited a high level of neutralising antibodies and protected mice against a lethal challenge (Talbot *et al.*, 1989). Its position is near the middle of the S2 subunit, between two potentially alpha helical regions which have been suggested to frame the peplomer stalk. Whether this region corresponds to a natural antigenic site remains to be determined.

The above observations support the proposal that the carboxy-terminal S2 subunit of MHV i) contains distinct major antigenic sites, ii) bears neutralisation epitopes, strain-specific epitopes and essential virulence determinants. Surprisingly, there is date, no published evidence of MAb binding to the S1 subunit of MHV. However studies based on the localisation of point mutants or deletions conferring neutralisation-resistance have clearly established the existence of major neutralisation sites on S1 (see articles by Gallagher *et al* and Parker *et al* in Chapter   of this volume).

IBV S Protein

In striking contrast, consistent evidence has been obtained that the S1 subunit of IBV is both the major inducer of neutralising MAbs and the major site of antigenic variation. Isolated S1 reacted with strongly neutralising MAbs (Mockett *et al.*, 1984) and elicited neutralising antisera (Cavanagh *et al.*, 1986). By comparing the amino acid sequences of different IBV strains it was found that most substitutions had occurred in the S1 subunit; S1 proteins can differ in upto 50% of their amino acids (Niesters *et al.*, 1986, Binns *et al.*, 1986, Kusters *et al.*, 1989). In particular, sequence alignments allowed the identification in Massachusetts serotype strains of two regions of clustered substitutions, the hypervariable regions, HVR1 (56-69) and HVR2 (117-133), which were suggested to contain neutralisation epitopes (Niesters *et al.*, 1986). Indeed a mutation which prevented neutralisation by two MAbs was localised in HVR1 by direct sequencing of the genomic RNA of the relevant escape mutants (Cavanagh *et al.*, 1988).

Whereas most neutralising MAbs investigated so far are reported to be directed against S1, the S2 subunit has been shown to react with MAbs having a weak neutralising activity (Koch *et al.*, 1986) Several overlapping conformation-independent epitopes recognised by such MAbs have been precisely localised in the 30 N-terminal residues of S2 through expression of random fragments of S using the pEX system (Lenstra *et al.*, 1989). At least some of these epitopes are conserved in several serotypes as judged by reactivity of the fusion protein with different antisera. In contrast none of the pEX expression products containing fragments of S1 reacted with MAbs suggesting that this subunit contains conformation-dependent epitopes.

The above findings lend support to the view that the major neutralisation domain of IBV resides on the amino-terminal S1 subunit and is composed mainly of serotype specific and conformation-dependent epitopes. Whether distinct regions of S1 are involved remains to be established. In addition at least one immunodominant site, defined by weakly-neutralising and broadly reactive MAbs, is present on the carboxy-terminal S2 subunit.

TGEV S Protein

Detailed epitope maps have defined 4 to 5 major antigenic sites on the TGEV S protein (Delmas *et al.*., 1986, Correa *et al.*, 1988). Most of the determinants critical for neutralisation were highly conserved among the strains and susceptible to denaturation (Laude *et al.*, 1986, Jimenez *et al.*, 1986). Recent data indicate that all of these sites are located in the amino-terminal half of the protein (see articles by Delmas *et al.* and Enjuanes *et al.* in this volume).

BCV S Protein

In the case of the BCV S protein all the neutralising antibodies characterised so far have been directed against gp100 which has recently been found to correspond to the S1 subunit of the S protein (Deregt & Babiuk, 1987, Vautherot *et al.*, this volume). These data are consistent with recent observations on the role of S1 in the neutralisation of MHV (see above) to which BCV is closely related (see Chapter 10 of this volume).

OTHER GLYCOPROTEINS

M Protein

The M glycoprotein is largely buried within the virus membrane or closely associated with its inner surface. Two adjacent epitopes recognised by polyclonal antibodies are located in the 15 carboxy-terminal residues of the MHV M protein as revealed by studies of fragments expressed in the pEX system. Proteolytic digestion abolished the binding of one MAb, presumably directed against the C-terminal region (Tooze & Stanley, 1986). Three overlapping epitopes have been mapped in the first 30 N-terminal residues of TGEV M protein, through localisation of amino acid substitutions in mutants resistant to complement-mediated neutralisation (Laude *et al.*, to be published). Thus in agreement with its predicted relationship with the virus envelope, the major antigenic sites of the M protein correspond to the short protruding hydrophilic domains located at each extremity of the molecule.

HE Protein

The HE protein, associated with a coronavirus subgroup including BCV, HEV and HCV-OC43, is responsible for the strong haemagglutinating activity of these viruses and is also able to elicit neutralising antibodies. Competition experiments between anti-BCV MAbs have defined at at least one major neutralisation site, not yet correlated with HE primary structure (Deregt & Babiuk, 1987).

CONCLUDING REMARKS

Despite significant advances in the physical mapping of B cell epitopes on coronavirus glycoproteins, the emerging picture is still incomplete. The published data mainly concern the peplomer proteins of MHV and IBV. However substantial information about the TGEV peplomer protein has been presented during the symposium. Moreover additional data reported on the MHV peplomer protein, which have established the presence of neutralisation sites on the S1 subunit, have reconciled the apparent discrepancy between MHV and other coronavirues. The difficulties inherent in the elucidation of antigenic structures on a polypeptide which is both very large and highly glycosylated such as the coronavirus peplomer protein should not be underestimated. Clearly, a single linear epitope is less difficult to map than a highly conformation-dependent antigenic site. In this context, methods other than bacterial expression of antigen fragments need to be employed. Moreover, the use of complementary approaches should be preferred whenever possible, since each of them contains its own pitfall. Finally, it should be noted that the role of carbohydrate sidechains in the expression of antigenicity has received very little attention so far.

Continuing investigation in this area is of obvious importance for coronavirologists. First, the resulting information is most helpful for the development of recombinant or synthetic vaccines. In this respect, T cell-recognised structures deserve increased attention in future research. Second, as epitopes often coincide with functional determinants, these studies provide a unique opportunity to explain in terms of molecular structure, fundamental virus processes such as neutralisation, cell receptor recognition and antigenic variation.

SELECTED LITERATURE

Cavanagh, D., Davis, P.J. and Mockett, A.P.A. (1988) Amino acids within hypervariable region 1 of avian coronavirus IBV (Massachusetts serotype) spike glycoprotein are associated with neutralisation epitopes. Virus Res., 11: 141-150.

Lenstra, J.A., Kusters, J.G., Koch, G. and van der Zeijst, B.A.M. (1989) Antigenicity of the peplomer protein of infectious bronchitis virus. Mol. Immunol., 26: 7-15.

Lutyes, W., Geerts, D., Posthumus, W., Meloen, R. and Spaan, W. (1989) Amino acid sequence of a conserved neutralising epitope of murine coronaviruses. J. Virol., 63: 1408-1412.

Makino, S., Fleming, J.O., Keck, J.G., Stohlman, S.A. and Lai, M.M.C. (1987) RNA recombination of coronaviruses: localisation of neutralising epitopes and neuropathogenic determinants on the carboxy terminus of peplomers. Proc. Natl. Acad. Sci. USA. 84: 6567-6571.

Talbot, P.J., Dionne, G. and Lacroix, M. (1988) Vaccination against lethal coronavirus-induced encephalitis with a synthetic decapeptide homologous to a domain in the predicted peplomer stalk. J. Virol., 62: 3032-3036.

Tooze, S.A., and Stanley, K.K. (1986) Identification of two epitopes in the carboxyterminal 15 amino acids of the E1 glycoprotein of mouse hepatitis virus A%9 by using hybrid proteins. J. Virol. 60: 928-934.

BINDING OF ANTIBODIES THAT STRONGLY NEUTRALISE INFECTIOUS BRONCHITIS

VIRUS IS DEPENDENT ON THE GLYCOSYLATION OF THE VIRAL PEPLOMER PROTEIN

G. Koch and A. Kant

Central Veterinary Institute
Dept. of Virology
Postbox 365, 8200 AJ Lelystad, The Netherlands

INTRODUCTION

Most of the biological properties of infectious bronchitis virus
(IBV) are associated with the S_1 glycoprotein (1) that together with the
S_2 glycoprotein forms the peplomer protein (2,3). Both glycoproteins bear
N-linked oligosaccharides (4).

In an earlier study, we mapped the antigenic domains of the peplomer
protein topographically and functionally using a competitive binding
assay. This article summarises the results of the competitive binding
experiments which will be described in detail elsewhere (Koch et al., submitted).

In the present article, we studied whether the binding of MAbs that
strongly neutralise IBV are dependent on glycosylation of the peplomer
protein. We conclude from the results of these experiments and the
biochemical characteristics of the MAbs that the antigenicity of antigenic
domains on IBV that induce virus-neutralising antibodies depends on the
tertiary structure of the peplomer glycoproteins.

MATERIALS AND METHODS

Virus, cell culture, and monoclonal antibodies

IBV strain D207 was used throughout this study. The growth and purification of virus, cell culture conditions, production of MAbs, and techniques used for the biochemical and biological characterisation of MAbs
have been described earlier (5, Koch et al, submitted).

Isolation of the S_1 subunit of the peplomer

The glycoprotein S_1 was isolated from allantoic fluid by precipitating proteins with polyethylene glycol 6000 followed by affinity chromatography with MAb CVI-IBVS$_1$-48.3 coupled to Sepharose.

Coronaviruses and Their Diseases
Edited by D. Cavanagh and T.D.K. Brown
Plenum Press, New York, 1990

Deglycosylation of virus and S₁ glycoprotein

Deglycosylation of virus and S_1 glycoprotein

Virus was deglycosylated with endoglycosidase F that contained glycopeptidase F, glycopeptidase-free endoglycosidase F, or endoglyco-sidase H (all purchased from Boehringer Mannheim GmbH, FRG). Samples of 240 μg of IBV or of 3-4 μg of purified S_1 in 100 μl Tris-HCl buffer pH 7.2 (10 mM Tris-HCl, 100 mM NaCl, 1 mM EDTA) were incubated for 44 h at 37 °C with 50 mU of either contaminated or purified endoglycosidase F, or with 10 mU of endoglycosidase H. At hours 16 and 44 of incubation, samples were collected and their reactivity with MAbs was tested in enzyme immunoassays and Western blotting.

Enzyme immunoassay

An indirect enzyme immunoassay (EIA) and a double-antibody sandwich (DAS) EIA were used to test whether MAbs against IBV reacted with endoglycosidase-treated IBV samples. The indirect EIA has been described earlier (5, Koch et al, submitted). The DAS-EIA was performed as follows. Microtiter plates were coated with 1 μg of the immunoglobulin fraction of various MAbs directed against viral proteins. MAb CVI-IBVS₁-69.3, which is directed against S_1, was labelled with peroxidase and used as conjugate.

Western blotting

Polyacrylamide gel electrophoresis was performed as described before (Koch et al, submitted) and Western blotting was performed by the method of (6). Blots were stained with Concanavalin A (Con A) (Pharmacia) and horseradish peroxidase to detect glycoproteins (7).

RESULTS

Antigenic topography of the peplomer

The antigenic map of the peplomer protein was determined by measur-ing the competitive binding of labelled and unlabelled MAbs. This approach was based on the premise that if two epitopes are either identical, over-lapping, or adjacent, the binding of MAb to one of the epitopes will ste-rically block the binding of MAb to the second epitope and *vice versa*. In

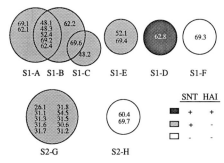

Fig. 1. Antigenic map of the peplomer protein of IBV. Circles represent antigenic domains of the peplomer protein. MAbs that define domains are indicated within circles. Biological functions of MAbs are indicated by hatched lines.

contrast, no blocking will occur if epitopes are sufficiently distant from each other. The results of the competitive binding studies are described and discussed in detail in another paper (Koch et al, submitted). Eight antigenic domains were identified on the peplomer protein, six on S_1 (S_1-A, -B, -C, -D, -E, and F) and two on S_2 (S_2-G and -H) (Fig. 1).

The MAbs with strong neutralising activity were directed against domains S_1-A, -B, -C, -D, and -E; one (MAb 31.1) was directed against domain S_2-G. Only domain S_1-D was associated with haemagglutination.

Effect of deglycosylation

To determine the nucleotide sequences encoding for the antigenic do-mains, we inserted peplomer gene fragments into a prokaryotic expression vector, pEX. Bacteria transfected with the vector produced hybrid proteins consisting of β-galactosidase and polypeptide fragments of the peplomer. Polypeptides were thus synthesised that together covered the whole peplo-mer protein (8,9). Only MAbs directed against the domains S_1-F and S_2-G bound to some of the hybrid proteins (MAbs directed against domain S_2-H were not tested). Since proteins synthesised by bacteria are rarely glycosylated, we questioned whether the binding of MAbs directed against other domains than these three were dependent on protein glycosylation. We therefore investigated whether MAbs directed against these antigenic domains also bound to deglycosylated virus and deglycosylated isolated S_1 glycoprotein.

IBV and purified S_1 were deglycosylated by incubating with a endogly-cosidase F that contained glycopeptidase F, glycopeptidase-free endoglyco-sidase F, or endoglycosidase H. The enzyme-treated virus or protein sam-ples were analysed by Western blotting. In untreated virus samples, only one 94K protein was stained by MAb 69.3 (directed against S_1). In contrast, in endoglycosidase-treated virus, proteins with apparent MW ranging from 65,000-92,000 were stained by MAb 69.3 (Fig. 2). Likewise, in untreated virus, MAb 26.1 (directed against S_2) stained a 275K protein and

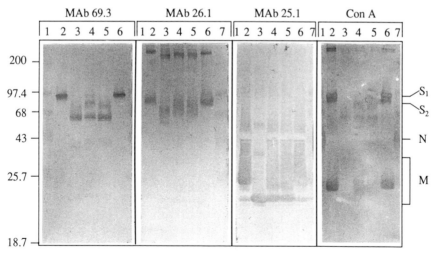

Fig. 2. Western blotting of endoglycosidase-treated IBV. Virus was incub-ated with endoglycosidase F containing glycopeptidase F (lane 3), purified endoglycosidase F (lane 4), endoglycosidase H (lane 5), or with buffer only (lane 2) at 37 °C for 44 h. Virus that was not incubated at 37 °C was electrophoresed in lane 6. Blots were stained with MAb directed against S_1 (MAb 69.3), against S_2 (MAb 26.1), or against the matrix protein (MAb 25.1) and stained for glycoproteins with Con A and peroxidase. Molecular weight markers were electrophoresed in lanes 1 and 7.

a 88K protein, whereas in treated virus, this MAb stained proteins with MW ranging from 61,000-92,000 and from 200,000-250,000. MAb 25.1 (directed against matrix protein) stained a 22K protein and proteins with a MW ranging from 24,000-36,000 in untreated virus. The amount of the latter proteins was decreased compared to the amount the 22K protein in enzyme-treated samples. Enzyme treatment of IBV had no affect on the MW of its nucleoprotein (data not shown). Con A stained all proteins that were stained by MAbs 69.3, 26.1, and 25.1 except the 200K-250K, 65K, 61k, and the 22K proteins.

When purified S_1 was treated with endoglycosidases, only a 65K protein was stained by MAb 69.3 in Western blots. Proteins with MWs ranging from 73,000-92,000 were very weakly stained by Con A only in virus samples which were treated with purified endoglycosidase F (Fig. 3, right panel).

Effect of deglycosylation on the binding of MAbs

Whether MAbs directed against IBV were also able to bind to deglycosylated virus was tested in an indirect EIA (Table 1) and in the DAS-EIA (data not shown). The binding of MAbs to coated, enzyme-treated virus was reduced compared to untreated virus, in particular, when treated with endoglycosidase F containing glycopeptidase F. Reduced binding resulted in a lower optical density. Incubating virus at 37 °C reduced the binding of MAb 62.8 to the virus even without enzyme.

The reactivity of MAbs with affinity-purified S_1 was determined in the DAS-EIA. All S_1 samples were diluted 1:240, except those that were added to wells coated with MAb 62.8. The latter samples were diluted 1:24, since at higher dilutions, MAb 62.8 did not bind to untreated S_1. Binding of S_1 was strongly reduced after deglycosylation. The binding was severely

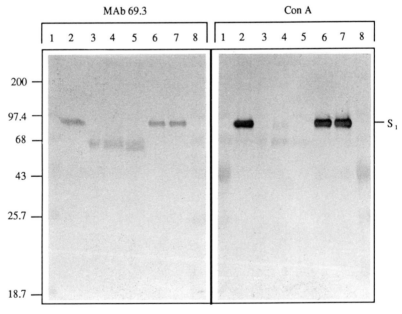

Fig. 3. Western blotting of endoglycosidase-treated S_1. Glycoprotein S_1 was incubated with endoglycosidase F and glycopeptidase F (lane 3); purified endoglycosidase F (lane 4); endoglycosidase H (lane 5); or with buffer only (lane 2). Untreated glycoprotein S_1 was electrophoresed in lane 6 and 7. Blots were stained by incubation with MAb directed against S_1 (left panel) and for glycoproteins with Con A and peroxidase (right panel). Molecular weight markers were electrophoresed in lanes 1 and 8.

Table 1. Effect of deglycosylation on the binding of MAbs directed against IBV proteins.

Treatment[a]	Optical densities[b] of IBV samples bound by monoclonal antibodies														
	69.1	62.1	48.1	48.3	52.4	69.2	62.4	62.2	48.2	62.8	52.1	69.3	26.1	25.1	26.2
endo F/ Glycopept. F	0.3	0.5	0.3	0.3	0.4	0.3	0.7	0.9	0.3	0.7	0.8	2.1	1.9	2.5	2.8
endo F	0.6	1.2	0.7	0.6	0.9	0.8	1.2	1.5	0.7	0.7	0.8	2.3	2.1	2.5	2.8
endo H	0.2	0.4	0.3	0.3	0.3	0.3	0.4	0.8	0.2	0.8	0.8	1.4	2.1	2.5	2.8
buffer	1.6	2.0	1.5	1.6	1.7	1.7	2.1	2.2	1.7	0.5	0.2	2.9	2.3	2.5	2.7
untreated	1.3	1.8	1.3	1.3	1.5	1.4	1.9	2.1	1.5	2.0	0.6	2.6	2.4	2.7	3.0

a. Virus strain D207 was incubated for 44 h at 37 0C with 50 mU of endoglycosidase F containing glycopeptidase, 50 mU of glycopeptidase-free endoglycosidase F, 10 mU of endoglycosidase H, or with buffer. Virus that was not incubated at 37 0C was used as positive control. Wells of microtitre plates were coated with 1 ug of treated or untreated samples and then incubated with monoclonal antibodies.
b. Wave length of 450 nm after incubation with optimal dilution of monoclonal antibodies.

147

Table 2. Effect of deglycosylation on the binding of MAbs directed against glycoprotein S_1.

Treatment[a] Optical densities[b] of IBV samples bound by monoclonal antibodies:

	69.1	62.1	48.1	48.3	52.4	69.2	62.4	62.2	48.2	62.8	52.1
endo F/ Glycopept. F	0.1[b]	0.2	0.2	0.2	0.1	0.1	0.1	0.2	0.1	0.4	0.2
endo F	0.3	0.8	0.2	0.3	0.5	0.3	0.7	1.0	0.3	1.1	0.4
endo H	0.2	0.4	0.2	0.2	0.3	0.2	0.4	0.6	0.2	1.0	0.4
buffer	3.0	3.0	2.4	2.4	3.0	3.0	3.0	3.0	3.0	0.8	2.2
untreated	2.1	3.0	1.6	1.6	2.6	2.4	2.8	3.0	2.3	0.7	0.6

a. Affinity purified S_1 of IBV strain D207 was incubated for 44 h at 37 °C with 50 mU of endoglycosidase F containing glycopeptidase F, 50 mU of glycopeptidase-free endoglycosidase F, 10 mU of endoglycosidase H, or buffer only. Wells of microtitre plates were coated with 1 µg of purified MAb and incubated with 1:240 diluted, enzyme-treated or untreated samples except for wells coated with MAbs 62.8 which was incubated with 1:24 diluted samples. Untreated S_1 was used as positive control. The plates were stained by incubation with peroxidase-labelled MAb 69.3 and substrate solution.
b. Optical density measured at a wave length of 450 nm.

reduced when S_1 was incubated with endoglycosidase F that contained glycopeptidase and with glycopeptidase H; binding was least reduced when S_1 was incubated with glycopeptidase-free endoglycosidase F (Table 2).

DISCUSSION

MAbs that had high neutralising titres bound to microtitre plates coated with virus and with affinity-purified S_1. In addition, when used as catching antibodies in the DAS-EIA, these MAbs bound S_1 in solution. However, when either virus or purified S_1 was deglycosylated by incubating it with endoglycosidases, the reaction of the MAbs with S_1 was severely reduced. Thus, binding of neutralising MAbs to the IBV peplomer is dependent on glycosylation of the virus.

Deglycosylation of IBV lowered the MW of its glycoproteins (Fig. 2). Like Stern (4) and Cavanagh (10), we found that IBV contains only N-linked oligosaccharides, to which type of oligosaccharides enzymes used for deglycosylation are specific. As a result of deglycosylation, the MW of S_1 and S_2 were reduced. Since the 65K protein was stained by a MAb directed against S_1, but not by Con A (Fig. 2 and 3), this protein was concluded to be the unglycosylated form of S_1 and out of similar reasoning the 61K protein the unglycosylated form of S_2. After oligosaccharides were removed from S_1 by endoglycosidase H, the MW of S_1 was estimated to be 64,000 (10) and MW of the total peplomer was calculated on basis of the nucleotide sequence to be 127,000 (11). Deglycosylation of S_1 was incomplete, because various proteins with MW ranging between 73,000 and 92,000 were both stained with MAb 69.3 and Con A. Deglycosylation may have been incomplete because we incubated S_1 with endoglycosidase under nonreducing and nondenaturating conditions. Protein conformation may have prevented the enzymes coming in contact with the oligosaccharides. Also, we may have used too little enzyme; it should be noted, however, that we used higher concentration (90 mU/ml) than Stern et al. (4) (32.5 mU/ml) and Cavanagh et al. (10) (25 mU/ml), and thus this possibility is highly unlikely. Nevertheless, these investigators detected complete deglycosylation using radio-labelled IBV.

We detected that IBV was best deglycosylated by endoglycosidase F containing glycopeptidase F. According to Tarrentino et al. (12), glyco-peptidase F hydrolyses N-linked oligosaccharides directly from the poly-peptide chain at the glycosylamine linking site. In contrast, endoglycosi-dase F and H cleave the oligosaccharide chain in such a way that a single N-acetylglucosamine residue bound to asparagine remains in the protein. Endoglycosidase F and H cleave different oligosaccharide substrates. Endo-glycosidase F cleaves N-linked high mannose and complex oligosaccharides (13), whereas endoglycosidase H cleaves N-linked high-mannose and hybrid type of oligosaccharides (14). The fact that endoglycosidase H deglyco-sylated better than glycopeptidase F-free endoglycosidase F suggests that the oligosaccharides on the IBV peplomer protein are mainly of the hybrid type.

Deglycosylation reduces the binding of neutralising MAbs to virus and to purified S_1 (Tables 1 and 2). Results of the Western blotting tests showed that less antibody was bound after oligosaccharides were removed from virus or from S_1 by treatment with a endoglycosidase F contaminated with glycopeptidase F than after treatment with glycopeptidase F-free endoglycosidase or with endoglycosidase H. In both immunoassays, the bind-ing that was detected, particularly when IBV was treated with endoglycosi-dase F, was probably caused by small amounts of glycoproteins, which remained after deglycosylation.

The effect of deglycosylation on the binding of MAb 62.8 could not be determined, since the binding of this MAb was reduced merely by incubation at 37 °C. The binding of MAb 62.8 was reduced by 50% when endoglycopeptid-ase F contaminated with glycopeptidase F but was unreduced when both other enzymes were used to deglycosylate S_1. Reduced binding cannot be explained by proteolytic degradation of deglycosylated S_1, because a single 65K pro-tein stained by a MAb directed against S_1, was detected by Western blot-ting. MAbs may be directed against the carbohydrate unit itself, but this possibility is highly unlikely, first, because oligosaccharide are immuno-genically weak and second, because the MAbs would then have cross-reacted with different IBV serotypes and with other avian viruses.

We conclude that the binding of neutralising MAbs to antigenic domains on IBV is dependent on glycosylation. Because the oligosaccharide unit of glycoprotein is important for the tertiary structure of proteins (15), removing this unit by deglycosylation probably results in changes of the protein conformation. Antigenic domains S_1-A, -B, -C, -D, and -E are probably dependent on protein conformation. In contrast, the antigenic domains S_1-F and S_2-G do not depend on protein conformation, since binding of MAbs directed against these domains was not affected by deglycosylation (Table 1, Fig. 2, and data not shown). Results of the Western blotting tests supported these conclusions; antigenic domains S_1-A, -B, -C, -D, and -E were destroyed under the denaturating conditions, whereas antigenic domains S_1-F and S_2-G were conserved.

The results of this study have important implications for vaccine development. In producing a vaccine, whether inactivated attenuated, sub-unit, or peptide vaccine, our results indicate that the conformation of the viral proteins must be conserved or mimicked. In producing a peptide vaccine, Geysen et al. (16) have described a procedure for mimicking the conformation of an epitope with a synthetic peptide. They have improved the binding of MAbs to a synthetic peptide by systematically replacing its amino acids. In producing an inactivated attenuated vaccine, any change in conformation caused by inactivation should be avoided. In production of viral sub-units, eukaryotic expression systems should be preferred to prokaryotic expression systems to ensure the glycosylation of subunits.

ACKNOWLEDGEMENT
    We thank L. Hartog and D. van Roozelaar for technical assistance,
G.F. de Boer and G. Wensvoort for critical reading, and V. Thatcher for
excellent editorial assistance.

REFERENCES

1. D. Cavanagh and P.J. Davis, Coronavirus IBV: Virus retaining spike
    glycopolypeptide S_2 but not S_1 is unable to induce virus-neutraliz-
    ing or haemagglutination-inhibiting antibody, or induce chicken
    tracheal protection, J. Gen. Virol. 67: 1435-1442 (1986).
2. D.F. Stern, L. Burgess, and B.M. Sefton, Structural analysis of virion
    proteins of the Avian Infectious Bronchitis Virus, J. Virology 42:
    208-219 (1982).
3. D. Cavanagh, Coronavirus IBV: structural characterization of the spike
    protein, J. Gen. Virol. 64: 2577-2583 (1983).
4. D.F. Stern and B.M. Sefton, Coronavirus proteins: Structure and func-
    tion of the oligosaccharides of the Avian Infectious Bronchitis Vi-
    rus glycoproteins, J. Virology 42: 804-812 (1982).
5. G. Koch, L. Hartog, A. Kant, D. van Roozelaar, and G.F. de Boer, Dif-
    ferentiation of IBV variant strains employing monoclonal anti-
    bodies, Isr. J. Vet. Med. 42: 89-97 (1986).
6. H. Towbin, T. Staehlin, and J. Gordon, Electrophoretic transfer of
    proteins from polyacrylamide gels to nitrocellulose sheets. Pro-
    cedure and some applications, Proc. Natl. Acad. Sci. 6: 4350-4354
    (1979).
7. R. Hawkes, Identification of Concanavalin A-binding proteins after
    sodiumdodecyl sulfate-gel electrophoresis and protein blotting,
    Anal. Biochem. 123: 143-146 (1982).
8. J.A. Lenstra, J.G. Kusters, G. Koch, and B.A.M. van der Zeijst,
    Antigenicity of the peplomer protein of infectious bronchitis
    virus, Mol. Immunol. 1: 7-15 (1989).
9. J.G. Kusters, E.J. Jager, J.A. Lenstra, G. Koch, W.P.A. Posthumus,
    R.H. Meloen, and B.A.M. van der Zeijst, Analysis of an immunodo-
    minant region of avian coronavirus IBV, J. Immunol., in press,
    (1989).
10. D. Cavanagh, Coronavirus IBV glycopeptides size of the polypetide
    moieties and nature of their oligosaccharides, J. Gen. Virol. 64:
    1187-1191 (1983).
11. M.M. Binns, M.E.G. Boursnell, D. Cavanagh, D.J.C. Pappin, and T.D.K.
    Brown, Cloning and sequencing of the gene encoding the spike
    protein of the coronavirus IBV, J. Gen. Virol., 66: 719-726 (1985).
12. Tarentino, A.L., C.M. Gómes, and T.H. Plummer, Deglycosylation of
    aspargine-linked glycans by peptide:N-glycosidase F, Biochem. 24:
    4665-4671 (1985).
13. J.H. Elder, and S. Alexander, Endo-β-acetylglucosaminidase F: Endo-
    glycosidase from Flavobacterium meningosepticum that cleaves both
    high-mannose and complex glycoproteins, Biochem. 79: 4550-4544
    (1982).
14. A.L. Tarentino, T.H. Plummer, and F. Maley, Purification and
    properties of an endo-N-acetylglucosaminidase H from Streptomyces
    griseus, J. Biol. Chem. 249: 811-817 (1974).
15. Rose, M.C., W.A. Voter, H. Sage, C.F. Brown, B. Kaufman, S. Basu, and
    B. Bartholomew, J. Biol. Chem. 259: 3167-3172 (1984).
16. H.M. Geysen, S.J. Rodda, and T.J.Mason, The delineation of peptides
    able to mimic assembled epitopes, In: "Synthetic peptides as anti-
    gens", Ciba Found. Symp. 119, J. Wiley & Sons, Chichester (1986).

ENTERIC CORONAVIRUS TGEV : MAPPING OF FOUR MAJOR ANTIGENIC

DETERMINANTS IN THE AMINO HALF OF PEPLOMER PROTEIN E 2

B. Delmas, M. Godet, J. Gelfi, D. Rasschaert, H. Laude

I.N.R.A.

Laboratoire de Virologie et d'Immunologie Moléculaires
Centre de Recherches de Jouy-en-Josas. France

INTRODUCTION

Transmissible gastroenteritis virus (TGEV) is an enteropathogenic coronavirus of swine which induces an acute diarrhea syndrome especially severe in newborn animals less than two weeks of age (15). The organisation of the TGEV genome has been established as well as the sequences of the genes encoding the structural and non structural proteins, except the polymerase (7, 9, 13, 14). TGEV virions are made of three proteins, a nucleoprotein (N, 47K) and 2 envelope glycoproteins : M (29K), an integral membrane protein, and S (220K), which forms the surface projections. The peplomer protein S is a 1431 amino acid long, highly glycosylated polypeptide, with a membrane anchoring domain near its carboxy terminus (14). This protein is responsible for the induction of neutralising antibodies (4, 8) and is presumably involved in the recognition of target cells. A minimum of four major antigenic sites have been delineated using monoclonal antibodies (1, 3, 6).

The correlation of these sites with the primary structure of the molecule might contribute to the identification of functional domains of importance with regard to the immunogenicity or pathogenicity of the virus. A combination of several approaches has enabled us to localise the four main antigenic sites A, B, C and D defined previously using our hybridoma library (3). The present paper briefly reports the main findings of this study.

MATERIALS AND METHODS

Viruses : The high passage Purdue-115 strain was used as a virus source. The propagation of the virus and the selection of neutralisation escape mutant have been described (3).

Monoclonal antibodies : The characteristics of the 23 anti TGEV-S MAbs used in this study have been reported (8).

Characterisation of immunoreactive proteolytic fragments : (^{35}S) cysteine-labelled cytosols were prepared as described (8), with some modifications (multiplicity of infection 50 PFU, 8 hr labelling at 3 h p.i., 100 µCi/ml). Proteolytic digestions were performed 2 hr at 37°C using one of these

Coronaviruses and Their Diseases
Edited by D. Cavanagh and T.D.K. Brown
Plenum Press, New York, 1990

endopeptidases : α-chymotrypsin, collagenase (*clostridium perfringens*), trypsin and V8 protease (200 to 600 μg/ml). Immunoprecipitations were performed as reported using hybridoma ascites fluids (5 μl for 50 μl of digested material) and protein A-Sepharose (8). Immunoreactive fragments were resolved on a 9-20% polyacrylamide gradient gel then fluorographed.

Amino-terminal sequencing of proteolytic fragments : Radiolabelled fragments were prepared as above using one of the following tritiated precursors : valine, threonine, isoleucine (0.5-1 mCi/ml). Appropriate fragments were excised from the gel, electroeluted, then subjected to microsequencing by Edman degradation in an automated gas-phase apparatus.

Production of bacterial fusion proteins : The pEX expression vectors were used to produce S fragments as a C-terminal extension of Cro-β-galactosidase, under control of the thermoinducible promotor λP$_r$ (16). The S-cDNA clones used were from a previous study (13). All experiments were carried out in the *E. coli* strain MC1061 transformed with the plasmid pCI. DNA constructs were made using standard protocols. DNA fragments and plasmids were purified using the Geneclean kit (NEB). A random sublibrary was produced from one of the obtained DNA inserts by sonication. A second sublibrary was generated following Bal31 nuclease resection ("slow form", IBI) of a linearised plasmid. Screening of epitope expressing transformed bacteria was performed by colony blot procedure (16) using 1:100 diluted MAb ascites fluids and (125I) protein A. The immunoreactivity of fusion proteins from positive colonies was examined after lysis of bacterial cells by lysozyme + Triton X100, SDS-PAGE resolution and Western blotting.

Sequencing procedures : Point mutations of escape mutants were localised by direct RNA sequencing of portions of the S gene. RNA matrixes were obtained by proteinase K-SDS treatment of virions semi-purified through a glycerol cushion, phenol-chloroform extraction and precipitation by LiCl 2M. (20-mer) oligonucleotides complementary to TGEV S gene sequence were used to prime reverse transcription of the RNA in the presence of a mixture of deoxy/dideoxynucleotides (1-2 μg RNA per sequence, AMV reverse transcriptase, (^{35}S)dATP). Determination of the S encoding sequences in the inserts from sublibraries was achieved by supercoiled dideoxy-sequencing. Plasmids prepared according to the alkali-SDS method were precipitated by PEG-NaCl and denatured by NaOH as reported (11). Appropriate primers homologous to pEX sequences were used to prime the elongation reaction.

RESULTS

Localisation of the site C

Seven partially overlapping cDNA restriction fragments covering the entire S gene except 110 nucleotides at the 5' end were subcloned into appropriate pEX vectors. Clones expressing a β-Gal chimaeric protein were then subjected to colony blot immunoscreening towards our panel of anti-S monoclonal antibodies (MAbs). None of the expression products was found to react with any of the MAbs directed against A, B and D sites or unrelated epitopes. In contrast, 3 overlapping expression products were recognised by each of the 3 MAbs defining the site C. One of the positive clones had a 0.7Kb long insert with its 5' end corresponding to the unique Xho I site of the S sequence. In order to localise the site C more accurately, a random pEX library was created using sonicated fragments - about 100 base pair long - of the latter insert. The S nucleotide sequence of 10 of the epitope-expressing clones obtained in this way was determined by direct sequencing using appropriate synthetic primers. As a striking feature, all the deduced S-specific amino acid sequences possessed the same N-terminus, thus delineating the amino-terminal limit of the site C. Fine mapping of the carboxy-terminal limit was achieved by analysing a third pEX library generated by Bal31 exonuclease resection of the smallest - 89 base pair long - random insert. As a final result, a fusion β-Gal protein having 9 amino acid residues was characterised, which was recognised by all site C MAbs in Western blotting. According to these data, the site C would stretch from residue 363 to 371 of the mature S protein (Fig. 1). Furthermore, 2 point mutations, leading to a non conservative amino acid change at position 367 and 368, were identified by direct RNA sequencing of mutants resistant to neutralisation by site C MAbs 3[b].5 and 10.4, respectively.

Localisation of the sites A and B

Their localisation was accomplished through the following two-step approach : i) fragmentation analysis of native S protein ; ii) microsequencing of the smallest fragment retaining immunoreactivity. S fragments were generated by controlled proteolytic cleavage using four separate endopeptidases (see Materials and Methods) then subjected to immunoprecipitation with anti-S MAbs. In general, the resulting profiles of cleavage products were typical of a given antigenic site. Fragmentation and competition experiments were thus in good agreement ; however, the sites A and B could not be distinguished in these experiments, which can be related to the fact that these sites share a common epitope, 48.1 (3).

Collagenase digestion led to the characterisation of a 26K fragment (CO-26K), which retained a strong reactivity towards all site A-B MAbs. Its mobility was identical in reductive and non reductive conditions, thus establishing that the antibody binding site was on the fragment itself. Then 3H-threonine or 3H-isoleucine labelled CO-26K precipitated by MAb 48.1 were purified and subjected to N-terminal sequencing. Determination of the position of the radioactive residues allowed us to align unambiguously the N-terminal extremity of CO-26K with the S amino acid sequence (Fig. 1). Its carboxy limit could be predicted on the basis of the fragment size and the presence of a potential collagenase cleavage site. According to the data, the A-B epitopes must be located within a ∿ 200 residue long segment starting at serine 506 of mature S.

In order to confirm this finding, we have searched the location of mutations in the S gene of relevant escape mutants. The sequence encoding the totality of the 26K region was determined by direct sequencing of genomic RNA. Mutants resistant to neutralisation by MAb 20.9 (site A) or 48.1 (sites A-B) were analysed. Each mutant had a single nucleotide change resulting in a non conservative amino acid substitution in the 26K region (Fig. 1).

Localisation of the D site

The approach followed for the localisation of this site was similar to that described above. Chymotrypsin digestion experiments have been shown to produce a 13K fragment (CT-13K) which was strongly recognised by all site D MAbs. Microsequencing of labelled CT-13K isolated using MAb 40.1 identified a unique sequence of valine, which allowed the determination of Asn 82 as the amino limit of the fragment. One of the 3 aromatic residues found at position 200-212 is candidate as the C-terminus of CT-13K (Fig. 1). The evidence for the location of site D was strengthened by direct RNA sequencing of MAb 40.1 escape mutants, which identified single amino acid changes at position 145, 147 and 149.

The presence of CT-13K as a minor band was observed in the chymotrypsin profiles obtained with most of the other anti-S MAbs, including site A, B and C MAbs, but not with anti-E1 or N MAbs. Partial amino

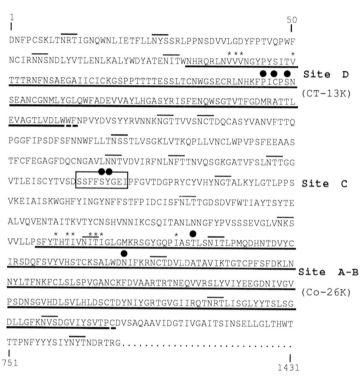

```
1                                              50
I                                              I
DNFPCSKLTNRTIGNQWNLIETFLLNYSSRLPPNSDVVLGDYFPTVQPWF
                                      ***              *
NCIRNNSNDLYVTLENLKALYWDYATENITWNHRQRLNVVVNGYPYSITV
                                          ● ● ●          Site  D
TTTRNFNSAEGAIICICKGSPPTTTTESSLTCNWGSECRLNHKFPICPSN
                                                       (CT-13K)
SEANCGNMLYGLQWFADEVVAYLHGASYRISFENQWSGTVTFGDMRATTL
EVAGTLVDLWWFNPVYDVSYYRVNNKNGTTVVSNCTDQCASYVANVFTTQ
PGGFIPSDFSFNNWFLLTNSSTLVSGKLVTKQPLLVNCLWPVPSFEEAAS
TFCFEGAGFDQCNGAVLNNTVDVIRFNLNFTTNVQSGKGATVFSLNTTGG
              ● ●
VTLEISCYTVSD[SSFFSYGEI]PFGVTDGPRYCYVHYNGTALKYLGTLPPS  Site  C
VKEIAISKWGHFYINGYNFFSTFPIDCISFNLTTGDSDVFWTIAYTSYTE
ALVQVENTAITKVTYCNSHVNNIKCSQITANLNNGFYPVSSSEVGLVNKS
          *  **   ***              *   ●
VVLLPSFYTHTIVNITIGLGMKRSGYGQPIASTLSNITLPMQDHNTDVYC
                                 ●
IRSDQFSVYVHSTCKSALWDNIFKRNCTDVLDATAVIKTGTCPFSFDKLN
                                                     Site  A-B
NYLTFNKFCLSLSPVGANCKFDVAARTRTNEQVVRSLYVIYEEGDNIVGV
                                                     (Co-26K)
PSDNSGVHDLSVLHLDSCTDYNIYGRTGVGIIRQTNRTLISGLYYTSLSG
DLLGFKNVSDGVIYSVTPCDVSAQAAVIDGTIVGAITSINSELLGLTHWT
TTPNFYYYSIYNYTNDRTRG.............................
I                                              I
751                                            1431
```

Fig. 1. The amino acid sequence of the amino half of TGEV S is shown (data from 14 ; potential N-glycosylation sites overlined). The underlines and box indicate the proposed location of the antigenic sites. Radioactive residues detected by microsequencing: *. Point mutations identified in neutralisation escape mutants: ●.

sequencing of CT-13K fragment prepared using MAb 20.9 (site A) also revealed Asn 82 as its N-terminus.

DISCUSSION

In this study, several approaches have been developed in order to correlate major antigenic sites of TGEV peplomer protein S with its primary structure. By combining proteolytic digestion of the native protein and microsequencing of immunoreactive cleavage products we were able to localise the sites A, B and D, whereas bacterial expression of large fragments of S failed to produce fusion proteins expressing these sites. A fourth antigenic site, C, could be mapped accurately through prokaryotic expression of short S fragments. The proposed location of these sites was confirmed by identification of point mutations in the S gene of relevant escape mutants.

Major antigenic sites have been mapped in the carboxy-terminal subunit of both MHV and IBV peplomer proteins (for references see H. Laude, this volume). In the case of TGEV, however, the four main antigenic sites delineated using our MAb library all cluster in the amino-terminal half of S, which is assumed to correspond to the globular part of the peplomer (Fig. 2). Such a picture is closer of that reported for several virus glycoproteins, like influenza virus (17).

The site C appears to be composed of potentially linear epitopes, lying in a short sequence of 9 contiguous amino acid residues (363-371). This site is defined by moderately or non neutralising MAbs, and exhibits a slight antigenic variation (3, 8). Thus, the British isolate FS 772/70 is not recognised by neutralising MAbs 3[b].5 and 10.4. Comparison of its sequence (P. Britton, personal communication) with that of Purdue strain actually revealed amino acid divergence at position 366, within the antibody binding site. Besides, two adjacent amino acid changes (365-366) have been noted in the homologous sequence of the feline coronavirus FIPV (strain 79-1146 ; 2), which does not react with any of our site C MAbs. These findings, together with those derived from the analysis of selected epitope mutants (see results) indicate that the residues Phe-Ser-Tyr 368 are critical for neutralisation by MAb 3[b].5 and 10.4, and Phe 365 for binding by MAb 11.20.

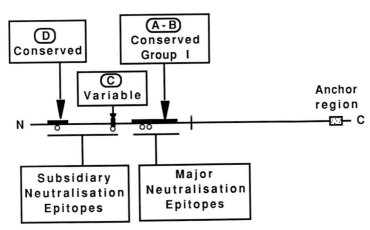

Fig. 2. Schematic view of the location of four major antigenic sites on the TGEV S polypeptide chain. The approximate position of residues critical for antibody binding is marked by an open circle. The minimal distance between A-B and D sites is 290 amino acids.

In contrast to site C, sites A, B and D have been shown to be highly conserved among TGEV strains. The spatially related sites A and B constitute the major neutralisation-mediating domain of S, and are immunodominant in the natural host species. Microsequencing of a collagenase 26K fragment specifically recognised by site A and B MAbs led us to conclude that this domain is contained within a ∿ 200 residue long region with residue 506 as its amino-terminal limit. The positions of amino acid substitutions confering neutralisation resistance were consistent with this location. The site D is not a major neutralisation site as only one (40.1) of the delineating MAbs is highly neutralising. Substantial evidence for the location of this site was obtained by alignment with the S sequence of a chymotrypsin 13K fragment, which was strongly - but not specifically - recognised by the relevant MAbs, and by identification of point mutations present on MAb 40.1 escape mutant.

Since there is no overlap between the 13K region (site D), the 26K region (A-B domain), and the 9 amino acid sequence (site C), the observed weak reactivity of non site D MAbs with the 13K cleavage product is an intriguing feature. The absence of binding when using anti-E1 or anti N MAbs indicated that this effect is S-specific. One explanation would be that the antibody binding sites for A, B and C MAbs also involve sequences of the 13K region. If so, all these epitopes would be of the assembled type. Alternatively, a non-covalent interaction of some stability might exist between the 13K region and another part of the S molecule ; as a consequence, the 13K fragment would be coprecipitated via larger S fragments.

The localisation of several major antigenic sites of TGEV S provides a molecular basis for the understanding of the relationships between TGEV and closely related viruses. We have shown in a separate study (10) that all site A and B MAbs do react with both FIPV and PRCV (a newly recognised respiratory variant of TGEV : 12), whereas site D MAbs exhibit no cross-reactivity. An optimal alignment of the predicted amino acid sequence corresponding to 26K and 13K regions of TGEV and FIPV revealed a level of homology of 92 and 25%, respectively. The clustering of most of the critical neutralisation epitopes within the highly homologous and immunodominant 26K region thus explains the high level of cross-neutralisation observed between the members of coronavirus group I, also including canine CCV (5). Such a conservation of the major neutralisation mediating domain raises the question of its biological function. On the other hand, it is tempting to speculate that determinants essential to the expression of the tropism or host specificity of this group of coronaviruses resides within the non conserved N terminal region of S, where the site D has been mapped.

REFERENCES

1. I. Correa, G. Jimenez, C. Sune, M.J. Bullido & L. Enjuanes (1988). Antigenic structure of the E2 glycoprotein from transmissible gastroenteritis coronavirus. Virus Res. 10 : 77-94 .
2. R.J. De Groot, J. Maduro, J.A. Lenstra, M.C. Horzinek, B.A.M. Van der Zeijst & W.J.M. Spaan (1987). cDNA cloning and sequence analysis of the gene encoding the peplomer protein of feline infectious peritonitis virus. J. Gen. Virol. 68 : 2639-2646.
3. B. Delmas, J. Gelfi & H. Laude (1986). Antigenic structure of transmissible gastroenteritis virus. II. Domains in the peplomer glycoprotein. J. Gen. Virol. 67 : 1405-1418 .
4. D.J. Garwes, M.H. Lucas, D.A. Higgins, B.V. Pike & S.F. Cartwright (1978-1979). Antigenicity of structural components from porcine transmissible gastroenteritis virus. Vet. Microbiol. 3 : 179-190 .
5. M.C. Horzinek, H. Lutz & N.C. Pedersen (1982). Antigenic relationships among homologous structural polypeptides of porcine, feline and canine coronaviruses. Infect. Immun. 37 : 1148-1155 .

6. G. Jimenez, I. Correa, M.P. Melgosa, M.J. Bullido & L. Enjuanes (1986). Critical epitopes in transmissible gastroenteritis virus neutralization. J. Virol. 60 : 131-139 .

7. P.A. Kapke & D.A. Brian (1986). Sequence analysis of the porcine transmissible gastroenteritis coronavirus nucleocapsid protein gene. Virology 151 : 41-49 .

8. H. Laude, J.M. Chapsal, J. Gelfi, S. Labiau & J. Grosclaude (1986). Antigenic structure of transmissible gastroenteritis virus. I. Properties of monoclonal antibodies directed against virion proteins. J. Gen. Virol. 67 : 119-130 .

9. H. Laude, D. Rasschaert & J.C. Huet (1987). Sequence and N-terminal processing of the transmembrane protein E1 of the coronavirus transmissible gastroenteritis virus. J. Gen. Virol. 68 : 1687-1693.

10. H. Laude, J. Gelfi, D. Rasschaert & B. Delmas (1988). Caractérisation antigénique du coronavirus respiratoire porcin à l'aide d'anticorps monoclonaux dirigés contre le virus de la gastro-entérite transmissible. Journées Rech. Porcine en France 20 : 89-94.

11. H.M. Lim & J.J. Pène (1988). Optimal conditions for supercoil DNA sequencing with *Escherichia coli* DNA polymerase I large fragment. Gene Anal. Techn. 5 : 32-39.

12. M. Pensaert, P. Callebaut & J. Vergote (1986). Isolation of a porcine respiratory, non-enteric coronavirus related to transmissible gastroenteritis. Vet. Quart. 8 (3) : 257-261.

13. D. Rasschaert, J. Gelfi & H. Laude (1987). Enteric coronavirus TGEV : partial sequence of the genomic RNA, its organization and expression. Biochimie 69 : 591-600 .

14. D. Rasschaert & H. Laude (1987). The predicted primary structure of the peplomer protein E2 of the porcine coronavirus transmissible gastroenteritis virus. J. Gen. Virol. 68, 1883-1890 .

15. L.J. Saif & E.H. Bohl (1986). Transmissible gastroenteritis. In : Diseases of swine (sixth edition). pp. 255-274. Edited by A.D. Leman, B. Straw, R.D. Glock, W.L. Mengeling, R.H.C. Penny & E. Scholl. Iowa State University Press .

16. K.K. Stanley & J.P. Luzio (1984). Constructions of a new family of high efficiency bacterial expression vectors : identification of cDNA clones coding for human liver proteins. EMBO J. 3 : 1429-1434.

17. D.C. Wiley, I.A. Wilson & J.J. Skehel (1981). Structural identification of the antibody-binding sites of Hong Kong influenza haemagglutinin and their involvement in antigenic variation. Nature 289 : 373-378 .

LOCATION OF ANTIGENIC SITES OF THE S-GLYCOPROTEIN OF

TRANSMISSIBLE GASTROENTERITIS VIRUS AND THEIR CONSERVATION IN

CORONAVIRUSES

L. Enjuanes[1], F. Gebauer[1], I. Correa[1],
M.J. Bullido[2], C. Suñé[1], C. Smerdou[1], C. Sánchez[1],
J.A. Lenstra[2], W.P.A. Posthumus[3], and R.H. Meloen[3]

(1) Centro de Biología Molecular
    CSIC-UAM, Facultad de Ciencias
    Universidad Autónoma
    Canto Blanco
    28049 Madrid, Spain

(2) Institute of Infectious Diseases and
    Immunology Veterinary Faculty, State
    University
    3508 TD Utrecht, The Netherlands

(3) Central Veterinary Institute
    P.O. Box 65
    8200 AB Lelystad
    The Netherlands

INTRODUCTION

Transmissible gastroenteritis virus (TGEV) has a single-stranded, positive-sense RNA genome of more than 20 kb (Brian et al., 1980; Rasschaert et al., 1987) and three structural proteins: S, N and M, with 1447, 382 and 262 amino acids, respectively (Kapke and Brian, 1986; Laude et al., 1987; Rasschaert and Laude, 1987; Jacobs et al., 1987).

The S glycoprotein is responsible for the induction of neutralizing antibodies (Garwes et al., 1978). On the S protein a minimum of four antigenic sites have been defined, site A being the major inducer of neutralizing antibodies (Jiménez et al., 1986). This site has been subdivided into three antigenic subsites (Correa et al., 1988). In the S glycoprotein we have defined 16 epitopes, of which 10 are involved in virus neutralization (Sánchez et al., 1989).

In this chapter, we locate the antigenic sites on the protein sequence by studying the binding of monoclonal antibodies (MAbs) to S-protein fragments and to recombinant products of pEX-TGEV vectors, and by identifying nucleotide sequence differences between TGEV genome and MAb resistant (mar) mutants. In addition, we studied the conservation of the antigenic sites in coronaviruses, and defined type, group and interspecies

TABLE 1

S-GENE[a] FRAGMENTS EXPRESSED BY pEX-TGEV RECOMBINANTS

FRAGMENT NUMBER	NUCLEOTIDE[b] FRAGMENT	S PROTEIN FRAGMENT
1	-8 - 1136	1 - 378
2	976 - 1674	326 - 558
3	1588 - 2021	530 - 673
4	1675 - 2021	559 - 673
5	1819 - 2238	607 - 746
6	2022 - 2760[c]	675 - (920)[c]
7	2622 - 3477	875 - 1159
8	3447 - 3717	1150 - 1239
9	3478 - 4255	1160 - 1418

a. The S-gene from TGE virus has 4341 nucleotides, encoding a protein of 1447 residues (Rasschaert et al., 1987; Jacobs et al., 1987).

b. Numbers are relative to the start of the coding sequence.

c. Insert 6 was derived from clone B1 (Jacobs et al., 1987) using the Pst I site from the polylinker. It was checked that contains the Hpa I site at nucleotide 2619. The S-fragment coded by this insert includes, at least, the residues 675-919.

epitopes, which permitted the differentiation between enteric and respiratory porcine coronaviruses, and to classify the human coronavirus (HCV) 229E in an antigenic cluster distinct from the one formed by TGEV, canine coronavirus (CCV), feline infectious peritonitis virus (FIPV), and feline enteric coronavirus (FECV).

MATERIALS AND METHODS

Viruses, cell lines, MAbs and mar mutants

The viruses, cell lines, MAbs, and mar mutants used, have been described previously (Jiménez et al., 1986; Correa et al., 1988; Bullido et al., 1989; Sánchez et al., 1989). The purification of the virus and the S-glycoprotein has been described elsewhere (Correa et al., 1989).

Analysis of peplomer fragments

S-protein was digested with **Staphylococcus aureus** V8 protease, and the fragments analyzed by immunoblotting or fractionated by HPLC on gel filtration columns (Correa et al., 1989). A 28-kDa fragment separated by HPLC was purified by polyacrylamide gel electrophoresis in the presence of SDS (SDS-PAGE). Antiserum to this fragment was produced in mice (Correa et al., 1989).

A peptide (Cys-Asp-Asn-Phe-Pro-Cys-Ser-Lys-Leu-Thr-Asn-Arg-Thr-Ile-Gly-Asn-Gln-Trp-Asn) with the sequence of the N-terminal 18 residues of the mature S protein of the TGEV strain PUR46.CC120-MAD (Gebauer et al., 1989) was synthetized and its recognition by serum analyzed by dot-blot as previously described (Correa et al., 1989).

Expression of S-gene fragments in pEX vectors

S-gene fragments were cloned in pEX expression plasmid (Stanley & Luzio, 1984; Lenstra et al., 1989). The cro-β-galactosidase hybrid proteins were extracted and analyzed by immunoblotting (Correa et al., 1989).

DNA and RNA sequencing

S-gene cDNA was cloned on Bluescript phagemid as described (Gebauer et al., 1989). Three DNA fragments, which included the nucleotides -8 to 1587, 1135 to 3329, and 3330 to 4628, of TGEV strain PUR46.CC120-MAD (Sánchez et al., 1989) were cloned. DNA purified from Bluescript plasmid, and RNA from purified virions were sequenced by oligodeoxynucleotide primer extension and dideoxy-nucleotide chain termination procedure (Sanger et al., 1977; Zimmern & Kaesberg, 1978). The sequence nucleotide differences between the PUR46.CC120.MAD **wt** and the **mar** mutants were detected using the primer complementary to nucleotides 1980 to 2000 of S-gene: 3'-TCTGTTGTATCACCCACATG-5'. Sequence data were assembled and analyzed by using the computer programs by Genetic Computer Group (Wisconsin University).

Binding of MAb to virus and antigenic homology

The binding of MAbs was determined by RIA, and the percentage of antigenic homology of a particular virus isolate, relative to the reference virus PUR46.CC120-MAD, was estimated by the formula $[(a + 2b)/2n]$ x 100, where a and b are the number of MAbs with binding percentage values equal to 31 to 50, and 51 to 100, respectively, for the considered virus isolate, and n=42, the total number of MAbs (García-Barreno et al., 1986; Sánchez et al., 1989).

RESULTS

Location of antigenic sites on S-protein fragments

S-protein was digested with **Staphyloccocus aureus V8** protease, the digestion products fractionated by gel filtration HPLC, and the antigenic sites located on the fragments by immunoblotting using MAbs as probes (**Figure 1**). Five fractions (a, b, c, d, and e) were separated by HPLC. Site-A and -C specific-MAbs recognized a peptide of 28-kDa (present in fraction d) and other partially digested peptides of higher molecular weight. Site-B specific-MAbs did not bind any peptide, while site-D specific-MAbs recognized a 50-kDa fragment (present in fraction c). The 28-kDa fragment selected by HPLC was separated from a 18-kDa component by polyacrylamide gel electrophoresis in the presence of sodium dodecyl sulphate (SDS-PAGE), and its homogeneity analyzed by reverse phase HPLC. A single protein band was detected, although the presence of a second component accounting for less than 10% of the total protein could not be excluded (not shown).

To locate the antigenic sites on S-protein, S-gene fragments (**Table 1** and **Figure 2**) were expressed by pEX-TGEV vectors. Nine overlapping inserts, numbered 1 to 9, accounted for

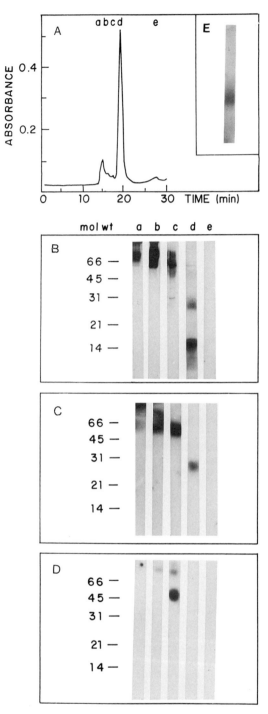

Fig. 1. Fractionation by HPLC of peptides from V8–protease digested S–protein. V8–protease fragments of S glycoprotein were separated by gel filtration HPLC on two Protein Pak columns (Fig. 1A). Five major fractions, a, b, c, d, and e, were analyzed by SDS–PAGE and silver staining (Fig. 1B), or by immunoblotting with site–A (Fig. 1C), or site–D (Fig. 1D) specific MAbs (1G.A7 and 1D.G3, respectively). Site–C specific MAbs gave the same pattern as the site–A specific MAbs (not shown). Figure 1E shows the 28–kDa fragment selected by preparative SDS–PAGE.

98% of S-gene. On immunoblots, the site-specific MAbs recognized only the expression products of inserts 1 and 2. **Figure 3** shows representative results of the binding of different MAbs to TGEV expression products. Four site-A specific MAbs (1G.A7, 1D.E7, 1A.F10, and 6A.C3) tested did not bind to the expression products. One site-B specific-MAb (1B.H11) and two site-C specific MAbs (5B.H1 and 6A.A6) bound to the product of insert 1. In contrast, two MAbs (1D.G3 and 8D.H8), which are site-D specific, recognized the product of plasmid containing insert 2, but not any of the other products.

The 28-kDa fragment was coded by the 5'-end of S-gene, as: i) polyvalent antiserum induced by this fragment(s) only recognized the product of insert 1 (**Figure 4A**), and ii) the antiserum to the 28-kDa fragment(s) recognized a synthetic peptide which included the 18 N-terminal amino acids, coupled to KLH, but not KLH alone, in a dot-blot assay (**Figure 4B**).

Amino acid sequence of a TGEV epitope present in serum proteins

The binding sequence of site-C specific-MAbs (Correa et al., 1988) has been identified using synthetic nonapeptides in a PEPSCAN and random pEX libraries (Enjuanes et al., submitted for publication; Geysen et al., 1984; Stanley and Luzio, 1984; Lenstra et al., 1989). Two sets of nonapeptides were recognized by site-C specific-MAbs (**Figure 5**), but residues 48-Pro-Pro-Asn-Ser-Asp-52 gave higher absorbance in the PEPSCAN, compared with residues 164-Pro-Ser-Asn-Ser-Glu-168. In addition, residues 48-53 have a higher surface probability based on Chou and Fasman algorithms (Enjuanes et al., submitted for publication). These data suggest that the sequence from residue 48 to 52 is the one recognized in the native virus. Interestingly, these sequences are present in proteins of sera from different species (Correa et al., 1988; Enjuanes et al., submitted for publication).

Nucleotide differences between the sequences of TGEV **wt** and **mar** mutants selected from this virus

The S-gene of TGEV strain PUR46.CC120-MAD and of the double **mar** mutant **dmar** 1B.B5-1B.B1 were cloned in the Bluescript vector. Three cDNA fragments covering the S-gene of each virus were inserted on the plasmid, using the strategy described previously (Gebauer et al., 1989). The first 1950 nucleotides of the 5'-end of each gene were sequenced on these plasmids. Three nucleotide differences were detected at the DNA level (**Table 2**), which corresponded to residues 538, 543 and 631 of the S-protein. To determine if these nucleotide differences were present in the consensus population of the genomic RNA, direct RNA sequencing of the **wt** virus, of four **dmar** mutants, and of 11 single **mar** mutants, selected by MAbs specific for the three antigenic subsites Aa, Ab and Ac, was performed. The sequence differences detected by DNA sequencing (**Table 2**) were confirmed by sequencing of consensus genomic RNA populations. All **mar** mutants selected with subsite-Aa specific-MAbs showed nucleotide differences which caused a change in residue 538 of S-protein. One **mar** mutant selected with a subsite-Ac specific-MAb had the two other residue changes (543 and 631), also detected in the two **dmar** mutants derived from it. The change in residue 631 may have been incidental during the cloning of the **mar** mutant 1B.B5, which was used to select the **dmar** 1B.B5-1B.B1 and **dmar** 1B.B5-1D.E7, as synthetic nonapeptides that contain residue 543 were recognized by the subsite-Ac specific-MAb 1A.F10 (L. Enjuanes, W.P.A. Posthumus, and R. Meloen, unpublished results). Two mutants (**mar** 1D.E7 and **mar** 1H.D2) selected with subsite-Ab specific-MAbs, one mutant (**mar**

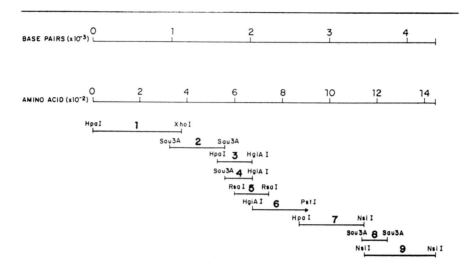

Fig. 2. S-gene fragments cloned in pEX vector. Location of the nine partially overlaping S-gene fragments named 1 to 9, from 5'-end to 3'-end, inserted in the expression vector pEX (Stanley and Luzio, 1984), using the indicated restriction endonuclease insertion sites. For insert 6, a **Pst** I site from the polylinker region of the cDNA clone B1 (Jacobs et al., 1987) was used.

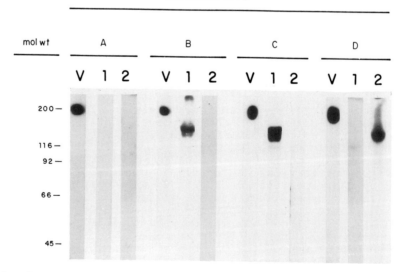

Fig. 3. Immunoblotting of pEX-TGEV expression products with MAbs. Lane V contains TGEV proteins; lanes 1 and 2 the expression products of insert 1 and 2, respectively. Antigens had been incubated in the presence of 2.5% SDS and 5% 2-ME. A, site-A specific MAbs (1G.A7, 1D.E7, 1A.F10, and 6A.C3); B, site-B specific MAb (1B.H11); C, site-C specific MAbs (5B.H1 and 6A.A6); and, D, site-D specific MAb (1D.G3).

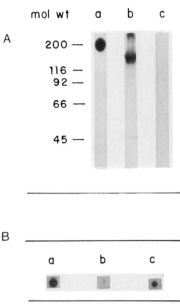

Fig. 4. Binding of antiserum against the 28-kDa S protein
fragment to pEX-TGEV expression products or to a synthetic
peptide from the N-terminal end of S protein. Figure 4A shows
an immunoblot of the TGEV proteins (lane a) or pEX-TGEV
expression products of insert 1 (lane b) and 2 to 9 (lane c),
incubated with a murine antiserum against the 28-kDa
fragment. Figure 4B shows an immunodot analysis of the 28-kDa
specific antiserum with TGEV (a), KLH (b), and with a
synthetic peptide containing the 18 N-terminal residues of
the S protein, conjugated to KLH (c).

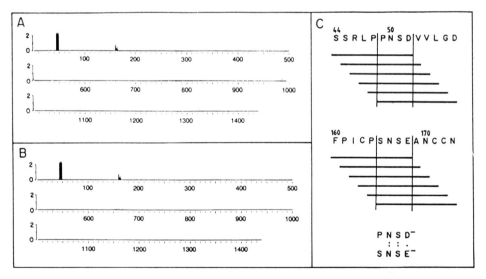

Fig. 5. PEPSCAN results of site-C specific MAbs tested on
overlapping nonapeptides covering the S-protein. Binding
activities of MAb 6A.A6 (A) and 5B.H1 (B), measured in an
ELISA, were plotted on the vertical axis and on the
horizontal axis the sequence position of the N-Terminal amino
acid of the peptide. The position and sequence of the two
sets of overlapping peptides recognized by both MAbs was the
same and it is shown in panel C.

1B.H6) that has altered subsites Aa and Ab, and three double
mutants (**dmar** 1B.B5-1D.E7, **dmar** 1D.E7-1G.A6, and **dmar**
1D.E7-1B.B1) have nucleotide differences at positions 586 or 591
(**Table 2**), indicating that these residues are involved in subsite
Ab.

Variability of the antigenic sites

The binding of 42 MAbs specific for the strain
PUR46.CC120-MAD of TGEV to 26 coronavirus strains (**Figure 6**)
indicated that TGEV, PRCV, FIPV, FECV, and CCV had conserved
determinants in the three major structural proteins. These
viruses had in common, in the peplomer protein, the antigenic
subsite Ac, an inducer of TGEV neutralizing antibodies. In
contrast, the antigenic sites B, C and D, showed a high
variability, particularly sites B and C, which were generally
present in TGEV isolates, were absent in PRCV strains, and in the
other coronaviruses analyzed. None of the 42 MAbs bound to HCV
229E, porcine epidemic diarrhea virus (PEDV), hemagglutinating
encephalomyelitis virus (HEV), and mouse hepatitis virus (MHV).

Five MAbs, three specific for antigenic subsite Ac an two
other site-A specific-MAbs, neutralized TGEV, PRCV, FIPV, FECV
and CCV (Sánchez et al., 1989). None of the 42 MAbs, including
those which recognized the conserved epitopes, neutralized either
the HVC 229E or the serologically unrelated coronaviruses: PEDV,
HEV and MHV (Sánchez et al., 1989).

Based on the percentage of antigenic homology of each
particular virus isolate, relative to the reference virus
(PUR46.CC120-MAD) (**Figure 1**), the studied coronaviruses could be
classified into four different clusters, with homology
percentages between 90-100, 69-83, 26-30, and 0, which included
the TGEVs, PRCVs, the canine and feline isolates, and the other
viruses, respectively. No antigenic relationship has been
described among the members of the fourth cluster. These results
(**Figure 1**, and Sánchez et al., 1989), defined: i) **type specific
epitopes**, which were common to enteric TGEV isolates -e.g., those
recognized by MAbs 1D.B12 and 8F.B3; ii) **group specific epitopes**,
which were common to enteric TGEV and respiratory PRCV isolates
-e.g., those defined by MAbs 1D.E8, 1D.E7 and 1H.D2; and, iii)
interspecies specific epitopes, which were the ones shared by
TGEV, PRCV, and coronaviruses from other species (feline and
canine), antigenically related to TGEV -e.g., MAbs 1B.B5, 1A.F10,
6A.C3, and 8B.E3.

As no TGEV-specific MAb recognized the HCV 229E, it was
studied if polyvalent antisera, specific for the structural
proteins of each virus, bound or neutralized to both viruses. The
results (Sánchez et al., 1989) showed that there was no
crossneutralization. Anti-TGEV serum did not bind to the HCV
229E. The anti-HCV 229E serum apparently bound to MHV and, into a
minor extent, to TGEV, but these reactivities were extensively
diminished by preadsorbing the serum with the cells used to grow
TGEV and HCV 229E.

In order to differentiate sera from animals infected with
TGEV or PRCV, two type specific MAbs, 1D.B12 and 8F.B3, could be
used in a competitive RIA, as these MAbs bound to all strains of
TGEV tested, but not to the PRCV isolates (Sánchez et al., 1989).

DISCUSSION

In this chapter, we describe a correlation between the

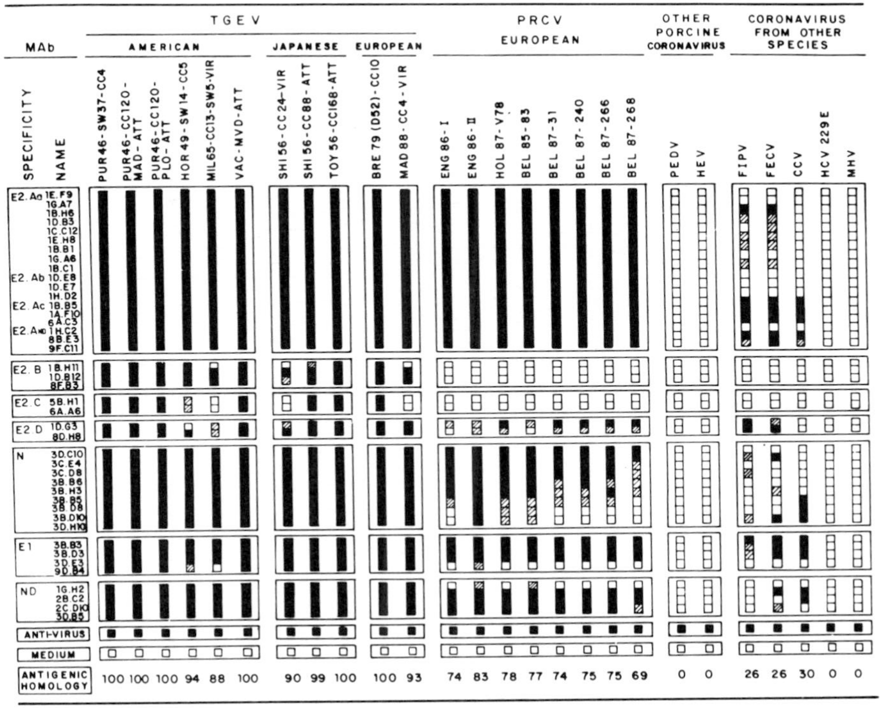

Fig. 6. Binding of MAbs to coronaviruses. The value of the MAb binding to the PUR46.CC120-MAD, determined by RIA, was taken as the reference value (100). The characteristics of the viruses used were summarized previously (Sánchez et al., 1989). The specificity of the MAbs is named according to Correa et al. (1988). Symbols □, 0 to 30; ▨, 31 to 50; ▧, 51 to 100. The antigenic homology of each virus isolate relative to the reference virus PUR46.CC120-MAD, was expresed in percentage. The anti-virus sera were TGEV specific in the case of TGEV, PRCV, FIPV, FECV, and CCV, and specific for the homologous virus, in the case of PEDV, HEV, HCV 229E, and MHV.

167

antigenic structure of the TGE virus S-protein with its physical map. MAbs specific for four antigenic sites were used to screen protein fragments, as well as the expression products of S-gene sequences. In addition, the sequencing of **mar** mutants, selected from TGEV stocks with site-A specific-MAbs was used to locate this site on S-gene. The antigenic homology among 26 coronavirus strains has been studied with a collection of 42 MAbs, which recognized a minimum of 25 epitopes, and polyvalent antisera. This analysis identified type, group and interspecies epitopes, provided MAbs which differentiate members of the TGEV antigenic types, particularly TGEV and PRCV isolates, and revealed that the inclusion of the HCV 229E in this taxonomic cluster should be reconsidered.

HPLC fractionation of the peptides obtained after degradating S-protein with staphyloccocal V8 protease, resulted in the isolation of a 28-kDa fragment, which was identified as being N-terminal, since an antiserum to this peptide, only reacted with the recombinant product of insert 1 (**Figure 4A**), and because of the recognition by this antiserum of a synthetic peptide containing the 18 N-terminal residues of S-protein (**Figure 4B**). The presence of a second 28-kDa fragment formed by residues different from the first 325 amino acids, which could have been copurified by HPLC and SDS-PAGE with the other 28-kDa fragment, can not be completely ruled out. Nevertheless, this possibility seems unlikely, since the polyvalent antiserum induced by the 28-kDa fragment recognized recombinant products of insert 1.

Figure 7 summarizes the location of the antigenic sites. Site A must be complex and discontinuous. To the formation of this site residues around positions 538, 543, 586, and 591, changed in the **mar** mutants selected with site-A specific-MAbs must be essential. The residue 538 must be implicated in the formation of subsite Aa (or influences its conformation), as seven **mar** mutants selected with MAbs specific for this subsite showed nucleotide differences in this residue. Amino acids 543 and 631 may be involved in the formation of subsite Ac, as these two residues were changed in **dmar** 1B.B5-1B.B1, **dmar** 1B.B1-1D.E7, and **mar** 1B.B5, from which the **dmars** were derived. Recognition of synthetic nonapeptides, that contain residue 543, by the subsite-Ac specific-MAb 1A.F10 (L. Enjuanes, W.P.A. Posthumus, and R. Meloen, unpublished results), suggests that the relevant residue difference which facilitated the escape of the **mar** 1B.B5 mutant from the neutralization by the corresponding MAb, is in position 543. The change in residue 631 may have been incidental during the cloning of **mar** 1B.B5 mutant. Subsite Ab must be formed by amino acids around residues 586 and 591, as nucleotide differences corresponding to either one of these residues were detected in two single mutants (**mar** 1D.E7 and **mar** 1H.D2), or in three double mutants (**dmar** 1B.B5-1D.E7, **dmar** 1D.E7-1G.A6, and **dmar** 1D.E7-1B.B1). In addition, site-A specific-MAbs bound to a 28-kDa fragment, identified as N-terminal, which suggest that amino acids within the first 325 residues may contribute to the formation of site A. The antigenic site A of TGEV may resemble one of the neutralization epitopes of foot-and-mouth-disease virus, shown recently to be formed by two separated antigenic regions (Thomas et al., 1988; Parry et al., 1989).

The precise location of site C was determined by PEPSCAN between residues 48 and 52, and we have also obtain data on the locations of site D by using the same technology (Posthumus et al., this volume), which confirmed the results presented here. Interestingly, the four antigenic sites A, B, C, and D, are in the 40% N-terminal residues of S-protein, and they are the target

TABLE 2

NUCLEOTIDE SEQUENCE DIFFERENCES BETWEEN TGEV-wt AND TGEV-mar MUTANTS

CLONE	NUCLEIC ACID SEQUENCED	ANTIGENIC SUBSITE SPECIFICITY OF MAb[c]	NUCLEOTIDE SEQUENCE IN wt VIRUS	IN mar MUTANT	BASE CHANGED	AMINO ACID CHANGE RESIDUE	FROM	TO
BLUESCRIPT.PUR46. dmar 1B.B5-1B.B1[a]	DNA	c/a	AAG	CAG	1612	538	Lys	Gln
			GGT	GAT	1628	543	Gly	Asp
			GTT	GCT	1892	631	Val	Ala
PUR46.dmar 1B.B5- 1B.B1[b]	RNA	c/a	AAG	CAG	1612	538	Lys	Glu
			GGU	GAU	1628	543	Gly	Asp
			GUU	GCU	1892	631	Val	Ala
PUR46.dmar 1B.B5- 1D.E7	RNA	c/b	GGT	GAT	1628	543	Gly	Asp
			GAC	AAC	1756	586	Asp	Asn
			GTT	GCT	1892	631	Val	Ala
PUR46.dmar 1D.E7- 1G.A6	RNA	b/a	CGA	CAA	1772	591	Arg	Gln
PUR46.dmar 1D.E7- 1B.B1	RNA	b/a	CGA	CAA	1772	591	Arg	Gln
PUR46. mar 1B.B5	RNA	c	GGU	GAU	1628	543	Gly	Asp
			GUU	GCU	1892	631	Val	Ala
PUR46. mar 1G.A7	RNA	a	AAG	AUG	1613	538	Lys	Met
PUR46. mar 1B.C1	RNA	a	AAG	ACG	1613	538	Lys	Thr
PUR46. mar 1D.B3	RNA	a	AAG	ACG	1613	538	Lys	Thr
PUR46. mar 1G.A6	RNA	a	AAG	ACG	1613	538	Lys	Thr
PUR46. mar 1C.C12	RNA	a	AAG	ACG	1613	538	Lys	Thr
PUR46. mar 1E.H8	RNA	a	AAG	ACG	1613	538	Lys	Thr
PUR46. mar 1E.F9	RNA	a	AAG	AUG	1613	538	Lys	Met
PUR46. mar 1D.E7	RNA	b	CGA	CAA	1772	591	Arg	Gln
PUR46. mar 1H.D2	RNA	b	CGA	CCA	1772	591	Arg	Pro
PUR46. mar 1B.H6[d]	RNA	a/b	GAC	AAC	1756	586	Asp	Asn

a. The sequences of the 5'-ends 2x10³ nucleotides of the PUR 46.Cl strain of TGE virus and of the double mar mutant dmar 1B.B5-1B.B1 were obtained using cDNAs cloned on the Bluescript plasmid.

b. RNA sequencing was performed on RNA from purified virions.

c. The antigenic subsites were defined as described by Correa et al. (1988).

d. mar 1B.H6 has altered part of both subsites a and b (Gebauer et al., 1989)

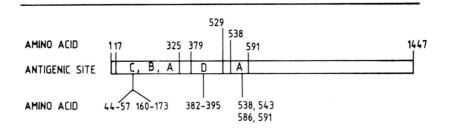

Fig. 7. Location of the antigenic sites of S glycoprotein. Site A is discontinuous and formed by residues around positions 538 to 591 and, probably, by residues between 1 and 325. Site B is located between 1–325. The precise position of site D has been determined by Posthumus et al. (This volume). The relative order of sites C and B and part of site A is not defined.

169

of 1015 independently derived TGE virus hybridomas selected in our laboratory (Correa et al., 1988). This indicates that the S-peplomer has a relatively small immunogenic area, which in the model of De Groot et al. (1987) is located in the globular part of the peplomer.

While antigenic site A is higly conserved, sites B, C, and D, showed variability. Particularly, sites B and C were not present in the respiratory isolates. The interspecies specific subsite Ac is conserved in porcine, feline and canine coronaviruses. Anti-idiotypic antibodies of the β-type, specific for MAb 6A.C3 which recognized this subsite, could have a role in protection against coronaviruses of the three species.

PRCV was detected for the first time in 1984 (Pensaert et al., 1986; Callebaut et al., 1988) and could be derived from TGEV, by recombination between this virus and other porcine (PEDV or HEV), feline (FIPV or FECV), or canine (CCV) coronaviruses, which would provide the modified antigenic sites B and C. This hypothesis is favoured, versus the accumulation of point mutations, as two antigenic sites are different between these viral strains, and mechanisms of genetic recombination have been demonstrated in coronavirus (Makino et al., 1986). The production of PRCV variants by deletion in sites B, C, and D, could also be the mechanism of PRCV generation, as the mRNA coding the S-protein of PRCV is 5% smaller than the corresponding mRNA of TGEV (P. Britton, personal communication). Since PRCV provides some protection against TGEV (Hooyberghs et al., 1988), it could be predicted that the presence of TGEV will decrease in countries where PRCV is present, while other transmissible gastroenteric coronaviruses serologically unrelated to TGEV will be prevalent.

HCV 229E has been previously included in the TGEV group (Mcnaughton, 1981), based on a weak crossreactivity of antisera against TGEV and HCV 229E with these viruses, detected by immunofluorescence. In contrast, none of the 42 MAbs tested, bound or neutralized HCV 229E. Furthermore, polyvalent antisera to TGEV or HCV 229E did not show an antigenic homology between the viral proteins, as the crossreactivity observed could be adsorbed by uninfected cells. There are two other issues which differentiate the TGEV group viruses, from HCV 229E. First, while TGEV related isolates have three major structural proteins, HCV 229E has two other proteins (Kemp et al., 1984). Secondly, while the peplomer protein is not processed in TGEV related coronaviruses, the S-protein of the HCV 229E is processed in certain cell lines (Schmidt and Kenny, 1982; Kemp et al., 1984). Althought a minor antigenic relationship among HCV 229E and TGEV related strains can not be excluded, based on some homology detected by genome sequencing (Schreiber et al., 1989), HCV 229E does not make a uniform antigenic cluster with TGEV, FIPV, FECV, and CCV, and we strongly suggest reconsidering the inclusion of the human virus in the same taxonomic group.

ANCKNOWLEDGEMENTS

This investigation was funded by grants from the Consejo Superior de Investigaciones Científicas and the Comisión Interministerial de Ciencia y Tecnología, in Spain, the Netherlands Foundation of Medical Research (MEDIGON, grant 900-515-002) in The Netherlands, and the European Economical Community (Project BAP 0464.E).

REFERENCES

Brian, D.A., Dennis, D.E., and Guy, J.S. 1980. Genome of porcine transmissible gastroenteritis virus. J. Virol., 34:410.

Bullido, M.J., Correa, I., Jiménez, G., Suñe, C., Gebauer, F., and Enjuanes, L. 1988. Induction of transmissible gastroenteritis coronavirus neutralizing antibodies "in vitro" by virus-specific T helper cell hybridomas. J. Gen. Virol., 40:659.

Callebaut, P., Correa, I., Pensaert, M., Jiménez, G., and Enjuanes, L. 1988. Antigenic differentiation between transmissible gastroenteritis virus of swine and a related porcine respiratory coronavirus. J. Gen. Virol., 69:1725.

Correa, I., Jiménez, G., Suñé, C., Bullido, M.J., and Enjuanes, L. 1988. Antigenic structure of the E2 glycoprotein from transmissible gastroenteritis coronavirus. Virus Res. 10:77.

Correa, I., Gebauer, F., Bullido, M.J., Suñé, C., Baay, M.F.D., Zwaagstra, K.A., Posthumus, W.P.A., Lenstra, J.A., and Enjuanes, L. 1989. Localization of antigenic sites of the E2 glycoprotein of transmissible gastroenteritis coronavirus. J. Gen. Virol., in press.

De Groot, R.J., Luytjes, W., Horzinek, M.C., Van der Zeijst, B.A.M., Spaan, W.J.M., and Lenstra, J.A. 1987. Evidence for a coiled-coil structure in the spike proteins of coronaviruses. J. Mol. Biol. 196:963.

Enjuanes, L., Posthumus, W.P.A., Correa, I., Erkens, J.H.F., Meloen, R., Lenstra, H.A., and Stanley, K.K. 1989. Amino acid sequence of a transmissible gastroenteritis coronavirus epitope present in serum proteins. Submitted.

García-Barreno, B., Sanz, A., Nogal, M.L., Viñuela, E., and Enjuanes L. 1986. Monoclonal antibodies of African swine fever virus: antigenic differences among field virus isolates and viruses passaged in cell culture. J. Virol., 58:385.

Garwes, D.J., Lucas, M.H., Higgins, D.A., Pike, B.V., and Cartwright, S.F. 1978. Antigenicity of structural components from porcine transmissible gastroenteritis virus. Vet. Microbiol. 3:179.

Gebauer, F., Correa, I., Bullido, M.J., Suñé, C., Smerdou, C., and Enjuanes L. 1989. Sequences of two major epitopes of Transmissible gastroenteritis coronavirus. Virology.

Geysen, H.M., Meloen, R.H., and Barteling, S.J. 1984. Use of peptide synthesis to probe viral antigens for epitopes to a resolution of a single amino acid. Proc. Nat. Acad. Sci. USA. 81:3998.

Hooyberghs, J., Pensaert, M.B., and Callebaut, P. 1988. Transmissible gastroenteritis: outbreaks in swine herds previously infected with a TGEV-like porcine respiratory coronavirus. 10th Int. Pig. Veter. Soc. Congress. Rio Janeiro, p.200.

Jacobs, L., De Groot, R., Van der Zeijst, B.A.M., Horzinek, M.C. and Spaan, W. 1987. The nucleotide sequence of the peplomer gene of porcine transmissible gastroenteritis virus (TGEV): comparison with the sequence of the peplomer protein of feline infectious peritonitis virus (FIPV). Virus Res. 8:363.

Jiménez, G., Correa, I., Melgosa, M.P., Bullido, M.J., and Enjuanes, L. 1986. Critical epitopes in transmissible gastroenteritis virus neutralization. J. Virol. 60:131.

Kapke, P.A., and Brian, D.A. 1986. Sequence analysis of the porcine transmissible gastroenteritis coronavirus nucleocapsid protein gene. Virology 151:41.

Kemp, M.C., Hierholzer, J.C., Harrison, A., and Burks, J.S. 1984. Characterization of viral proteins synthesized in 229-E infected cells and effect(s) of inhibition of glycosylation and glycoprotein transport. **Adv. Exp. Med. Biol.** 173:65.

Laude, H., Rasschaert, D., and Huet, J.C. 1987. Sequence and N-terminal processing of the transmembrane protein E1 of the coronavirus transmissible gastroenteritis virus. **J. Gen. Virol.** 68:1687.

Lenstra, J.A., Kusters, J.G., Koch, G., and Van Der Zeijst, B.A.M. 1989. Antigenicity of the peplomer protein of infectious bronchitis virus. **Mol. Immunol.** 26:7.

Macnaughton, M.R. 1981. Structural and antigenic realtionships between human, murine and avian coronaviruses. **Adv. Exp. Med. Biol.** 142:19.

Makino, S., Stohlman, S.A., and Lai, M.M.C. 1986. Leader sequences of murine coronavirus RNA can be freely reassorted. Evidence for the role of free leader RNA in transcription. **Proc. Natl. Acad. Sci. USA**, 83:4204.

Parry, N.R., Barnett, P.V., Ouldridge, E.J., Rowlands, D.J., and Brown, F. 1989. Neutralizing epitopes of type O foot-and-mouth disease virus. II. Mapping three conformational sites with synthetic peptide reagents. **J. Gen. Virol.** 70:1493.

Pensaert, M., Callebaut, P., and Vergote, J. 1986. Isolation of a porcine respiratory, non-enteric coronavirus related to transmissible gastroenteritis. **Vet. Quart.** 8, 257.

Rasschaert, D., Gelfi, J. and Laude, H. 1987. Enteric coronavirus TGEV: partial sequence of the genomic RNA, its organization and expression. **Biochimie**, 69:591.

Rasschaert, D., and Laude, H. 1987. The predicted primary structure of the peplomer protein E2 of the porcine coronavirus transmissible gastroenteritis virus. **J. Gen. Virol.**, 68:1883.

Sánchez, C., Jiménez, G., Laviada, M.D., Correa, I., Suñé, C., Bullido, M.J., Gebauer, F., Smerdou, C., Callebaut, P., Escribano, J.M., and Enjuanes, L. 1989. Antigenic homology among coronaviruses related to transmissible gastroenteritis virus. **Virology.**

Sanger, F., Nicklen, S., and Coulson, A.R. 1977. DNA sequencing with chain-terminating inhibitors. **Proc. Natl. Acad. Sci. USA**, 74:5463.

Schmidt, O.W., and Kenny, G.E. 1982. Polypeptides and functions of antigens from human coronaviruses 229E and OC43. **Infect. Immun.**, 35:515.

Schreiber, S., Kamahora, T., and Lai, M.M.C. 1989. Sequence analysis of the nucleocapsid protein gene of human coronavirus 229E. **Virology** 169:142.

Stanley, K.K., and Luzio, J.P. 1984. Construction of a new family of high efficiency bacterial expression vectors: identification of cDNA clones coding for human liver proteins. **EMBO J.**, 3:1429.

Sturman, L.S., and Holmes, K.V. 1983. The molecular biology of coronaviruses. **Adv. Virus Res.**, 28:35.

Thomas, A.A., Woortmeijer, R.J., Puijk, W., and Barteling, S.J. 1988. Antigenic sites of foot-and-mouth disease virus type A10. **J. Virol.**, 62:2782.

Zimmern, D., and Kaesberg, P. 1978. 3'-Terminal nucleotide sequence of encephalomyocarditis virus RNA determined by reverse transcriptase and chain-terminating inhibitors. **Proc. Natl. Acad. Sci. USA.**, 75:4257.

TOPOLOGICAL AND FUNCTIONAL ANALYSIS OF EPITOPES ON THE S(E2) AND HE(E3)

GLYCOPROTEINS OF BOVINE ENTERIC CORONAVIRUS

J.F. Vautherot, M.F. Madelaine, and J. Laporte

I.N.R.A.

Laboratoire de Virologie et d'Immunologie Moléculaires. C.R.J.J.,
Domaine de Vilvert, 78350- Jouy-en-Josas. France

SUMMARY

Monoclonal antibodies (Mabs) were selected which reacted with bovine enteric coronavirus S and HE. Mabs to S were used to identify 2 cleavage products of S, S/gp105 and S/gp90. Monoclonals to S/gp105 and HE neutralised the virus; only Mabs to the latter inhibited haemagglutination and acetyl-esterase activity. Topological distribution of epitopes was studied on these 3 glycoproteins by means of competition binding experiments. Two independent epitopes were characterised on HE, 4 on S/gp105, and 2 on S/gp90. Neutralising Mabs defined one major site on both S/gp105 and HE; however a minor neutralisation epitope was also delineated on S/gp105. Functional mapping using neutralisation-resistant mutants confirmed the topological distribution of epitopes on S/gp105.

INTRODUCTION

Bovine enteric coronavirus (BCV) is a well characterised enteric virus which causes enteritis in newborn calves (1), as well as chronic shedding (1) and/or acute diarrhoea in adult cows (2). BCV has 4 major structural proteins, a nucleoprotein {N}, a trans-membrane protein {M } and 2 N-glycosylated proteins, S and HE, which constitute the peplomers (3,4,5). S is a large complex protein, processed from an intracellular precursor (gp170) which is further glycosylated to yield a transient gp190 (5), which, in turn, is proteolytically cleaved into glycoproteins with Mr of 90 to 105 kD (5). One of the cleavage products, gp105 (6) or gp100/E2 (5) was reported to elicit neutralising antibodies (6-7). HE, the haemagglutinin (8-9), is a disulphide-linked dimer (3,4,5), also recognised by neutralising Mabs(7), and recently shown to be responsible for the receptor-destroying activity of BCV(10).
The aims of the present investigation were i)to assess the specificity of Mabs to the different glycoproteins, with a particular concern for the cleavage products of S, ii) to characterise the viral functions inhibited by these Mabs, iii) to present an epitope map of the different glycoproteins and compare these maps with the results of functional and antigenic analyses.

MATERIAL AND METHODS

Viruses and cell-lines

Isolation and characterisation of the different BCV isolates (11), as well as their cultivation (3,6,11), titration (12), and purification from infected HRT 18 cells (3) have been described.

Coronaviruses and Their Diseases
Edited by D. Cavanagh and T.D.K. Brown
Plenum Press, New York, 1990

173

Production, purification (13), initial characterisation (6) of Mabs and their titration by neutralisation, ELISA, or haemagglutination-inhibition (HAI) (4,6,9,11), have also been reported.

Immune precipitation and Western Blotting

Isotopic labelling and immune precipitation of viral proteins were performed as previously described (6-14). For Western Blotting, virus proteins were first separated by PAGE (6), and transferred to a nitrocellulose sheet by transverse electrophoresis (15) in a Milliblot SDE electroblotting apparatus {Millipore} at 2,5 mA /cm^2 for 30 min. Mabs reacting with denatured virus proteins were detected using a sheep anti-mouse IgG conjugated to alkaline phosphatase {Biosys} and BCIP/NBT {Gibco-BRL} as substrate.

Selection of BCV mutants resistant to neutralisation by Mabs

The procedure followed was essentially similar to the one described for the selection of TGEV neutralisation escape mutants (14). Mutants resistant to neutralisation by their selecting Mab after 3 subcloning experiments were tested in a virus neutralisation test (V.N.T) using a panel of neutralising Mabs.

Labelling of monoclonal antibodies

Purified Mabs were either conjugated to horseradish peroxidase (HRPO), using the glutaraldehyde two-step method (16), or biotinylated (17).

ELISA for binding and competition binding of monoclonal antibodies

Binding assays for HRPO or biotin-labelled Mabs were performed in conditions that were similar to those of ELISA for unlabelled Mabs (11). Detection of biotinylated Mabs necessitated an additionnal step i.e. incubation with HRPO-labelled streptavidin {Amersham}, and 3 washs before incubation with the HRPO substrate { T.M.B Microwell Peroxidase System- Kirkegaard and Perry Lab.}.
Competition binding assays between Mabs were performed as described (14), except that detection of bound labelled Mabs was based on an enzymatic assay.

RESULTS

Specificity and biological functions of monoclonal antibodies

Biological functions relevant to each specificity were determined by testing Mabs in neutralisation, HAI and inhibition of acetyl-esterase assays.

Monoclonal antibodies to HE.
All Mabs to HE precipitated a 125 kD glycoprotein which was resolved in two monomers of 65 kD in the presence of reducing agents (fig. 1, lanes C and L). None of these Mabs recognised the denatured protein in Western Blotting. Six of the 14 anti-HE Mabs displayed a complement independent neutralising activity (Table 1). All neutralising and 6 non-neutralising Mabs inhibited haemagglutination of rat red blood cells (RRBC) by BCV (Table 1). Mabs were also tested in a rapid acetyl-esterase inhibition assay for their ability to protect a synthetic substrate of acetyl-esterase {para-nitrophenyl-acetate-PNPA; Aldrich} from cleavage by HE. Mab A12, a non-neutralising Mab, had a significant inhibitory effect on the enzymatic activity (data not shown).

Monoclonal antibodies to S.
Mabs to S were separated in two classes according to their immune precipitation pattern and reactivity in Western Blotting.
Mabs to S/gp105 precipitated gp105 together with its precursor gp170 from infected cell lysates (Fig.1, lanes A, B, and D), and gp105 alone from labelled virus disrupted with non-ionic detergents. Some Mabs of this specificity were also able to react with gp105 after denaturation with SDS alone (Mabs I16, P11, I7, I9, I11), or SDS and 2-ME (Mab I16).

Mabs to S/gp90 precipitated a 90 kD species together with the precursor gp170 and high Mr products from infected cell-lysates (Fig.1, lanes E,I,M). Four Mabs reacted with the denatured reduced gp90 in Western Blotting (data not shown). Expression in pUEx vector of a stretch of 109 amino-acids (aa) covering the N terminus part of S2 {carboxy-end cleavage fragment} and 28 aa at the C-terminus of S1 {Amino-end cleavage fragment}, yielded a ß-galactosidase fusion protein (P.Boireau and N. Woloszin, unpublished results) which was recognised by Mabs to S/gp90 (Table 1, subsite B2). A majority of Mabs to S/gp105 could neutralise BCV, but none of the anti S/gp90 had any effect on the viral replication in HRT 18 cells (Table 1).

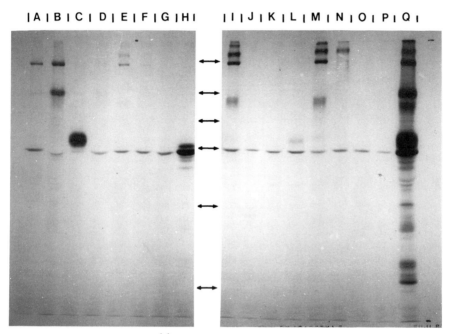

Fig. 1. PAGE analysis of ^{14}C labelled polypeptides immunoprecipitated from HRT 18 cells infected with BCV G110 isolate. In lanes A, B, D, Mabs C13, B5, and F15 precipitated gp170 and S/gp105. Lanes C and L, Mabs A12 and J10 reacted with gp65, the HE monomer. Mabs H3, J22, and G4, in lanes E, I, M respectively, precipitated S/gp90, gp170, and high Mr products.. Lane Q, precipitation of viral polypeptides by a rabbit hyperimmune antiserum. Molecular mass markers migrated to positions identified by double arrows, and were, from top to bottom, 170 kD, 97,4 kD, 68 kD, 55 kD, 36,5 kD, and 21,5 kD.

Delineation of epitopes

Competitive binding ELISA.

Labelling of Mabs had no major adverse effect on the antibody binding characteristics (except for 2 anti-S/gp90 Mabs), when binding curves of labelled and unlabelled Mabs were compared. A sequential competition binding assay against saturating amounts of homologous unlabelled Mab showed that the binding of a majority of Mabs was inhibited from 65 to 98%. Mabs which competed poorly in the sequential assay were retested in a simultanous assay and gave satisfactory results (self competition at 70 to 99%).

Table 1. Characterisation of monoclonal antibodies to S and HE

Specificity	Site or subsite	Number	Neutralisation	HAI	Western Blotting		Antigenic analysis
					SDS	SDS/2ME	
HE(E3)	A1	6	+	+	–	–	BCV
	A2	7	–	+	–	–	BCV
	B	1	–	–	–	–	BCV
S/gp105	A	1	+	–	–	–	BCV
	B1	1	+	–	+	–	BCV
	B2	4	+	–	+	–	BCV
	B3	6	+	–	–	–	BCV
	B4	2	+a	–	–	–	BCVb
	C	2	–	–	–	–	BCV & OC43
	D	1	–	–	+	+	BCV, OC43, & HEV
S/gp90	A	2	–	–	–	–	BCV & HEV
	B1	1	–	–	–	–	BCV & MHV
	B2	4	–	–	+	+	BCV,OC43,HEV, &MHV

a Mab A9 only neutralised the virus
b NCDCV (Mebus isolate) was not recognised by B4 Mabs

On HE, 2 independent epitopes (A, B) were delineated using 14 biotin-labelled Mabs. Non reciprocal competitions between Mabs of site A (Table 1) were observed. These may reflect differences in Mab avidity as well as conformational modifications of HE upon binding with neutralising Mabs. Epitope B was unequivocally delineated by Mab B22 which was only self-competing and had no effect on the binding of the other Mabs.

On S/gp90, two epitopes were identified using 6 biotin-labelled Mabs. Epitope B was further subdivided according to the reactivity of Mabs to denatured S/gp90 (subgroup B1 and B2 in Table 1).

On S/gp105, 4 independent sites were defined by using 18 Mabs (Fig.2). Site A was defined by Mab C13, a neutralising monoclonal antibody. All other neutralising Mabs mapped in site B, which could also be further subdivided on the basis of competition binding results (Fig.2).

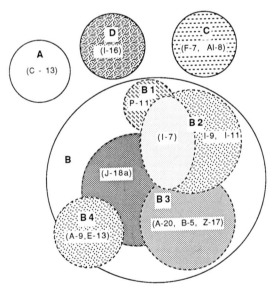

Fig. 2. Epitope map showing the 4 independent sites on S/gp105. Mabs delineating the different sites and subsites are indicated in brackets.

Subsite B1 was defined by Mab P11 which reciprocally competed by 40 to 50% with Mabs in subsite B2 (I7, I9, I11), but not with the other Mabs in site B.

Subsite B2 and B3 were differentiated on the basis of their reactivity to Mabs P11 and E11. Mabs of subsites B1 and B2 enhanced the fixation of labelled Mab E11, whereas Mabs of B3, together with E11 and J18a competed strongly with E11.

Subsite B4 was delineated by Mab A9 which competed reciprocally and strongly with Mab J18a only. Mab E13, a non-neutralising Mab, also mapped in this subsite, but did not reciprocally compete with Mab J18a.

Sites C and D were characterised as independent epitopes defined by non-neutralising Mabs F7 and Alfa8 (site C), and I16 (site D) (Fig.2).

Selection of neutralisation resistant mutants and functional mapping of S/gp105.

Neutralisation epitopes were further characterised by selecting a library of mutants that were resistant to neutralisation by anti S/gp105 Mab. These mutants were tested in a virus neutralisation test against anti-S/gp105 neutralising Mabs. Mutants which were selected by Mab I7, I11, I9, and J17a (subsite B2 as defined by competition binding experiments) were resistent to neutralisation by these Mabs. However some discrepancies were observed in the reactivity of J17a mutants which were neutralised by Mab I7 (Table 2). G19 mutants were only partially sensitive to neutralisation by Mabs I7 and I11 (Table 2), as both Mabs neutralised the 3 G19 mutants tested at a lower titre than the original virus (data not shown). Resistance to neutralisation by Mab J18a was the only common feature of mutants G19, J18a, B5, and A20, which progressively lost their resistance to Mab I9 (B5 mutants), G19 and J17a (A20 mutants), while acquiring resistance to Mabs B5 and A20. Mutants selected by Mabs A9, Z17, and C13 were found to resist only to their selecting Mab.

Table 2. Resistance to neutralisation of BCV mutants

ANTIGENIC MUTANTS

NEUTRALIZING ANTIBODY	I-7	I-11	I-9	J-17a	G-19	J-18a	B-5	A-20	A-9	Z-17	C-13
I - 7	▓	▓	▓	▓	░						
I - 11	▓	▓	▓	▓	░						
I - 9	▓	▓	▓	▓	▓	▓					
J -17a	▓	▓	▓	▓	▓	▓					
G -19	▓	▓	▓	▓	▓						
J - 18a					▓	▓	▓	▓			
B - 5						▓	▓	▓			
A - 20							▓	▓			
A - 9									▓		
Z - 17										▓	
C - 13											▓

▓ Total resistance to neutralization

░ Partial resistance to neutralization

☐ Total neutralization of all the mutants tested

177

Monoclonal antibodies were tested in an indirect immunofluorescence assay (11) for their reactivity with different BCV isolates and OC43, HEV and MHV (Table 1).

Mabs to S/gp105 delineating sites A and B reacted with BCV specific determinants. Futhermore Mabs mapping in site B4 did not recognise the NCDCV isolate of BCV (11), thus confirming the results of competition binding experiments. Anti-site C and D Mabs reacted also with OC43 (Mab F7 and Alfa8, site C) or with OC43 and HEV (Mabl16, site D).

Mabs to S/gp90 reacted with antigenic determinants which were found on BCV and HEV (site A Mabs), BCV and MHV (subsite B1 Mabs), and all the coronaviruses tested in antigenic group 2(subsite B2) (Table 1).

Anti-HE Mabs reacted with all the BCV isolates so far tested, and Mabs Y16 and H17 also recognised HEV and OC43.

DISCUSSION

Bovine enteric coronavirus has two large envelope glycoproteins, S and HE, which form the viral spikes and interact with the cellular receptor(s), thus mediating the entry of the virion in the sensitive cells (10) and modulating the immune response (18).

Monoclonal antibodies reacting with S identified the 2 cleavage products of this glycoprotein, S/gp105 and S/gp90. By comparison between the Mr of the immuneprecipitation products and the molecular masses predicted from sequence data (P.Boireau et al, in the press),we suggest that S/gp105 corresponds to S1 (amino terminus of S)and S/gp90 to S2 (carboxyl terminus of S). Expression in a procaryotic vector of a set of overlapping fragments covering the entire S2 showed that the antibody binding region of Mab to S/gp90 (subsite B2) mapped in a stretch of 109 aa extending from position 741 to 850. As this fragment contains 28 aa of S1, additionnal work is needed to remove the 28 N terminal aa in order to ascertain that binding of these Mabs is restricted to the S2 subunit. The linear epitope defined by these antibodies appears to be different from the one delineated on the S2 of MHV (19); the latter extends from aa 848 to aa 856, corresponding to aa 899 to 907 on BCV S2 (P.Boireau , personnal communication). Work is in progress to map more precisely the antibody binding sites of Mabs defining linear epitopes on S1 and S2.

Virus neutralisation was mediated by anti-S1/gp105 and anti-HE Mabs, but HAI and inhibition of acetyl-esterase activity were displayed by anti-HE Mabs only. The finding that all neutralising epitopes so far delineated on the S glycoprotein of BCV presumably map in the S1 subunit is in good correlation with results obtained for the characterisation of neutralising Mabs against IBV (20), and antibody binding sites on TGEV S glycoprotein (Delmas et al-this volume).

Competition binding experiments enabled us to define 2 non-overlapping epitopes on HE, 4 on S1/gp105, and 2 on S2/gp90. Epitopes defined on HE were SDS sensitive and functional analysis did not allow further differentiation of site A Mabs. All neutralising Mabs to S1/gp105 mapped in two sites, A and B, whereas sites C and D were defined by non-neutralising Mabs. Site B could be subdivided according to the results of competition binding experiments. These results were in good correlation with the analysis of SDS resistance of epitopes, and antigenic relationships. Functional mapping of S1/gp105 confirmed the importance of site B and the differences between subsites B2 and B3. For S2/gp90 also, the combination of the results of competition binding experiments with the antigenic analysis and SDS resistance of epitopes allowed us to confirm the topological map and to subdivide site B in two subsites, B1 and B2.

Previous publications reported the existence of 2 independent neutralising epitopes on gp100/E2 (S1/gp105) and 4 overlapping epitopes on E3 (HE) (7). In this report we describe a more complex epitope distribution for S1/gp105. By using a large panel of Mabs in competition binding experiments and functional analysis, it was possible to define a major neutralisation site which could be subdivided in 4 , a minor neutralisation epitope, and 2 additional independent sites defined by non-neutralising Mabs.

Mapping of antibody binding sites will be indispensable in unambiguously identifying the amino-acid sequences recognised by neutralising Mabs on S and HE.

REFERENCES

1. L.A. Babiuk, M. Sabara and G.R. Hudson, Rotavirus and coronavirus infections in animals, Progress in Veterinary Microbiology and Immunology 1: 80-120 (1985).

2. E. Takahashi, Y. Inaba, K. Sato, Y. Ito, H. Kurogi, H. Akashi, K. Satoda and T. Omori, Epizootic dirhoea of adult cattle associated with a coronavirus-like agent,.Vet.Microbiol. 5:151-154 (1980).

3. J. Laporte and P. Bobulesco, Polypeptide structure of bovine enteric coronavirus : comparison between a wild strain purified from feces and a HRT 18 cell-adapted strain, in: "Biochemistry and Biology of Coronaviruses," V. ter Meulen, S. Siddel and H. Wege ed. , Plenum Publishing Corp.,New-York (1981).

4. B. King and D.A. Brian, Bovine coronavirus structural proteins, J. Virol. 42(2): 700 (1982).

5. D.Deregt, M. Sabara and L.A. Babiuk, Structural proteins of bovine coronavirus and their intracellular processing, J. Gen. Virol. 68: 2863-2877 (1987).

6. J.F. Vautherot, J. Laporte, M.F. Madelaine, P. Bobulesco and A. Roseto, Antigenic and Polypeptide structure of bovine enteric coronavirus as defined by monoclonal antibodies, in: "Molecular Biology and Pathogenesis of Coronavirus"P.J.M. Rottier, B.A.M. van der Zeijst and W.J.M. Spaan,ed., Plenum Publishing Corp., New-York (1984).

7. D. Deregt and L.A. Babiuk, Monoclonaml antibodies to bovine coronavirus : Characteristics and topographical mapping of neutralising epitopes on the E2 and E3 glycoproteins, Virology 161:410-420 (1987).

8. B. King, B.J. Potts and D.A. Brian, Bovine coronavirus hemagglutinin protein, Virus Research 2:53-59 (1985).

9. M.D. Parker, G.J. Cox, D. Deregt, D.R. Fitzpatrick and L.A. Babiuk, Cloning and in-vitro expression of the gene for the E3 haemagglutinin glycoprotein of bovine coronavirus, J. Gen. Virol. 70: 155-164 (1989).

10. R. Vlasak, W. Luytjes, J. Leider, W. Spaan and P. Palese, The E3 protein of bovine coronavirus is a receptor-destroying enzyme with acetylesterase activity, J. Virol. 62(12): 4686-4690 (1988).

11. J.F. Vautherot and J. Laporte, Utilization of monoclonal antibodies for antigenic characterization of coronaviruses, Ann. Rech. Vet. 14(4): 437-444 (1983).

12. J.F. Vautherot, Plaque assay for titration of bovine enteric coronavirus, J. Gen. Virol. 56: 451-455 (1981).

13. B. Delmas, J. Gelfi and H. Laude, Antigenic structure of transmissible gastro-enteritis virus : II. Domains in the peplomer glycoprotein, J. Gen. Virol. 67:1405-1418 (1986).

14. H.Laude, J.M. Chapsal, J. Gelfi, S. Labiau and J. Grosclaude, Antigenic structure of transmissible gastro-enteritis virus . I. Properties of monoclonal antibodies directed against virion proteins, J. Gen. Virol. 67:119-130 (1986).

15. H. Towbin, T. Staehelin and J. Gordon, Electrophoretic transfer of proteins from polyacrylamide gels to nitrocellulose sheets : procedure and some applications, P.N.A.S. 76(9): 4350-4353 (1979).

16. S. Avrameas and T. Terninck, Peroxidase-labelled antibody and Fab conjugates with enhanced intracellular penetration, Immunochemistry 8:1175-1179 (1971).

17. J.L. Guesdon, T. Terninck and S. Avrameas, The use of Avidin Biotin interaction in immunoenzymatic techniques, J. Histochem. Cytochem. 27:1131-1139 (1979).

18. H. Wege, R. Dörries and A. Wege, Hybridoma antibodies to the murine coronavirus JHM : Characterization of epitopes on the peplomer protein (E2), J. Gen. Virol. 65:1931-1942 (1984).

19. W. Luytjes, D. Geerts, W. Posthumus, R. Meloen and W. Spaan, Amino-acid sequence of a conserved neutralizing epitope of murine coronavirus,J. Virol. 63:1408-1412 (1989).

20. A.P.A. Mockett, D. Cavanagh and T.D.K. Brown, Monoclonal antibodies to the S1 spike and membrane proteins of avian infectious bronchitis coronavirus strain Massachusets M41, J. Gen. Virol. 65:2281-2286 (1984).

LINEAR NEUTRALIZING EPITOPES ON THE PEPLOMER PROTEIN OF CORONAVIRUSES

Willem P.A. Posthumus and Rob H. Meloen
Central Veterinary Institute, P.O. Box 65, 8200 AB Lelystad
The Netherlands

Luis Enjuanes and Isabel Correa
Centro de Biologia Molecular (CSIC-UAM), Facultad de Ciencias
Universidad Autonoma, Canto Blanco, 28049 Madrid, Spain

Anthonie P. van Nieuwstadt and Guus Koch
Central Veterinary Institute, Department of Virology
P.O. Box 365, 8200 AJ Lelystad, The Netherlands

Raoul J. de Groot, Johannes G. Kusters, Willem Luytjes, Willy
J. Spaan, Bernard A.M. van der Zeijst, and Johannes A. Lenstra
University of Utrecht, Department of Bacteriology, Veterinary
Faculty, P.O. Box 80165, 3508 TD Utrecht, The Netherlands

Introduction

Three years ago, we reported a comparison of the primary structures of the S peplomer proteins of three coronaviruses - mouse hepatitis virus (MHV, strain A59), infectious bronchitis virus (IBV, strain M41), and feline infectious peritonitis virus (FIPV, strain 79-1146) - which represent the three antigenic clusters in the coronavirus family (De Groot et al., 1987a, b). A periodicity in the C-terminal part of the S sequence indicated the presence of a coiled-coil structure, which forms the stalk of the peplomer. The non-conserved N-terminal sequence probably forms the bulbous part of the peplomer.
In the work reported here, we used the sequence information to locate epitopes that mediate virus neutralization. We will report the results of an approach that focuses on linear epitopes, i.e., epitopes that depend only on the sequence and not on the native conformation of the protein.

Approach

The large size of the peplomer proteins (1162 to 1452 residues) clearly prohibits classical methods of synthesizing peptides to search for antigenic sequences. Instead, we used a combination of two methods, prokaryotic expression and PEPSCAN peptide synthesis. Insertion of peplomer cDNA fragments into the prokaryotic expression plasmid pEX (Stanley & Luzio, 1984) leads to an attachment of a peplomer fragment to the C terminus of a cro-β-galactosidase hybrid protein. The fragments were generated by restriction enzymes (Correa et al., 1989; De Groot et al., unpublished; Kusters et al., 1989b; Lenstra et al., 1989; Luytjes et al., 1989), by random action of DNase I (Lenstra et al., 1989), or by synthetic oligonucleotides (Kusters et al., 1989b). The antigenicity of the expression products was assayed by Western blotting. With only a few exceptions, antibodies that recognized the peplomer protein on a Western blot also bound to one of the hybrid proteins.

Coronaviruses and Their Diseases
Edited by D. Cavanagh and T.D.K. Brown
Plenum Press, New York, 1990

181

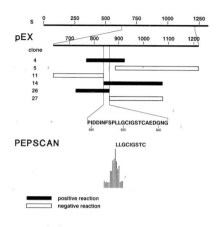

Figure 1. Binding of MAb 19.2 to pEX expression and PEPSCAN products of MHV.

S: The 1324 amino acids of the MHV-A59 peplomer protein.

pEX: Antigenicity of pEX expression products of clones 4, 5, 11, 14, 26, and 27, which delineate the epitope to the residues 839-862.

PEPSCAN: Analysis of nonapeptides from the S region 839-862, synthesized on a solid support and tested in an ELISA. Vertically is plotted the extinction, measured at 405 nm. The positive binding narrows down the epitope to nine amino acids (Luytjes et al., 1989).

The length of the identified antigenic sequences varied from 6 to 200 residues. Within such an antigenic sequence, the localization of the epitope was narrowed down by PEPSCAN analysis (Geysen et al., 1984). A few antibodies (see below) did not bind to any of the peptides, probably because of the unusual length of the epitopes.

Mouse hepatitis virus

Five antigenic sites were identified on the S peplomer protein of MHV (Talbot et al., 1984b; Talbot & Buchmeier, 1985). Three sites, designated A, B, and C, are involved in neutralization. Site A was found to be conformation independent (Talbot et al., 1984a) and is thought to be involved in cell-to-cell fusion (Collins et al., 1982). Various cDNA restriction fragments were expressed in pEX (Luytjes et al., 1989) and the epitope of the site A-specific MAb 19.2 was located within the sequence 839-862, 121 residues from the N terminus of the S2 subunit (Fig. 1, pEX). PEPSCAN analysis of nonapeptides from this region (Fig. 1, PEPSCAN) delineated the epitope within the 848-856 sequence.

Figure 2. Binding of MAbs to pEX expression and PEPSCAN products of IBV. The listed sequence of the S protein from strain D207 (residues 544-574) spans the junction of the two subunits between the residues 545 and 546. From strains D1466 and M41 the differences with D207 are indicated. The horizontal bars indicate the S sequence fragments synthesized by expression of cDNA fragments from strain D207 (pXD207-Rsa and -XP), D1466 (pXD1466- B, -NB, and -SN), and M41 (pXM41- 13.4, -15.1, and -2.1) or by expression of synthetic oligonucleotides (pXOligo-1 to -7). Dashed ends indicate continuation beyond the listed sequence. Vertical lines indicate the delineation of the epitopes. The PEPSCAN figure (analysis as described in Fig. 1) shows the binding of MAb 54.5 and 30.6 to nonapeptides from the region 550-578 (Kusters et al., 1989). In the SUMMARY figure dashed ends indicate that epitope boundaries were not located exactly.

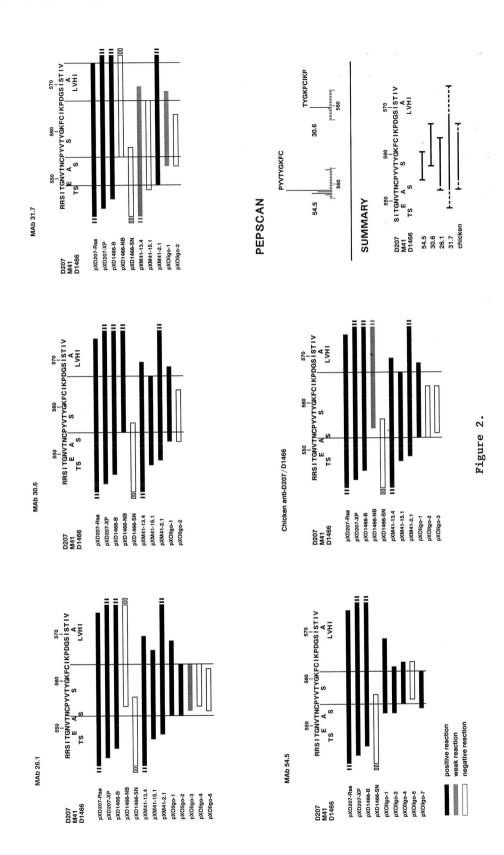

Figure 2.

183

Infectious bronchitis virus

The peplomer protein of IBV contains two subunits - S1 consisting of the residues 1-545 (Kusters *et al.*, 1989a) and S2 containing the residues 546-1180 (Kusters *et al.*,1989c). The S1 subunit contains most of the epitopes that are involved in neutralization (Cavanagh *et al.*, 1986). By mutual competition of monoclonal antibodies, Koch *et al.*, (1986, 1989) identified four antigenic sites. Three sites, located on S1, are conformation-dependent and induce the serotype-specific neutralizing response. The fourth site (site D) is located on S2; judged from the recognition of the antigen on Western blots it is conformation-independent. Antibodies specific for site D are not serotype-specific and have a weak but significant neutralizing activity (Koch *et al.*, 1986, 1989). Further, Lenstra *et al.* (1989) reported that this site is recognized strongly by rabbit, mouse, and chicken antisera. Restriction enzyme fragments as well as random DNase fragments from IBV strain M41 were used to generate hybrid proteins in pEX (Lenstra *et al.*, 1989) and to locate site D within the 37 N-terminal residues from S2. Subsequently, Kusters *et al.* (1989b) made a detailed map of the site D epitopes by testing the antigenicity of (i) expression products of cDNA fragments from the strains D207, M41, and D1466; (ii) expression products of synthetic oligonucleotides that encoded the epitope sequence (Fig. 2); and (iii) peptides of different lengths synthesized by the PEPSCAN method. This dissection of the antigenic site revealed the location of overlapping epitopes with lengths varying from 6 to at least 17 residues (Fig. 2, SUMMARY).
Despite extensive sequence divergence in both the S1 and the S2 subunits, the antigenic sequences has been conserved among the different serotypes (Kusters *et al.*, 1989b, c). Antibodies specific for site D bound to denatured virus, to pEX expression products, and to synthetic peptides. This indicates a segmental mobility on the peplomer surface (Westhof *et al.*, 1984). Presumably, the same mobility is essential for a specific molecular recognition during one of the stages of the virus life cycle.

Transmissible gastroenteritis virus and feline infectious peritonitis virus

Transmissible gastroenteritis virus (TGEV) and FIPV, both representatives of the third antigenic cluster, are generally recognized by the same antibodies. Three groups of investigators (Correa *et al.*, 1988; Delmas *et al.*, 1986; Garwes *et al.*, 1986) have inventoried the antigenic sites on the TGEV peplomer protein, using mutually competing monoclonal antibodies. For the sake of clarity we designated the sites found by Correa *et al.*, (1988) and Delmas *et al.*, (1986) by roman numerals (Table 1). Sites I and V contain most determinants mediating virus neutralization. The monoclonal antibody COR5 raised against FIPV (S.A. Fiscus, unpublished) neutralized both FIPV and TGEV and probably bound to a sixth antigenic site.
Antibodies specific for site I did not bind to any pEX products or peptides. Monoclonal antibody 1D.B12, which is specific for site II, can discriminate between TGEV and the closely related porcine respiratory coronavirus (PRCV) and bound to a hybrid protein from a pEX-TGEV recombinant containing the 1-

Table 1. Noncompetitive groups of MAbs directed against TGEV.

This paper	Correa *et al.*, 1988.	Delmas *et al.*, 1986.
I	A	A
II	B	D
III	C	
IV	D	C
V		B

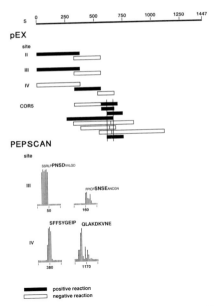

Figure 3. Binding of MAbs to TGEV/pEX and PEPSCAN products.
S : The 1447 amino acids of the TGEV peplomer protein.
pEX: Antigenicity of MAbs of group II, III, and IV with pEX expression products of cDNA clones (TGEV: Correa *et al.*, 1989; FIPV: De Groot *et al.*,
unpublished).
PEPSCAN: Analysis is as described in Fig 1. For MAbs of site III the common
amino acids from the recognized nonapeptides from the regions 40- 60 and
140-160 are indicated in bold. For MAb 57.57, a representative for MAbs of
site IV, the sequence of the most antigenic nonapeptide from the regions
370-390 and 1160-1180 (Posthumus *et al.*, 1989) is indicated.

378 sequence (Correa *et al.*, 1989), but not to any fragment of the sequence
326-1449 (Fig. 3, pEX). This indicates a location of the epitope within the
N-terminal region 1-325. Because the PEPSCAN pattern derived with nonapeptides from the TGEV peplomer sequence was inconclusive (not shown), the epitope is probably longer than nine residues. Site III is not involved in neutralization and cross-reacts with components of nonimmune porcine serum
(Correa *et al.*, 1988). Recognition by MAbs, specific for site III, of pEX
hybrid proteins and PEPSCAN peptides (Fig. 3) led to the identification of
the tetrapeptide motive P/S-N-S-E/D, which occurs not only twice in the
peplomer protein (residues 49-52 and 165-168) but also in several serum
proteins (Posthumus *et al.*, 1989b). Thus, the epitope mapping may explain
the cross-reaction with serum components.
Site IV is recognized by neutralizing as well as non-neutralizing monoclonal
antibodies (Delmas *et al.*, 1986; Correa *et al.*, 1988; Van Nieuwstadt *et al.*,
1989). MAb 57.57 and all other antibodies specific for site IV recognized
nonapeptides around residue 380 (Fig. 3, PEPSCAN). Only neutralizing antibodies specific for site IV bound to a second group of peptides around residue 1180 (Posthumus *et al.*, 1989). However, only the 380 region was antigenic
when tested as part of a pEX hybrid protein. Further, antisera against a
peptide with the sequence 377-390 were positive in a virus-ELISA and TGEV
neutralization assay, but antisera against a 1176-1184 peptide were not
(Posthumus *et al.*, 1989). We propose that site IV is complex and that the
recognition of nonapeptides from the region 1176-1193 (and nonapeptides with
a similar amino acid composition) reflects the surrounding of the region
380-388 in the tertiary structure of the peplomer. Thus, the neutralizing
MAbs specific for site IV may bind to a linear part of a discontinuous
epitope.

The epitope of COR5 was located in the region 607-660 (in the numbering of the TGEV sequence) by using pEX-FIPV and pEX-TGEV recombinants (Fig. 3, pEX; De Groot, unpublished). The region encoding this epitope appeared to encompass three restriction enzyme cleavage sites at positions corresponding to the amino acid residues 629, 640 and 648. These data indicate that the linear epitope of COR5 is unusually long and probably can explain the negative results obtained with PEPSCAN peptides.

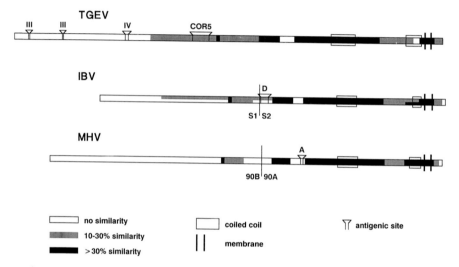

Figure 4. Linear antigenic sites on aligned peplomer sequences.

Survey of linear epitopes of the peplomer proteins

Fig. 4 shows a schematic alignment of the amino acid sequences (De Groot et al., 1987a, b) of the peplomer proteins from MHV, IBV and TGEV/FIPV with the locations of the linear epitopes. The length of the epitopes varied from 5 (TGEV site III) to at least 20 (COR5) residues. Antigenic sites appear to be located in regions without or with only moderate sequence similarity. In contrast to the finding with homologous picornaviruses (Rossman et al., 1985), no homology is observed with regard to the locations of the epitopes. For instance, in IBV nearly all linear epitopes of monoclonal antibodies (and most of the linear epitopes of polyclonal antibodies, Lenstra et al., 1989) are mapped in site D, but different patterns are observed for MHV and TGEV/FIPV. If the linear epitopes are located within relatively flexible surface

186

loops (Westhof *et al.*, 1984), our observations demonstrate the degree of structural divergence of the peplomer proteins of the different coronaviruses. This divergence is probably caused by differences in host range. It would be interesting to extend these observation to conformation-dependent epitopes. However, this awaits not only the localization of these epitopes by analyzing mutants that escape neutralization, but also a convincing alignment of the regions with a low apparent sequence similarity (de Groot *et al.*, 1987a).

Acknowledgments

We thank Wouter C. Puijk and Henk H. Plasman for synthesizing the PEPSCAN peptides, Douwe Kuperus and Hans H. Westra for performing the ELISA assays, Kornelisje A. Zwaagstra and Marc F.D. Baay for constructing of the pEX recombinants and performing the Western blot analyses. Part of this work was supported by a grant from the Netherlands Foundation for Medical Research (Medigon, grant 900-515-02) with financial aid from the Netherlands Organization for Scientific Research (NWO).

Literature cited

Cavanagh, D., P.J. Davis, D.J.C. Pappin, M.W. Binns, M.E.G. Boursnell, and T.D.K. Brown., 1986, Coronavirus IBV: partial amino terminal sequencing of spike protein S2 identifies the sequence Arg-Arg-Phe-Arg-Arg at the cleavage site of the spike precursor propolypeptide of IBV strain Beaudette and M41. *Virus Res.* 4:133-143.

Collins, A.R., R.L. Knobler, H. Powell, and M.J. Buchmeier., 1982, Monoclonal antibodies to murine hepatitis virus-4 (strain JHM) define the viral glycoprotein responsible for attachment and cell-cell fusion. *Virology* 119:358-371.

Correa, I., G. Jimenez, C. Sune, M.J. Bullido, and L. Enjuanes., 1988, Antigenic structure of the E2 glycoprotein from transmissible gastroenteritis coronavirus. *Virus Res.* 10:77-94.

Correa, I., M.J. Bullido, C. Sune, F. Gebauer, M.F.D. Baay, K.A. Zwaagstra, W.P.A. Posthumus, J.A. Lenstra, and L. Enjuanes., 1989, Correlation between physical and antigenic structure of transmissible gastroenteritis coronavirus E2-glycoprotein. *J. gen. Virol.*, in press.

Delmas, B., J. Gelfi, and H. Laude., 1986, Antigenic structure of transmissible gastroenteritis virus. II. Domains on the peplomer glycoprotein. *J. gen. Virol.* 67:1405-1418.

Garwes, D.J., F. Steward, and C.J. Elleman., 1987, Identification of epitopes of immunological importance on the peplomer of porcine transmissible gastroenteritis virus. In: *Coronaviruses*, Adv. Exp. Med. Biol. 218, p.509-515, M.M.C. Lai and S.A. Stohlman ed., Plenum Press, New York/London.

Geysen, H.M., R.H. Meloen, and S.J. Barteling., 1984, Use of peptide synthesis to probe viral antigens for epitopes to a resolution of a single amino acid. *Proc. Natn. Acad. Sci. U.S.A.* 81:3998-4002.

De Groot, R.J., W. Luytjes, M.C. Horzinek, B.A.M. van der Zeijst, W.J.M. Spaan, and J.A. Lenstra., 1987a, Evidence for a coiled-coil structure in the spike proteins of coronaviruses. *J. Mol. Biol.* 196:963-966.

De Groot, R.J., J.A. Lenstra, W. Luytjes, H.G.M. Niesters, M.C. Horzinek, B.A.M. van der Zeijst, and W.J. Spaan., 1987b, Sequence and structure of the coronavirus peplomer protein. In: *Coronaviruses*, Adv. Exp. Med. Biol. 218, p.31-38, M.M.C. Lai and S.A. Stohlman ed., Plenum Press, New York/London.

Koch, G., L Hartog, A. Kant, D. Van Roozelaar, and G.F. De Boer., 1986, Antigenic differentiation of avian bronchitis virus variant strains employing monoclonal antibodies. *Isr. J. Ved. Med.* 42:89-97.

Koch, G., L Hartog, A. Kant, and D. Van Roozelaar., 1989, Antigenic domains on the peplomer protein of avian infectious bronchitis virus: correlation with biological functions. *J. gen. Virol.*, submitted.

Kusters, J.G., H.G.M. Niesters, J.A. Lenstra, M.C. Horzinek, and B.A.M. van der Zeijst., 1989a, Phylogeny of antigenic variants of avian coronavirus IBV. *Virology* 169:217-221.

Kusters, J.G., E.J. Jager, J.A. Lenstra, G. Koch, W.P.A. Posthumus, R.H. Meloen, and B.A.M. van der Zeijst., 1989b, Analysis of an immunodominant region of avian coronavirus IBV. *J. Immunol.* 143.

Kusters, J.G., E.J. Jager, and B.A.M. van der Zeijst., 1989c, Sequence evidence for in vivo recombination in avian coronavirus IBV. Submitted.

Lenstra, J.A., J.G. Kusters, G. Koch, and B.A.M. van der Zeijst., 1989, Antigenicity of the peplomer protein of infectious bronchitis virus. *Molec. Immun.* 26:7-15.

Luytjes, W., D. Geerts, W. Posthumus, R. Meloen, and W. Spaan., 1989, Amino acid sequence of a conserved neutralization epitope of murine coronaviruses. *J. Virol.* 63:1408-1412.

Posthumus, W.P.A., J.A. Lenstra, W.M.M. Schaaper, A.P.K.M.I. van Nieuwstadt, B.A.M. van der Zeijst, and R.H. Meloen., 1989, Antigenic peptides of the E2 peplomer protein of transmissible gastroenteritis virus. Submitted.

Rossmann, M.G., E. Arnold, J.W. Erickson, E.A. Frankenberger, J.P. Griffith, H.J. Hecht, J.E. Johnson, G. Kamer, M. Luo, A.G. Mosser, R.R. Rueckert, B. Sherry, and G. Vriend., 1985, Structure of a human common cold virus and functional relationship to other picornaviruses. *Nature* (London) 317:145-153.

Stanley, K.K. and J.P. Luzio., 1984, Construction of a new family of high efficiency bacterial expression vectors: identification of cDNA clones coding for human liver proteins. *EMBO J.* 3:1429-1434.

Talbot, P.J. and M.J. Buchmeier., 1985, Antigenic variation among murine coronaviruses: evidence for polymorphism on the peplomer glycoprotein, E2. *Virus Res.* 2:317-328.

Talbot, P.J., R.L. Knobler, and M.J. Buchmeier., 1984a, Western and dot immunoblotting analysis of viral antigens and antibodies: applications to murine hepatitis virus. *J. Immunol. Meth.* 73:177-188.

Talbot, P.J., A.A. Salmi, R.L. Knobler, and M.J. Buchmeier., 1984b, Topographic mapping of epitopes on the glycoproteins of murine hepatitis virus-4 (strain JHM): correlation with biological activities. *Virology* 132:250-260.

Van Nieuwstadt, A.P., J. Boonstra, and J. Cornelissen., 1989, Differentiation between transmissible gastroenteritis virus and the related porcine respiratory coronavirus using monoclonal antibodies against transmissible gastroenterites virus. *J.Virol.*, in press.

Westhoff, E., D. Altschuh, D. Moras, A.C. Bloomer, A. Mondragon, A.A. Klug, and H.M.V. Van Regenmortel., 1984, Correlation between segmental mobility and the location of antigenic determinants in proteins. *Nature* (London) 311:123-126.

THE NUCLEOCAPSID PROTEIN OF IBV COMPRISES IMMUNODOMINANT

DETERMINANTS RECOGNIZED BY T-CELLS

Annemieke M. H. Boots, Johannes G. Kusters,
Bernard A. M. van der Zeijst and Evert J. Hensen

Institute of Infectious Diseases and Immunology
Fac. of Vet. Medicine, University of Utrecht, P.O.
Box 80.165, 3508 TD Utrecht, The Netherlands

INTRODUCTION

Infectious bronchitis virus (IBV), the type species of
the coronaviridae, is the causative agent of an acute
respiratory disease in chickens. The positive stranded RNA
genome of IBV encodes three major structural proteins: two N-
glycosylated envelope proteins, E1 and E2, and a non-
glycosylated nucleocapsid protein (N). The E2 protein, or
spike protein, consists of two or more copies of structurally
unrelated subunits (S1 and S2) with relative molecular masses
of 90 and 84 kd, respectively. The E1 protein, or matrix
protein, occurs in several forms (27 to 36 kd). The
phosphorylated basic nucleoprotein (56 kd) is closely
associated with the viral RNA.

IBV strains show a wide spectrum of serologically defined
differences. Based on cross neutralization studies, the Dutch
IBV strains have been classified into five different serotypes
(A to E)[3]. The occurrence of these serotypes and, more
specifically, the emergence of new serotypes are a problem in
vaccination programs[3].

A vaccine, should ensure reactivation of the immune
response at time of challenge. Therefore it should contain
virus-specific antigenic determinants recognized by T-cells in
addition to determinants recognized by B-cells. Thus, to study
protective immunity against the virus both T- and B-cell
responses have to be analyzed. So far, a number of
conformation independent B-cell epitopes have been precisely
located on the E2 protein[5]. To our knowledge, no data are
available on the contribution of T-cells in the response to
IBV. This study is focused on the characterization of
antigenic determinants recognized by T-cells.

MATERIALS AND METHODS

Virus strains

All strains, unless otherwise mentioned, were obtained
from the Poultry Health Institute in Doorn, The Netherlands.
Strains and serotypes are summarized in Table I. New Castle

disease virus (NCDV) was used as a control virus. All virus stocks were obtained by gradient-purification of egg-grown virus as described by Niesters et al.[7]. The M42 laboratory strain[13] was grown on Vero cells (m.o.i. 0.1) and the supernatant of the infected cells was harvested after 36 hours. Gradient-purified mouse hepatitis virus (MHV) strain A59 and Feline infectious peritonitis virus (FIPV) strain 79-1146 were kindly donated by Dr. W. Spaan (University of Utrecht, Utrecht, The Netherlands). Gradient-purified transmissible gastro-enteritis virus TGEV strain Purdue-46 was kindly donated by Dr. L. Enjuanes (Centro di Biologica Molecular, Madrid, Spain).

Generation of IBV specific T-cell hybridomas

Two Balb/c mice, 6 to 8 weeks old, were immunized intraperitoneally with a gradient-purified UV-inactivated M41 preparation (100 ug mixed with RIBI; Immunochemical Research, Inc. Hamilton, USA) Three weeks later the mice were boosted (100 ug M41 +RIBI). Six weeks thereafter the mice were killed to obtain the spleens. Spleen cells ($2x10^6$/ml) were weekly restimulated with antigen (M41 4ug/ml) in the presence of syngeneic spleen cells as antigen presenting cells (APCs) to generate responding T-cells. Three days after the last stimulation with antigen the remaining viable cells (10^7) of this T-cell line were fused with an equal number of cells from a T-cell lymphoma line, (W/Fu(C58NT)D[2.10.14]. After fusion, cells were plated in flat-bottomed microtiter plates; $5x10^4$ cells /well in 200 ul HAT selection medium (15% fetal calf serum Boehringer, Mannheim). Within 14-28 days, growth positive wells were scored and hybrid cells were cultured in HT medium (without aminopterine). Hybrids responsive to M41 were repeatedly subcloned to ensure monoclonality.

Selection and characterization of IBV specific hybridomas

Hybridomas were screened for their ability to produce IL-2 in the presence of antigen and APCs. Hybrid cells (10^4/well) were cultured in 200 ul of medium in flat-bottomed microtiter plates with $2x10^5$ irradiated (2500 rad) APCs per well and 0.5-1.0 ug UV-inactivated M41 antigen. After 24 to 48 h, 100 ul of the supernatant of this culture was harvested and assayed for IL-2 by the addition of $5x10^3$-10^4 IL-2-dependent CTLL cells. After a further 24 h, ^{3}H-thymidine (0.4 uCi/well, SA 1.0 Ci/mmol) was added and the incorporated radioactivity was measured 18 h later. Results are presented as counts per minute (c.p.m.) and/or stimulation indices (SI = antigen specific c.p.m. / control c.p.m.).

IBV specific hybridomas (MJB100 and MJB101), and control: C58 (fusion partner) were tested for the expression of L3T4 (CD4) and Ly 2 (CD8). Monoclonal antibodies from Becton Dickinson (California, USA): anti-L3T4 phycoerytrine conjugate and anti Ly 2 conjugated to FITC were used in a direct staining protocol. Cells (10^6) were incubated in a 1:50 dilution of the antibody conjugates for 30 min. at 4 °C., washed 3 times and analyzed with the FACSCAN (Becton Dickinson).

Construction of the IBV nucleocapsid pEX clone

In the pEX expression system, foreign gene fragments are inserted at the end of a cro-Lac Z expression vector[12]. Expression of the gene is under control of the lambda P_R promotor and induced by activation of the temperature

sensitive cI857 repressor at 42 °C. The resulting hybrid
protein containing the expression product precipitates inside
the cell. After solubilization it can be easily isolated.

The DNA encoding the nucleocapsid protein was isolated
from the IBV M41 cDNA library described by Niesters[7]. E. coli
pop 2136 was used as host strain for the pEX plasmids.
Recombinant plasmids were introduced into the cells via the
CaCl$_2$ transformation procedure. Recombinants were screened by
polyacrylamide gel electrophoresis of their expression
products. Clones synthesizing hybrid proteins of the expected
molecular weight were selected for further characterization.
Plasmid DNA isolated from these clones was digested with
various restriction enzymes and the insert sizes were
determined as additional controls. Clones of interest were
grown to isolate the hybrid protein containing the IBV
nucleocapsid protein sequences.

Immunogenicity of the pEX hybrid protein

Balb/c mice were immunized, subcutaneously, in the
axillary region, with a mixture of dimethyl dioctadecyl
ammonium bromide[11] (DDA, Kodak, 25 ug per immunization site)
and 0.25 ug of the nucleocapsid expression product. Six days
later the regional lymphnodes were isolated. Lymphnode cells
(10^4-$5x10^4$) were co-cultured with antigen (UV-inactivated
whole virus; M41, M42 or TGEV: 0.5-1.0 ug/well) in round-
bottomed microtiter plates over 3 to 4 days. Lymphocyte
proliferation was measured after the addition of ^{3}H-thymidine
(18 h).

Results

Selection and characterization of IBV-specific T-cell hybridomas

After fusion, 384 wells were seeded and within 4 weeks 28
wells contained hybridomas. Two of these 28 showed an antigen-
specific IL-2 response in the CTLL assay (SI values of 2.5).
These hybridomas, MJB100 and MJB101, were subcloned. The
positive subclones exhibited drastically increased IL-2
production upon antigenic stimulation with SI values of 25-27.
The hybridomas were specific for IBV (Fig. 1). Both IBV
strains, M41, the original antigen, and M42, a closely related
strain, induced a response. No response was found after
stimulation with uninfected allantoic fluid, the non-related
NCDV (grown and purified in the same way as M41), murine
coronavirus (MHV strain A59), feline coronavirus (FIPV) or
porcine coronavirus (TGEV).

Twelve well-characterized IBV strains with different
serotypes were tested for their capacity to induce an antigen-
specific response in both hybridomas. The results are shown in
Table I. MJB100 clearly recognized strains M41, M42, H52, H120
(all serotype A), strains V1259, V1385 (unidentified serotype)
strain V1397 (serotype A/C) and strain D3128 (serotype D). The
isolates D207 (B), D274 (B/E), D212 (C) and D1466 (C) were not
recognized. MJB101, compared to MJB100, shows a different
reaction pattern in both intensity and specificity. IBV
strains recognized by MJB101 are M41, M42, H52, V1259, V1385
and strain D3128.

The response of the two T-cell hybridomas was MHC-
restricted; only APCs from syngeneic mice were capable of
inducing the response (not shown).

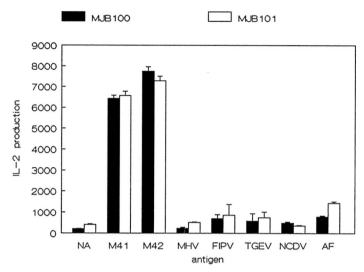

Fig. 1. IBV specific IL-2 response of T-cell hybridomas MJB100 and MJB101. Antigens were used at a concentration of 1 ug/well.
NA: no antigen. AF: allantoic fluid. NCDV: New Castle disease virus. MHV: mouse hepatitis virus. FIPV: feline infectious peritonitis virus. TGEV: transmissible gastroenteritis virus.

Table 1. IL-2 response (in SI) of MJB100 and MJB101 to several IBV strains with different serotypes. Approximately one ug of antigen per well was used. Passage history and serotype of IBV strains have been described[3].

| IBV strain | SI values of | | serotype |
	MJB100	MJB101	
M41	53.6	52.6	A
M42	53.3	46.3	A
H52	32.0	18.1	A
H120	6.0	$\pm$ 1.0	A
V1259	35.9	20.0	?
V1385	29.8	10.4	?
V1397	12.4	$\pm$ 1.0	A/C
D207	$\pm$ 1.0	$\pm$ 1.0	B
D274	$\pm$ 1.0	$\pm$ 1.0	B/E
D212	$\pm$ 1.0	$\pm$ 1.0	C
D1466	$\pm$ 1.0	$\pm$ 1.0	C
D3128	16.0	10.5	D

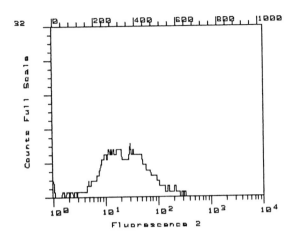

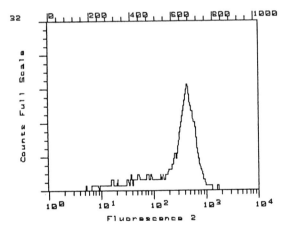

Fig. 2. FACS profile of MJB100 (upper) and MJB101 (lower) after staining with the anti-CD4 antibody (fluorescence 2).

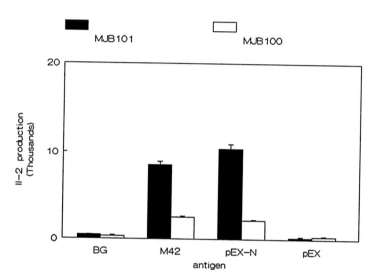

Fig. 3. IL-2 response of MJB100 and MJB101 to IBV strain M42,
the pEX nucleocapsid protein expression-product (pEX-N) and to
the bacterial beta-galactosidase protein (pEX expression
protein without insert). One ug of antigen per well was used.
BG: no antigen.

FACS analysis showed that MJB100 and MJB101 cells stained with the anti CD4 (T-helper) monoclonal antibody (Fig. 2), whereas the C58 and 2C4E9 cell lines were negative for CD4.

Specificity of MJB100 and MJB101

We determined which of the IBV structural components was recognized by the T-cell hybridomas. Initially, we fractionated the virus and thereafter purified the individual structural components. It appeared that both hybridomas were responsive to the nucleocapsid protein of IBV. Therefore, we cloned the gene encoding the nucleocapsid protein into pEX and the expression product was tested for the induction of an antigen-specific IL-2 response in both T-cell hybridomas. MJB100 and MJB101 were both responsive to the expression product but not to the bacterial beta-galactosidase (Fig. 3).

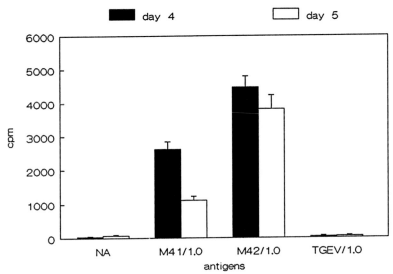

Fig. 4. Lymphocyte proliferative response of lymphnode cells after immunization with the nucleocapsid expression protein. Proliferation measured at day 4 and 5 after isolation of lymphnode cells is shown. One ug per well of the following antigens was used. IBV (M41, M42) and TGEV. NA: no antigen.

Immunogenicity of the pEX expression product

After immunization with the pEX nucleocapsid expression product the lymphocyte proliferation test showed a response to IBV strain M41 and M42 (gradient-purified) over two consecutive days. No stimulation was found with TGEV (Fig. 4).

Immunization with peplomer protein pEX fragments[5] showed no induction of cellular immune responses in the lymphocyte proliferation test.

DISCUSSION

It is generally accepted that for the induction of B-cell responses, e.g. antibody production, T-helper cell responses are obligatory. At time of challenge, viral glycoprotein fragments comprising virus neutralizing determinants have to be recognized in the presence of relevant, virus-specific, determinants recognized by T-cells. For that reason antigenic determinants eliciting cellular immune responses have to be studied. Until now, cellular immune responses to avian coronavirus have been neglected and no data are available on the role of T-cells in the response to IBV. In this paper we describe two T-cell hybridomas with specificity for IBV, generated from a mouse T-cell line which had been repeatedly stimulated in vitro. After fractionation of the virus and thereafter purification of the individual structural proteins, T-hybridoma reactivity appeared to be directed at the nucleocapsid protein. This was proven after cloning this protein into the expression vector pEX.

After repetitive stimulation in vitro with whole virus antigen it appeared that, in the conditions used, the "immunodominant" determinants recognized by T-cells were located on the nucleocapsid protein. Further evidence for the presence of determinants recognized by T-cells was found after immunization with the expression product. Strong cellular immune responses to the whole virus antigen could be induced. Earlier immunizations with peplomer protein pEX expression products did not show elevated responses to whole virus antigen in the lymphocyte stimulation test. Findings in other viral model systems, e.g. influenza, hepatitis B and rabies virus, have shown also that the immune system deals with the viral particle as a physical entity[1,4,6,8,9]. In the studies mentioned, strong primary cellular immune responses to the viral core protein ensured adequate antibody responses to several viral surface proteins when challenged. The elegant studies of Milich et al.[6] have given insight into the mechanism of protection induction. A peptide of the hepatitis B virus core antigen (p120-140) comprising only one determinant recognized by T-cells was capable of priming T-helper cells. After administration of the whole virus, antibody production to several hepatitis B surface proteins was shown.

Early observations have shown that protection to IBV in chickens could be induced after immunization and challenge with heterologous IBV strains[15]. The strains which induced cross protection belong to the so-called protectotypes. Our finding of T-cell reactivity to strains of different serotype indicates a sharing of antigenic determinants recognized by T-cells among IBV strains and could be the basis of protection by protectotypes.

This study suggests that antigenic determinants of the nucleocapsid protein might be necessary components for the induction of an adequate protective immune response.

ACKNOWLEDGEMENTS

We would like to thank Drs. P. Breedenbeek (University of Utrecht, Utrecht, The Netherlands) for isolation of the nucleocapsid gene from the cDNA library.

LITERATURE

1. B. Dietzschold, H. Wang, C. E. Rupprecht, E. Celis, M. Tollis, H. Ertl, E. Heber-Katz and H. Koprowski. 1987. Induction of protective immunity against rabies by immunisation with rabies virus ribonucleoprotein. Proc. Natl. Acad. Sci. USA 84, 9165-9169.

2. S. Fazekas de St. Groth, and D. Scheidegger. 1980. Production of monoclonal antibodies stratology and tactics. J. Immunol. Meth. 35, 1.

3. J. G. Kusters, H. G. M. Niesters, N. M. C. Bleumink-Pluym, F. G. Davelaar, M. C. Horzinek and B. A. M. van der Zeijst. 1987. Molecular epidemiology of infectious bronchitis virus in the Netherlands. J. gen. Virol. 68, 343-352.

4. J. R. Lamb, J. N. Woody, R. J. Hartzman and D. C. Eckels. 1982. In vitro influenza-specific antibody production in man: antigen specific and HLA-restricted induction of helper activity mediated by cloned human T-lymphocytes. J. Immunol. 129, 1465-1470.

5. J. A. Lenstra, J. G. Kusters, G. Koch and B. A. M. van der Zeijst. 1989. Antigenicity of the peplomer proteins of infectious bronchitis virus. Mol. Immunol. 1, 7-15.

6. D. R. Milich, A. McLachlan, G. B. Thornton and J. L. Hughes. 1987. Antibody production to the nucleocapsid and envelope of the hepatitis B virus primed by a single synthetic T-cell site. Nature 329, 547-549.

7. H. G. M. Niesters, J. A. Lenstra, W. J. M. Spaan, A. J. Zijderveld, N. M. Bleumink Pluym, F. Hong, G. J. M. van Scharrenburg, M. C. Horzinek and B. A. M. van der Zeijst. 1986. The peplomer protein sequence of the M41 strain of Coronavirus IBV and its comparison with Beaudette strains. Virus Res. 5, 253-263.

8. S. M. Russell, and F. Y. Liew. 1979. T-cells primed by influenza virion internal components can cooperate in the antibody response to heamagglutinin. Nature 280, 147-148.

9. P. A. Scherle, and W. Gerhard. 1988. Differential ability of B cells specific for external vs. internal influenza virus proteins to respond to help from influenza virus specific T-cell clones in vivo. Proc. Natl. Acad. Sci. USA 85, 4446-4450.

10. A. Silva, H. R. MacDonald, A. Conzelmann, P. Corthesy and M. Nabholz. 1983. Rat X Mouse T-cell hybrids with inducible specific cytolytic activity. Immunol. Rev. 76, 105-129.

11. R. H. Smith, and B. Ziola. 1986. Cyclophosphamide and dimethyl dioctadecyl ammonium bromide immuno-potentiate the delayed type hypersensitivity response to inactivated enveloped viruses. Immunol. 58, 245-250.

12. K. K. Stanley, and J. P. Luzio. 1984. EMBO J. 3, 1429-1434.

13. D. F. Stern, and B. M. Sefton. 1984. Coronavirus multiplication: locations of genes for virion proteins on the avian infectious bronchitis virus genome. J. Virol. 50, 22-29.

14. W. van Eden, A. Noordzij, E. J. Hensen, R. van der Zee, J. D. A van Embden and R. Meloen. 1989. A modified method for the rapid identification and characterization of T-cell epitopes in protein antigens. Modern approaches to new vaccines including prevention of AIDS. Cold Spring Harbor Laboratory, Cold Spring Harbor 33-36.

15. R. W. Winterfield, and A. M. Fadly. 1972. Some characteristics of isolates of infectious bronchitis virus from commercial vaccines. Avian Dis. 16, 746-755.

Chapter 4

Expression and Immunogenicity
of the Structural Proteins

BACKGROUND PAPER

PROGRESS TOWARDS A CORONAVIRUS RECOMBINANT DNA VACCINE

Willy J.M. Spaan

Institute of Infectious Diseases and Immunology
Department of Virology
Veterinary Faculty
State University of Utrecht
The Netherlands

During the last decade recombinant DNA technology has been successfully applied to the development of 'new' vaccines. Although there are many examples of successful vaccines which have been developed using the 'classical approach' e.g. inactivated, attenuated and subunit vaccines, the demand for a new generation of vaccines is evident. The risk of the escape of a pathogen from a vaccine production facility, the difficulties associated with the production of viral subunits, the high mutation frequency observed in many RNA viruses and the possibility of genetic reassortment and recombination have stimulated researchers to explore new avenues of vaccine biotechnology.

With the cDNA cloning of several genes this approach has now also become feasable for coronaviruses. The aim of this chapter is to summarize recent advances towards the development of recombinant DNA vaccines against coronavirus induced diseases.

Which antigens should be chosen for the development of (bio)synthetic vaccines? Coronaviruses possess three major structural proteins: a nucleocapsid protein (N), a small integral membrane glycoprotein (M) and a large spike glycoprotein (S). While all coronaviruses contain these proteins, a subset (the MHV strains JHM and S, HEV, HCV-OC43 and BCV) is now recognized to possess an additional glycopolypeptide (gp65 or HE) which is unrelated to S or M. The candidate antigen for a vaccine is often predicted on the basis of *in vitro* neutralization assays and passive transfer of antibodies followed by a virus challenge. However, a detailed understanding of both the humoral and cellular immune response in the natural disease is necessary to select the most effective antigen.

S and HE induce virus neutralizing antibody and in addition some anti-M antibodies neutralize virus in the presence of complement. The M protein of TGEV not only induces antibody which neutralizes in the presence of complement, but also induces the release of interferon by peripheral blood lymphocytes. Two anti-M MAbs were able to inhibit this induction.

Does *in vitro* neutralizing activity correlate with protection? Passive transfer of Mabs to animals followed by a challenge infection can give additional information on immune status. Some anti-M Mabs and anti-S MAbs, and a non-neutralizing anti-N Mab, were able to passively protect mice against lethal challenge. Complement does not play a role *in vivo* during protection mediated by passive transfer of an anti-M Mab since mice deficient in the C5 complement component were also protected and depletion of the C3 component did not affect the protective activity of this Mab.

A few attempts to protect animals using purified antigens from whole virus have been reported, but with limited success. Mice which had been inoculated intraperitoneally with purified S, but not N or M, from MHV-3 were protected from lethal challenge. The low level of protection induced by inactivated IBV was abolished after the removal of Sl by urea treatment. A subunit, with a M_r of approximately 25K released from TGEV by sonication induced neutralising antibodies in pigs. This material protected against challenge with virulent TGEV and induced antibody in gilts which, when transferred to suckling offspring, resulted in reduced morbidity and mortality after challenge. Further characterization of the 25K entity has not been published.

Thus there is substantial evidence that the S protein can evoke a protective immune response. However in the case of feline infectious peritonitis (FIP), which is a progressive debilitating condition affecting domestic and wild Felidae, one must also consider the fact that S can induce a severe immunological reaction. The presence of antibody directed against FIP proteins often leads to an accelerated, fulminating course of the disease, i.e. clinical signs and lesions develop earlier and the mean survival time is significantly reduced ('early death'). These findings may be explained by antibody dependent enhancement (ADE) of virus infection, a phenomenon previously described for representatives of the flaviviridae, alphaviridae, bunyaviridae, poxviridae, rhabdoviridae, herpesviridae and reoviridae. Binding of antibody results in the formation of infectious virus-antibody complexes, which attach to the surface of the macrophage (via Fc-receptors) with higher efficiency than virus without antibody. Experimental evidence has recently been obtained that this mechanism is also involved in FIP. In a recent comparison of feline coronaviruses it was shown that virulent strains infect more macrophages, producing higher titers, and spread more readily to other macrophages; in addition, their infectivity was enhanced by antibody from sensitized cats (Stoddart 1988, personal communication). Immune enhancement is central to FIP pathogenesis and is due to anti-peplomer responses, as has been proven *in vivo* with the aid of a vaccinia virus recombinant (see article by Vennema *et al.*).

Research towards a recombinant DNA coronaviral vaccine is now conducted in several laboratories. Delineation of B-cell epitopes (see article by Laude *et al.*) and possibly in the near future also of T-cell epitopes will form the basis for the development of synthetic peptide, antigen and chimeric viral vaccines. The latter approach in which an epitope is genetically engineered into a carrier protein or carrier particle looks especially promising since the immunogenicity of these antigens is much better than a synthetic peptide chemically coupled to a carrier protein. Vaccination with synthetic peptides homologous to residue 993-1002 and 848-856 of the MHV S protein protected mice against lethal coronavirus-induced encephalitis. Although domain 848-856 of S of MHV binds to one neutralizing Mab, antibodies raised against the synthetic peptide did not neutralize MHV *in vitro*. Hence, protection against disease does not correlate with *in vitro* neutralization.

Mapping of B-cell epitopes and strain comparison on the level of the amino acid sequence of field isolates will also provide necessary data concerning antigenic variation. Immunological escape due to point mutations and/or recombination will certainly hamper the development of a vaccine against IBV. This problem may be solved by the identification of conserved B and T-cell epitopes.

A wide variety of expression systems have been developed for the production of antigens. Since the coronavirus spike gene encodes a highly glycosylated protein, eucaryotic expression systems have to be used to obtain recombinant protein that closely resembles the viral protein. Recombinant FIPV S protein isolated from a transformed mouse fibroblast cell line which was obtained after transfection with a bovine papilloma virus expression vector expressing the FIPV S gene under the control of the heat shock promoter, was fusogenic and induced neutralizing antibodies in mice. Experiments using virus-based transient expression systems like baculovirus recombinants (production in insect cells) and vaccinia virus recombinants (production in mammalian cells) are in progress, and some of the data are presented in other chapters (Taguchi *et al.*; Vennema *et al.*; Parker *et al.*).

The application of vectored live virus vaccines has been limited to vaccinia virus. Vaccinia virus recombinants expressing the IBV and FIPV S gene evoke an *in vitro* neutralizing immune response in chickens and kittens, respectively. The immunized chickens were only partially protected (50%), whereas immunized kittens became sensitized (see above). Future research will focus on the use of DNA carrier viruses with a narrow host range e.g. fowlpox for protection against IBV, canine adenovirus for protection against canine coronavirus and feline herpesvirus for the protection against FIPV. Often a long-lasting immunity can only be achieved using a live attenuated virus vaccine. The main reason is that replicating immunogens evoke a broad spectrum of immune responses including local immunity. However, because of genetic instability the vaccine virus can regain virulence. The genetic stability of attenuated vaccines can possibly be increased by deletion mutagenesis. For RNA viruses this approach is only possible if an infectious cDNA clone is available and will certainly be an important area of future coronavirus research.

PROTECTION OF MICE FROM LETHAL CORONAVIRUS MHV-A59 INFECTION

BY MONOCLONAL AFFINITY-PURIFIED SPIKE GLYCOPROTEIN

Claude Daniel and Pierre J. Talbot

Virology Research Center
Institut Armand-Frappier, Université du Québec
531, boulevard des Prairies
Laval, Québec, CANADA H7N 4Z3

ABSTRACT

Numerous studies have provided indirect evidence that the spike glycoprotein of coronaviruses (E2 or S) bears determinants for pathogenesis and the induction of protective immunity. In order to directly evaluate its immunogenicity, the E2 glycoprotein of the murine hepatitis virus, strain A59, was purified by immunoaffinity chromatography. High titers of neutralizing and fusion inhibiting antibodies were induced in mice vaccinated with purified E2/S in Freund's adjuvant, which were protected from an intracerebral challenge with 10 LD_{50} of MHV-A59. This study provides a direct demonstration of the importance of the coronavirus spike glycoprotein in the induction of a protective immune response.

INTRODUCTION

The E2/S glycoprotein, which contitutes the characteristic surface projections (spike or peplomer) of the coronaviruses, mediates many of the biological properties of the virus. Indeed, attachment of murine hepatitis virus (MHV) to cell receptor[1] and spread of infection by virus-induced cell to cell fusion, which is activated by cleavage of the whole glycoprotein (180 kDa) into two subunits of 90 kDa[2], have been related to E2/S.

Several studies have also demonstrated indirectly the importance of E2/S in antiviral immunity, such as in the production of virus-neutralizing complement-independent antibodies[1,3,4,5], as a target for passive antibody protection[3,6] and in cell-mediated immunity[7,8]. Recently, neutralizing antibodies and protection were induced by immunization with a synthetic decapeptide of E2/S[9]. In order to directly evaluate the involvement of the whole glycoprotein in a protective immune response against murine coronaviruses, the MHV-A59 E2/S glycoprotein was purified by affinity chromatography and its immunogenicity ascertained in mice.

METHODS

Cells and virus

The A59 strain of MHV (MHV-A59), obtained from the American Type Culture Collection (Rockville, MD, U.S.A.), was plaque-purified twice and passaged four times at a multiplicity of infection (MOI) of 0.01 on DBT cells[10].

Antigen preparation

Virus was produced as described previously[10] in culture medium containing 1% (v/v) FCS. DBT cell monolayers were infected with MHV-A59 at an MOI of 0.01 and medium was harvested 16 hrs post-infection. Cell debris were pelleted and virus concentrated by precipitation with 10% (w/v) polyethyleneglycol in 0.5 M NaCl. Viral antigens were resuspended and dialyzed against TMEN buffer (0.1 M Tris-acid-maleate, pH 6.2, 0.1 M NaCl, 1 mM EDTA), and kept at -70°C until used. In some experiments, virus was labeled by adding 4 mCi of $[^{35}S]$methionine (ICN Biochemicals Canada, Ville St-Laurent, PQ, Canada) to culture medium at 6 hrs post-infection.

Affinity chromatography

The E2/S-immunoadsorbent was prepared by coupling five milligrams of purified MAb 7-10A[11] to 1 g of CNBr-activated Sepharose 4B (Pharmacia, Dorval, PQ, Canada), all steps performed according to manufacturer's instructions. For affinity chromatography, concentrated virus was solubilized with 2% (v/v) Nonidet P-40 (NP-40) for 2 hrs at room temperature (RT), and soluble proteins were mixed with the 7-10A-Sepharose gel and incubated end-over-end for 16 hrs at 4°C. The gel specificity was determined by immuno-adsorption of radiolabeled antigen, extensive washing with 0.1% (v/v) NP-40 (in 0.2 M phosphate buffer, pH 6.2, 0.1 M NaCl, 1mM EDTA), and elution of adsorbed proteins into electrophoresis sample buffer. Otherwise, the gel was poured into a column and washed until the absorbance at 280 nm had dropped to baseline level, after which the column was washed with 4 gel volumes of the same buffer containing 0.1% (w/v) of octylglucoside for detergent replacement. Elution was carried out by adding 3 M ammonium isothiocyanate to the latter solution. Fractions of 1 ml were collected and dialyzed against 0.05 M ammonium bicarbonate, pH 7.4. A sample of each fraction was lyophilized, resuspended in electrophoresis sample buffer, and analyzed on a 7-15% linear polyacrylamide gel, prior to fluorography with Enlightning® (Dupont Canada, Lachine, PQ, Canada) for radiolabeled antigen or silver staining[12]. Fractions containing purified E2/S were pooled and used for immunological studies.

Immunization experiments

Eight MHV-seronegative female 6-week-old BALB/c mice were inoculated intraperitoneally with approximately 1 µg of purified E2/S, or an equivalent volume of TMEN, emulsified in complete (day 0) or incomplete (day 25) Freund's adjuvant. At day 40, immunized and control mice were given an intracerebral (i.c.) challenge with 10 LD_{50} of MHV-A59 (5×10^5 PFU). Mice were bled from the retroorbital plexus with heparinized capillary tubes on days 0, 25, and 40, and these plasma samples were analyzed for their ability to neutralize either 50-100 PFU or 30-300 $TCID_{50}$ of MHV-A59, in which residual infectivity was assayed by either a plaque assay[10] or CPE assay[11], respectively. In the latter assay, neutralizing titers were evaluated by the method of Karber. The capacity of plasma samples to prevent the formation of syncytia was also assayed[11].

RESULTS AND DISCUSSION

Production and characterization of anti-E2/S MAbs

Two cloned hybridoma lines, named 7-10A and 4-11G, which secreted anti-E2/S monoclonal antibodies (MAbs) were obtained and selected for further study[11]. Their specificity was determined by immunoprecipitation, in which they showed reaction with the 180 kDa form of E2/S. These MAbs were also able to neutralize virus infectivity and virus-induced cell-to-cell fusion *in vitro* , and passively protect mice *in vivo*. Epitopes recognized by both MAbs are overlapping, as shown by partial reciprocal competition between these MAbs in ELISA[11]. Furthermore, these epitopes were shown to be conformational by the loss of reaction of corresponding MAbs with viral antigen after denaturation by SDS (Table

1). However, they were differently sensitive to denaturation by the chaotropic agent ammonium isothiocyanate, as shown by the different reactivity of each determinant in dot blots after treatment of viral antigen with this agent (Table 1). These results demonstrated that a conformational antigenic site may be formed of various structures in which different molecular interactions are involved. Since the chaotropic salts act mainly on hydrophobic bonds[13,14], this type of interaction seems therefore essential to the 7-10A epitope conformation.

Table 1. Sensitivity of two E2/S epitopes to protein denaturation

Antigen treatment	MAb reactivity	
	4-11G	7-10A
NP-40[a]	+	+
NH4SCN[b]	+	-
SDS[c]	-	-

[a] Concentrated viral antigen solubilized with 2% (v/v) NP-40 for 2 hrs at RT.
[b] Treated with 4 M NH4SCN for 5 min at RT.
[c] Treated with 1% (w/v) SDS for 2 min at 100°C.

Evaluation of the immunoadsorbent specificity

The specificity of the 7-10A-Sepharose gel was determined by immunoprecipitation of [^{35}S]methionine-labeled antigen. Figure 1 shows the electrophoretic profile of the proteins specifically retained on the gel, which reacted specifically with the dimeric form of the E2/S glycoprotein (180 kDa). The purity of this protein, evaluated by densitometry, was estimated to be 87%.

Moreover, two polypeptides of molecular masses of 87 and 96 kDa, which could be monomeric forms of E2/S, were also reproducibly observed in immunoadsorption and purification experiments. Ricard et. al.[15] have showed that cleavage of E2/S, through virion maturation, results in the production of two subunits which both had a molecular mass of 90 kDa. The sizes that we observed for these subunits could correlate to those estimated from the nucleotide sequence of the MHV-A59 E2/S gene[16]. From this sequence, the molecular mass estimates for the subunits are 66 and 79.8 kDa, both derived from an apoprotein of 146 kDa. If the remaining 34 kDa of carbohydrates residues are added equivalently to each subunit, which both possess 10 potential N-glycosylation sites, the subunits obtained should have molecular masses of 83 and 97 kDa, which is consistent with those obtained in our experiments. The use of gradient gels may have allowed the separation of closely migrating species, such as E2/S monomers. It is also possible that these different subunits have arisen from a glycosylation pattern different in DBT cells than in L2 cells, the cell substratum used in these previous studies.

Purification and immunogenicity of E2/S glycoprotein

The E2/S glycoprotein used for immunogenicity studies was purified from viral antigens concentrated from 1.8 liters of culture medium from MHV-A59-infected DBT cells. Fractions eluted after immunoaffinity chromatography were analyzed by SDS-PAGE and silver staining. Figure 2 shows that the dimeric and monomeric forms of E2/S were purified without detectable contamination from other viral proteins. However, a contaminant (30 kDa), which was probably of cellular origin, was reproducibly observed. The purified glycoprotein was partially denatured, as confirmed by its loss of reactivity with the MAb 7-10A (data not shown).

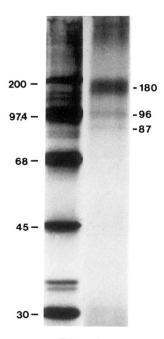

Fig. 1. Immunoadsorption of [^{35}S]methionine-labeled antigen on 7-10A-Sepharose gel. Lane M, molecular mass markers (kDa); Lane 1, proteins eluted from the affinity gel.

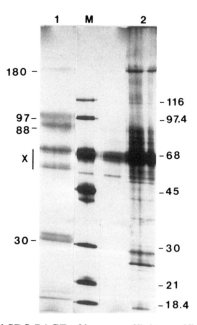

Fig. 2. Silver-stained SDS-PAGE of immunoaffinity-purified E2 glycoprotein. Lane M, molecular mass markers (kDa); Lane 1, proteins eluted from the affinity gel; Lane 2, antigen applied on gel. The unnumbered lane contains only PAGE sample buffer and shows some artefactual bands (X) reproducibly observed in our silver-stained reducing SDS-PAGE.

We also developed an antigen-capture ELISA specific to E2/S for evaluating the efficiency of the purification method. We found that one third of E2/S remained insoluble after treatment with NP-40. Increasing the NP-40 concentration to 4% (v/v) or adding 2% (w/v) sodium deoxycholate did not improve solubilization[11].

Plasma samples from mice immunized with purified E2/S or TMEN buffer were collected and pooled. Animals immunized with E2/S showed neutralizing titers of 1/1600 in plaque assay and 1/230 in CPE assay, whereas control mice showed titers less than 1/15 in both assays. These plasma samples were also able to inhibit the formation of syncytia by 50% at a dilution of 1/40. Moreover, the lack of competition between immune plasma samples and MAb 7-10A confirmed the denaturation of this epitope on purified E2/S, whereas the epitope recognized by MAb 4-11G was conserved, as showed by competition between immune plasma and this MAb[11].

Mice immunized with either E2/S or TMEN buffer were challenged i.c. with 10 LD_{50} of MHV-A59. Control mice died from MHV-A59 infection within five days, whereas all of the E2/S-immunized mice were protected. However, some clinical signs of infection (ruffled fur, apathy, hunched position) were initially observed in protected mice, which recovered a few days later.

The biological importance of the peplomer glycoprotein of coronaviruses in their biological activities, including interaction with the immune system, has been indirectly demonstrated by numerous studies, but few have reported direct evidence of it. The surface projections of MHV-3, purified by ultracentrifugation, were shown to protect mice against infection with the same virus[17]. Mockett[18] has also shown that affinity-purified spike glycoproteins of infectious bronchitis virus were able to induce neutralizing antibodies. Thus, our results confirm directly the biological importance of the peplomer protein in the immune response against a neurotropic murine coronavirus.

However, The E2/S glycoprotein should not be considered as the unique mediator of the anti-viral immune response. Recent studies have shown that the N protein[19] and the E1/M glycoprotein[20], which induced protective immunity, could also have some importance in the immune response against the virus and its pathogenicity. The relative contribution of these viral proteins and their *in vivo* interactions will therefore need to be clarified in order to better understand the molecular basis of coronavirus pathogenesis.

ACKNOWLEDGMENTS

This work was supported by grants UO-387 and MT-9203 to P.J. Talbot from the Natural Sciences and Engineering Research Council (NSERC) and the Medical Research Council of Canada (MRC), respectively. Studentship (C. Daniel) and scholarship (P. J. Talbot) support from NSERC is gratefully acknowledged. The authors thank the excellent technical assistance of Francine Lambert.

REFERENCES

1.   A. R. Collins, R. L. Knobler, H. Powell, and M. J. Buchmeier, Monoclonal antibodies to murine hepatitis virus-4 (strain JHM) define the viral glycoprotein responsible for attachment and cell-cell fusion, Virology 119: 358 (1982).

2.   L. S. Sturman, C. S. Ricard, and K. V. Holmes, Proteolytic cleavage of the E2 glycoprotein of murine coronavirus: activation of cell-fusing activity of virions by trypsin and separation of two different 90K cleavage fragments, J. Virol. 56: 904 (1985).

3.   H. Wege, D. Dorries, and H. Wege, Hybridoma antibodies to the murine coronavirus JHM: characterization of epitopes on the peplomer protein (E2), J. Gen. Virol. 65: 1931 (1984).

4.   P. J. Talbot, A. A. Salmi, R. L. Knobler, and M. J. Buchmeier, Topographical mapping of epitopes on the glycoproteins of murine hepatitis virus-4 (strain JHM): correlation with biological activities, Virology 132: 250 (1984).

5.   W. Gilmore, J. O. Fleming, S. A. Stohlman, and L. P. Weiner, Characterization of the structural proteins of the murine coronavirus strain A59 using monoclonal antibodies, Proc. Soc. Exp. Biol. Med. 185: 177 (1987).

6.   M. J. Buchmeier, H. A. Lewicki, P. J. Talbot, and R. L. Knobler, Murine hepatitis virus-4 (strain JHM)-induced neurologic disease is modulated *in vivo* by monoclonal antibody, Virology 132: 261 (1984).

7.   K. V. Holmes, R. M. Welsh, and M. V. Haspel, Natural cytotoxicity against mouse hepatitis virus-infected target cells. I. Correlation of cytotoxicity with virus binding to leucocytes, J. Immunol. 136: 1446 (1986).

8.   S. A. Stohlman, G. K. Matsushima, N. Casteel, and L. P. Weiner, *In vivo* effects of coronavirus-specific T cell clones: DTH inducer cells prevent a lethal infection but do not inhibit virus replication, J. Immunol. 136: 3052 (1986).

9.   P. J. Talbot, G. Dionne, and M. Lacroix, Vaccination against lethal coronavirus-induced encephalitis with a synthetic decapeptide homologous to a domain in the predicted peplomer stalk, J. Virol. 62: 3032 (1988).

10.   C. Daniel, and P. J. Talbot, Physico-chemical properties of mouse hepatitis virus, strain A59, Arch. Virol. 96: 241 (1987).

11.   C. Daniel, and P. J. Talbot, (submitted for publication, 1989).

12.   B. R. Oakley, D. R. Kirsh, and N. R. Morris, A simplified ultrasensitive silver stain for detecting proteins in polyacrylamide gels, Anal. Biochem. 105: 361 (1980).

13.   D. H. von Hippel, and K.- Y. Wong, Neutral salts: the generality of their effects on the stability of macro-molecular conformations, Science 145: 577 (1964).

14.   Y. Hatefi, and W. G. Hanstein, Solubilization of particulate proteins and non-electrolytes by chaotropic agents, Proc. Natl. Acad. Sci. USA 62: 1129 (1969).

15.   C. S. Ricard, and L. S. Sturman, Isolation of the subunits of the coronavirus envelope glycoprotein E2 by hydroxyapatite high-performance liquid chromatography, J. Chromato. 326: 191 (1985).

16.   W. Luytjes, L. S. Sturman, P. J. Bredenbeek, J. Charite, B. A. M. van der Zeijst, M. C. Horzinek, and W. J. M. Spaan, Primary structure of the glycoprotein E2 of coronavirus MHV-A59 and identification of the trypsin cleavage site, Virology 161: 479 (1987).

17.   H. J. Hasony, and M. R. Macnaughton, Antigenicity of mouse hepatitis virus strain 3 subcomponents in C57 strain mice, Arch. Virol. 69: 33 (1981).

18.   A. P. A. Mockett, Envelope proteins of avian infectious bronchitis virus: purification and biological properties, J. Virol. Methods 12: 271 (1985).

19.   J. Lecomte, V. Cainelli-Gebara, G. Mercier, S. Mansour, P. J. Talbot, G. Lussier, and D. Oth, Protection from mouse hepatitis virus type 3-induced acute disease by an anti-nucleoprotein monoclonal antibody, Arch .Virol. 97: 123 (1987).

20.   J. O. Fleming, R. A. Shubin, M. A. Sussman, N. Casteel, and S. A. Stohlman, Monoclonal antibodies to the matrix (E1) glycoprotein of mouse hepatitis virus protect mice from encephalitis, Virology 168: 162 (1989).

EXPRESSION OF THE SPIKE PROTEIN OF MURINE CORONAVIRUS JHM USING A BACULOVIRUS VECTOR

Fumihiro Taguchi[1] Sayaka Yoden[1], Stuart Siddell[2], and Tateki Kikuchi[1]

National Institute of Neuroscience, NCNP, 4-1-1
Ogawahigashi, Kodaira, Tokyo 187, Japan[1]
Institute of Virology, University of Würzburg, Versbacher strasse 7
8700 Würzburg, Federal Republic of Germany[2]

INTRODUCTION

Coronaviruses are enveloped RNA viruses with single positive stranded genomic RNA of approximately 32 kilobases which encodes at least 3 structural proteins; a nucleocapsid protein (N), a matrix glycoprotein (M) and a spike glycoprotein (S), as well as several non-structural proteins (1). The S protein forms the projecting spikes or peplomers on the surface of the virus particle (2). This protein is considered to be involved in the attachment of virus to susceptible cells, the induction of cell-to-cell fusion, and the induction of neutralizing antibodies (3,4). It is also believed that the S protein is important for determining the pathogenic potential of murine coronaviruses (5,6). For more detailed structural and functional analyses of S protein, we need to have large quantities of S protein uncontaminated with other viral proteins. For this purpose, we have sought to express the S gene product in a baculovirus expression vector. The *Autographa californica* nuclear polyhedrosis virus (AcNPV) insect baculovirus vector was chosen because of the high levels of foreign gene expression obtained using the AcNPV polyhedrin promoter (7). Also, translational modifications such as glycosylation, phosphorylation, and cleavage of the signal peptide are known to occur in this system. In this paper, we describe the expression of the MHV strain JHM (JHMV) S protein by recombinant baculovirus in insect cells, characterization of the protein and analysis of epitopes existing on the S protein.

RESULTS

Isolation of a recombinant baculovirus containing the JHMV S gene

To construct the baculovirus transfer vector containing the S gene of JHMV, the cDNA prepared from mRNA3 of JHMV (8) was inserted into the Bam H1 site of the transfer vector pAcYM1 (pAcYM1-S) in the correct orientation. Sequence analysis of the transfer vector has shown that the AUG codon of the S gene was located to be 75 bases downstream of the linker region. In order to obtain recombinant baculovirus containing the S gene, pAcYM1-S DNA and infectious AcNPV DNA were co-transfected into insect Sf cells as described previously (9). Plaques produced by the progeny viruses from the transfection were screened for a polyhedrin-negative phenotype as well as S protein production in Sf cells by immunofluorescence. Among 4 polyhedrin-negative clones, 3 were shown to be recombinant viruses, since they produced S protein in Sf cells.

Expression of the S protein by recombinant baculovirus in insect cells and characterization of the polypeptide

Firstly the time course of synthesis of S protein by the recombinant baculovirus was examined by ELISA. Extracts of Sf cells infected with the recombinant baculovirus 1 to 4 days before were adsorbed to microplates, and then the amount of expressed S protein was determined by anti-JHMV serum. As a control, wild-type AcNPV-infected cell extracts were employed. The results showed that immunoreactive S protein could be detected as early as two days post-infection and that the amount of S protein was maximal at three days post-infection. Radiolabelled S protein expressed in insect cells was initially detected at 24 hours post-infection, and its synthesis was still detectable at 72 hours post-infection.

The size of the protein expressed by recombinant baculovirus was determined in a pulse-label experiment (Fig. 1A). Sf cells infected with baculoviruses or mock-infected cells were labelled with ^{3}H-leucine for 30 min at 24 hours post-infection. Cell lysates were electrophoresed in SDS-polyacrylamide gels. As shown in Fig. 1A, the recombinant virus synthesized a protein that migrated with an estimated molecular weight of 150K, similar to that of the co-translationally glycosylated JHMV S protein synthesized in infected DBT cells. A protein of this molecular weight was not observed in cells infected with wild-type AcNPV or mock-infected Sf cells. The 150K protein was examined by immune precipitation with polyclonal anti-JHMV mouse serum. As shown in Fig. 1B, the 150K protein was precipitated from cells infected with the recombinant virus by anti-JHMV antibodies. As expected, the anti-JHMV serum also precipitated the 60K mol. wt. N protein synthesized in JHMV-infected cells (Fig. 1B). In wild-type AcNPV infected Sf cells, a strong band with a molecular weight of 33K was detected, which has been shown to be non-specifically precipitated polyhedrin protein resulting from incomplete solubilization of the occlusions in the immunoprecipitation buffer (Fig. 1B). These data indicate that a protein indistinguishable in terms of electrophoretic pattern from S protein produced in JHMV-infected DBT cells was produced by recombinant baculovirus in insect cells.

In order to determine whether carbohydrate chains were attached to S protein produced in insect cells, Sf cells infected with recombinant virus were treated with various concentration of tunicamycin and immunoprecipitated with anti-JHMV serum. As shown in Fig. 2, the molecular weight of the S protein expressed in the presence of 10 µg/ml of tunicamycin was reduced to approximately 130K, which was also observed in DBT cells infected with JHMV. These results indicated that glycosylation of S protein was carried out in insect cells after recombinant virus infection. To assess proteolytic cleavage of the S protein expressed in insect cells, Sf cells infected with the recombinant virus were pulse-chase labelled with ^{3}H-leucine and cell lysates were immunoprecipitated with anti-JHMV serum. Although cleavage of the S protein produced in mouse cells infected by JHMV occurs within 180 minutes, no cleavage products were detected in the insect cells during a 4-hour chase. The localisation of the S protein expressed in insect cells was studied by immunofluorescence. Sf cells were infected with the recombinant virus and 3 days later, cells were fixed with acetone. The fixed cells were incubated with anti-JHMV antibodies and stained with FITC-conjugated anti-mouse IgG. The S protein expressed in insect cells could be localized on the cell surface. No JHMV-related antigen was detected within the AcNPV-infected cells or mock-infected cells. The surface location of the S protein found in cells infected with the recombinant virus was confirmed by immunofluorescence using unfixed cells.

Production and characterisation of antisera to expressed S protein in rats

To see whether the S protein produced by the recombinant baculovirus elicited antibodies, rats and mice were immunized with sucrose gradient-purified material. A lysate of Sf cells infected with recombinant baculovirus was loaded onto a 10 to 50% (w/w) sucrose gradient and centrifuged. The fractions with high ELISA titres were pooled; the pool was shown to have an ELISA titre of 1:625 and a protein concentration of 3 mg/ml. Sera collected from the animals immunized with this material were serologically tested. Rats immunized with the S protein produced antibodies which reacted by immunoprecipitation with the S protein synthesized in DBT cells infected with JHMV (Fig. 3). In immunofluorescence DBT cells infected with JHMV were stained by the antisera. However in the plaque reduction assay the antisera failed to neutralize the infectivity of JHMV (neutralization titre <1:5). Since mice immunized with partially purified S protein did not produce detectable levels of antibodies against S protein in immunofluorescence or immunoprecipitation, alternative immunizations were carried out, i.e., immunization with the intact Sf cells carrying expressed S protein or the lysate of Sf cells infected with the recombinant baculovirus. However, none of these immunizations stimulated detectable antibody production in mice.

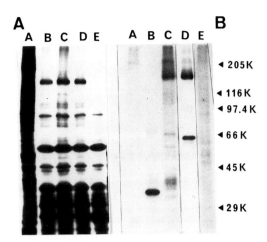

Fig. 1. Expression of S protein in Sf cells by recombinant baculovirus. A. The protein synthesized in Sf cells infected with three recombinant baculoviruses (B, C, D), Sf cells infected with wild-type baculovirus (E), or mock-infected Sf cells (A) were labelled with ^{3}H-leucine. Cell lysates were analysed by 10% SDS-PAGE. B. Immunoprecipitation with anti-JHMV serum of ^{3}H-leucine-labelled proteins from Sf cells infected with recombinant baculovirus (C), Sf cells infected with wild-type baculovirus (B), mock-infected Sf cells (A), JHMV-infected DBT cells (D) and mock-infected DBT cells (E). Immune precipitates were analysed by 10% SDS-PAGE.

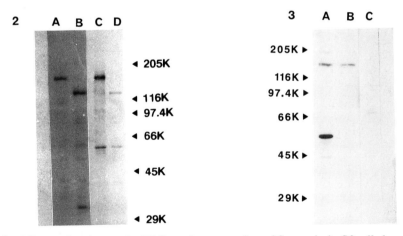

Fig. 2. Effects of tunicamycin (TM) on the expression of S protein in Sf cells by recombinant baculovirus. Sf cells infected with recombinants were treated with 0 (A) or 10 μg/ml (B) of TM and cell lysates were immunoprecipitated with anti-JHMV serum. As a control, JHMV-infected DBT cells treated with 0 (C) or 4 μg/ml of TM were similarly immunoprecipitated. Precipitates were analysed by 10% SDS-PAGE.

Fig. 3. Detection of anti-S antibodies in rat serum immunized with S protein expressed in Sf cells by a recombinant baculovirus. The lysates from JHMV-infected (A, B) and mock-infected DBT cells (C) were immunoprecipitated with the serum of immunized rat (B, C) and with anti-JHMV mouse serum (A). Immune precipitates were analysed by 10% SDS-PAGE.

Table 1

Reactivity of monoclonal antibodies to S1 and S2 proteins expressed by recombinant baculoviruses[1]

Monoclonal Ab	NT[2] on virus isolates		Immunofluorescence against proteins expressed by baculovector			
	cl-2	sp4	S	S1	S2	Mock[3]
32-4	+	+	+	+	-	-
110-3	+	+	+	+	-	-
75-4	+	+	+	+	-	-
8-1	+	+	+	+	-	-
141-3	-	-	+	+	-	-
104-2	-	-	+	+	-	-
29-6	-	-	-	-	+	-
80-1	+	-	-	-	-	-

1. All monoclonal antibodies were shown to recognize S protein of cl-2 by immunofluorescence.
2. Neutralization test.
3. Sf cells infected with wild type baculovirus.

Expression of S1 and S2 proteins by recombinant baculoviruses.

Since we could not detect cleavage products of S protein in insect cells, we cut the cDNA with Cla I, which gives 2 cDNA fragments. The fragment from the 5' half encodes a protein which is 13 amino acids larger than the deduced cleavage product of JHMV and is designated S1. The other fragment derived from the 3' half encodes a polypeptide 12 amino acids shorter than the other deduced cleavage product and was named S2. Recombinant baculoviruses containing these fragments were isolated and the properties of S1 and S2 expressed in insect cells by the recombinants were examined. Using immune precipitation, S1 and S2 proteins with molecular weights of 95K and 63K, respectively, were shown to be produced in insect cells by the recombinants. S1 was shown to be glycosylated using tunicamycin. However, S2 was not glycosylated probably because the protein lacks a signal peptide. These two proteins were used in an attempt to elicit antibodies in rats. High titred antibodies from rats against S2 were detected by immunofluorescence and immunoprecipitation. However, no antibodies recognizing S1 were detected. Since these 2 proteins were well precipitated by anti-JHMV mouse serum, it seems likely that these proteins retain the antigenicity of S protein. We therefore used these proteins to study the localization of epitopes recognized by the monoclonal antibodies (McAbs) produced by immunizing with cl-2 virus which contains an S protein larger than that encoded by the cDNA clone used in these experiments (10). As shown in Table 1, among 8 McAbs examined, 80-1 could not react with S, S1 or S2 and was probably specific to the large S protein of cl-2 as reported previously (11). Of the 7 McAbs, 6 reacted to S1 as well as S by immunofluorescence. All McAbs with neutralizing activity to sp-4 reacted with S1 but not S2. These data suggest that the majority of epitopes which elicit neutralizing antibodies are located in the N-terminal half of S protein.

DISCUSSION

In the present paper, we have demonstrated high level expression of the JHMV S protein in insect cells infected with recombinant baculoviruses. The S protein expressed by recombinant baculovirus in insect cells was shown to correspond in size and antigenicity to the glycosylated S protein produced in mouse cells infected with JHMV and to be expressed on the cell surface as was observed in JHMV-infected mouse cells. However, the post-translational processing of the S protein expressed in insect cells was shown to be different from that in JHMV-infected mouse cells. For example, proteolytic cleavage, which is believed to be a prerequisite for the fusogenic activity of the JHMV S protein was not observed. Also further studies will be necessary to determine if the complex post-translational processing of the JHMV S carbohydrate components is identical in insect and mouse cells.

Rats immunized with the S protein expressed in insect cells produced antibodies against the S protein. In previous reports, antibodies raised against viral surface glycoproteins expressed in the baculovirus system have been shown to neutralize infectivity of the virus (12). Unexpectedly, the antibodies which we obtained failed to neutralize the infectivity of JHMV, although these antibodies bound to the S protein produced in mouse cells. There are several possible explanations. Firstly, as suggested above, there might be differences in the carbohydrate structure between the S protein expressed in insect cells and that produced in mouse cells. Such differences may influence epitopes involved in eliciting neutralizing antibodies. Secondly the uncleaved form of the S glycoprotein might not be able to induce neutralizing antibodies in animals. Thirdly, it is possible that the S cDNA clone used (or the RNA molecule from which it was produced) acquired mutations critical to the epitopes responsible for eliciting neutralizing antibodies. We consider this possibility unlikely, because of 6 different monoclonal antibodies directed against the S protein, four of which are neutralizing antibodies, all reacted well with the S protein expressed in insect cells. The last possibility is that the antibodies obtained after immunization with S protein were mostly against epitopes residing in the C terminal half of the S protein. This is supported by the observtion that the immunogenicity of S1, the N terminal half of the S protein, was shown to be very weak, while that of S2 was fairly strong as shown by the cDNA fragment experiments, and that with monoclonal antibody analysis, the majority of neutralising epitopes were suggested to reside in S1. In our view many of these questions can be further investigated by expressing the S glycoprotein in mouse cells using the vaccinia virus system.

ABSTRACT

The spike (S) protein of murine coronavirus JHM strain (JHMV) has been expressed in insect cells using a recombinant baculovirus vector. The expressed S protein was shown to be glycosylated and expressed on the cell surface, and to be similar in size and antigenic properties to the S protein produced in mouse cells infected by JHMV. However, no proteolytic cleavage was detected in insect cells. The sera from rats immunised with S protein derived from insect cells reacted in immunoprecipitation and immunofluorescence with the S protein produced in JHMV-infected mouse cells. However, the antisera failed to neutralize the infectivity of JHMV. The studies on two proteins expressed by recombinant baculoviruses, corresponding to the cleavage products S1 and S2, and a panel of monoclonal antibodies suggest that the majority of epitopes which elicit the neutralizing antibodies are present in the N terminal half of the S protein.

ACKNOWLEDGEMENTS

The authors thank Mrs. H. Hirano for technical assistance. This work was partly supported by the Grant-in-aid from Ministry of Health and Welfare of Japan.

REFERENCES

1. Siddell, S., Wege, H. and ter Meulen, V. (1983) The biology of coronaviruses. J. gen. Virol. 64, 761-776.
2. Sturman, L.S. and Holmes, K.V. (1983) The molecular biology of coronaviruses. Adv. Virus Res. 18, 35-112.
3. Holmes, K.V., Doller, E.W. and Behnke, J.N. (1981) Analysis of the function of coronavirus glycoprotein by differential inhibition of synthesis with tunicamycin. Adv. Exp. Med. Biol. 142, 133-142.
4. Collins, A.R., Knobler, R.L., Powell, H. and Buchmeier, M. (1982) Monoclonal antibodies to murine hepatitis virus-4 (strain JHM) define the viral glycoprotein responsible for attachment and cell-cell fusion. Virology, 119, 358-371.
5. Fleming, J.O., Trousdale, M.D., El-Zaatari, F.A.K., Stohlman, S.A. and Weiner, L.P. (1986) Pathogenicity of antigenic variants of murine coronavirus JHM selected with monoclonal antibodies. J. Virol. 58, 869-875.
6. Wege, H., Winter, J. and Meyermann, R. (1988) The peplomer protein E2 of coronavirus JHM as a determinant of neurovirulence: Definition of critical epitopes by variant analysis. J. gen. Virol. 69, 87-98.
7. Luckow, V.A. and Summers, M.D. (1988) Trends in the development of baculovirus expression vectors. Bio/Technology, 6, 47-55.

8. Schmidt, I., Skinner, M. and Siddell, S. (1987) Nucleotide sequence of the gene encoding the surface projection glycoprotein of coronavirus JHV-JHM. <u>J. gen. Virol.</u> 68, 47-56.

9. Matsuura, Y., Possee, R.D., Overton, H. and Bishop, D.H. (1986) Expression of the S-coded genes of lymphocytic choriomeningitis arenavirus using baculovirus vector. <u>J. gen. Virol.</u> 67, 1515-1529.

10. Taguchi, F., Siddell, S., Wege, H. and ter Meulen, V. (1985) Characterisation of a variant virus selected in rat brains after infection by coronavirus mouse hepatitis virus JHM. <u>J. Virol.</u> 54, 429-435.

11. Taguchi, F. and Fleming, J.O. (1989) Comparison of six different murine coronavirus JHM variants by monoclonal antibodies against the E2 glycoprotein. <u>Virology</u>, 169, 233-235.

12. Kuorda, K., Hauser, C., Rudolf, R., Klenk, H.-D and Doerfler, W. (1986) Expression of the influenza virus haemagglutinin in insect cells by a baculovirus vector. <u>EMBO J.</u> 5, 1359-1365.

IMMUNOGENICITY OF RECOMBINANT FELINE INFECTIOUS

PERITONITIS VIRUS SPIKE PROTEIN IN MICE AND KITTENS

Harry Vennema, Raoul J. de Groot, David A. Harbour[1], Mieke
Dalderup, Tim Gruffydd-Jones[1], Marian C. Horzinek and
Willy J.M. Spaan

Department of Virology, Faculty of Veterinary Medicine
State University of Utrecht, Yalelaan 1, P.O. Box 80.165
3508 TD Utrecht, The Netherlands
[1]Department of Veterinary Medicine, Langford House
University of Bristol, Langford, Bristol BS18 7DU, England

SUMMARY

The gene encoding the fusogenic spike protein of the coronavirus
causing feline infectious peritonitis (FIPV) was recombined into the genome
of vaccinia virus, strain WR. The recombinant induced spike protein
specific, in vitro neutralizing antibodies in mice. When kittens were
immunized with the recombinant, low titers of neutralizing antibodies were
obtained. After challenge with FIPV, these animals succumbed earlier than
the vWR-immunized control group ("early death syndrome").

INTRODUCTION

Feline infectious peritonitis (FIP) is a progressive, debilitating,
highly fatal disease in wild and domestic Felidae. In the pathogenesis of
FIP the infection of cells of the monocyte/macrophage lineage appears to be
of central importance (3, 4, 9, 10). The causative agent, FIPV, has been
identified as a member of the family Coronaviridae (7). Thus far attempts
to vaccinate against FIPV have failed. Protective immunity was obtained in
some kittens after immunization with low-virulence FIPV strains or
sublethal amounts of virulent FIPV; others, however, developed disease or
became sensitized resulting in early death after challenge (1). Early death
in experimental FIP has been demonstrated following passive transfer of
anti-FIPV antiserum (11), suggesting that early death is caused by antibody
dependent enhancement (ADE) of infectivity (6).

The viral proteins involved in protective immunity and early death
have not been identified. The FIPV virion is composed of an RNA genome of
about 30kb and three protein species: the 45kD nucleocapsid protein N, the
25-32kD membrane glycoprotein M and the 200kD spike glycoprotein S (7). The
latter mediates attachment of the virus to the cell receptor, triggers
membrane fusion and elicits virus neutralizing antibodies.

In this report we show that a challenge infection with FIPV of kittens
previously immunized with a recombinant vaccinia virus expressing the major
surface glycoprotein of FIPV results in early death.

Coronaviruses and Their Diseases
Edited by D. Cavanagh and T.D.K. Brown
Plenum Press, New York, 1990

METHODS AND RESULTS

Immunogenicity of recombinant FIPV spike protein in mice. The gene
encoding the S protein of FIPV strain 79-1146 was inserted into the
vaccinia virus genome by homologous recombination. Details of the isolation
of the recombinant vaccinia virus, designated vFS, and demonstration of
biological activity e.g. cell-cell fusion have been presented (see Vennema
et al., this volume). After metabolic labelling in vitro with [³⁵S]-
methionine a protein which comigrated with the FIPV spike protein was
specifically immunoprecipitated from lysates of cells infected with vFS,
using a polyvalent anti-FIPV antiserum (Fig. 1a).

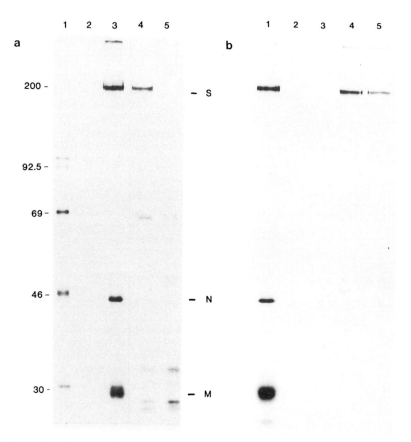

FIG. 1a. In vitro analysis of the recombinant spike protein of
          FIPV. Lysates of metabolically labelled mock (lane 2),
          FIPV (lane 3), vFS (lane 4) and vWR (lane 5) infected
          cells were used in a radio immunoprecipitation (RIP) assay
          with ascitic fluid (A36) of a field case of FIP.
FIG. 1b. Immunoprecipitation analysis of pooled sera of recombinant
          vaccinia virus immunized mice. Pooled sera of five mice
          immunized with vFS, collected on the day of booster (lane
          3) and 2 (lane 4) or 4 (lane 5) weeks after the booster,
          were used in a RIP assay with labelled FIPV proteins.
          Pooled sera of five mice immunized with recombinant
          vaccinia virus vIS, collected 2 weeks after the booster
          served as negative control (lane 2). As a positive control
          RIP was carried out with A36 (lane 1). FIPV structural
          proteins are indicated.

To evaluate the immunogenicity of the recombinant S protein, vFS was used to immunize mice. Five male Balb/c mice were injected intraperitoneally (i.p.) with 5×10^7 PFU of recombinant vFS. Recombinant vaccinia virus expressing the infectious bronchitis virus (IBV) S protein (see Vennema et al., this volume) was used for the immunization of five control mice. Three weeks later a second i.p. immunization of 2×10^8 PFU was given. Sera were collected 2, 4 and 8 weeks after the second immunization. The sera from mice immunized with vFS neutralized FIPV infectivity in vitro up to a 500-fold dilution in a neutralization assay and specifically immunoprecipitated the FIPV S protein (Fig. 1b). Sera obtained from control mice neither neutralized FIPV infectivity in vitro nor immunoprecipitated FIPV S protein.

Immunization of kittens with vFS; early death syndrome. In order to study the role of the S protein in early death syndrome, the recombinant vFS was used to immunize kittens prior to challenge with FIPV. Five 13-14 week old specific pathogen-free kittens were injected subcutaneously with a total of 10^8 PFU of vFS; a second group of five kittens immunized with the same dose of wild type vaccinia virus strain WR (vWR) served as controls. A second immunization was given after three weeks. All kittens developed pox lesions at the site of primary inoculation; no lesions were observed after the second immunization, suggesting an effective immune response to the primary vaccinia virus infection. Two weeks after the second immunization all kittens were challenged orally with 5×10^5 PFU of FIPV strain 79-1146. Once daily, kittens were examined clinically and rectal temperatures were measured. Euthanasia was carried out when the kittens became prostrate and a full post-mortem examination was performed.

Apart from minor pyrexia shortly after the primary vaccinia virus immunization, temperatures were normal during the period before challenge. The mean rectal temperature curves after challenge were similar to those presented previously (11). Briefly, temperatures in both groups rose to a peak on PCD 3. This peak was slightly higher in the vFS immunized group than in the control kittens. In the vFS immunized kittens body temperatures remained elevated. In the control group temperatures dropped and reached normal values on PCD 7 and remained normal until PCD 14. Thereafter, the temperature rose again in 4 out of 5 control kittens and remained high for an extended period. Only 1 of the 4 recovered from this second fever.

Survival times after challenge (Table 1) were reduced significantly ($P<0.05$) in the group immunized with vFS, as tested by the Mann-Whitney procedure. Mean survival times ±SEM after challenge were 8.2 ±1.1 days and 29.0 ±1.7 days for vFS and vWR-immunized kittens respectively. Two kittens of the control group survived challenge.
Histological studies on tissues taken at post-mortem examination showed that the vFS-immunized kittens had suffered from a form of FIP much more severe than naturally occurring FIP, even though no gross changes were observed. The vFS-immunized kittens had multiple lesions in liver, spleen and brain. Mesenteric lymph nodes and Peyer's Patches of the small intestine showed a histiocytic response. The lesions in the vFS-immunized kittens largely represent histiocytic infiltration and proliferation. The presence of multiple small lesions in many organs is atypical of naturally occurring FIP. The diseased kittens of the control group had gross lesions and peritoneal exudate characteristic of effusive FIP. In one cat the brain had focal lymphoid cell infiltrates, in another the liver showed multiple foci of necrosis and the third cat had focal pyogranulomatous lesions in spleen, small intestinal serosa and mesenteric lymph nodes.

Humoral immune response to FIPV spike protein. Serum samples were taken on the days of primary and secondary immunization, on the day of challenge and on PCD 3, 9, 17, 24 and 31 or on the day when euthanasia in extremis was performed. Sera were tested for FIPV neutralizing activity in vitro by

Table 1. Survival times after challenge and neutralizing antibody
          titers of vaccinia virus immunized, FIPV challenged
          kittens.

immunized with vaccinia virus:	kitten	survival time in days	titer[a] PCD 0	titer[b] PCD 9(*=7)	titer[b] PCD 17
vFS	G62	7	32	2455*	
	G67	9	4	725	
	G72	7	10	727*	
	G76	9	4	305	
	118	9	10	610	
vWR	G63	31	<4	77	8192
	G68	>400	<4	75	258
	G73	28	<4	299	2907
	119	>400	<4	150	867
	123	28	<4	<10	514

[a]   reciprocal of the serum dilution that gave 50% plaque
      reduction of 250 PFU of FIPV on fcwf cells.
[b]   reciprocal of the serum dilution that gave 50% CPE
      reduction of 100 $TCID_{50}$ on fcwf cells in a standard
      microtitre assay.

reduction of plaque formation or by inhibition of viral CPE (see footnotes
Table 1). On the day of challenge vFS-immunized kittens had low titers of
neutralizing antibodies, detectable only in a plaque reduction assay (Table
1). No neutralizing antibodies were detectable in sera of the control kittens
(Table 1). Titers remained unchanged on PCD 3 but by PCD 7 or 9 all sera had
increased neutralizing activity (Table 1). Except for kitten G76 all kittens
immunized with vFS had significantly higher titers than control kittens.

The sera were then used in a RIP assay with labelled FIPV proteins.
Figure 2 shows the results for one representative kitten of both groups. No
response was detected in this assay with sera from PCD 3 and before. Serum
from vFS-immunized kitten G76 of PCD 9 precipitated the S protein but none of
the other structural proteins. Using the standard RIP assay which detects only
IgG antibodies, the PCD 9 serum from control kitten G73 did not show an FIPV
specific response. Hence, the antibodies in this serum detected in the
neutralization assay, were probably of IgM isotype, as would be expected in a
primary response. Immunoprecipitation of all structural proteins was obtained
with sera from the control kitten from PCD 17 onwards. Similar patterns were
found for all kittens (manuscript submitted).

DISCUSSION

The data presented here show that immunization of kittens with a
recombinant vaccinia virus, expressing the FIPV spike protein resulted in
early death after challenge with FIPV. From the analysis of the humoral immune
response we conclude that immunization with vFS led to an S protein specific
priming and a low level of in vitro neutralizing antibodies. The S antigen
produced in the initial rounds of replication boosted the primed S response to

a relatively high level of IgG antibodies early in infection. The early death syndrome was probably caused by a combination of these factors, through a mechanism consistent with ADE. The demonstration of early death in experimental FIP following passive transfer of anti-FIPV antiserum (11) supports the hypothesis that early death can be caused by ADE. Furthermore, ADE of FIPV infectivity in vitro in cultured feline macrophages has recently been reported (8). The data presented here show that an immune response against the viral spike protein alone can trigger early death syndrome after challenge with FIPV.

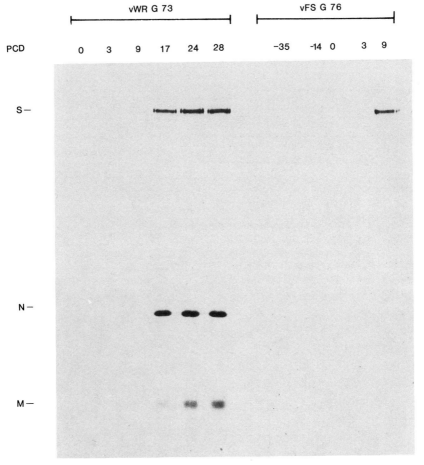

FIG. 2.   Immunoprecipitation analysis of sera of experimentally infected kittens. Sera of vaccinia virus immunized kittens were tested in a RIP assay with labelled FIPV proteins. The vaccinia virus used for immunization, vFS or vWR, and the code number for the kitten are indicated at the top of the panels. Above each lane the post challenge day on which the serum was taken has been indicated.

ACKNOWLEDGEMENTS

We thank P.J. Brown and G.R. Pearson for the post-mortem examination, A. Boots for immunizations of mice, H. Egberink and E.D. Chirnside for reviewing the manuscript and B. Moss for vaccinia virus insertion vector pGS20. Supported by a grant from Duphar BV, Weesp, the Netherlands.

LITERATURE CITED

1. Pedersen, N.C., and J.W. Black. 1983. Attempted immunization of cats against feline infectious peritonitis, using avirulent live virus or sublethal amounts of virulent virus. Am. J. Vet. Res. 44:229-234.

2. Pedersen, N.C., and J.F. Boyle. 1980. Immunologic phenomena in the effusive form of feline infectious peritonitis. Am. J. Vet. Res. 41:868-876.

3. Pedersen, N.C., J.F. Boyle, K. Floyd, A. Fudge, and J. Barker. 1981. An enteric coronavirus infection of cats and its relationship to feline infectious peritonitis. Am. J. Vet. Res. 42:368-377.

4. Pedersen, N.C., J.F. Evermann, J. Alison, A.J. McKeirnan, and R.L. Ott. 1984. Pathogenicity studies of feline coronavirus isolates 79-1146 and 79-1683. Am. J. Vet. Res. 45:2580-2585.

5. Pedersen, N.C., and K. Floyd. 1985. Experimental studies with three new strains of feline infectious peritonitis virus: FIPV-UCD2, FIPV-UCD3, FIPV-UCD4. Compend. Contin. Educ. Pract. Vet. 7:1001-1011.

6. Porterfield, J.S. 1986. Antibody-dependent enhancement of viral infectivity. Adv. Virus Res. 31:335-355.

7. Spaan, W., D. Cavanagh, and M.C. Horzinek. 1988. Coronaviruses: Structure and genome expression. J. Gen. Virol. 69:2939-2952.

8. Stoddart, C.A., and F.W. Scott. 1989. Intrinsic resistance of feline peritoneal macrophages to coronavirus infection correlates well with in vivo virulence. J. Virol. 63:436-440.

9. Weiss, R.C., and F.W. Scott. 1981. Pathogenesis of feline infectious peritonitis: pathologic changes and immunofluorescence. Am. J. Vet. Res. 42:2036-2048.

10. Weiss, R.C., and F.W. Scott. 1981. Pathogenesis of feline infectious peritonitis: nature and development of viremia. Am. J. Vet. Res. 42:382-390.

11. Weiss, R.C., and F.W. Scott. 1981. Antibody-mediated enhancement of disease in feline infectious peritonitis: comparisons with Dengue hemorrhagic fever. Comp. Immun. Microbiol. Infect. Dis. 4:175-189.

EXPRESSION OF TGEV STRUCTURAL GENES IN VIRUS VECTORS

D. J. Pulford, P. Britton, K. W. Page and D. J. Garwes

AFRC Institute for Animal Health, Compton Laboratory
Compton, Newbury, Berkshire, RG16 0NN, U.K.

INTRODUCTION

TGEV is a coronavirus that causes gastroenteritis in pigs, resulting in a high mortality of neonates. The TGEV virion contains three major structural polypeptides; a surface glycoprotein (spike or peplomer protein) with a monomeric M_r 200000, a glycosylated integral membrane protein observed as a series of polypeptides of M_r 28000-31000 and a basic phosphorylated protein (the nucleoprotein) of M_r 47000 associated with the viral genomic RNA (1). The genes encoding TGEV nucleoprotein (NP), integral membrane protein (E1) and peplomer (E2) have been cloned and sequenced from an avirulent laboratory strain, Purdue (2, 3, 4, 5) and a virulent British field isolate, FS772/70 (6, 7).

TGEV antigens may be produced by gene expression in a eukaryotic vector system. Vaccinia viruses (VV) and baculoviruses have the potential for transporting, processing and folding foreign eukaryotic gene products correctly. Many heterologous genes have been expressed in these viral vector systems and are antigenically and functionally identical to their original gene product (8, 9). VV is a poxvirus, a large DNA (186 kpb) pleomorphic virus capable of carrying a 25 kb insert of foreign DNA, providing the potential to express all three coronavirus structural genes simultaneously. Wild-type and recombinant vaccinia viruses (RVV) have a wide host range, capable of infecting most mammalian species and inducing humoral and cell mediated immune responses. Utilisation of the VV $P_{7.5K}$ promoter enables modest expression of foreign genes during early and late infection. The insect baculovirus <u>Autographa</u> <u>californica</u> nuclear polyhedrosis virus (AcNPV) has a large DNA genome 126-129 kbp that can incorporate relatively large segments of foreign DNA. The virus is nonpathogenic and incapable of replication in vertebrate cells, making the vector inherently safe, but limiting its potential for expressing antigen to the immune system. The polyhedrin gene is a nonessential segment of the viral genome regulated by a strong late P_{33K} promoter. There is no evidence for cryptic RNA splicing and by utilising the strong late P_{33K}, very large amounts of a foreign gene product can be expressed with most post-translational modifications.

In this paper we describe the construction of recombinant viruses containing the TGEV NP, E1 and E2 genes and compare the products expressed with TGEV structural proteins to evaluate a suitable TGEV protein candidate for providing immunity.

Coronaviruses and Their Diseases
Edited by D. Cavanagh and T.D.K. Brown
Plenum Press, New York, 1990

METHODS AND MATERIALS

Viruses and cells

Transfections and growth of wild-type VV (WR strain) and recombinant vaccinia viruses (RVV) were performed as in Mackett et al. (10). AcNPV and recombinant baculovirus stocks were grown and assayed according to the procedures of Brown and Faulkner (11) on Spodoptera frugiperda cells (Sf9) at 28°C with Graces Insect medium (Flow Labs.) containing 10% FCS. TGEV (FS772/70) was grown on adult pig thyroid (APT/2) cell monolayers (12) for neutralisation assays. TGEV antigens were isolated from infected LLC-PK1 cells (13).

Construction of plasmid insertion vectors

Recombinant plasmids pGSN1, pGSIM1 and PGSP1 were constructed by ligating the NP, E1 and E2 BamHI gene cassettes from plasmids pBNP5 (6), pBIM3 (7), and pPBP1 respectively into the BamHI site of pGS20 (14). The E1 BamHI gene cassette was ligated into the baculovirus insertion vector pAcRP23 BamHI site to generate pAcI6.

Production of recombinant viruses

RVV containing only one TGEV gene cassette were constructed by the methods of Mackett et al. (10, 14). Recombinant baculoviruses were generated by cotransfecting pAcI6 plasmid DNA with infectious AcNPV DNA (15) on Sf9 cells (16). Plaques not containing visible occlusion bodies were recovered from agarose overlays of infected monolayers.

Extraction and characterisation of viral DNA

Wild-type and recombinant vaccinia virus DNA was prepared as by Merchlinsky and Moss (17). Recombinant and wild-type AcNPV virions were isolated from infected cell culture medium as in Matsuura et al. (16) and DNA prepared as by Merchlinsky and Moss (17).

Immunofluorescence

Cultures of HTK⁻ cells on glass coverslips were infected with recombinant vaccinia viruses at m.o.i. = 1 and incubated for 24 h. The infected cells were fixed in cold 80% acetone and probed with mouse monoclonal antibodies (mAbs) DA3 (18) and 3BB3 (19) specific to TGEV NP and E1 respectively, and a cocktail of mouse anti-TGEV E2 mAbs, including 1B6, 5A5, 6A6, 8A4, 3C1 and 6D4 (20) all diluted 1/500. Bound antibody was detected with fluorescein-conjugated rabbit anti-mouse IgG antiserum (Nordic Immunology).

Immunoblot analysis

Infected cell cultures were lysed in 0.1M Tris-HCl pH 8.0, 0.1M NaCl, 0.5% Nonidet P40, 0.1% Aprotinin (Sigma), and proteins transferred onto nitrocellulose membrane (BA85, Schleicher and Schuell) using a Biorad Dot Blot apparatus or after SDS polyacrylamide gel electrophoresis.

Immunoprecipitations

Infected cells were lysed with RIPA buffer as described by Garwes et al. (20) and supernatants containing TGEV polypeptides were preabsorbed with formalin-fixed Staphylococcus aureus (Sac) cells (Cowan strain, Immunoprecipitin, BRL) before incubating with antisera for 1 h and precipitating with washed Sac cells and analysed as in Britton et al. (21).

Animal inoculations

Partially purified recombinant and wild-type VV were prepared by pelleting stock virus through an equal volume of 36% w/v sucrose in 10 mM Tris-HCl, 1 mM EDTA pH 8.8 in a 55.5 swing-out rotor (Kontron Instruments) at 25,000 x g for 80 min at 4°C. Pelleted virus was resuspended in phosphate buffered saline (PBS 10 mM potassium phosphate, 150 mM NaCl, pH 7.2) for inoculation into animals.

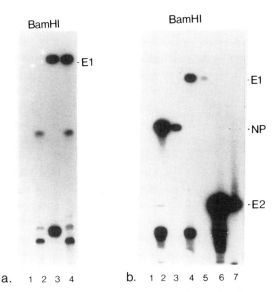

Fig. 1. Identification of TGEV genes in recombinant virus genomes by Southern blot with high molecular weight fragments at the bottom. Plasmid and viral DNA was digested with BamHI for 4 h and DNA fragments separated by electrophoresis on a 0.8% agarose gel. Denatured DNA was transferred onto a Biodyne filter and probed. Fig. 1a Lane (1) contained pAcRP23, (2) vAcNPV, (3) pAcI6, (4) vAcI2 DNA probed with ^{32}P-labelled E1 BamHI gene cassette. Fig. 1b Lane (1) contained wt VV, (2) pGSN1, (3) vTN1, (4) pGSI1, (5) vTI1, (6) pGSP1, (7) vTP1 DNA probed with ^{32}P-labelled NP, E1 and E2 BamHI gene cassettes.

TGEV neutralisation assay

Mouse and pig anti-recombinant vaccinia sera were heat treated at 55°C for 30 mins to destroy any complement activity before being serially diluted and mixed with 100 pfu of TGEV in an equal volume of M199 medium (Medium 199 (Flow Laboratories), supplemented with 50 mM HEPES, 0.14% sodium bicarbonate, 2.5% calf serum and antibiotics) for 1 h at 37°C. Residual virus activity was assayed in triplicate by plaque reduction using APT/2 cells incubated with a M199/0.6% agarose overlay. After 3 days the plaques were detected with a neutral red overlay and the neutralising titres were expressed as the reciprocal of the serum dilution that reduced 50% of the plaques.

RESULTS AND DISCUSSION

Construction and DNA analysis of recombinant viruses

All three complete TGEV structural protein genes were inserted downstream of the vaccinia early/late $P_{7.5K}$ promoter in the plasmid insertion
vector pGS20. The TGEV NP gene was contained in a BamHI cassette (6),
which also included a second small open reading frame (ORF4), and was used
to generate RVV vTN1. The TGEV E1 gene was inserted into vaccinia and
baculovirus genomes as a BamHI gene cassette (7). The E1 gene was regulated
by the early/late $P_{7.5K}$ promoter in RVV vTI1 and by the strong late P_{33K}
polyhedrin promoter in vAcI2. The E2 gene was constructed as a 4657 bp
BamHI gene cassette (unpublished result) and used to generate a recombinant
vaccinia virus vTP1. The recombinant viral genomes were analysed by
Southern blot to confirm the integration of the TGEV structural genes (Fig.
1).

Recombinant virus expression of nucleoprotein

The gene products have been characterised by immune blotting and
immunoprecipitation of recombinant VV infected cell lysates. vTN1 infected
cell lysates contained a polypeptide M_r 47000, recognised by DA3 and polyclonal cat anti-feline infectious peritonitis virus (FIPV) serum, a
serologically related coronavirus. The recombinant NP comigrated with the
TGEV nucleoprotein (Fig. 2) implying that it was the same as the TGEV
product. The last 20 residues of the NP carboxyl-terminus have been
identified as containing the epitope site for the DA3 mAb (J. M. Alonso
Martin, personal communication). A smaller NP species of M_r 42000 has
been observed in TGEV infected cells using polyclonal antiserum (13), but
is not detected with DA3. A potential trypsin cleavage site, KRK, has been
identified at the carboxyl-terminus of the nucleoprotein that could result
in the deletion of the last 39 amino acids, containing the DA3 epitope,

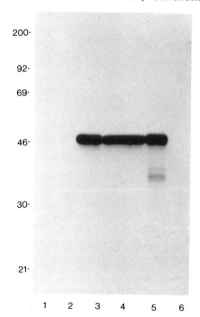

Fig. 2. Cell lysates from uninfected (1) WR infected (2) vTN1 24 h (3) and
48 h (4) post infected HTK⁻ cell lysates; TGEV infected (5) and
uninfected (6) LLC PK1 cells were separated by electrophoresis on
a 10% SDS PAGE gel, transferred onto nitrocellulose and probed
with DA3.

resulting in the truncated form of the nucleoprotein. Immunoprecipitation of radiolabelled TGEV antigen with DA3 can co-precipitate the M_r 42000 species with the M_r 47000 species, indicating that these two species of NP can associate. Smaller species of NP from vTN1 infected cells have also been detected with FIPV polyclonal antiserum, but not with DA3, and may be progressive degradation products. Breakdown products are found in TGEV infected cells when using DA3 (Fig. 2, lane 5) indicating that degradation may also occur from the N-terminus.

By indirect immunofluorescence (IIF), NP appeared to aggregate into complexes in the cell cytoplasm, at 24 h post infection with vTN1 (Fig. 4a) and by 8 h in TGEV infected cells. No recombinant or TGEV NP has been seen at the cell surface of unfixed infected cells.

Recombinant virus expression of integral membrane protein (E1)

Sequence analysis of the protein has identified three potential N-glycosylation sites at Asn [32], [55] and [251] each potentially adding 2000 daltons onto the M_r 29459 polypeptide (7). vTI1 infected cells produce a single species polypeptide of M_r 30000 but vAcI2 infected Sf9 cells produce two species of E1, an abundant M_r 30000 protein and a less common M_r 28000 species (Fig. 3). Cells infected with either vTI1 or vAcI2 in the presence of tunicamycin only express the M_r 28000 species. These observations support the theory that only one E1 N-glycosylation site, Asn [32], is occupied. The other two potential N-glycosylation sites occur in hydrophobic areas of the molecule and are thought to be hidden in the viral membrane. Larger but minor species of E1 have been observed in TGEV

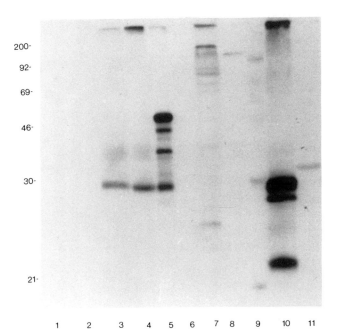

Fig. 3. Cell lysates from uninfected (1), WR infected (2), vTI1 24 h (3) and 48 h (4) post infected HTK⁻ cell lysates; TGEV infected (5) and uninfected (6) LLC PK1 cells; pURIM2 transfected (7) and pUR290 (8) transfected E. coli JM101 cell lysates [7, 21]; protein high molecular weight markers (9); vAcI2 (10) and vAcNPV (11) infected cell lysates were electrophoresed on a 10% SDS PAGE gel, transferred onto nitrocellulose and probed with cat anti-FIPV serum.

infected cells (1) but have not been detected in either recombinant virus infections. The immunogenicity of the unglycosylated form of the E1 molecule appears unaffected as it is recognised by both FIPV polyclonal and 3BB3 monoclonal antiserum.

By IIF, E1 usually has a polar distribution within the cytoplasm of TGEV and vTI1 infected cells (Fig. 4b), consistent with the hypothesis that E1 is associated with the endoplasmic reticulum (ER) and golgi apparatus. The distribution of E1 in Sf9 cells was generally cytoplasmic (Fig. 4d). Contrary to earlier observations, TGEV E1 was not found on the cell surface of TGEV or recombinant virus infected cells, supporting the evidence that the E1 molecule has its own targeting and anchoring transport signals which restrict it to the endoplasmic reticulum and golgi apparatus.

Sequence analysis of the TGEV peplomer

The E2 gene is an ORF of 4341 bp coding for 1447 amino acids contained within the TGEV 8.4 kb mRNA subgenomic species. The sequence context, (AC)ACCATGA, of the peplomer gene is favourable for initiation by eukaryotic ribosomes ((CC)ACCATGG) (22, 23). The peplomer gene is terminated by the codon TAA which is also the terminator of the nucleoprotein and integral membrane protein genes. The first 16 amino acids of the peplomer poly-peptide fulfil the criteria of being a eukaryotic signal sequence, with the potential cleavage site between the glycine [16] and aspartic acid [17] residues. The cleavage site of the peplomer signal sequence has been confirmed (5), from the avirulent Purdue strain of TGEV, as being between residues 16 and 17 by N-terminal amino acid sequencing of the peplomer isolated from virions. Following cleavage of the signal sequence the

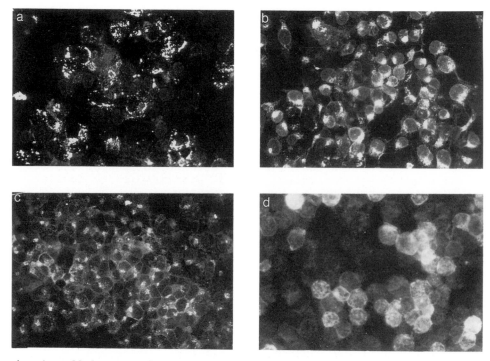

Fig. 4. Cellular location of TGEV structural proteins in recombinant virus infected cells by indirect immunofluorescence. NP was detected using DA3 (a), E1 using 3BB3 (b), and E2 using a mAb cocktail (c). E1 was also detected in fixed vAcI2 infected Sf9 cells with 3BB3 at 48 h post infection (d).

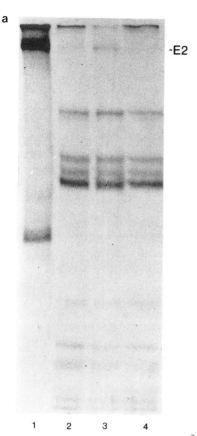

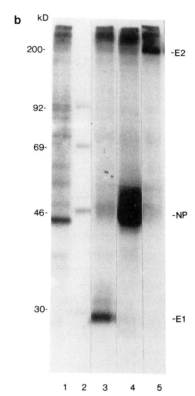

Fig. 5a. Immunoprecipitation of [^{35}S]-methionine labelled E2 protein from
TGEV infected LLC PK1 cells (1); vTP1 (2), (3) and WR (4) infected
HTK$^-$ cells with cat anti-FIPV serum (1), (3), (4), and 3C1 (2) a
major neutralising E2 monoclonal antibody.

Fig. 5b. Immunoprecipitation of [^{35}S]-methionine labelled TGEV polypeptides
with mouse anti-vTI1 (3), anti-vTN1 (4) and anti-vTP1 (5) antiserum. Lane (1) contains whole cell lysate diluted 1:100 and
(2) protein high molecular weight markers.

primary structure of the peplomer would be 1433 amino acids with a M_r
157891. There are 33 potential N-linked glycosylation sites providing the
TGEV peplomer monomer with an overall M_r 226000. The monomeric molecular
weight of the TGEV peplomer, by SDS PAGE, is M_r 200000 (1) implying that
most of the potential N-linked glycosylation sites must be occupied.

Recombinant virus expression of peplomer (E2)

The E2 antigen is sensitive to reduction by 2-mercaptoethanol. E2
expressed by RVV can be detected by immunoblotting in non-reducing conditions, but is best observed by immunoprecipitation (Fig. 5a), where it
comigrated with the peplomer protein of TGEV M_r 200000. The amount of RVV
expressed E2 is poor compared with TGEV. A recombinant vaccinia virus
expressing TGEV E2 cloned from the Miller strain has been previously
published (24). This E2 gene construct had a deletion at the 3' end which
resulted in the loss of the last 190 amino acids, which included part of
the stalk and all of the anchor region. This observation was obtained from

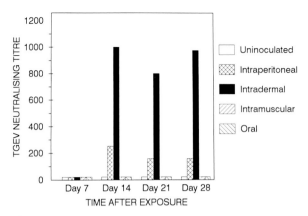

Fig. 6. The effect of inoculation route at inducing TGEV neutralising
antibodies in vTP1 infected gnotobiotic piglets.

our sequencing analysis and was confirmed by other data (5) for the Purdue
strain of TGEV.   The truncated form of E2 was capable of inducing low level
TGEV neutralising antibody, but could not be detected on the cell surface
by IIF probably due to the deletion of the anchor region.

Analysis, by IIF, showed that the E2 from RVV vTP1 reacted with all
the peplomer competition mAb groups (20) indicating that the immunogenicity
of the expressed E2 is preserved.   Fixed and unfixed infected cells had a
diffuse cytoplasmic staining with occasional polar concentrations on the
cell perimeter.   Fine points of fluorescence, probably capped protein,
appeared around the cell perimeter of unfixed vTP1 infected cells suggesting
that the E2 is exported to the cell membrane.   No specific staining was
observed for unfixed WR infected and uninfected cells using E2 mAbs.   Antisera raised in mice to all three RVV were analysed by immunoprecipitation
and neutralisation assay.   All mouse anti-RVV serum specifically immunoprecipitated a single TGEV structural protein product (Fig. 5b).   No

Table 1.   TGEV neutralisation assay using mouse anti-RVV serum

Vaccinia virus	Single dose	Hyperimmunisation
vTN1	10	10
vTN2	10	60
vTI1	<10	40
vTI2	<10	<10
vTP1	490	1120
vTP2	160	430
WR	<10	<10

significant TGEV neutralisation was detected with mouse anti-vTN1 or vTI1 serum (Table 1), though it has been reported that anti-E1 mAbs in the presence of guinea pig complement can enhance TGEV neutralisation (25). Only mouse anti-vTP1 serum and hyperimmune vTP-1 serum contained neutralising antibody titred at 490 and 1120 respectively in a 50% TGEV plaque reduction assay, demonstrating that the recombinant product can induce TGEV neutralising activity (Table 1). The efficacy of vTP1 inducing neutralising antibody was studied in gnotobiotic piglets. Animals were given a standard inoculum of vTP1 (2×10^5 pfu) by the intramuscular, intraperitoneal, oral (by feeding through a stomach tube), intradermal (scarification) and control (uninoculated) routes (Fig. 6). Only two routes induced TGEV neutralising serum antibody. Intraperitoneal inoculation induced a titre of 250 at 14 days post infection but diminished by 28 days. Intradermal inoculation induced a neutralising titre of 950 which remained constant up to 28 days post infection. Work is in progress to determine if vTP1 serum antibodies can protect the piglet from a TGEV infection.

ACKNOWLEDGEMENTS

This research was supported by the Biotechnology Action Programme of the European Communities (Contract No. BAP-0235-UKHI)). We would like to thank Dr. R. D. Possee from the NERC Institute of Virology, Oxford for the plasmid pAcRP23 and Sf9 cells, Mrs A. Waite for animal supervision, Dr. L. Enjuanes from the Centro de Biologia Molecular, Madrid for the mAb 3BB3 and Dr. D. Harbour, Department of Veterinary Medicine, University of Bristol for the cat anti-FIPV serum.

REFERENCES

1. D. J. Garwes and D. H. Pocock, The polypeptide structure of transmissible gastroenteritis virus. J. Gen. Virol., 29:25-34 (1975).
2. P. A. Kapke and D. A. Brian, Sequence analysis of the porcine transmissible gastroenteritis coronavirus nucleocapsid protein gene. Virology, 151:41-49 (1986).
3. P. A. Kapke, F. Y. C. Tung, D. A. Brian, R. D. Woods and R. Wesley, Nucleotide sequence of the porcine transmissible gastroenteritis coronavirus matrix protein, Adv. Exp. Med. Biol., 218: 117-122 (1987).
4. H. Laude, D. Rasschaert and J. C. Huet, Sequence and N-terminal processing of the transmembrane protein E1 of the coronavirus transmissible gastroenteritis virus, J. Gen. Virol., 68:1687-1693 (1987).
5. D. Rasschaert and H. Laude, The predicted primary structure of the peplomer protein E2 of the porcine coronavirus Transmissible Gastroenteritis Virus, J. Gen. Virol., 68:1883-1890 (1987).
6. P. Britton, R. S. Carmenes, K. W. Page, D. J. Garwes and F. Parra, Sequence of the nucleoprotein gene from a virulent British field isolate of transmissible gastroenteritis virus and its expression in Saccharomyces cerevisiae, Mol. Microbiol., 2: 89-99 (1988).
7. P. Britton, R. S. Carmenes, K. W. Page and D. J. Garwes, The integral membrane protein from a virulent isolate of transmissible gastroenteritis virus: Molecular characterisation, sequence and expression in Escherichia coli, Mol. Microbiol., 2:497-505 (1988).
8. B. Moss and C. Flexner, Vaccinia virus expression vectors, Ann. Rev. Immunol., 5:305-324 (1987).

9. W. Doerfler, Expression of the Autographa californica Nuclear Polyhedrosis virus genome in insect cells: Homologous viral and heterologous vertebrate genes - the Baculovirus vector system, Current
Topics in Microbiol. and Immunol., 131:51-65 (1986).

10. M. Mackett, G. L. Smith and B. Moss, The construction and characterisation of vaccinia virus recombinants expressing foreign genes.
in: "DNA Cloning, a Practical Approach, Vol. II", D. M. Glover, ed.,
IRL Press (1985).

11. M. Brown and P. Faulkner, A plaque assay for nuclear polyhedrosis
viruses using a solid overlay, J. Gen. Virol., 36:361-364 (1977).

12. D. H. Pocock and D. J. Garwes, The influence of pH on the growth and
stability of transmissible gastroenteritis virus in vitro, Arch.
Virol., 49:239 (1985).

13. D. J. Garwes, L. Bountiff, G. C. Millson and C. J. Elleman, Defective
replication of porcine transmissible gastroenteritis virus in a
continuous cell line, Adv. Exp. Med. Biol., 178:79-93 (1984).

14. M. Mackett, G. L. Smith and B. Moss, General method for production and
selection of infectious vaccinia virus recombinants expressing
foreign genes, J. Virol., 49:857-864 (1984).

15. G. E. Smith and M. D. Summers, Analysis of baculovirus genomes with
restriction endonucleases, Virology, 89:517-527 (1978).

16. Y. Matsuura, R. D. Possee, H. A. Overton and D. H. L. Bishop, Baculovirus expression vectors: The requirements for high level expression
of proteins, including glycoproteins, J. Gen. Virol., 68:1233-1250
1987).

17. M. Merchlinsky and B. Moss, Resolution of vaccinia virus DNA concatamer
junctions requires late-gene expression, J. Virol., 63:1595-1603
(1989).

18. D. J. Garwes, F. Stewart, S. F. Cartwright and I. Brown. Differentiation of porcine coronavirus from transmissible gastroenteritis
virus, Vet. Rec., 122:86-87 (1988).

19. G. Jimenez, I. Correa, M. P. Melgosa, M. J. Bullido and L. Enjuanes,
Critical epitopes in transmissible gastroenteritis virus neutralisation, J. Virol., 60:131-139 (1986).

20. D. J. Garwes, F. Stewart and C. J. Elleman, Identification of epitopes
of immunological importance on the peplomer of porcine transmissible
gastroenteritis virus, Adv. Exp. Med. Biol., 218:509-516 (1987).

21. P. Britton, D. J. Garwes, K. W. Page and J. Walmsley, Expression of
porcine transmissible gastroenteritis virus genes in E. coli as β-
galactosidase chimaeric proteins, Adv. Exp. Med. Biol., 218:55-64
(1987).

22. M. Kozak, Comparison of initiation of protein synthesis in prokaryotes,
eukaryotes and organelles, Microb. Rev., 47:1-45 (1983).

23. M. Kozak, Point mutations define a sequence flanking the AUG initiator
codon that modulates translation by eukaryote ribosomes, Cell,
44:283-293 (1986).

24. S. Hu, J. Bruszewski and R. Smalling, Infectious vaccinia virus
recombinant that expresses the surface antigen of porcine transmissible gastroenteritis virus (TGEV), in: "Vaccinia Viruses as
Vectors for Vaccine Antigens," Quinnan, ed., Elsevier Science
Publishing Co., the Netherlands (1985).

25. R. D. Woods, R. D. Wesley and P. A. Kapke, Complement-dependent
neutralisation of Transmissible Gastroenteritis Virus by monoclonal
antibodies, Adv. Exp. Med. Biol., 218:493-500 (1987).

Chapter 5

The Nucleocapsid (N) Protein

BACKGROUND PAPER

FUNCTIONS OF THE CORONAVIRUS NUCLEOCAPSID PROTEIN

Paul S. Masters and Lawrence S. Sturman

Wadsworth Center for Laboratories and Research
New York State Department of Health
Albany
NY 12201-0509
USA

In 1962 Caspar and Klug conjectured that self-assembly of equivalent or quasi-equivalent protein subunits and viral nucleic acid produces either icosahedral or helical structures according to the biological functions required (1). Some 15 years later Wengler introduced the terms "transcription helices" and "translation helices" to describe the relationship between helical ribonucleoprotein (RNP) structure and genome function for animal viruses containing single-stranded RNA (2). In transcription helices the RNA genome is transcribed into complementary nucleic acid, without permanent disassembly of the RNP. In translation helices the RNA is liberated from the RNP and translated into protein. To account for the fact that no examples of enveloped viruses containing translation helices had been described, Wengler speculated that "the forces exerted on the viral RNP during budding necessitate the design of a helical RNP of such high stability that RNA cannot be released for translation *in vivo*. Therefore, translation helices will not be present in viruses which obtain a viral membrane by budding".

Today we know this prediction to be wrong: at least one family of viruses, coronaviruses, contains translation helices. However, Wengler's analysis still provides a useful framework for considering some aspects of the molecular biology of these interesting viruses. Most centrally, we do not presently understand how the interactions between the nucleocapsid (N) protein and the viral genome allow the coronavirus RNP to stably acquire its envelope during the maturation process but yet permit the RNA to be released for translation during the early stages of infection. In this overview we will attempt to briefly summarize what is known about coronavirus N proteins and what are the more pertinent outstanding questions.

N PROTEIN STRUCTURE

To date, the deduced amino acid sequences of the N proteins of at least six coronaviruses (MHV, BCV, HCV-OC43, TGEV, HCV229E, and IBV) have been reported (3-5). All have comparable general physical properties. They range from 382 - 455 amino acids in length (M_r 43 - 50,000) and have isoelectric points of 10.3 - 10.7, reflecting a preponderance of basic residues (58 - 72 lysine plus arginine) over acidic residues (44 - 53 glutamate plus aspartate). The basic residues have some degree of localization but are not as densely clustered as in certain viral and cellular nucleic acid binding proteins. The coronavirus N proteins have a 7 - 10% serine content, and many of these residues are clustered. In contrast to the overall basic character of the N molecules, their carboxy termini are markedly acidic: the 45 C-terminal amino acids of each have isoelectric points of 4.5 - 5.3. It is interesting that all of the characteristics noted to this point are also shared by the nucleocapsid proteins of influenza viruses.

Coronaviruses and Their Diseases
Edited by D. Cavanagh and T.D.K. Brown
Plenum Press, New York, 1990

Despite their mutual resemblance, the amino acid sequences of the coronavirus N proteins are generally not very similar. The notable exception to this is a region of 64 - 67 residues, falling within the N-terminal one-third of each molecule, which exhibits a high amount of sequence identity among all the N proteins. The meaning of such a striking degree of conservation is unknown, but it implies that an important function may be assigned to this segment of the molecule.

RNA BINDING

The most salient feature of the N proteins is that they bind to RNA. As such, however, they bear no obvious resemblance to any well-characterized cellular RNA binding protein. In particular, none of the coronavirus N sequences contain regions homologous to the consensus RNA binding sequences common to the family of cellular proteins that includes poly(A) binding proteins, nucleolin and many snRNP proteins (6). A better analogy may be found by comparison with viral RNA binding proteins, specifically the N (or NP) proteins of other single-stranded RNA viruses having helical nucleocapsids. These seem to fall into two classes. The N (NP) proteins of the rhabdoviruses and the paramyxoviruses are neutral or even slightly acidic in their amino acid composition. The complexes they form with their RNA genomes are very stable to conditions of high ionic strength and are highly resistant to the action of RNase. In contrast to these are the N (NP) proteins of the coronaviruses and the orthomyxoviruses. In addition to the above-mentioned physical similarities between the coronavirus and influenza virus N (NP) proteins, both of these form RNPs which are more easily disrupted at high salt concentrations and which afford their RNA genomes relatively little protection against RNase.

Robbins *et al.* developed an RNA overlay protein blot assay (ROPBA) which demonstrated *in vitro* the RNA binding properties of the N protein of MHV but was not specific for viral RNA (7). Stohlman *et al.* made the ROPBA specific for labeled viral RNA by competing out the nonspecific binding of labeled cellular RNA with a large excess of unlabelled cellular RNA (8). These experiments were then extended using synthetic RNA substrates to identify a potential nucleation site for the binding of N to nucleotides 56-65 of the MHV genome and subgenomic RNAs. Interestingly, this region falls within a potential RNA hairpin loop. It remains to be seen whether this will be the only high affinity binding site on the viral RNA. Conversely, the domain(s) of the N protein which participate in RNA binding also have not been determined.

N:N INTERACTIONS

There are potentially two forms of interactions between N molecules in the helical nucleocapsid. The first would be between adjacent monomers bound along the length of the RNA strand. There is presently no evidence for such interactions, although any RNA binding model of nucleation followed by cooperative encapsidation seems to require that they occur. However, one possible interpretation of the relative RNase sensitivity of the coronavirus RNP is that there exists little or no contact between adjacent N monomers. The second type of N:N interaction would be between monomers that become adjacent per each helical turn of the RNP. It is difficult to see how the nucleocapsid could have a helical structure without this sort of interaction. In their study of RNA binding, Robbins *et al.* detected a disulfide-linked multimeric form of the MHV N protein, possibly a dimer or trimer (7). This species, then, may represent one of these types of N:N interaction.

N:M INTERACTIONS

The assembly of coronaviruses is thought to be driven by interactions between the N protein in the RNP and the large cytoplasmic domain of the M protein, which may act in a manner analogous to the matrix proteins of rhabdoviruses and paramyxoviruses. Sturman *et al.* found that in NP40-disrupted MHV virions a temperature-dependent association between M and the RNP could be demonstrated *in vitro* (9). However, much work remains to be done to define the regions of the N and M proteins which participate in viral maturation.

PHOSPHORYLATION

The N proteins of coronaviruses are known to be phosphorylated both intracellularly and in assembled virions. Moreover, for MHV a virion-associated protein kinase has been described by Siddell *et al.* which can transfer additional phosphate from ATP to the N protein *in vitro* (10). This enzyme appears to be cyclic AMP-independent and may be of either viral or host origin. The phosphate linkage, *in vitro* and *in vivo*, has been shown to be to serine residues, and this has prompted comment about the high serine content of the coronavirus N proteins. However, an HPLC analysis of the tryptic phosphopeptides of MHV N proteins suggests that, despite the large number of potential target residues, N phosphorylation may occur at only some small number of sites (1 - 3) (11). The exact number and location of the N protein phosphoserines and the identity of the responsible protein kinase(s) are open questions at present.

Perhaps more intriguing is the related question of the function of N protein phosphorylation. Stohlman *et al.* have shown that the MHV N protein is phosphorylated in the cytoplasm of infected cells within 10 to 20 minutes of its synthesis and it concomitantly becomes associated with a membrane fraction of the cells (12). It has been speculated by a number of workers that N phosphorylation may govern the tightness of the association between N and RNA, and it may thus be a regulator of assembly. However, there is as yet no evidence that bears on this possibility.

PARTICIPATION IN RNA SYNTHESIS

Compton *et al.*, working with an *in vitro* RNA synthesizing system prepared from MHV-infected cells, found that RNA synthesis was greater than 90% inhibited by antibodies to N (13). This implies a critical role for N protein in the transcription and replication of viral RNA. N may act in one or both of two capacities: firstly, by encapsidation, as an antiterminator or protector of the nascent RNA strand; secondly, as a component of the template, associating with the proteins that constitute the viral RNA polymerase. Compton *et al.* have shown that the RNA product synthesized in their *in vitro* system is encapsidated by N protein (13). However, the data of Perlman *et al.* indicate that the pools of free N protein in infected cells are quite large, and thus free N may not be rate limiting for MHV RNA synthesis even though it clearly participates in the process (14).

Since most newly synthesized coronavirus RNA is of positive polarity, then N protein must be directly associated with the negative-stranded antigenome if N functions as an essential template component. At present, it has not been established that this is the case. Baric *et al.* have shown, contrary to expectations, that monoclonal antibodies to N coprecipitate <u>all</u> intracellular viral RNAs of MHV, including positive-stranded subgenomic messages, leaders larger than 65 nucleotides and the negative-stranded antigenome (15). In the latter case, however, the negative-stranded RNA may be coprecipitating by virtue of its association with genome in a double-stranded RNA replicative form. In the modified ROPBA of Stohlman *et al.* N protein failed to bind to a 1.1 kb RNA complementary to the 5' end of the MHV genome (8). Thus it is uncertain whether N directly participates as part of the transcription template in a manner similar to that observed with rhabdoviruses, paramyxoviruses and orthomyxoviruses.

OTHER N PROTEIN FUNCTIONS

A few other aspects of coronavirus N protein function warrant mention because they may point to additional potentially exciting areas of research. First, the finding by Baric *et al.* that N is complexed to at least part of all MHV mRNAs (15) raises the possibility that it plays some role in translation. N protein cannot be strictly required for translation since naked coronavirus RNA is infectious. Nevertheless, N may in some way act as a translational enhancer. Second, many coronavirus N genes encode other polypeptides in internal overlapping reading frames. However, it is not known whether any of these proteins are actually expressed *in vivo* and, if so, what may be their functions. Finally, the N protein of MHV has been shown to migrate to the nucleus of infected cells. This translocation is not essential to a productive infection because MHV is capable of replicating in enucleated cells. Nuclear migration may mean, however, that the N protein plays some modulatory role in host cell gene expression. In conclusion, then, it is clear that the molecular biology of coronavirus N proteins contains numerous areas deserving much further exploration.

REFERENCES

1. D.L.D. Caspar and A. Klug, Physical principles in the construction of regular viruses, Cold Spring Harbor Sympos. Quant. Biol., 27: 1 (1962).
2. G. Wengler, Structure and function of the genome of viruses containing single-stranded RNA as genetic material: the concept of transcription and translation helices and the classification of these viruses into six groups, Current Topics Microbiol. and Immunol., 70: 239 (1977).
3. W. Spaan, D. Cavanagh, and M.C. Horzinek, Coronaviruses: structure and genome expression, J. Gen. Virol., 69: 2939 (1988).
4. S.S. Schreiber, T. Kamahora, and M.M.C. Lai, Sequence analysis of the nucleocapsid protein of human coronavirus 229E, Virology, 169: 142 (1989).
5. T. Kamahora, L.H. Soe, and M.M.C. Lai, Sequence analysis of the nucleocapsid gene and leader RNA of human coronavirus OC43, Virus Res., 12: 1 (1989).
6. C.C. Query, R.C. Bentley, and J.D. Keene, A common RNA recognition motif identified within a defined Ul RNA bindingdomain of the 70K Ul snRNP protein, Cell, 57: 89 (1989).
7. S.G. Robbins, M.F. Frana, J.J. McGowan, J.F. Boyle, and K.V. Holmes, RNA binding proteins of coronavirus MHV: detection of monomeric and multimeric N protein with an RNA overlayprotein blot assay, Virology, 150: 402 (1986).
8. S.A. Stohlman, R.S. Baric, G.W. Nelson, L.H. Soe, L.M. Welter, and R.J. Deans, Specific interaction between coronavirus leader RNA and nucleocapsid protein, J. Virol., 62:4288 (1988).
9. L.S. Sturman, K.V. Holmes, and J. Behnke, Isolation of coronavirus envelope glycoproteins and interaction with the viral nucleocapsid, J. Virol. 33:449 (1980).
10. S.G. Siddell, A. Barthel, and V. Ter Meulen, Coronavirus JHM: a virion-associated protein kinase, J. Gen. Virol., 52: 235 (1981) .
11. S.M. Wilbur, G.W. Nelson, M.M.C. Lai, M. McMillan, and S.A. Stohlman, Phosphorylation of the mouse hepatitis virus nucleocapsid protein, Biochem. Biophys. Res. Commun., 141: 7 (1986).
12. S.A. Stohlman, J.O. Fleming, C.D. Patton, and M.M.C. Lai, Synthesis and subcellular localization of the murine coronavirus nucleocapsid protein, Virology, 130: 527 (1983).
13. S.R. Compton, D.B. Rogers, K.V. Holmes, D. Fertsch, J. Remenick, and J.J. McGowan, In vitro replication of mouse hepatitis virus strain A59, J. Virol., 61: 1814 (1987).
14. S. Perlman, D. Ries, E. Bolger, L.-J. Chang, and C.M. Stoltzfus, MHV nucleocapsid synthesis in the presence of cycloheximide and accumulation of negative strand MHV RNA, Virus Res., 6: 261 (1987).
15. R.S. Baric, G.W. Nelson, J.O.Fleming, R.J. Deans. J.G. Keck, N. Casteel, and S.A. Stohlman, Interactions between coronavirus nucleocapsid protein and viral RNAs: implications for viral transcription, J. Virol., 62: 4280 (1988).

STRUCTURE AND FUNCTION STUDIES OF THE NUCLEOCAPSID

PROTEIN OF MOUSE HEPATITIS VIRUS

Paul S. Masters*, Monica M. Parker*, Cynthia S. Ricard*, Cynthia Duchala**, Mark F. Frana**, Kathryn V. Holmes** and Lawrence S. Sturman*

*Wadsworth Center for Laboratories and Research
New York State Department of Health
Albany, NY 12201-0509

**Uniformed Services University of the Health Sciences
Bethesda, MD 20854

Coronaviruses, like virtually all single-stranded RNA viruses, contain a nucleocapsid (N) protein in close structural association with their genomes.[1] Knowledge of the structure and functions of N proteins would be fundamental to an understanding of the viral life cycle and pathogenesis. We have undertaken a study of the N protein of mouse hepatitis virus (MHV) in an attempt to learn the roles of this protein in viral assembly, transcription and translation. Specifically, we would like to examine: (i) the nature of the interaction between N protein and the genome RNA; (ii) the nature of the interactions between adjacent and more distant pairs of N monomers in the helically symmetric viral nucleocapsid; and (iii) the location and purpose of the phosphoserine residue(s) known to occur in the N molecule.[2,3] To date, we have pursued three approaches to these questions: (i) a comparison of the sequences of the N proteins of different, independently isolated strains of MHV; (ii) the examination of an N protein mutant of MHV-A59, Albany-4; and (iii) the in vitro expression and functional assay of N protein and of engineered mutants of N protein. Our results suggest that the MHV N protein has three structural domains, at least two of which may be functionally distinct.

METHODS

The N genes of MHV-A59, the Albany-4 mutant of MHV-A59, MHV-1, MHV-3 and MHV-S were cloned from polyA(+) RNA from infected 17Cl1 cells, essentially by the method of Gubler and Hoffman,[4] and were sequenced by the dideoxy chain termination technique[5] using synthetic oligonucleotide primers. The N genes of MHV-A59 and of the Albany-4 mutant were inserted in either orientation into the SP6/T7 transcription vector pGEM3Zf(-) (Promega), and these constructs were used as templates for the in vitro synthesis of capped full-length and 3'-terminal truncated mRNAs. The messages so produced were translated in a micrococcal nuclease-treated rabbit reticulocyte lysate (Amersham); (^{35}S)methionine-labeled protein products were analyzed by both sodium dodecylsulfate polyacrylamide gel electrophoresis (SDS-PAGE) and nondenaturing PAGE followed by autoradiography, as described previously.[6]

RESULTS AND DISCUSSION

The sequences of the genes encoding the N proteins of three independently isolated strains of MHV were determined in order to examine the structural constraints maintained on this molecule throughout evolution. It has been reported previously that the sequences of the N proteins of MHV-A59 and MHV-JHM are highly homologous, having ca. 94% amino acid identity, but that positions of nonidentity are not distributed randomly over the molecule.[7] To extend this pairwise comparison, we cloned and sequenced cDNAs to the N mRNAs of MHV-1, MHV-3 and MHV-S. The amino acid sequences deduced for these proteins showed that they, too, were highly similar to the previously determined N sequences. As shown schematically in Fig. 1, amino acid changes among the five proteins were clustered in two small regions of the N molecule: between residues 140-162 and between residues 381-404. These two loci also have the greatest density of changes at the nucleotide level. For the most divergent pair of sequences, the N proteins of MHV-A59 and MHV-JHM, 19 of the 30 amino acid differences between the two are concentrated in these regions, while the other nonidentical residues are scattered throughout the remaining 90% of the molecule. These results show that the N protein has undergone very little evolutionary drift among these five strains, implying that few structural changes can be tolerated by the molecule without impairing its function. This raises the possibility, then, that the highly variable amino acid clusters merely act as spacers, having little sequence specificity, but connecting the more conserved regions of the molecule. Thus, we have tentatively divided the N molecule into three structural, and possibly functional, domains (I, II and III) tethered to each other by the putative spacers A and B (Fig. 1). Domains I and II each contain regions with a large excess of positively charged residues, accounting for the overall basic character of the N molecule. By contrast, domain III is the most acidic portion of the molecule, having an excess of negatively charged residues.

Further support for the notion that at least one of the spacers is dispensible for N protein function came from the examination of a mutant of MHV-A59 designated Albany-4. This mutant is temperature-sensitive, forming tiny plaques on 17C11 or L2 cells at the nonpermissive temperature, 39°, but showing no significant reduction in growth at 33°. Albany-4 is also thermolabile, i.e., extended incubation at the nonpermissive temperature produces at least 100-fold greater loss of infectious titer in this virus than in its heat-resistant parent.[8] This implies that the lesion in this mutant is in one of the three structural proteins of the MHV virion. Furthermore, it was noted that the N protein of Albany-4 had a greater electrophoretic mobility on SDS-PAGE than did its parent virus counterpart, whereas the E1 and E2 proteins of parent and mutant migrated identically.[8] This raised the possibility that the alteration in the mutant resided in the N gene. In order to directly test this idea, the N gene of Albany-4 was cloned, and its sequence was compared to the N gene of the heat-resistant parent. Such an analysis showed that the Albany-4 N gene was everywhere identical to the parent N gene with the exception of a deletion of 87 nucleotides in the distal portion of the gene. This resulted in a 29 amino acid in-phase deletion of residues 380 through 408, almost exactly encompassing the region we have designated as spacer B (Fig. 1).

Evidence presented below shows that this deletion in Albany-4 produces some reduction in the ability of the N protein to bind to RNA. However, it must be noted that the finding of an alteration of the N protein in Albany-4 does not prove it to be the lesion responsible for the temperature-sensitivity or thermolability of the mutant virus. Moreover, it has not been established that the temperature-sensitive and thermolabile phenotypes are due to the same mutation. Nevertheless, the data allow us to conclude, at a minimum, that the complete excision of spacer B from the N molecule does not lethally impair the function of N since Albany-4 is completely viable at the permissive temperature and even partially viable at the nonpermissive temperature.

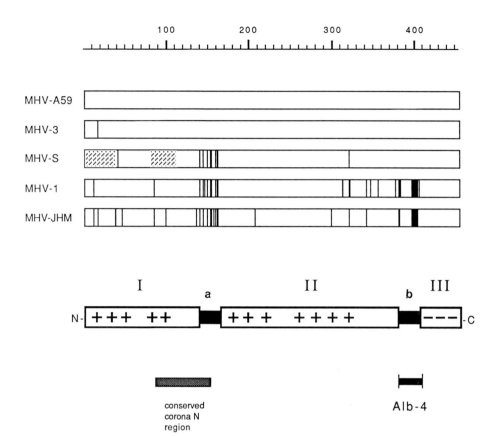

Fig. 1. Strain sequence comparison and model of the N protein of MHV. For each strain of MHV, a vertical line denotes an amino acid change in the N sequence at that position; the number line at the top indicates amino acid residues. The shaded portions of the MHV-S sequence have not yet been determined. The MHV-JHM sequence is from reference 7. The three domain model of the MHV N protein is shown beneath. At the bottom are indicated a region of sequence which is highly conserved among all coronavirus N proteins sequenced to date [9,10] and the region of N which is deleted in the Albany-4 mutant.

In order to attempt to functionally dissect the N protein in vitro, the N gene of MHV-A59 was inserted into a plasmid vector adjacent to the promoter for the RNA polymerase of either bacteriophage T7 or SP6. This allowed the in vitro synthesis of N mRNA, which was then used to program protein synthesis in a rabbit reticulocyte lysate. The (^{35}S)methionine-labeled translation product was analyzed by gel electrophoresis. As shown in Fig. 2A, the synthetic N mRNA was translated into a protein which ran as a single major band on SDS-PAGE. This polypeptide had a mobility indistinguishable from that of N protein translated from RNA isolated from MHV-A59-infected 17Cl1 cells (data not shown). When the same translation product was analyzed by nondenaturing PAGE, a significant fraction of it entered the running gel, forming a discrete band with a mobility of ca. 0.25 relative to bromphenol blue (Fig. 2B). Initially this was surprising because the N protein, which would be expected to have a large net positive charge, was migrating toward the positive pole during electrophoresis. This suggested either (i) that the conformation of the N molecule was such that most of its lysine and arginine residues had extremely altered pK$_a$'s, (ii) that the N molecule underwent extensive posttranslational modification resulting in its having a net negative charge, or (iii) that the N molecule was tightly complexed to some polyanionic molecule which was carrying N into the nondenaturing gel as it migrated toward the positive pole.

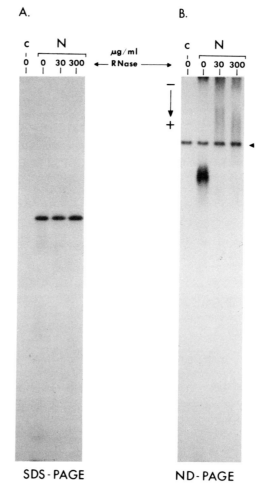

Fig. 2. SDS-PAGE and nondenaturing PAGE of in vitro translated parent virus N protein. In each panel, C indicates a control lane of a translation mix with no added mRNA. In panel B, the arrow on the left indicates the direction and polarity of electrophoresis; the arrowhead on the right denotes an endogenous (^{35}S)methionine-labeled band in the reticulocyte lysate.

The latter alternative was shown to be the case, since treatment of the translated N protein with RNase A abolished its ability to enter the nondenaturing gel (Fig. 2B) without altering the integrity of the N molecule as monitored by SDS-PAGE (Fig. 2A).

At present we have not identified the RNA to which the N protein is binding in vitro. Preliminary experiments with labeled N mRNA suggest that N protein is not binding to its own message. Thus, the bound species may be some endogenous RNA in the reticulocyte lysate. The binding appears to be specific, since the labeled protein migrates to a single position, forming a discrete band instead of the heterogeneous smear that might be expected if N were nonspecifically binding to any available RNA. In addition, N protein translated from total RNA from infected cells migrates identically in nondenaturing gels, indicating that the unknown RNA species is not appreciably competed out by viral RNA species. Thus, in spite of the unresolved nature of the RNA involved, the ability of the N protein to enter a nondenaturing gel constitutes an assay for RNA binding which could then be used to characterize mutants of N.

A set of carboxy-terminal truncated forms of N protein were next generated by the digestion of the MHV N gene T7 (or SP6) transcription templates with restriction enzymes that have unique sites in the distal portion of the cDNA copy of the N gene. The enzymes AccI, BsmI, ScaI, EcoRI and SpeI yielded DNA fragments which, when transcribed and translated, produced N proteins with carboxy-terminal deletions of 56, 77, 94, 118 and 148 amino acids, respectively. In addition, the Albany-4 N gene was inserted into transcription vectors, and this 425 amino acid mutant N protein was expressed by the same strategy.

Analysis by SDS-PAGE of the N/AccI, N/Albany-4, N/ScaI and N/EcoRI translated proteins is shown in Fig. 3. All four of these species have the expected relative sizes and are not grossly altered by incubation with RNase A. There was some heterogeneity of the band for N/AccI; this has been seen consistently in a number of experiments, and we do not presently know if it was due to post-translational processing or to some limited proteolytic breakdown of this species.

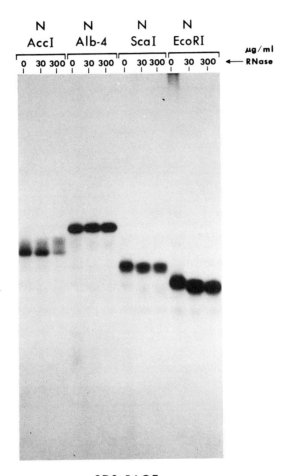

SDS-PAGE

Fig. 3. SDS PAGE of four N protein mutants translated in vitro.

The analysis of the same four N protein deletion mutants by nondenaturing PAGE is shown in Fig. 4. Two of these N variants, N/AccI and N/Albany-4, were seen to be able to enter the nondenaturing gel in an RNase-sensitive fashion, having slightly higher mobilities than the parent N protein (each ca. 0.28 relative to bromphenol blue). Thus, these two proteins retained a significant ability to bind to RNA. By contrast, two other N variants, N/ScaI and N/EcoRI, were not able to enter the nondenaturing gel to any appreciable extent. Only upon a much longer exposure of the autoradiogram in Fig. 4 was a faint band seen for each of these species (each with a mobility of ca. 0.49 relative to bromphenol blue). An additional two N variants, N/BsmI and N/SpeI also failed to enter nondenaturing gels (data not shown). The extent of truncation from the carboxy termini of these N mutants, then, had almost completely abolished their ability to bind RNA. This result also argued for the specificity of the RNA binding seen with the parent N protein and the N/AccI and N/Albany-4 variants. If the N protein - RNA complexes observed in nondenaturing gels were due simply to nonspecific electrostatic interactions, then species like N/ScaI and N/EcoRI would be expected to bind RNA as well as or better than the parent N species because they are even more basic due to the elimination of the negatively charged carboxy terminus of the molecule. That they were largely unable to bind to RNA suggests that a specific domain of the N molecule is involved in RNA binding and that the deletions in these variants have either removed or altered the conformation of that domain.

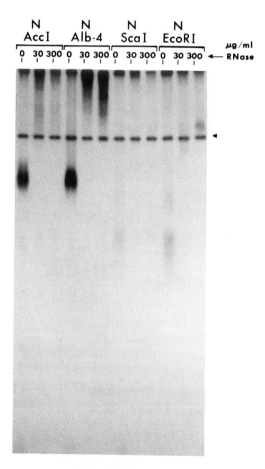

ND-PAGE

Fig. 4. Nondenaturing PAGE of four N protein mutants translated in vitro. The arrowhead on the right denotes an endogenous (^{35}S)methionine-labeled band in the reticulocyte lysate.

The ability of the various N mutants to bind to RNA was quantitated by excising the bands from a number of gels similar to those in Fig. 2-4 and comparing the ratios of cpm in the nondenaturing PAGE band to the cpm in the SDS-PAGE band. These results, as well as a representation of the locations of the deletions in the N variants, are summarized in Fig. 5. From the N/AccI mutant it is clear that removal of the entirety of domain III of the N molecule has little effect on the ability of the molecule to bind to RNA. Thus, the putative domain III appears to be a truly distinct protein domain, both functionally as well as structurally. Although it appears to be dispensable with respect to one aspect of N protein function, RNA binding, domain III likely plays an important role since it is one of the most conserved regions of the molecule (Fig. 1).

The N/Albany-4 mutant also retained significant RNA binding activity: sufficient to produce viable virions in vivo, but less than that of N/AccI. This reduction in binding may have been due to either (i) an alteration in the conformation of N brought about by the too close juxtaposition of domains II and III, or (ii) the entry of the left boundary of the deletion in N/Albany-4 into a portion of domain II which may be essential for RNA binding. Indeed, the N/BsmI mutant, the truncation in which extended just a few amino acids further into domain II, had lost almost all ability to bind to RNA. Further truncation of N (as in N/ScaI, N/EcoRI and N/SpeI) similarly reduced RNA binding to insignificant levels. These results, then, define the right-most boundary of the portion of the N protein which, directly or indirectly, is required for the ability to bind to RNA. The construction of additional N mutants is underway in order to define the minimal RNA-binding domain of the N molecule.

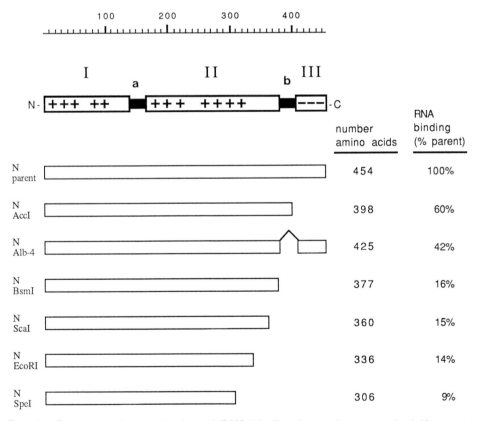

Fig. 5. Summary of quantitation of RNA binding for carboxy-terminal N protein mutants. The extent of each deletion is represented with respect to the three domain model and the number line at the top indicating amino acid residues. The values in the column at the right are the average of four (N parent, N/AccI, N/Albany-4, N/ScaI, N/EcoRI) or two (N/BsmI, N/SpeI) independent experiments.

ACKNOWLEDGEMENTS

We are grateful for the skilled secretarial assistance of Kathleen Cavanagh. This work was supported by grants GM31698 and AI18997 from the National Institutes of Health The opinions or assertions contained herein are the private views of the authors and should not be construed as official or necessarily reflecting the views of the Uniformed Services University of the Health Sciences or the Department of Defense.

REFERENCES

1. L.S. Sturman and K.V. Holmes, The molecular biology of coronaviruses, Adv. Virus Res. 28:35 (1983).

2. S.G. Siddell, A. Barthel and V. Ter Meulen, Coronavirus JHM: a virion-associated protein kinase, J. Gen. Virol. 52:235 (1981).

3. S.M. Wilbur, G.W. Nelson, M.M.C. Lai, M. McMillan and S.A. Stohlman, Phosphorylation of the mouse hepatitis virus nucleocapsid protein, Biochem. Biophys. Res. Commun. 141:7 (1986).

4. U. Gubler and B.J. Hoffman, A simple and very efficient method for generating cDNA libraries, Gene 25:263 (1983).

5. F. Sanger, S. Nicklen and A.R. Coulson, DNA sequencing with chain terminating inhibitors, Proc. Natl. Acad. Sci. USA 74:5463 (1977).

6. P.S. Masters and A.K. Banerjee, Resolution of multiple complexes of phosphoprotein NS with nucleocapsid protein N of vesicular stomatitis virus, J. Virol. 62:2651 (1988).

7. M.A. Skinner and S.G. Siddel, Coronavirus JHM: nucleotide sequence of the mRNA that encodes the nucleocapsid protein, Nucl. Acids Res. 11:5045 (1983).

8. L.S. Sturman, C. Eastwood, M.F. Frana, C. Duchala, F. Baker, C.S. Ricard, S.G. Sawicki and K.V. Holmes, Temperature-sensitive mutants of MHV-A59, Adv. Exp. Med. Biol. 218:159 (1987).

9. M.E.G. Boursnell, M.M. Binns, I.J. Foulds and T.D.K. Brown, Sequences of the nucleocapsid genes from two strains of avian infectious bronchitis virus, J. Gen. Virol. 66:573 (1985).

10. P.A. Kapke and D.A. Brian, Sequence analysis of the porcine transmissible gastroenteritis coronavirus nucleocapsid protein gene, Virology 151:41 (1986).

MHV LEADER RNA SECONDARY STRUCTURE AFFECTS BINDING TO THE

NUCLEOCAPSID PROTEIN

Lisa M. Welter[1], Stephen A. Stohlman [1,2], and Robert J. Deans[*1]

Department of Microbiology[1] and Neurology [2]
University of Southern California School of Medicine
Los Angeles, California 90033

INTRODUCTION

Leader RNA is found at the 5' end of the mouse hepatitis virus (MHV) genomic RNA, at the 5' end of the seven viral mRNAs, and free in the cell. Leader RNA is synthesized by a transcriptional activity separate from the activities that synthesize both (-) sense genomic length RNA and the virus mRNAs[1]. It is believed to function as a primer, binding to complementary intergenic sites, on (-) sense template, situated 5' of each of the initiation sites for viral mRNAs[2]. Using monoclonal antibodies specific for the nucleocapsid (N) protein, immunoprecipitations of RNA/protein complexes from infected cells indicate that the N protein is complexed to: 1) genomic RNA; 2) viral mRNAs; and 3) even free leader containing RNA fragments as small as 60 nucleotides in length[3]. Northwestern blot analysis showed that the viral N protein exhibits RNA binding activity that is specific for viral leader containing RNA when expressed in the (+) sense[4,5]. However, this system has several limitations. First, in denaturing conditions, RNA/protein interactions which require the interaction of multiple protein subunits cannot be studied, and second, it is not possible to quantify relative affinities and binding characteristics.

The gel retardation assay (GRA) was used to define the N protein interaction with leader RNA. The advantages of this technique are: 1) the detection of weak nucleic acid/protein interactions; 2) the use of crude protein extracts thereby eliminating the requirement of purification of a single binding protein; 3) the visualization of multiple protein interactions with a single nucleic acid species; and 4) the nucleic acid protein interactions are able to occur freely in solution.

To study the RNA-protein interactions of MHV and to understand how N interactions with free leader, mRNA, or genomic RNA are related to viral assembly, we have used the GRA to define a high affinity interaction between leader RNA and the N protein. In this study we show the resolution of a high affinity RNA-protein complex formed in the presence of in vitro radiolabelled leader RNA transcripts, using MHV infected cell lysates as a source of N protein, and non-radiolabelled uninfected cytoplasmic RNA as a non-specific competitor. The specific RNA-protein complex is observed only with infected but not uninfected cell lysates. Through the use of the GRA we have been able to map the location of this binding activity to a proximal stem loop structure of leader RNA.

Coronaviruses and Their Diseases
Edited by D. Cavanagh and T.D.K. Brown
Plenum Press, New York, 1990

MATERIALS AND METHODS

In Vitro Transcript Preparation

The in vitro RNA transcripts used in this study were derived from Bluescribe (+), (BS+) plasmids (Stratagene, La Jolla, CA) containing a BamHI/DdeI fragment from the 5' end of mRNA from gene F of the A59 strain of MHV, inserted at the BamHI site of the BS+ plasmid[6]. A schematic map of these plasmids, and the in vitro transcripts produced are depicted in Figure 1. This construct, pBSL contains the 72 base leader plus 15 nucleotides extending into the E1 coding region[4]. Transcripts containing the 3' nucleotide sequences of leader RNA, starting at nucleotide 24, were derived by deleting the sequences between SmaI and SnaBI sites of pBSL. This plasmid is designated pBSL-SSΔ. Plasmid F82D was obtained from Dr. Michael Lai. This cDNA clone of genomic RNA initiates at nucleotide 56 of leader. Transcripts containing viral genomic sequences from 56 to 180, are obtained by digesting with the restriction endonuclease NarI which cleaves interval genomic sequences. Recombinant pT7 plasmids were first linearized with one of the restriction enzymes shown in Figure 1 to allow synthesis of transcripts of different lengths. Transcription was carried out as previously described[4].

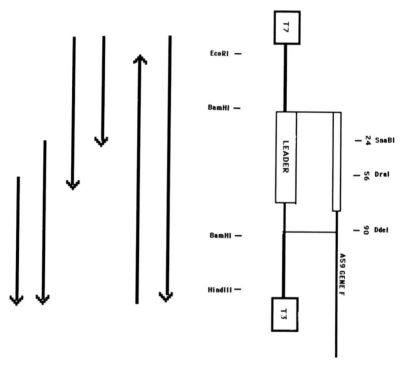

Figure 1. Schematic map of leader plasmids. The RNA transcripts containing leader sequences I-24, I-56 or all 72 nucleotides were derived from pBSL digested with SnaBI, DraI or HindIII respectively. RNA transcripts containing leader sequences beginning at nucleotide 24 of leader were derived from pBSL-SSΔ digested with HindIII. RNA transcripts beginning at nucleotide 56 of leader was derived from plasmid F82D digested with NarI.

Preparation of Protein Extracts

Cellular lysates containing the N protein were prepared from DBT cells infected with the A59 strain of MHV, as previously described[4,7]. N protein was also obtained by electroelution following resolution by SDS-polyacrylamide gel electrophoresis. Protein lysates, prepared as described above, were electrophoresed on 10% polyacrylamide gels[4]. Exterior lanes were loaded with ^{32}P labelled protein lysates of infected cells. Following electrophoresis, the ^{32}P-labelled N protein was identified by autography using the wet gel. A slice of gel containing the unlabelled N was removed and N was isolated by electroelution in a Schleicher and Schuell electroeluter using 25 mM Tris, 0.165 M glycine, pH 8.0 buffer as described[8]. Protein was quantitated by the Branford colorimetric microassay[9]. The identity of purified N was confirmed by Western blot analysis using the anti-N monoclonal antibody designated A1.10[2].

RNA Gel Retardation Assay

Binding reactions and gel conditions are a modification of those described by Schneider et al. (10). A typical 20 ul binding reaction contained 25 mM HEPES pH 7.5, 1 mM EDTA, 150 mM NaCl, 5 mM DTT, 0.5 mM PMSF, 10% glycerol, and 5 ug of total cytoplasmic mouse liver RNA as a nonspecific competitor. Prior to their addition, RNA transcripts were boiled for 1 minute and quenched on ice. The final reaction mixture contained 20-30 ng of ^{32}P labeled RNA transcript and 10-20 ug of the appropriate protein extract in the presence or absence of cytoplasmic liver RNA as a non-specific competitor. After incubation at room temperature for 10 minutes, 5 ul of loading dye containing 50% glycerol, 0.05% bromophenol blue and 10 mM DTT was added. 7% acrylamide gels (made from a 44% acrylamide: 0.8% w/v bisacrylamide stock) containing 5% glycerol in Tris-glycine buffer (50 mM Tris base, 0.33 M glycine, pH 8.5) were equilibrated overnight by storing them in Tris-glycine buffer. Prior to loading, gels were pre-run at 25 mAmps until constant current was obtained. Fresh running buffer was added prior to addition of the samples. Samples were then electrophoresed at room temperature for 2-4 hours at 25 mAmps (until the bromophenol blue reached the bottom of the gel).

RESULTS

Identification of Specific RNA/Protein Interactions in Infected Cell Lysates

The GRA was used to resolve specific RNA-protein interactions between MHV leader RNA sequences, and the proteins from viral infected cells or purified N protein. Prior to addition, ^{32}P-labeled in vitro transcripts were heated to 100°C for 1 minute, quenched on ice, and then incubated at 25°C with the appropriate protein. Figure 2 shows that the RNA transcript containing 72 nucleotides of (+) sense viral leader RNA migrates as a retarded heterogeneous population when incubated with infected cell lysate. Mouse liver RNA had previously been demonstrated by Northwestern blot analysis to be an effective competitor of non-specific RNA/protein interaction[4]. Figure 2 shows that the retarded population is resolved into a discrete band with the addition of nonspecific competitor.

Two lines of evidence indicated that the N protein is required for formation of the leader RNA/protein complex. First, the persistence of the discrete complex formed in the presence of competitor RNA is only seen with extracts prepared from infected cells and not with extracts from uninfected cells. In addition, we have confirmed that N protein, which has been isolated by elution from 10% SDS-polyacrylamide gels, generates the leader specific protein complex (Figure 3).

COMPETITOR   - - + - +
PROTEIN   - + + + +
PROBE   + + + + +

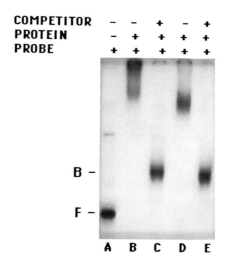

B -

F -

A B C D E

Figure 2.   GRA of infected cell lysates binding to leader-containing transcripts,
derived from pBSL digested with HindIII. The migration of transcript
alone is shown in lane A.   Radiolabeled in vitro transcripts were
incubated at room temperature with 40 ug (lanes B and C) or 20 ug
(lanes D and E) of infected cell lysate either alone (lanes B and D), or
in the presence of 5 ug of liver RNA as a nonspecific competitor
(lanes C and E).

COMPETITOR   - - + - +
PROTEIN   - + + +[a] +[b]
PROBE   + + + + +

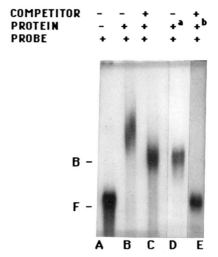

B -

F -

A B C D E

Figure 3.   GRA of uninfected cell lysates or purified N protein.   In vitro
transcripts derived from pBSL, digested with HindIII, were incubated
incubated with 20 ug of infected cell lysates (lanes B and C) in the
absence (lane B) or presence (lane C) or 5 ug of liver RNA as a
nonspecific competitor. Lane D shows the transcript incubated with
7.8 µg of purified N.   Lane E shows the transcript incubated with
40 µg of unifected cell lysate and 5 µg of liver RNA as nonspecific
competitor.

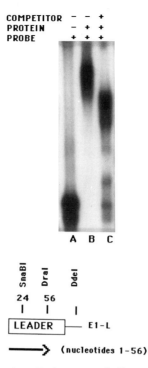

COMPETITOR   −   −   +
PROTEIN   −   +   +
PROBE   +   +   +

A   B   C

SnaBI   DraI   DdeI

24   56

LEADER ├── E1−L

⟶⟩ (nucleotides 1−56)

Figure 4.   GRA of infected cell lysates binding to transcripts containing nucleotides I-56 of leader derived from pBSL digested with DraI. The migration of transcript alone is shown in lane A. Radiolabeled in vitro transcripts were incubated at room temperature with 20 ug of infected cell lysate (lanes B and C), in the absence (lane B), or in the presence of 5 ug of liver RNA as a nonspecific competitor (lane C).

Sequence Specificity Involved in Complex Formation

Three lines of evidence confirm the sequence specificity of the leader RNA/N-protein interaction. First, an in vitro transcript consisting solely of plasmid sequences is unable to form a specific complex. Secondly, there is no specific complex formation when 5S RNA is used as a probe. Finally, the MHV leader transcript in the (-) sense in the presence of nonspecific competitor, does not form a specific RNA-protein complex (data not shown). These results confirm that the RNA/protein interaction is specific for leader sequences in the (+) sense[11].

Mapping Binding Regions of Leader RNA

We have used the GRA to map the N protein binding region of MHV leader RNA. This was accomplished by testing RNA transcripts containing partial sequences of MHV leader RNA. RNA transcripts containing nucleotides 1 to 24 (data not shown), nucleotides 24 to 90 (Figure 6) or nucleotides 56 to 180 (Figure 5) did not exhibit specific binding. However, RNA transcripts containing nucleotide sequences from 1 to 56 (Figure 4) and from 1 to 90 (Figure 2) do exhibit specific binding activity. This data is summarized in Figure 7.

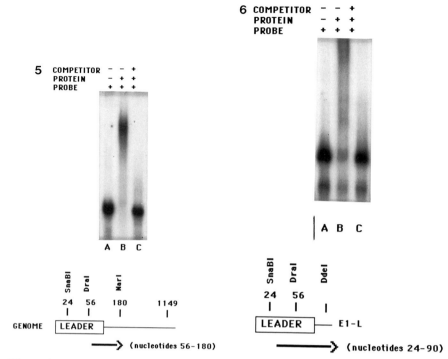

Figure 5.   GRA of infected cell lysates binding to transcripts beginning at leader nucleotide 56, derived from pF82D digested with NarI. The migration of transcript alone is shown in lane A. Radiolabeled in vitro transcripts were incubated at room temperature with 20 ug of infected cell lysate (lanes B and C), in the absence (lane B), or in the presence of 5 ug of liver RNA as a nonspecific competitor (lane C).

Figure 6.   GRA of infected cell lysates binding to leader-containing transcripts, derived from pBSL-SSΔ digested with HindIII. The migration of transcript beginning at nucleotide 24 of leader alone is shown in lane A. Radiolabeled in vitro transcripts were incubated at room temperature with 20 ug of infected cell lysate (lanes B and C), in the absence (lane B), or in the presence of 5 ug of liver RNA as a nonspecific competitor (lane C).

Secondary Structure Predictions of Leader RNA

We performed a computer analysis of potential secondary structure of free leader RNA (Zuker[12]) and this predicts a proximal stem loop structure (Figure 7). This structure is conserved between transcripts containing leader nucleotides 1 to 56 and 1 to 90. These RNAs exhibit specific binding (Figures 2 and 4). In contrast, the RNAs in which the stem loop structure is absent did not exhibit specific binding (Figures 5 and 6).

DISCUSSION

These experiments were initiated from our interest in studying the RNA/protein interactions involved in viral morphogenesis. The RNA binding property of the viral N protein has been previously demonstrated by the use of Northwestern blotting techniques and these data show specificity of binding for the leader RNA sequences

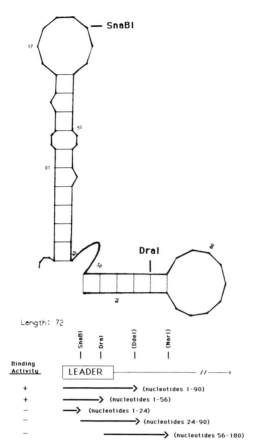

Figure 7. Summary of binding activity and predicted secondary structure of A59 leader sequences (I-72). The predicted secondary structure was generated by computer analysis using the program by Zuker[12]. Below is a summary of transcript binding activity observed in the gel retardation assay.

expressed in a (+) sense configuration[4,5]. We have also previously shown that monoclonal antibodies specific for the N protein could immunoprecipitate RNA/protein complexes[3]. These studies demonstrated that not only free viral leader RNA, but also viral genomic and mRNAs, which have leader sequences at their 5'-ends, are complexed with the N protein[3,4], consistent with the findings that all (+) sense encoded virus RNA species contain leader sequences at their 5' ends[13].

Virus subgenomic mRNAs are not packaged into mature virions at a detectable level, and hence other signals may be involved in directing genomic RNA into the assemble pathway. Examination of specific MHV leader RNA/N protein interactions will allow definition of the role of the N protein during the lytic cycle and persistence phases of MHV infection. For example, RNA sequences found on genomic RNA but absent from mRNA may control the cooperativity of N protein binding, such that RNA is appropriately presented or packaged into virions. Protein/protein interactions between the N protein complexed to free leader RNA and the viral polymerase may also be required for viral transcription. In addition, N may be involved in binding (+) sensed genomic RNA and mRNAs during replication and/or transcription in order to prevent anti-sense inhibition of gene expression.

The data presented in this report confirm our previous description of the specificity of the binding of MHV leader RNA in the (+) sense configuration to the MHV encoded N protein[4]. Our mapping data using RNA transcripts containing various leader sequences demonstrates that the leader RNA/N interactions may depend on secondary structure as well as specific nucleotide sequences, since only those transcripts exhibiting the secondary structure comparable to free leader exhibit specific binding.

We are presently constructing plasmids that contain mutations in the stem or loop site of the predicted conserved secondary structure. These mutations will determine if primary sequences are the sole determinant, or the extent to which these sequences in the correct context of secondary structure are required for recognition. Recently we have conducted competition experiments using purified N protein and the previously described RNA transcripts as homologous competitors. Those results confirm our mapping data in which only those transcripts with the designated secondary structure are able to compete for binding activity (data not shown). In addition, testing of the predicted secondary structure is being determined through the use of specific chemical modifications and cleavage, as well as using various ribonucleases whose activity are sensitive to secondary structure. The ability to isolate RNA complexes by GRA is also well suited for the application of in situ chemical cleavage and footprinting analysis, such as has been described by Murakawa et al.[14] and Nielsen et al.[15]. We are currently using these approaches to map the specific nucleotides of leader RNA which interact with the MHV N protein.

ACKNOWLEDGEMENTS

This work was supported by grant DMB-17148 from the National Science Foundation (SAS); GM 40146 from the N.I.H. (RJD) and a grant from the Medical and Life Insurance Foundation (RJD).

REFERENCES

1. P. R. Brayton, M. M. C. Lai, C. D. Patton and S. A. Stohlman, J. Virol. 42:847-853 (1982).
2. R. S. Baric, C. -K. Shieh, S. S. Stohlman and M. M. C. Lai, Virol. 156:342-354 (1987).
3. R. S. Baric, G. W. Nelson, J. Q. Fleming, R. J. Deans, J. G. Keck, N. Casteel and S. A. Stohlman, J. Virol. 62:4280-4287 (1988).
4. S. A. Stohlman, R. S. Baric, G. W. Nelson, L. H. Soe, L. M. Welter and R. J. Deans, J. Virol. 62:4288-4295 (1988).
5. S. G. Robbins, M. F. Frana, J. J. McGowan, J. F. Boyle and K. W. Holmes, Virol. 150:402-410 (1986).
6. J. Armstrong, S. Smeeken and P. Rottier, Nucl. Acids Res. 11:883-891.
7. M. M. C. Lai and S. A. Stohlman, J. Virol. 26:236-242 (1978).
8. E. Jacobs and A. Clad, Anal. Biochem. 154:583-589 (1986).
9. M. Bradford, Anal. Biochem. 72:248 (1976).
10. R. Schneider, I. Gander, U. Miller, R. Mertz and E. L. Wennacher, Nucl. Acids Res. 14, 1303-1317.
11. L. M. Welter, G. Nelsen, S. A. Stohlman and R. J. Deans, Submitted to Nucl. Acids Res. (1986).
12. M. Zuker and P. Stiegler, NAR 9:133-148 (1981).
13. M. M. C. Lai, Baric, R. S., Brayton, P. R. and Stohlman, S. A. Proc. Natl. Acad. Sci. USA 81:3626-3630 (1984).
14. G. J. Murakawa, B. C. Chen, M. D. Kuwabara, D. P. Nierlich and D. S. Sigman, Nucl. Acids Res. In Press.
15. P. E. Nielsen, C. Jeppesen and O. Buchardt, FEBS Letters 235:122-124 (1988).

IN VIVO AND IN VITRO MODELS OF DEMYELINATING DISEASE: A PHOSPHOPROTEIN PHOSPHATASE IN HOST CELL ENDOSOMES DEPHOSPHORYLATING THE NUCLEOCAPSID PROTEIN OF CORONAVIRUS JHM

D.V. Mohandas and S. Dales

Cytobiology Group
Department of Microbiology and Immunology, London
Ontario, Canada   N6A 5C1

Coronavirus JHM (JHMV) shows specific tropism for oligodendrocytes of the CNS.[1] Primary oligodendrocytes induced to differentiate using agents like dibutyryl cyclic AMP (dbcAMP) develop resistance to JHMV infection.[1,2] Several studies suggest that the virus enters the host cell through receptor mediated endocytosis.[3,4] Earlier studies also found that the nucleocapsid protein (NC) of JHMV is reduced in molecular weight (MW) from a 56K to a 50K component during the early stages of infection.[5] A change in the molecular weight of this magnitude with phosphorylated proteins can be accounted for by dephosphorylation.[6] The reversible phosphorylation-dephosphorylation of a capsid polypeptide-nucleic acid binding protein has been shown to influence the binding of nucleic acid in a retrovirus.[7] This information suggests that a phosphoprotein phosphatase (PPPase) dephosphorylating the NC of JHMV effects the uncoating of the RNA genome during the early stages of infection. Here we present evidence for such a dephosphorylating activity in neural and other cells which are hosts for JHMV.

[32P]-labelled NC protein was prepared from JHMV infected L-2 mouse fibroblasts labelled with [32P] orthophosphate using conventional biochemical methods. The final product, isolated from preparative SDS-PAGE, was examined and confirmed to be pure by autoradiography and Western blotting. The assay mixture for PPPase consisted of 25 mM Tris-maleate buffer (pH 7.0), 1 mM $MnCl_2$, 0.1% Triton X-100 and [32P]-labelled NC protein in a total volume of 100 ul. The reaction was terminated after 90 min. at 30°C by precipitating on ice with 25% TCA. The [32P] released from the substrate was determined by scintillation counter according to Maene and Greengard.[8] To separate the NC as a band the reaction mixture was boiled in Laemmli's dissociation buffer and subjected to SDS-PAGE[9] and autoradiography.

Coronaviruses and Their Diseases
Edited by D. Cavanagh and T.D.K. Brown
Plenum Press, New York, 1990

Modulation of the 56K Nucleocapsid Protein

Addition of phosphate was made to infected L-2 cell
monolayers, when about 10% of cells had formed syncytia. Upon
completion of syncytia formation the cells were harvested,
disrupted, centrifuged at 7,000 x g for 15' and the supernatant
treated with 0.5% NP-40. Separation by 10% SDS-PAGE gel and
Western blotting with anti-NC monoclonal antibody revealed the
homogeneity of the NC component. Following exposure of L-2
cell monolayers infected with JHMV to varying concentrations of
phosphate two MW species of NC of 56 and 50K were evident in
the cell extracts. The proportion of each MW type present
depended on the phosphate concentration applied (Figure 1).
The results, shown as relative percentage of NC antigen, are
calculated from densitometer scanning of the 56K and 50K bands
in the Western blots. As shown in Figure 1, the amount of 50K
protein decreased in relation to increasing phosphate
concentrations, being completely absent at 5 mM phosphate.
These data imply that phosphate concentration in the growth
medium determines the amount of 56K NC protein which is
produced presumably in relation to the phosphorylation of the
50K protein.

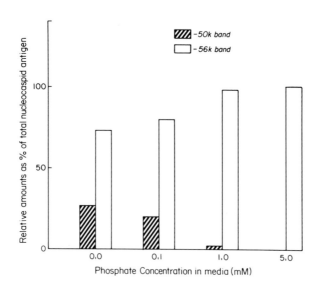

Figure 1. Relationship between phosphate
concentration (mM) added to the NM and relative
percentage of 56K and 50K nucleocapsid antigen.
Following inoculation and incubation to allow virus
replication virus-cell complexes were disrupted and
the larger cell organelles were removed by
centrifugation. The remaining supernatant material
was treated with detergent NP-40, prior to separation
of the components by SDS-PAGE. The 50K and 56K NC
antigens were detected by immunoblotting. Relative
antigen concentrations were determined by
scanning densitometer.

Subcellular Localization of PPPase Acting on 56K NC Protein

The presumed association of inoculum JHMV with endosomes during early cell-virus interactions led us to isolate an endosomal fraction from host L-2 cells. For this purpose the method of Merion and Poretz[10] was followed, using a two step centrifugation through percoll gradients. The individual fractions collected from the gradients were identified by contents of marker enzymes (data not shown). Some of these results on one enzyme activity within various cellular fractions are summarized in Table 1. After addition of Triton X-100 to the reaction mixture, specific activity of the PPPase with a neutral pH optimum was enhanced more than 3-fold, indicating that this PPPase is membrane associated. The neutral PPPase was found to be concentrated in the endosomal fraction of L-2 cells, since in this cell fraction a 25-fold increase in specific activity was evident, compared to that in the homogenate (Table 1).

Table 1. Subcellular distribution of a 'neutral' phospho-protein phosphatase from L-2 cells, active on JHMV nucleocapsids

Cell fraction	Specific activity units/mg protein	Amplification in Sp. activity relative to homogenate
Total homogenate with 0.1% Triton X-100	65	1.0
Total homogenate without detergent	19	0.3
Nuclear pellet	162	2.5
Post-nuclear supernatant	96	1.5
Lysosomal	333	5.1
Cytosolic	288	4.5
Endosomal/prelysosomal	1,660	25.5

For comparative purposes specific PPPase activity is a measure of the percentage of [^{32}P] released from NC, one unit being equivalent to release of 1% [^{32}P] dpm from the NC substrate. The representative data shown are from one of several such experiments.

Table 2. Characteristics of PPPase

1. pH optimum	7.0
2. Cation requirement	Mn^{++}, 1 mM
3. Effect of 30 mM NaF inhibition	30%
4. Effect of commercial acid and alkaline phosphatase on the NC substrate	No activity
5. Effect of PPPase on [^{32}P]-labelled Casein and Histone	Active

Partial Characterization of the Neutral PPPase

In order to define the endosomal PPPase further, partial characterization was undertaken. A summary of the findings is presented in Table 2. The pH optimum for the PPPase activity was found at about neutrality, in line with characteristics of other phosphoprotein phosphatases.[11] This finding suggests that the PPPase under study is more likely to function in the prelysosomal/endosomal subpopulations termed 'early endosomes'[12] which have been shown to contain a milieu at pH of about 6.5. Divalent cation requirement for Mn^{++} is also in line with characteristics of other protein phosphatases.[13] Exposure to 30 mM NaF inhibited the endosomal PPPase by only 30%, distinguishing it from the acid phosphatase activity present in the same cell material, which was inhibited by over 95% with NaF, when acting on the non-specific substrate p-nitrophenyl phosphate (pNPP). Commercial acid phosphatase from potato and alkaline phosphatase from E. coli were inert against the NC protein as substrate when used at concentrations which caused comparable dephosphorylation of pNPP to that obtained with phosphatases in the endosomal extract, indicating that the endosomal PPPase activity is distinguishable from that of the acid and alkaline phosphatases. PPPase in the endosomal extracts was able to dephosphorylate [^{32}P]-labelled -casein and histone when used as substrates, implying that the neutral endosomal PPPase activity acts on phosphorylated serine or threonine residues in the NC protein.

Characterization of the endosomal PPPase was made on the abundantly available L-2 murine fibroblasts because of the difficulty in obtaining sufficient quantities of primary oligodendrocytes. Presence of a neutral PPPase in neural tissue was determined with brain homogenates from Wistar Furth rat neonates and homogenates from cultured primary oligodendrocytes. The neural material possessed higher specific activities than homogenates of L-2 cells (Figure 2). the closest comparison between L-2 cells and oligodendrocytes which could be undertaken by us utilized endosomes isolated from Roc-1 cells, a hybrid C_6 astrocytoma x primary oligodendrocyte cell line (a kind gift from Dr. F.A. McMorris, The Wistar Institute, PA). It is evident from Figure 2 that Roc-1 cell endosomes possess a neutral PPPase activity comparable to that of L-2 cell endosomes.

SUMMARY

We have identified a phosphoprotein phosphatase which dephosphorylates efficiently the NC protein of coronavirus JHM. The activity was found in L-2 murine fibroblasts, Wistar Furth rat neonatal brain extracts, Wistar Furth rat oligodendrocyte primary cells and in Roc-1 cells, an oligodendrocytic hybrid cell line. In both L-2 cells and Roc-1 cells the enzyme was found to be localized predominantly in the endosomal fraction. The enzyme is optimally active at pH 7.0 and has a requirement for Mn^{++} ions. This PPPase activity is distinguishable from acidic and alkaline phosphatases. In view of the specificity

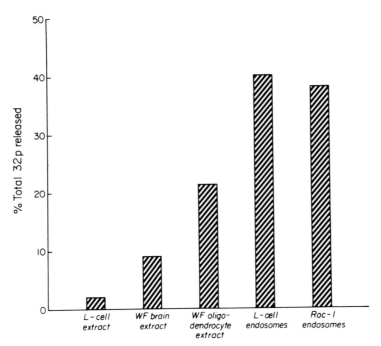

Figure 2. Comparison of specific activity of 'neutral' PPPase in brain tissue and neural cells with that of L-2 cells. The representative data are expressed from one of several such experiments as percent dephosphorylation of $[^{32}P]$-NC by enzyme in samples containing 50 ug protein during 90 min reaction at $30^{\circ}C$.
WF = Wistar Furth rats.

of the endosomal PPPase for the phosphory-lated NC protein it is hypothesized that this enzyme may have a function during early stages of coronavirus infection.

REFERENCES

1. S. Beushausen, and S. Dales, In vivo and in vitro models of demyelinating disease XI. Tropism and differentiation regulate the infectious process of coronaviruses in primary explants of the rat CNS, Virology 141:89 (1985).
2. S. Beushausen, S. Narindrasorasak, B.D. Sanwal, and S. Dales, In vivo and in vitro models of demyelinating disease: Activation of the adenylate cyclase system influences JHM virus expression in explanted rat oligodendrocytes, J. Virol. 61:3795 (1987).
3. K. Krzystyniak, and J.M. Dupuy, Entry of mouse hepatitis 3 into cells, J. Gen. Virol. 65:227 (1984).

4. L. Mizzen, S. Hilton, S. Cheley, and R. Anderson, Attenuation of murine coronavirus infection by ammonium chloride, _Virology_ 142:378 (1985).

5. M. Coulter-Mackie, R. Adler, G. Wilson, and S. Dales, _In vivo_ and _in vitro_ models of demyelinating diseases. XII. Persistence and expression of corona JHM virus functions in RN2-2 schwannoma cells during latency, _Virus Res_. 3:245 (1985).

6. C.L. Smith, C. Debouck, M. Rosenberg, and J.S. Culp, Phosphorylation of serine residue 89 of human adenovirus E1A proteins is responsible for their characteristic electrophoretic mobility shifts, and its mutation affects biological function, _J. Virol_. 63:1569 (1989).

7. J. Leis, S. Johnson, L.S. Collins, and J.A. Traugh, Effects of phosphorylation of avian retroviruses nucleocapsid protein pp12 on binding of viral RNA, _J. Biol. Chem_. 259:7726 (1984).

8. H. Maeno, and P. Greengard, Phosphoprotein phosphatases from rat cerebral cortex. Subcellular distribution and characterization, _J. Biol. Chem_. 247:3269 (1972).

9. U.K. Laemmli, Cleavage of structural proteins during the assembly of the head of bacteriophage T_4, _Nature (London)_ 227:680 (1970).

10. M. Merion, and R.D. Poretz, The resolution of two populations of lysosomal organelles containing endocytosed _Wistario floribunda_ agglutinin from murine fibroblasts, _J. Supramol. Struct. Cell. Biochem_. 17:337 (1981).

11. T.S. Ingebristen, and P. Cohen, Protein phosphatases: properties and role in cellular regulation, _Science_ 221:331 (1983).

12. R. Fuchs, S. Schmid, and I. Mellman, A possible role for Na^+, K^+-ATPase in regulating ATP-dependent endosome acidification, _Proc. Natl. Acad. Sci. U.S.A_. 86:539 (1989).

13. D.L. Brantigan, and C.L. Shriner, Methods to distinguish various types of protein phosphatase activity, _Methods in Enzymology_ 159:339 (1988).

IN VIVO AND IN VITRO MODELS OF DEMYELINATING DISEASE. POSSIBLE
RELATIONSHIP BETWEEN INDUCTION OF REGULATORY SUBUNIT FROM cAMP
DEPENDENT PROTEIN KINASES AND INHIBITION OF JHMV REPLICATION IN
CULTURED OLIGODENDROCYTES

G.A.R. Wilson, D.V. Mohandas, and S. Dales

Cytobiology Group, Dept. of Microbiology and
Immunology, Univ. of Western Ontario
London, Ontario, Canada   N6A 5C1

Among the parameters controlling coronavirus (CV)
replication within the nervous system of rodents is the state
of glial-cell maturation.[1,14] Thus differentiation of primary
cultures of oligodendrocytes with dibutyryl cAMP (dbcAMP)
effectively results in a restriction of CV-JHMV replication.
Treatment of cells with dbcAMP, which directly raises the
intracellular concentration of cAMP, stimulates the adenylate
cyclase system. In primary rat oligodendrocytes stimulation of
the adenylate cyclase system results in an induction of the
regulatory subunit (R) of cAMP-dependent protein kinase type 1
(PK_1).[2] It is conceivable that the function of increase in
free R_1 within host-cells may be related to inhibition of
phosphoprotein phosphatases (PPPase), as previously
demonstrated in rabbit skeletal muscle with R_2 from PK_2.[6,7].
Evidence from our studies indicates that a PPPase may
participate in the early stages of CV infection, perhaps during
traverse through endosomes of the host.[12] The present study
was undertaken to ascertain whether the R protein plays any
role in restricting JHMV replication in mature glial cells by
inhibiting an endosomal PPPase.

Inhibition of Endosome PPPase Activity with the R_1 Protein

Purified endosomes, obtained through percoll gradient
fractionation of L-2 mouse fibroblasts[12] were used in an in-
vitro PPPase assay to detect phosphoserine phosphatase activity
against purified preparations of [^{32}P]-labeled JHMV
nucleocapsid (NC) protein. This assay has previously been
shown to result in the specific dephosphorylation of labeled NC
preparations.[12]

Briefly, reactions were initiated containing 25 mM Tris-
maleate pH 7.0, 10 mM 3':5' cAMP, 25 mM $MgCl_2$, 1% Triton X-
100, 25 ug of endosomes and varying quantities of affinity-

purified R and catalytic (C) subunits or the PK holoenzyme. After incubation at 30°C for 30 min the $[^{32}P]$-NC protein substrate was added to the reaction mixture and incubation continued for 90 min. at 30°C. Reactions were terminated by addition of 1% BSA and 25% TCA and the contents analysed either for $[^{32}P]$ released or, following dissociation in 3x Laemmli's buffer for NC polypeptide by means of SDS-PAGE. The amount of $[^{32}P]$ released into the supernatant was determined,[9] permitting us to calculate the amount of NC dephosphorylation.

The data in Figure 1 indicate that as little as 1 ug of free R_1 protein is capable of inhibiting NC protein dephosphorylation due to the endosome PPPase by 32%. With increasing concentration of R_1 there was a corresponding increase in PPPase inhibition up to a maximum of 50% when 12 ug of R_1 were added. Since the reaction was not affected appreciably at concentrations of R_1 above 3 ug, this concentration was employed in all subsequent experiments. Inhibition of PPPase by R_1 could be visualized after separating the $[^{32}P]$-NC protein by 10% SDS-PAGE and employing autoradiography (Figure 2). The results demonstrate a substantial reduction of the $[^{32}P]$-signal following the PPPase reaction (lane 2) as compared to the control sample (lane 1). Upon addition of 3 ug R_1 to the PPPase reaction less dephosphorylation occurred (lane 3) corresponding to approximately a 40% inhibition of PPPase activity, as determined by densitometric scanning of the autoradiogram. From these findings it is concluded that (1) the endosomal PPPase activity possesses specificity for the NC protein of JHMV and (2) R_1 subunit of PK can inhibit the endosomal PPPase, albeit incompletely.

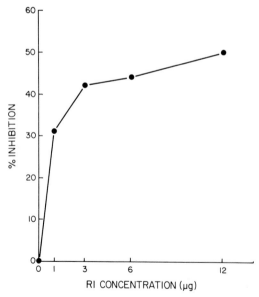

Figure 1. Effects of increasing R_1 concentration on PPPase activity: % inhibition of NC protein dephosphorylation as a function of increasing R_1 concentration.

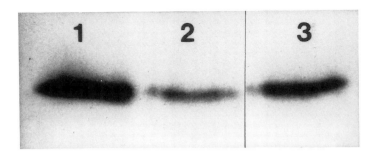

Figure 2. Autoradiogram of PPPase assay. Lane 1, undephosphorylated NC protein. Lane 2, NC protein dephosphorylated using L cell endosomes. Lane 3, NC protein dephosphorylation using L cell endosomes and 3 ug R_1 protein.

Specificity of PPPase Inhibition with R_1 Protein

Additional assays were undertaken using PK_1 and PK_2 holoenzymes as well as isolated catalytic subunits to determine if the PPPase inhibition was specific for the regulatory subunit. The results (Table 1) show the inability of catalytic subunits to inhibit PPPase activity as compared with R_1 subunit. Holoenzyme preparations of PK_1 and PK_2 were inert. However, upon addition of 10 mM 3':5' cAMP to promote R and C dissociation, small but significant PPPase inhibition was observed. This result further draws attention to the specificity of R in suppressing the endosomal PPPase. The present findings are supported by previous studies demonstrating inhibition by R_2 of a PPPase from rabbit skeletal muscle.[6,7] Our data and those from the cited articles draw attention to other functions of R_1 and R_2, such as inhibition of PPPases, apart from that of controlling the phosphorylation by the catalytic subunits.

Effects of NC dephosphorylation on nucleic acid binding potential

Previous evidence with the P56 protein of CV A59 and JHMV has indicated the affinity for binding nucleic acid by this protein.[2,13] The question of an altered nucleic acid binding capacity following dephosphorylation has significance for trying to understand the sequence of events which occur during CV uncoating process which may involve the endosome.

The procedure was essentially as previously described.[2] Following incubation of NC protein with endosomal PPPase the material was separated by 10% SDS-PAGE, then transferred to nitrocellulose paper. Blots were probed with [^{32}P]-labeled CV-A59 g344 plasmid DNA,[3] washed and subjected to autoradiography. The dephosphorylated NC protein had a greatly reduced ability

Table 1. Dephosphorylation of NC protein by an endosomal PPPase in the presence of PK and R or C enzyme subunits

Addition	Activity in Units/mg endosomal[1] protein	% Inhibition[2]
none	1,440 (9)	
PK_1 holoenzyme	1,480 (4)	0
PK_2 holoenzyme+cAMP	1,240 (5)	14 ± 3.2
PK_2 holoenzyme	1,480 (2)	0
PK_2 holoenzyme+cAMP	1,120 (4)	22 ± 2.6
R_1 3 ug	960 (3)	33 ± 2.7
R_1 3 ug+cAMP	760 (9)	47 ± 7.0
C_1 5 ug+cAMP	1,680 (4)	0

[1] Data from a representative experiment repeated the number of times shown in brackets. One unit of activity is defined as 1% of [^{32}P] released in 90 min at 30°C.

[2] Average values with standard error of the mean.

to bind the nucleic acid probe (data not shown). This, as yet preliminary, evidence indicates that NC protein dephosphorylation reduces its binding capacity for nucleic acids. This observation implies that normal uncoating may require NC dephosphorylation. Therefore, differentiation of oligodendrocytes associated with elevation of R_1 creates an intracellular environment in which dephosphorylation of the NC by an endosomal PPPase is inhibited, thereby affecting the uncoating process.

SUMMARY

The results in this study suggest a unique possible association between inhibition of JHMV replication and the induction of R_1 proteins in differentiating oligodendrocytes, involving inhibition of a PPPase found in the endosome fractions of cells. Free R_1 protein appears to prevent the dephosphorylation of purified JHMV-NC substrate thereby possibly blocking the normal sequence of events necessary for NC release of viral genomes. Inhibition of host-cell endosome PPPase's may have relevance to controlling JHMV infection since CV particles adsorbing to cell surface receptors are believed to penetrate via clathrin coated pits into endosomes.[4,5,8,10,11] Thus, the early stages of CV infection, including dephosphorylation of NC protein within endosomes, provide a possible site for controlling the initial stages of viral infection.

REFERENCES

1. S. Beushausen and S. Dales, In-vivo and in-vitro models
        of demyelinating disease XI. Tropism and
        differentiation regulate the infectious process
        of coronaviruses in primary explants of the rat
        CNS, Virol. 141:89-101 (1985).
2. S. Beushausen, S. Narindrasorasak, B. D. Sanwal, and S.
        Dales, In-vivo and in-vitro models of
        demyelinating disease: Activation of the
        adenylate cyclase system influences JHM virus
        expression in explanted rat oligodendrocytes, J.
        Virol. 61:3795-3803 (1987).
3. C. J. Budzilowicz, S. P. Wilczynski, and S. R. Weiss,
        Three intergenic regions of coronavirus mouse
        hepatitis virus strain A59 genome RNA contain a
        common nucletide sequence that is homologous to
        the 3' end of the viral mRNA leader sequence, J.
        Virol. 53:834-840 (1985).
4. M. Coulter-Mackie, R. Adler, G. A. R. Wilson, and S. Dales,
        In-vivo and in-vitro models of demyelinating
        diseases. XII. Persistence and expression of
        corona JHM virus functions in RN2-2 schwannoma
        cells during latency, Virus Res. 3:245-261
        (1985).
5. J. F. David-Ferreira and R. A. Manaker, An electron
        microscope study of the development of a mouse
        hepatitis virus in tissue culture cells, J. Cell
        Biol. 24:57-58 (1965).
6. S. R. Jurgensen, P. B. Chock, S. Taylor, J. R. Vandenheede,
        and W. Merlevede, Inhibition of the Mg(II)-ATP-
        dependent phosphoprotein phosphatase by the
        regulatory subunit of cAMP dependent protein
        kinase. Proc. Natl. Acad. Sci. USA 82:7565-
        7569.
7. B. S. Khatra, R. Printz, C. E. Cobb, and J. D. Corbin,
        Regulatory subunit of cAMP-dependent protein
        kinase inhibits phosphoportein phosphatase.
        Biochem. Biophys. Res. Comm. 130:567-573 (1985).
8. K. Krzystyniak and J. M. Dupuy, Entry of mouse hepatitis
        virus 3 into cells, J. Gen. Virol. 65:227-231
        (1984).
9. H. Maeno and P. Greengard, Phosphoprotein phosphatases
        from rat cerebral cortex. Subcellular
        distribution and characterization, J. Biol. Chem.
        247:3269-3277 (1972).
10. L. Mallucci, Effect of chloroquine on lysosomes and on
        growth of mouse hepatitis virus (MHV$_3$), Virol.
        28:355-362 (1986).
11. L. Mizzen, A. Hilton, S. Cheley, and R. Anderson,
        Attenuation of murine coronavirus infection by
        ammonium chloride, Virol. 142:378-388 (1985).
12. D. V. Mohandas and S. Dales, In-vivo and in-vitro models of
        demyelinating disease. An endosomal
        phosphoprotein phosphatase active on the
        nucleocapsid protein of a murine coronavirus.
        Submitted for publication.

13. S. G. Robbins, M. F. Frana, J. J. McGowan, J. F. Boyle,
    and K. V. Holmes, RNA-binding proteins of
    coronavirus MHV: Etection of monomeric and
    multimeric N protein with an RNA overlay in
    protein blot assay, <u>Virol</u>. 150:402-410 (1986).
14. G. A. R. Wilson, S. Beushausen, and S. Dales, In-vivo and
    in-vitro models of demyelinating disease. XV.
    Differentiation in primary explants of mouse CNS,
    <u>Virol</u>. 151:253-264 (1986).

Chapter 6

The Polymerase and other Non-Structural Proteins

A RIBOSOMAL FRAMESHIFT SIGNAL IN THE POLYMERASE-ENCODING REGION

OF THE IBV GENOME

S.C. Inglis, N. Rolley and I. Brierley

Division of Virology, Department of Pathology
University of Cambridge, Tennis Court Road, Cambridge, U K

INTRODUCTION

Nucleotide sequencing studies on the genomic RNA of infectious bronchitis virus (IBV) has revealed the presence, at its 5' end of two very large open reading frames (ORFS) termed F1 and F2 (Boursnell *et al.*, 1987). The 5' proximal ORF, F1 has the capacity to encode a polypeptide of approximately 440K, while the distal ORF, F2, which overlaps F1 by about 40 nucleotides (ntds) in a different (-1) reading frame, can encode a 300K polypeptide. Our previous work has indicated that both these open reading frames can be expressed as a single polypeptide from genomic mRNA by ribosomal frame-shifting within the overlap region (Brierley *et al.*, 1987, 1989). This conclusion was based on experiments which showed that sequences from the F1-F2 junction region, when introduced into a heterologous mRNA could direct efficient ribosomal frame-shifting during translation *in vitro* and *in vivo*. Thus the primary translation products of IBV genomic RNA in the infected cell consists of a 440K product, corresponding to the F1 ORF, and an additional 740K 'read-through' product representing fusion of the F1 and F2 ORFs (Figure 1).

Fine mapping of the frame-shift signal

Recently we have begun to map sequences around the F1/F2 junction in IBV RNA which contain the signal for this ribosomal frameshift event by site-directed mutagenesis (Brierley *et al.*, 1989). The essence of this work is that a minimum sequence of approximately 86 ntds

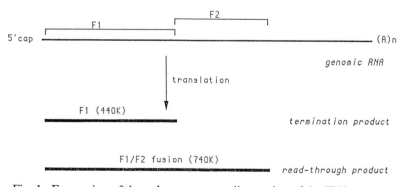

Fig. 1. Expression of the polymerase-encoding region of the IBV genome.

Coronaviruses and Their Diseases
Edited by D. Cavanagh and T.D.K. Brown
Plenum Press, New York, 1990

pFS7.13   UAC

slip site   V   PK1   PK2   PK3   PK4

UAUUUAAAGGGUACGGGGUAGCAGUGAGGCUCGGCUGAUACCCCUUGCUAGUGGAUGUGAUCCUGAUGUUGUAAAGCGAGCCUUU

Construct	slip site	PK1	PK2	PK3	PK4
pFS7.1	C				
pFS7.12					UCCGA
pFS7.14	U				
pFS7.15			UCGGA		
pFS7.16			UCGGA		UCCGA
pFS7.17	C				
pFS7.18		CCCCAU			
pFS7.19				AUGGGG	
pFS7.20		CCCCAU		AUGGGG	
pFS7.22	(deletion)				
pFS8.5	UGA				

Construct	Frame-shift efficiency	Construct	Frame-shift efficiency
pFS7.1	–	pFS7.18	–
pFS7.12	–	pFS7.19	–
pFS7.13	–	pFS7.20	++
pFS7.14	–	pFS8.5	++
pFS7.15	–	pFS7.14	–
pFS7.16	++	pFS7.22	–

Fig. 2. Effect on frameshifting activity of specific nucleotide substitutions within the F1/F2 frameshift signal. Sequences from the F1/F2 junction were cloned into a reporter gene, altered by site-drected mutagenesis, and assayed for frameshifting by *in vitro* transcription and translation as described (Brierley *et al.*, 1989).

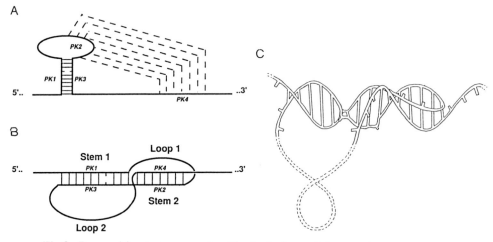

Fig.3. Base-pairing between nucleotides in the loop of the stem-loop structure and a region downstream (A) results in the formation of an extended double helix, shown schematically (B), consisting of two helical regions (S1 and S2) connected by two single stranded loops (L1 and L2). An artist's impression of this structure is shown (C).

from the junction region is in itself sufficient to direct high efficiency frame-shifting in a heterologous context (Figure 2). Positioned at the 5' end of this sequence is a 7 nucleotide 'slippery sequence', UUUAAAC, similar to those described in retrovirus RNA frame-shifting signals (Jacks *et al.*, 1988a). By analogy with the situation in retroviruses (Jacks and Varmus, 1988a,b) this is likely to be the point at which frame-shifting actually occurs by a simultaneous "slippage" mechanism in which tRNAs decoding the UUA codon (occupying the ribosomal P site) and the AAC codon (occupying the A site) slip back on the mRNA to form mismatched (2 out of 3) pairings with UUU and AAA triplets. This model is strongly supported by the observation that introduction of a termination codon in the F1 reading frame immediately after the slippery site does not affect frame-shifting (Figure 2, pFS8.5). Thus frame-shifting must occur before this triplet is read, and since nucleotides upstream of the predicted slip site are dispensable, it seems highly likely that the UUUAAAC is indeed the site of frame-shifting. Also consistent with this is the observation that single nucleotide substitutions in the slippery sequence that would disrupt pairing in the slipped position are inhibitory to frame-shifting (Figure 2, pFS7.1, 7.14, 7.17).

In addition to the slippery site however, downstream sequences are required for efficient frame-shifting, and our mutational analysis (Brierley *et al.*, 1989) has shown that these downstream sequences fold to form an RNA tertiary structure (Figure 3), which has been termed a pseudoknot (Pleij *et al.*, 1981; Puglisi *et al.*, 1988) and which is an essential element of the signal. This structure consists essentially of a stem loop in which certain of the nucleotides in the loop are in fact paired with nucleotides provided by a downstream sequence, creating 2 stems (S1 & S2) which are stacked on top of each other and linked by two connecting loops (L1 & L2). Evidence in favour of this kind of model comes from the creation of complementary base mutations in each strand of both proposed stems (Figure 2). These changes, which would destabilise the proposed pseudoknotted structure, are highly inhibitory to frame-shifting (e.g. mutants pFS7.18, 7.19 for stem 1 and pFS 7.12, 7.15 for stem 2). However, when double mutations are made to restore potential base-pairing, creating complementary changes in both strands of each proposed stem, frame-shifting is restored to wild-type efficiency (pFS 7.20 and pFS 7.16).

The results strongly suggest that the proposed base-pairing does occur and that a pseudoknot is an essential element of the ribosomal frame-shifting signal. Although we cannot be sure, we believe the most likely structure for the pseudoknot to be that shown in Figure 4. In this structure, stem 1 consists of a 11 base pair helix, with 9 Watson-Crick pairs plus one G:U and one 'wobble' A:G pair. Stem 2 consists of a 6 base pair helix continuous with, and coaxially stacked on top of stem 1. The shorter of the connecting loops, L1, bridges the major groove of the stem 2 helix and is only 2 nucleotides long, the minimum number required to span the distance (about 11Å) between the top of stem 1 and the top of stem 2. The longer, L2, is 32 nucleotides in length, which is more than sufficient to bridge the distance (about 42Å) between the base of stem 1 and the base of stem 2.

From the model shown it is possible to make predictions about the effect of certain kinds of mutations on the pseudoknot structure and function, and to test these readily by mutagenesis (Figure 4). One obvious prediction is that much of loop 2 is redundant, and indeed 24 nucleotides can be removed from L2 without affecting frame-shifting (pFS 8.2). Similarly, insertion of an additional 6 ntds has no effect (pFS 8.1). Another prediction is that nucleotides in L1 can be changed to their complements without effect, and once again this is the case (pFS 8.7). On the other hand, making complementary changes in the proposed stems should be inhibitory. For stem 1 this is demonstrated clearly by mutants pFS 8.4 and pFS 8.6 in which the top 3 nucleotides in each strand of stem 1 have been altered; in each case frame-shifting is dramatically reduced, but in the double mutant, pFS 8.12, once again it is restored to wild type efficiency. Changing only the top nucleotide of this trio (pFS 8.11) similarly has a drastic inhibitory effect. In stem 2 conversion of a central G residue to a C is highly inhibitory (pFS 7.23), and destabilisation of the nucleotide pair immediately above also reduced frame-shifting, although in this case the reduction was much less dramatic. This may indicate a lower contribution of this nucleotide pair to the overall stability of the structure, which would be consistent with its position at the very end of stem 2. Surprisingly however, changing a G residue at the base of stem 2 to a C (pFS 8.10) had no effect on frame-shifting, suggesting that the proposed G:U pairing may not occur. It is possible however that in this mutant, the U residue normally opposing the wild type G could be displaced from the structure by the adjacent

G on the end of loop 2, creating a new base pair with the mutated C. This would create an even more stable pseudoknot, and indeed this mutant displayed slightly more efficient frameshifting than did the wild type sequence. An alternative explanation however is that the G residue in the wild type structure is in reality unpaired and 'bulges' out of the helix without affecting its overall structure or stability.

So far then our experimental observations support the proposed model, but clearly confirmation will require direct structural analysis using a range of biochemical and biophysical techniques.

Role of the pseudoknot in frame-shifting

It is not yet clear how the pseudoknot causes ribosomes to change reading frame during mRNA translation. The most obvious possibility is that the necessity to unwind the knot slows or stalls the ribosome as it passes through the frame-shift region, such that there is an increased chance of slippage at the slippery site. In such a situation presumably the position of the knot with respect to the slip site would be critical, and indeed insertion or deletion of 3 nucleotides between the two (Figure 2) severely inhibits frame-shifting. However it is equally possible that a protein factor recognises the knotted RNA, and that somehow this interaction could promote frame-shifting. Further experiments will be required to distinguish between these possibilities.

Significance of frame-shifting for IBV gene expression

Our data suggest that translation of IBV genomic RNA in infected cells leads to the production of a 440K F1 product and a 740K F1-F2 read-through product, in a ratio of about 3:1. As yet we know very little about the nature of these proteins other than that the primary translation products are almost certainly cleaved.proteolytically to produce a number of smaller polypeptides (Brierley *et al*. this volume). Since IBV genomic RNA alone is infectious

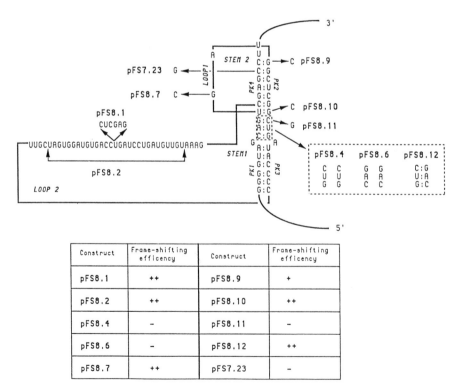

Construct	Frame-shifting efficency	Construct	Frame-shifting efficency
pFS8.1	++	pFS8.9	+
pFS8.2	++	pFS8.10	++
pFS8.4	-	pFS8.11	-
pFS8.6	-	pFS8.12	++
pFS8.7	++	pFS7.23	-

Fig. 4. Testing of predicted pseudoknot structure through site-directed mutagenesis of specific nucleotides. Mutated frameshift sites were constructed and assayed for frameshifting as before.

(Schochetman *et al.*, 1977) one can assume also that among the F region translation products there is a virus RNA-dependent RNA polymerase, although as yet the activity has not been identified.

Why then is ribosomal frame-shifting required for expression of the F region? One possibility is that it provides a mechanism by which a defined ratio of products may be synthesised from the upstream F1 and downstream F2 ORF. This kind of explanation has been advanced for retrovirus *gag-pol* expression which occurs by a similar mechanism. However whereas for the retroviruses RSV and HIV, the ratio of gag to gag-pol product is about 20:1 (Jacks *et al.*, 1985, 1988a), for IBV the F1:F2 ratio would be only 3:1. It is difficult to imagine therefore why such a relatively crude control mechanism would be favoured by the virus. Another explanation is that the frame-shift signal simply provides a mechanism for creating two different protein products from the same genomic region. Thus successful virus replication might require a protein consisting of the terminal region of F1 alone, and another consisting of fused sequences from both F1 and F2. This end is achieved in other ways by other viruses. For example in the picornaviruses, incomplete proteolytic cleavage at particular sites can generate alternative protein products (Kitamura *et al.*, 1981), and in the alphavirus Sindbis, a similar result arises from the presence of a "leaky" stop codon (Strauss *et al.*, 1983, Lopez *et al.*, 1985) in the non-structural coding region of the genomic RNA. Ribosomal frame-shifting therefore may represent yet another variation on this theme.

Acknowledgements

This work was supported by an AFRC "Link" grant, LRG171, awarded to SCI. We are grateful to members of the Institute of Animal Health, Houghton Laboratory, and in particular Mike Boursnell for useful discussion

References

Boursnell, M.E.G., Brown, T.D.K., Foulds, I.J. Green, P.F., Tomley, F.M. and Binns, M.M., 1987, Completion of the sequence of the genome of the Coronavirus Avian Infectious Bronchitis Virus, J. Gen. Virol., 68: 57.

Brierley, I., Boursnell, M.E.G., Binns, M.M., Bilimoria, B., Blok, V.C., Brown, T.D.K. and Inglis, S.C., 1987, An efficient ribosomal frame-shifting signal in the polymerase-encoding region of the coronavirus IBV, EMBO J., 6: 3779.

Brierley, I., Digard, P. and Inglis, S.C., 1989, Characterisation of an efficient coronavirus ribosomal frameshifting signal: Requirement for an RNA pseudoknot, Cell, 57: 537.

Jacks, T. and Varmus, H.E., 1985, Expression of the Rous sarcoma virus *pol* gene by ribosomal frameshifting, Science, 230: 1237.

Jacks, T., Madhani H.D., Masiarz, F.R., and Varmus, H.E., 1988a, Signals for ribosomal frameshifting in the Rous sarcoma virus *gag-pol* region Cell, 55: 447.

Jacks, T., Power, M.D., Masiarz, F.R., Luciw, P.A., Barr, P.J. and Varmus, H.E., 1988b, Characterisation of ribosomal frameshifting in HIV-1 *gag-pol* expression, Nature, 331: 280.

Kitamura, N., Semler, B.L., Roth, P.G., Larsen, G.R., Adler, C.J., Dorner, A.J., Emini, E.A., Hanecak, R., Lee, J.J., van der Werf, S., Anderson, C.W. and Wimmer, E., 1981, Primary structure, gene organisation, and polypeptide expression of poliovirus RNA Nature, 291: 547.

Lopez, S., Bell, J.R., Strauss, E.G. and Strauss, J.H., 1985, The nonstructural proteins of Sindbis as studied with an antibody specific for the C-terminus of the nonstructural read-through polyprotein, Virology, 141: 235.

Pleij, C.W.A., Rietveld, K. and Bosch, L., 1985, A new principle of RNA folding based on pseudoknotting, Nucl. Acids Res., 13: 1717.

Puglisi, J.D., Wyatt, J.R. and Tinoco, I., 1988, A pseudoknotted RNA oligonucleotide, Nature, 331: 283.

Schochetman, G., Stevens, R.H. and Simpson, R.W., 1977, Presence of infectious polyadenylated RNA in the coronavirus avian infectious bronchitis virus, Virology, 77: 772.

Strauss, E.G., Rice, C.M. & Strauss, J.H., 1983, Sequence coding for the alphavirus nonstructural proteins is interrupted by an opal termination codon, Proc. Natl. Acad. Sci. USA, 80: 5271.

PRODUCTS OF THE POLYMERASE-ENCODING REGION OF THE CORONAVIRUS IBV

I. Brierley, M.E.G. Boursnell*, M.M. Binns*, B. Bilimoria, N.J. Rolley, T.D.K. Brown , and S.C. Inglis

Division of Virology, Department of Pathology, University of Cambridge, Tennis Court Road, Cambridge, CB2 1QP; and *Houghton Poultry Research Station, Houghton, Huntingdon, Cambs., PE17 2DA

INTRODUCTION

The avian coronavirus infectious bronchitis virus (IBV) has a single-stranded, polyadenylated, positive-sense RNA genome some 27.6 Kb in length (Boursnell et al., 1987). IBV replication almost certainly proceeds by the same mechanism that occurs in the more intensively studied coronavirus, mouse hepatitis virus (MHV). Genomic RNA is first translated to produce the viral RNA-dependent RNA polymerase, which transcribes the genomic RNA to generate a negative-stranded full-length copy of the virion RNA. This copy RNA then serves as a template for the production of a nested set of 3′-co-terminal transcripts from which virus polypeptides are translated (reviewed in Spaan et al., 1988). These transcripts include a genomic-sized RNA (mRNA 1) and five subgenomic RNAs (mRNAs 2-6) of which mRNA 6 is the smallest (Stern and Kennedy, 1980). Almost all detailed analysis of IBV gene function to date has concentrated on the products of mRNAs 2, 4 and 6 which encode the viral structural proteins spike, membrane and nucleocapsid respectively (see Figure 1). Together, these mRNAs account for less than 30% of the genomic coding capacity; most of the remaining information is in two large, overlapping open-reading frames (ORFs) 1a and 1b, encoded by mRNA 1. These ORFs could potentially produce some 740 kD of protein and must encode the RNA polymerase (Boursnell et al., 1987). A number of associated activities predicted to be involved in viral replication are also suspected to be encoded by mRNA 1 (Gorbalenya et al., 1989). To date, however, the only product of this RNA that has been detected in coronavirus-infected cells is a 28 kD MHV polypeptide (p28) of unknown function (Denison and Perlman, 1987) which is derived from the 5′-end of the MHV genome (Soe et al., 1987).

In this study, we have investigated expression of the 1a and 1b ORFs of IBV by using a panel of monospecific antisera raised against portions of the two ORFs. A number of polypeptides encoded by each ORF have been identified in infected cells and are likely to have arisen as a result of processing of larger precursor translation products. This is the first identification of products encoded by the polymerase-encoding region of IBV.

METHODS AND RESULTS

Expression of RNA 1 ORFs in bacteria

Our approach to the identification of polypeptides encoded by RNA 1 has been to prepare antisera against regions of ORFs 1a and 1b through expression of portions of these ORFs in bacteria, and to use these sera as probes for the analysis of infected cells.

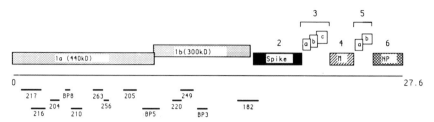

Figure 1. Organisation of the IBV genome. The boxes represent open reading frames and are numbered (1-6) with respect to the particular subgenomic mRNA from which they are expressed. Regions of the 1a and 1b ORFs which have been cloned into the pEX expression system are indicated by black bars and are numbered with respect to the original cDNA clone from which they were derived.

Our strategy was based on the pEX series of plasmids developed by Stanley and Luzio (1984), which allows the expression of "foreign" sequence information as a C-terminal fusion with β-galactosidase. Expression of the fusion protein is under the control of the bacteriophage lambda repressor; in bacterial cells containing a temperature sensitive repressor, expression is induced by raising the temperature (from 30oC to 42oC). Following induction, harvested bacteria are lysed and a Triton-insoluble pellet obtained which contains the crude fusion protein. The genomic position of each of the regions expressed in this study is shown in Figure 1 and the precise sequence information in Figure 2a. Each construct was numbered with reference to the original cDNA clone from which the IBV information was derived (detailed in Boursnell *et al.*, 1987). In total, some 65% of the 1a and 45% of the 1b coding regions were cloned and expressed in *E. coli*. Figure 2b shows the proteins synthesized in bacteria harbouring either wild-type (pEX1) or recombinant pEX plasmids following a one hour induction. All of the constructs expressed high levels of fusion protein (10-40 mg/litre) with the exception of constructs pEX256 and pEX205. The fusion proteins were purified by preparative SDS-polyacrylamide gel electrophoresis and electroelution from gel slices, and used to immunize rabbits. Animals were inoculated initially with approximately 0.1 mg of purified protein emulsified in Freund's Complete Adjuvant by intramuscular injection and at monthly intervals were boosted by the same route, using similar amounts of material in Freund's Incomplete Adjuvant.

Products of mRNA 1 ORFs 1a and 1b

We have investigated expression of mRNA 1 *in vivo* by testing the ability of the antisera raised against regions of ORFs 1a and 1b to recognize IBV-specified polypeptides in infected cell lysates in Western blotting experiments. Confluent chick kidney (CK) or VERO cell monolayers were inoculated with the Be-42 strain of IBV (at a multiplicity of infection of 1, 90 minutes at 37oC) and the cells harvested at various times post infection. Viral replication was essentially completed by about 16 hours post-infection in CK cells and some 24 hours post-infection in VERO cells. Samples were prepared for Western blot analysis as follows. Mock-infected or infected cell pellets were resuspended in phosphate-buffered saline (PBS) (at 5×10^6 cells/ml), mixed with an equal volume of twice-strength Laemmli's sample buffer (Laemmli, 1970), sonicated for 30 seconds in the presence of 1mM phenylmethylsulphonylfluoride and boiled for 4 minutes. Aliquots were loaded onto 4-20% gradient SDS-polyacrylamide gels and following electrophoresis, proteins were transferred to nitrocellulose by electroblotting (Bio-Rad Transblot). Following transfer, filters were probed with 1% solution of the relevant antiserum in 5% low-fat milk, 1% foetal calf serum in PBS, and bound antibodies detected using ^{125}I-labelled Staphylococcus protein A.

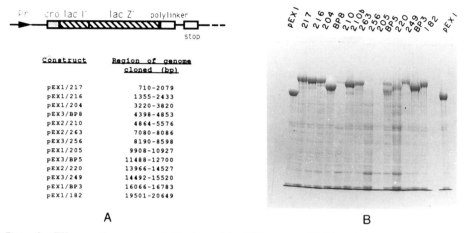

pEX System

Construct	Region of genome cloned (bp)
pEX1/217	710-2079
pEX1/216	1355-2433
pEX1/204	3220-3820
pEX3/BP8	4398-4853
pEX2/210	4864-5576
pEX2/263	7080-8086
pEX3/256	8190-8598
pEX1/205	9908-10927
pEX3/BP5	11488-12700
pEX2/220	13966-14527
pEX3/249	14492-15520
pEX1/BP3	16066-16783
pEX1/182	19501-20649

A   B

Figure 2. pEX expression system. A. Regions of the IBV genome which have been cloned into the pEX polylinker and expressed in *E. coli* are shown. B. Expression of β-galactosidase-IBV fusion proteins in *E. coli*. Bacteria harbouring wild-type (pEX1) or recombinant pEX plasmids were grown for 2 hours and 30°C then induced for 1 hour at 42°C. Following lysis, a Triton-insoluble pellet was obtained and a small aliquot ran on a 7.5% SDS-polyacrylamide gel. Proteins were stained with Coomassie brilliant blue R. The major product in each track is the fusion protein.

In Figure 3, a western blot experiment is shown in which both CK and VERO mock-infected or infected cell lysates from varying times post-infection have been probed with antiserum 216 (α-216), a serum raised against a 5'-proximal region of 1a. In CK cells, a large number of non-specific bands common to both mock-infected and infected cells were seen. However, two proteins were detected which were unique to infected cells and accumulated during viral replication, one of 75 kD, the other 220 kD. In IBV-infected VERO cells, the 75 kD and 220 kD products were also detected, although the 220 kD product was less abundant. Two additional low-abundance proteins of 90 kD and 180 kD were detected in VERO cells. No specific bands were seen when similar filters were probed with pEX 216 pre-immune serum or an irrelevant hyperimmune serum raised against the influenza PA protein (not shown). Because of the background of non-specific bands associated with CK cells, the investigation was continued with VERO cells only.

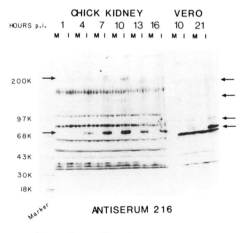

Figure 3. Detection of 1a expression products with antiserum 216. IBV-infected (I) or mock-infected (M) chick kidney or Vero cells from various times post-infection were probed in a Western blot with antiserum 216. Products unique to infected cells are indicated by arrows.

The western blot in Figure 4 shows the products seen in infected VERO cells when filters were probed with antisera α204 and α210, sera raised against central portions of 1a. The patterns of reactivity seen were highly similar; four specific proteins of approximate molecular weights 62kD, 80kD, 140kD and 180kD were detected by both antisera. Antiserum α210 recognised, in addition, a 40kD protein. The regions of cDNA from which α204 and α210 were raised are closed spaced on the IBV genome; it is likely, therefore that the sera are recognising the same group of polypeptides. When an identical filter was probed with pEX210 pre-immune serum (at four times the immune serum concentration), no specific products were recognised. This was also the case for pre-immune serum from pEX204 (not shown). Our preliminary analysis of 1a expression, therefore, suggests strongly that the primary translation product of the ORF is processed to yield a number of cleavage products which accumulate during infection. Whether the proteins detected in these experiments represent the final products of processing is not yet clear since this type of immunological analysis enables only the detection of accumulated products of ongoing viral replication.

ANALYSIS OF 1a

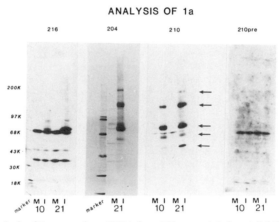

Figure 4. Further analysis of 1a expression. IBV-infected (I) or mock-infected (M) Vero cells were probed with antiserum 216, 204, 210 or with 210 pre-immune sera in a Western blot experiment.

Prior to this study, the only product that had been detected from the polymerase-encoding region of a coronavirus was a 28kD polypeptide of MHV expressed from the extreme 5'-end of the 1a coding sequence (Denison and Perlman, 1987; Soe *et al.*, 1987). We have attempted to determine whether a similar protein is expressed in IBV-infected cells by using antiserum α217. This serum was raised against a 1.4kb region at the extreme 5'-end of the IBV 1a ORF. As yet, however, we have no evidence that p28 is produced in IBV-infected cells, since the α217 serum did not detect any specific proteins. The most likely explanation for the lack of reactivity seen, however, is that the pEX217 immunization has failed to produce a suitable immune response in the experimental animals. As the α217 serum was raised against a cDNA which overlapped considerably with that used to raise antiserum α216, we expected that the α217 serum would recognise the 75kD and 220kD proteins seen with α216. Thus expression of the extreme 5' end of the IBV 1a ORF remains to be characterized.

In addition to the 1a analysis, we have also carried out a preliminary analysis of 1b expression in a similar manner. Mock-infected or IBV-infected VERO cells harvested at twenty hours post-infection were blotted and probed with three anti-1b sera, α220, α249 or α182. As can be seen in Figure 5, no high molecular weight proteins were detected with any of the three 1b antisera tested. The most C-terminal serum, α182 detected three specific proteins of approximate molecular weights 30kD, 34kD and 36kD. Antisera α220 and α249 recognised only a single polypeptide of 49kD. As these antisera were raised against overlapping 1b cDNAs, the sera are probably recognising the same polypeptide. It therefore appears that the primary translation of 1b is also processed post-translationally.

ANALYSIS OF 1b

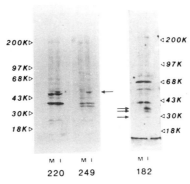

Figure 5. Detection of 1b expression products. IBV-infected (I) or mock-infected (M) Vero cells 21 hours post infection were probed with antiserum 220, 249 or 182 in a Western blot experiment. Products unique to infected cells are indicated by arrows.

DISCUSSION

The complete sequence of IBV (Boursnell *et al.*, 1987) has revealed that the 'unique' region of the genomic RNA contains two extremely large, briefly overlapping ORFs 1a and 1b, which have a 740kD protein coding capacity. In this study we have prepared a panel of 13 monospecific antisera against selected portions of the two ORFs and used a number of these in Western blots to identify products in infected cells. Our results indicate that the primary translation products of the two ORFs appear to be processed proteolytically, giving rise to a number of polypeptides in infected cells. The largest abundant species identified was a 220kD protein encoded within 1a. Recent *in vitro* work on the mechanism of 1a/1b expression has suggested that *in vivo*, 1b is probably expressed as a fusion with the overlapping 1a ORF following a ribosomal frameshift event during translation of the genomic RNA (Brierley *et al.*, 1987;1989; Inglis *et al.*, this volume). Thus the predicted primary translation products are a 440kD product corresponding to 1a, and a 740kD product corresponding to a 1a-1b fusion protein. In this study, we were not able to detect proteins of such size in any quantity. Longer exposures of the 1a blots, however, did reveal a number of minor species with molecular weights considerably in excess of 220kD. These may represent intermediates produced early in a cleavage pathway.

A more rigorous analysis of mRNA 1 expression has been hindered by our inability to detect reproducibly products by radioimmuneprecipitation. The reason for this is uncertain, but may reflect the method of production of the sera, since rabbit antibodies were raised against denatured protein in this study. Nevertheless, when the regions of cDNA used in the pEX constructs were cloned into SP6-based transcription vectors, and synthetic mRNAs derived from these vectors translated *in vitro*, a number of the sera were able to specifically immunoprecipitate the relevant target antigen (not shown). Thus the problem may simply be one of sensitivity.

As the genomic RNA of IBV is infectious (Schochetman *et al.*, 1977) the RNA-dependent RNA polymerase(s) of the virus is almost certainly encoded by 1a/1b; indeed a region in the 1b coding sequence has been predicted to encode an RNA polymerase activity based on a sequence homology with the RNA polymerases of other positive-stranded RNA viruses (Hodgman, 1988; Gorbalenya *et al.*, 1989). To date, no RNA polymerase activity has been detected in IBV-infected cells. However, such an activity has been reported in MHV-infected (Brayton *et al.*, 1982; Mahy *et al.*, 1983) and in transmissible gastroenteritis virus (TGEV)-infected cells (Dennis and Brian, 1982).

279

Recent sequence analysis of MHV (Bredenbeek *et al.*, this volume) has revealed that MHV, like IBV, has two large overlapping ORFs in the unique region of the genomic RNA and, in addition, the RNA polymerase 'homology' sequence found in IBV, is conserved in MHV. In our preliminary analysis of IBV 1a/1b expression described here, two antisera (α220 and α249) which were raised against the region of the genome containing this polymerase homology region reacted with a 49kD protein in infected VERO cells. Whether this protein has any polymerase activity remains to be determined.

ACKNOWLEDGEMENTS

This work was supported by the Agriculture and Food Research Council.

REFERENCES

Boursnell, M.E.G., Brown, T.D.K., Foulds, I.J., Green, P.F., Tomley, F.M. and Binns, M.M., 1987, Completion of the sequence of the genome of the coronavirus avian infectious bronchitis virus, J. gen. Virol., 68:57-77.

Brayton, P.R., Lai, M.M.C., Patton, D.F. and Stohlman, S.A., 1982, Characterisation of two RNA polymerase activities induced by mouse hepatitis virus, J. Virol., 42:847-853.

Brierley, I., Boursnell, M.E.G., Binns, M.M., Bilimoria, B., Blok, V.C., Brown, T.D.K. and Inglis, S.C., 1987, An efficient ribosomal frame-shifting signal in the polymerase-encoding region of the coronavirus IBV, EMBO J., 6:3779-3785.

Brierley, I., Digard, P. and Inglis, S.C., 1989, Characterisation of an efficient coronavirus ribosomal frameshifting signal: requirement for an RNA pseudoknot, Cell, 57:537-547.

Denison, M. and Perlman, S., 1987, Identification of a putative polymerase gene product in cells infected with murine coronavirus A59, Virology, 153:565-568.

Dennis, D.E. and Brian, D.A., 1982, RNA-dependent RNA polymerase activity in coronavirus-infected cells, J. Virol., 42:153-164.

Gorbalenya, A.E., Koonin, E.V., Donchenko, A.P. and Blinov, V.M., 1989, Coronavirus genome: prediction of putative functional domains in the non-structural polyprotein by comparative amino acid sequence analysis, Nucl. Acids Res., 17:4847-4860.

Hodgman, T.C., 1988, A new superfamily of replicative proteins, Nature, 333:22-23.

Laemmli, U.K., 1970, Cleavage of structural proteins during the assembly of the head of bacteriophage T4, Nature, 227:680-685.

Mahy, B.W.J., Siddell, S., Wege, H. and ter Meulen, V., 1983, RNA dependent RNA polymerase activity in murine coronavirus infected cells, J. gen. Virol., 64:103-111.

Schochetman, G., Stevens, R.H. and Simpson, R.W., 1977, Presence of infectious polyadenylated RNA in the coronavirus avian infectious bronchitis virus, Virology, 77:772-782.

Soe, L.H., Shieh, C.K., Baker, S.C., Chang, M.F. and Lai, M.M.C., 1987, Sequence and translation of the murine coronavirus 5'-end genomic RNA reveals the N-terminal structure of the putative RNA polymerase, J. Virol., 61: 3968-3976.

Spaan, W., Cavanagh, D. and Horzinek, M.C., 1988, Coronaviruses: structure and genome expression, J. gen. Virol., 69:2939-2952.

Stanley, K.K. and Luzio, J.P., 1984, Construction of a new family of high efficiency bacterial expression vectors: identification of cDNA clones coding for human liver proteins, <u>EMBO J</u>, 3:1429-1434.

Stern, D.F. and Kennedy, S.I.T., 1980, Coronavirus multiplication strategy. I. Identification and characterisation of virus-specified RNA, <u>J. Virol.</u>, 34:665-674.

MURINE CORONAVIRUS GENE 1 POLYPROTEIN CONTAINS AN AUTOPROTEOLYTIC ACTIVITY

Susan C. Baker, Nicola La Monica, Chien-Kou Shieh and
Michael M.C. Lai

Department of Microbiology
University of Southern California, School of Medicine
Los Angeles, CA 90033

SUMMARY

The 5' most gene of the murine coronavirus genome, gene 1, is presumed to encode the viral RNA-dependent RNA polymerase. cDNA clones representing this gene encompass more than 22 kilobases, suggesting that this region may encode multifunctional polyprotein(s). It has previously been shown that the N-terminal portion of this gene product is cleaved into a protein of 28 kilodaltons (p28). To identify possible functional domains of gene 1 and further understand the mechanism of synthesis of the p28 protein, cDNA clones representing the 5'-most 5.3 kilobases of the murine coronavirus mouse hepatitis virus strain JHM were subcloned into pT7 vectors from which RNAs were transcribed and translated in vitro. Although p28 is encoded from the first 1 kilobase at the 5'-end of the genome, translation of in vitro transcribed RNAs indicated that this protein was not detected unless the product of the entire 5.3 kilobase region was synthesized. This result suggests that the region close to 5.3 kilobases from the 5'-end of the genomic RNA is essential for the proteolytic cleavage and may contain an autoproteolytic activity. Addition of the protease inhibitor $ZnCl_2$ blocked cleavage of the p28 protein. Site-directed mutagenesis of Cys residue 1137 significantly reduced the cleavage of the p28 protein, indicating that this residue, probably in conjuction with a downstream domain, plays an essential role in the cleavage of p28. This Cys residue may be part of a papain-like autoprotease encoded by gene 1.

INTRODUCTION

Mouse hepatitis virus (MHV) contains an RNA genome of more than 6×10^6 molecular weight (15, 27). Upon infection of a susceptible cell, the viral genomic RNA is first translated, producing the viral RNA-dependent RNA polymerase. This polymerase transcribes the virion genomic RNA into a negative-stranded RNA, which is, in turn, transcribed into a positive-sensed genomic RNA and six subgenomic mRNAs (2, 3, 12, 14). These mRNAs form a nested-set structure and contain an identical 5'-end leader sequence of approximately 72 nucleotides, which is derived by a unique leader-primed transcription mechanism (13, 19, 21, 24).

In vitro translation studies of MHV mRNAs revealed three viral structural proteins which are the nucleocapsid protein, N, and two glycoproteins, M and S. Several small, nonstructural proteins are also encoded by subgenomic mRNAs (17, 22). The largest mRNA, which is of genomic length, is thought to encode the viral RNA-dependent RNA polymerase. Sequencing of the entire genome of another coronavirus, avian infectious bronchitis virus (IBV), suggests that this gene has a capacity to encode two very large proteins of larger than 300 kilodaltons (kDa) (1, 6). In vitro translation studies of murine coronavirus genomic RNA indicated that a large polyprotein of 250 kDa is synthesized and cleaved to 28 kDa and 220 kDa proteins (7, 23). The p28 protein has been detected in MHV-infected cells (8). Previous sequencing and translation studies had established that the p28 protein represents the N-terminal portion of the presumed RNA polymerase precursor (7, 23). To further elucidate the structure and mechanism of synthesis of the potential RNA-dependent RNA polymerase of MHV, cDNA clones representing the 5'-end 5.3 kilobase (kb) region of genomic RNA were translated in vitro. Translation studies of in vitro synthesized RNA derived from these cDNA clones showed that this protein may contain an autoproteolytic activity which is responsible for the cleavage of the p28 protein. The protein domain essential for this proteolytic activity is located in the region from 3.9 to 5.3

Coronaviruses and Their Diseases
Edited by D. Cavanagh and T.D.K. Brown
Plenum Press, New York, 1990

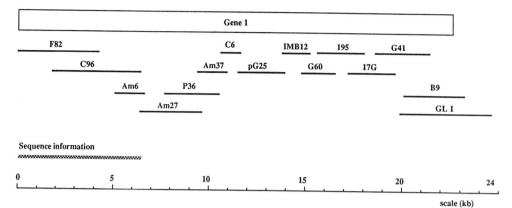

Fig. 1. Schematic diagram of cDNA clones representing MHV-JHM gene 1. Lengths are expressed in kilobase pairs (kb).

kb from the 5'-end of the genomic RNA. Site-directed mutagenesis of this cDNA suggests that Cys 1137 interacts with this domain and is essential for the cleavage of p28.

MATERIALS AND METHODS

cDNA Clones. cDNA clones representing the entire genome of MHV-JHM were generated by priming for first-strand cDNA synthesis with specific oligodeoxyribonucleotides as previously described (21, 23). Fig. 1 shows the positions of the cDNA clones relative to MHV-JHM genomic RNA.

In vitro transcription and translation. Plasmids pT7-NH, pT7-N2H, and pT7-NBgl consist of MHV-JHM gene 1 sequence from the Nar I site (nucleotide 187) to the first Hind III site (nucleotide 1989), the second Hind III site (nucleotide 3880), and the Bgl II site (nucleotide 5273), respectively, inserted downstream from the T7 polymerase promoter (26). DNA was linearized in the polylinker region following the MHV sequence by digestion with restriction enzyme Eco RI and transcribed in vitro with T7 RNA polymerase as previously described (23). The resulting RNA was translated in an mRNA-dependent rabbit reticulocyte lysate (Promega Biotech) under conditions optimized for MHV RNA translation (7).

Immunoprecipitation of in vitro translated proteins. Anti-p28 serum was generated in rabbits directed against a synthetic peptide representing amino acids 78-93 (NH_3-R-D-I-F-V-D-E-D-P-Q-K-V-E-A-S-T-COOH) of the p28 protein (23). Immunoprecipitation was performed by the method of Kessler (11) and proteins were analyzed by electrophoresis on 5 to 12.5% SDS-polyacrylamide gels (18).

Mutagenesis of plasmid pT7-NBgl. Site-directed mutagenesis was accomplished following the procedure of Higuchi et al using oligonucleotides containing specific mismatches and the polymerase chain reaction to amplify mutated DNA (10). Briefly, oligo #98 (5'-GTGAGGCATGCGACAGGGAA-3'), encompassing the unique Sph I site at nucleotide 3339, and oligo #99 (5'-CGAAGCCAAGAATTAGTACG-3') containing a mismatch at nucleotide 3624, were used to prime DNA synthesis from plasmid pT7-NBgl in the polymerase chain reaction (PCR). Likewise, oligo #101 (5'-CGCTCTTAACTAGTTTGTCC-3'), encompassing a unique Spe I site at nucleotide 3743 and oligo #100 (5'-CGTACTAATTCTTGGCTGCG-3') also containing a mismatch at nucleotide 3624 were used to prime DNA synthesis from pT7-NBgl. The product DNAs from these two reactions were then mixed, denatured and reassembled, and oligos #98 and #101 added to again prime DNA synthesis by PCR. The resulting PCR product DNA consisted of MHV genomic cDNA sequence from nucleotide 3334 to 3756 with a specific mutation (G to C) at nucleotide 3624 which would result in an amino acid change from cysteine to serine at residue 1137. The DNA was digested with Sph I and Spe I and inserted into the Sph I to Spe I site of pT7-NBgl and the resultant plasmid designated pT7-NB.1. The specific mutation was confirmed by sequencing the double stranded plasmid DNA using the Sequenase system (US Biochemicals).

RESULTS

cDNA cloning of MHV-JHM. To understand the structure and biochemical properties of the probable RNA polymerase of MHV, cDNA clones representing the entire gene were prepared (Fig. 1). From preliminary sequence information, we estimate the size of gene 1 to be greater than 22 kilobases, making the genomic RNA

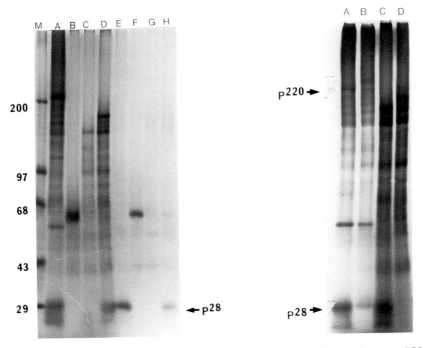

Fig. 2. Translation and immunoprecipitation of MHV-JHM gene 1 polypeptides (left). Capped RNA was synthesized from linearized plasmids pT7-NH, pT7-N2H, and pT7-NBgl with T7 RNA polymerase. The RNA was translated in vitro in rabbit reticulocyte lysates in the presence of (^{35}S)-methionine. The protein products were analyzed on a 3 to 12.5% gradient SDS-polyacrylamide gel. Lanes A, B, C, and D, respectively, show translation products of MHV-JHM genomic RNA, pT7-NH generated RNA, pT7-N2H generated RNA, and pT7-NBgl generated RNA. Lanes E, F, G and H show the products of immunoprecipitation with antiserum to p28. Lane M contained (^{14}C)-labeled marker polypeptides; molecular masses are given in kilodaltons on the left.

Fig. 3. Effects of ZnCl$_2$ on cell-free translation of gene 1 RNA (right). Zinc Chloride (1 mM) was added to the reticulocyte lysate before the addition of RNA, and translation reactions were incubated for 90 min in the presence of (^{35}S)-methionine. Lanes: A, control translation of MHV-JHM genomic RNA; B, with ZnCl$_2$; C, translation of pT7-NBgl-generated RNA; D, with ZnCl$_2$.

of murine coronavirus approximately 32 kb. The sequence of the 5'-most 2.0 kb region encoding the p28 protein has been reported previously (23). We have further extended the sequence for an additional 4.5 kb downstream (data not shown).

 Translation and processing of the MHV Gene 1 protein products. In vitro translation studies of MHV genomic RNA have revealed two primary protein products, p28 and p220 (7). It has previously been shown that p28 is an amino-terminal cleavage product of the MHV gene 1 protein (23). To obtain more information on the translation and processing of gene 1 protein products, we subcloned into pT7 vectors various fragments of cDNA clones containing gene 1 sequences. These plasmids represent gene 1 sequences starting from nucleotide 187, which is just upstream of the initiator AUG (nucleotide 215), and extend to 2.0, 3.9, and 5.3 kb from the 5'-end of the genome. RNA was transcribed from linearized plasmids and translated in the presence of (^{35}S)-methionine in rabbit reticulocyte lysates. The protein products were analyzed by polyacrylamide gel electrophoresis as shown in Fig. 2. In vitro translation of MHV-JHM genomic RNA resulted in the synthesis of the p28 and p220 proteins (Fig. 2, lane A), in agreement with the previously published results (7, 23). The identity of p28 was confirmed by its precipitation by an antiserum specific to a peptide of p28 (Fig. 2, lane E). In contrast, translation of an RNA representing the first 2.0 kb of gene 1 yielded only a primary translation product of approximately 65 kDa (Fig. 2, lane B). Translation of an RNA extending 3.7 kb into the gene 1-coding region resulted in the translation of a primary protein product of approximately 135 kDa (Fig. 2, lane C). No p28 was detected in either of these two translation reactions even though both primary translation products are predicted to contain p28 sequence. However, translation of an RNA extending to 5.3 kb of the gene 1 sequence yielded a translation product of approximately 160 kDa and the p28 protein (Fig. 2, lane D). The identity of p28 was confirmed by its precipitation by the specific antiserum against the peptide of p28

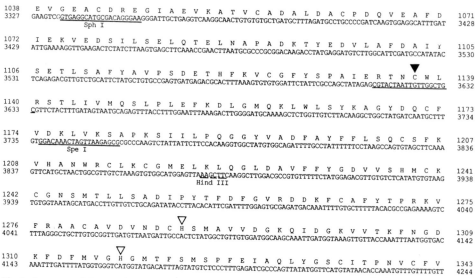

Fig 4. Sequence of the putative protease domain of MHV-JHM gene 1. A translation of the long open reading frame is shown in single-letter amino acid code. The cysteine residue proposed to be essential for protease activity is indicated by the filled triangle. Histidine residues which may be important for protease activity are indicated by open triangles. Sequences used to generate oligonucleotides used for site-directed mutagenesis are underlined.

(Fig. 2, lane H). These data indicated that the translation of a region between 3.9 kb and 5.3 kb from the 5'-end of the genomic RNA is required for the cleavage of the N-terminal portion, p28, from the primary gene 1 protein. The estimated molecular mass of the primary translation products of the three in vitro transcribed RNAs is 66 kDa, 136 kDa, and 186 kDa, respectively. This is in close agreement with the estimated molecular mass of the translation products detected on the gels: 65 kDa for pT7-NH, 135 kDa for pT7-N2H, and 160 kDa plus 28 kDa for pT7-NBgl.

Interestingly, the 65 kDa protein from the pT7-NH-generated translation reaction was precipitated by p28-specific serum (Fig. 2, lane F), while the 135 kDa protein from the pT7-N2H translation reaction was not (Fig. 2, lane G), indicating that the p28 epitope is either unavailable for binding or absent from that protein. As predicted, p160 was not precipitated since it does not contain the p28 sequence. The above data indicated that the cleavage of the p28 protein occurred only after the translation of a region more than 3.9 kb from the 5'-end of the viral RNA. This suggests that the region between 3.9 and 5.3 kb may contain an autoproteolytic activity or that it induces a conformational change in the protein which allows cleavage of p28.

To identify the primary translation product of pT7-NBgl RNA, we performed in vitro translation in the presence of protease inhibitors. As has been shown previously (7), the cleavage of p28 from the primary translation product (250 kDa) of MHV genomic RNA could be inhibited by addition of 1 mM ZnCl$_2$ to the translation reaction (Fig. 3, lane B). When the pT7-NBgl RNA was translated in the presence of 1 mM ZnCl$_2$, a protein of 185 kDa, but no p28, was obtained (Fig. 3, lane D). This result is in agreement with the predicted molecular weight of the primary translation product of this open reading frame.

Identification of a putative protease domain. Analysis of the amino acid sequence of the gene 1 polyprotein revealed a homology to the thiol family of proteases (Gorbalenya, A. E. and E. V. Koonin, personal communication). Thiol proteases such as papain, act by the juxtaposition of a cysteine (Cys) and a histidine (His) residue brought together by secondary structure to form a catalytic site. For MHV gene 1 polyprotein, Cys 1137 and either His 1288 or His 1317 were identified as the probable amino acids that may be involved in the protease activity (Gorbalenya, A.T. and Koonin, E.V. personal communication). The positions of these amino acids are shown in Fig. 4. The Hind III site at the end of plasmid pT7-N2H falls between the Cys and His residues. The failure of pT7-N2H polyprotein to cleave p28 suggests that both Cys and His residues are required for the catalytic site. Site-directed mutagenesis was used to directly test the role of Cys 1137 in the protease activity of the gene 1 polyprotein. Mutagenesis of this residue in pT7.NBgl was accomplished by the method of Higuchi (10), using synthetic oligonucleotides and polymerase chain reaction as described in the Materials and Methods section. Nucleotide 3625, G, was converted to C, resulting in the amino acid change at position 1137 from Cys to serine (Ser). The mutant plasmid was designated pT7-NB.1. Mutagenesis was confirmed by sequencing the region of the mutation in both the parent and mutant plasmids (Fig. 5).

A

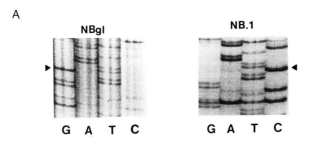

```
        NBgl                    NB.1

   G    A    T   C        G    A    T   C
```

B

```
             T  N  C  W  L

   NBgl:   ACTAATTGTTGGCTG


             T  N  S  W  L

   NB.1:   ACTAATTCTTGGCTG
```

Fig. 5. Sequence of region encompassing the Cys to Ser mutation in plasmid pT7-NB.1. (A) DNA sequence of plasmids pT7-NBgl and pT7-NB.1 from nucleotide 3619 to 3632. (B) Translation of the open reading frame is shown in single-letter amino acid code. The G to C change is underlined.

In vitro translation of RNA synthesized from pT7-NB.1 resulted in the synthesis of a large primary product of approximately 185 kDa (Fig. 6, lane B) in contrast to the pT7-NBgl-generated RNA which yield a smaller protein, p160, likely representing the processed protein (Fig. 6, lane A). As expected, when these translation reactions were precipitated with p28-specific antiserum, p28 was detected in the translation products of pT7 NBgl but not pT7-NB.1. Interestingly, the large primary protein product of 185 kDa was also precipitated from the pT7-NB.1 translation product (Fig. 6, lane D). This indicated that the conformation of this protein was such that the p28 epitope was available to bind to the antibody. Cys residue 1137 may be essential for both a conformational and catalytic role in the protease activity of the gene 1 polyprotein.

DISCUSSION

Theoretical considerations suggest that the 5'-most gene of the RNA genome of MHV, gene 1, codes for MHV-specific RNA-dependent RNA polymerases (23). We estimate the size of this genetic region to be greater than 22 kb; so far, only the amino-terminal protein, p28, of the potential gene product has been detected in virus-infected cells (8). This large genetic region is probably expressed as a single protein since there is only one mRNA species corresponding to gene 1. According to the nested-set structure of coronavirus mRNAs (12), only one translation initiation site at the 5'-end of each mRNA is utilized and, thus, only one functional protein is probably expressed from this entire gene. Significantly, the sequence of the avian coronavirus IBV genome reveals the presence of two overlapping ORFs in this region, which are likely translated into a polyprotein by a ribosomal frameshifting mechanism (4, 5). The exceptionally large size of this gene product suggests that the protein may have many different functional domains. Alternatively, the primary product of this large gene may undergo post-translational processing into smaller proteins. This possibility is comparable to other positive-stranded RNA viruses in which several nonstructural proteins are generated from post-translational cleavage of a single polyprotein (20, 25). Indeed, it has been shown that the 28 kDa protein is the N-terminal cleavage product of the gene 1 polyprotein (7, 23). The data presented in this report further show that this polyprotein may contain an autoproteolytic activity which is responsible for the cleavage of p28 from the primary translation product.   A potential papain-like protease domain was identified, which corresponds to approximately 3.6 to 4.2 kb from the 5'-end of the genomic RNA. Interestingly, IBV also contains a papain-like protease region at 4.3 to 4.9 kb from the 5'-end of the genomic RNA (1). The presence of an autoprotease activity may be a common feature for all coronaviruses.

Mutagenesis of Cys residue 1137 indicated that it was essential for the autoprotease activity. This Cys residue probably interacts with a downstream region, since the 135 kDa protein containing amino acids 1-1222 is unable to cleave p28 (Fig. 2). Cys 1137 may also be important for maintaining the conformation of

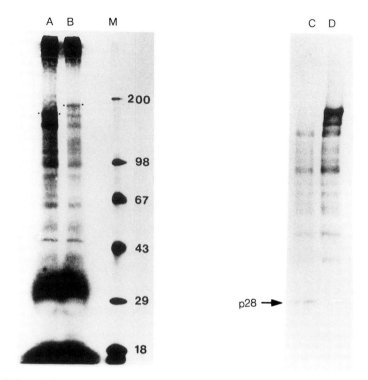

Fig. 6. Translation and immunoprecipitation of pT7-NBgl and pT7-NB.1 polypeptides. Capped RNA was synthesized from linearized plasmids pT7-NBgl and pT7-NB.1 with T7 RNA polymerase. The RNA was translated in vitro in rabbit reticulocyte lysates in the presence of (^{35}S)-methionine. The protein products were analyzed on a 3 to 12.5% gradient SDS-polyacrylamide gel. Lanes A and B, respectively, show translation products of pT7-NBgl and pT7-NB.1 generated RNA. Lanes C and D show the products of immunoprecipitation with antiserum to p28. Lane M contained (^{14}C)-labeled marker polypeptides; molecular masses are given in kilodaltons.

the protein. The primary translation product p135 was not precipitated by anti-p28 serum, indicating that the epitope was unavailable. In contrast, the pT7-NB.1 translation product, p185, which had a Ser at 1137, was precipitated with anti-p28 serum.

The gene 1 product of MHV may be a polyprotein analogous to that of picornaviruses, alphaviruses or flaviviruses (20, 25). In these viruses, the proteases are an integral part of the polyprotein and cleave the polyprotein at several sites. It is likely that the proteolytic activity of the MHV gene 1 product may also cleave itself at several additional sites. These cleavage products may perform various functions directly or indirectly involved in RNA synthesis. Each cleavage product of the gene 1 polyprotein may belong to a separate complementation group (16). By computer analysis of the IBV gene 1 sequence, it has been suggested that this protein may contain different domains for RNA polymerase, helicase, nucleotide binding activities and several proteases (9). Indeed, the complex mechanism of MHV RNA synthesis may require all of these enzymatic activities. The approach demonstrated in this paper may help us identify the enzymatic activities associated with these proteins. We are currently working to determine the role of His residues in the proteolytic activity and to identify the minimal region of the protease domain.

ACKNOWLEDGMENTS

This work was supported by Public Health Service research grants AI19244 and NS18146 from the National Institute of Health. S.C.B. is a postdoctoral fellow of the Arthritis Foundation. N.L.M. is a postdoctoral fellow of the National Multiple Sclerosis Society.

LITERATURE CITED

1. Boursnell, M. E. G., T. D. K. Brown, I. J. Foulds, P. F. Green, F. M. Tomley, and M. M. Binns. 1987. Completion of the sequence of the genome of the coronavirus avian infectious bronchitis virus. J. Gen.Virol. 68:57-77.

2. Brayton, P. R., M. M. C. Lai, C. D. Patton, and S. A. Stohlman. 1982. Characterization of two RNA polymerase activities induced by mouse hepatitis virus. J. Virol. 42:847-853.

3. Brayton, P. R., S. A. Stohlman, and M. M. C. Lai. 1984. Further characterization of mouse hepatitis virus RNA dependent RNA polymerases. Virology 133:197-201.

4. Brierly, I., M.E.G. Boursnell, M.M. Binns, B. Bilimoria, V.C. Blok, T.D.K. Brown and S.C. Inglis. 1987. An efficient ribosomal frame-shifting signal in the polymerase-encoding region of the coronavirus IBV. EMBO 6:3779-3785.

5. Brierley, I. P. Digard and S. C. Inglis. Characterization of an efficient coronavirus ribosomal frameshift signal: requirement for an RNA pseudoknot. Cell 57: 537-547.

6. Brown, T. D. K., M. E. G. Boursnell, M. M. Binns, and F. M. Tomley. 1986. Cloning and sequencing of 5' terminal sequences from avian infectious bronchitis virus genomic RNA. J. Gen. Virol. 67:221-228.

7. Denison, M. R., and S. Perlman. 1986. Translation and processing of mouse hepatitis virus virion RNA in a cell-free system. J. Virol. 60:12-18.

8. Denison, M. R., and S. Perlman. 1987. Identification of a putative polymerase gene product in cells infected with murine coronavirus A59. Virology 157:565-568.

9. Gorbalenya, A. E., E. V. Koonin, A. P. Donchenko, and V. M. Blinov. 1989. Coronavirus genome: prediction of putative functional domains in the non-structural polyprotein by comparative amino acid sequence analysis. Nuc. Acids Res. 17:4847-4861.

10. Higuchi, R., B. Krummel, and R. K. Saiki. 1988. A general method of in vitro preparation and specific mutagenesis of DNA fragments: study of protein and DNA interactions. Nuc. Acids Res. 16: 7351-7367.

11. Kessler, S. W. (1981). Use of protein A bearing staphylococci for the immunoprecipitation and isolation of antigens from cells. In "Methods in Enzymology" (J.J. Longone and H. Van Vunakis, Eds.), Vol. 73, pp. 442-459. Academic Press, New York.

12. Lai, M. M. C. 1988. Replication of Coronavirus RNA. In "RNA Genetics." (E. Domingo, J.J. Holland, and P. Ahlquist, Eds.), Vol. I, pp. 115-136. CRC Press, Inc., Boca Raton, Florida.

13. Lai, M. M. C., R. S. Baric, P. R. Brayton, and S. A. Stohlman. 1984. Characterization of leader RNA sequences on the virion and mRNAs of mouse hepatitis virus-a cytoplasmic RNA virus. Proc. Natl. Acad. Sci. USA 81:3626-3630.

14. Lai, M. M. C., P. R. Brayton, R. C. Armen, C. D. Patton, C. Pugh, and S. A. Stohlman. 1981. Mouse hepatitis virus A59: mRNA structure and genetic localization of the sequence divergence from hepatotropic strain MHV-3. J. Virol. 39:823-834.

15. Lai, M. M. C., and S. A. Stohlman. 1978. RNA of mouse hepatitis virus. J. Virol. 26:236-242.

16. Leibowitz, J. L., J. R. DeVries, and M.V. Haspel. 1982. Genetic analysis of murine hepatitis virus strain JHM. J. Virol. 42:1080-1088.

17. Leibowitz, J. L., S. R. Weiss, E. Paavola, and C. W. Bond. 1982. Cell-free translation of murine coronavirus RNA. J. Virol. 43:905-913.

18. Maizel, J. 1971. Polyacrylamide gel electrophoresis of viral proteins. Methods Virol. 5:176-246.

19. Makino, S., S. A. Stohlman, and M. M. C. Lai. 1986. Leader sequences of murine coronavirus mRNAs can be freely reassorted: evidence for the role of free leader RNA in transcription. Proc. Natl. Acad. Sci. USA 83:4204-4208.

20. Semler, B. L., R. J. Kuhn, and E. Wimmer. 1988. Replication of the poliovirus genome. In "RNA Genetics." (E. Domingo, J.J. Holland, and P. Ahlquist, Eds.), Vol. I, pp. 23-48. CRC Press, Inc., Boca Raton, Florida.

21. Shieh, C.-K., L.H. Soe, S. Makino, M.-F. Chang, S. A. Stohlman, and M. M. C. Lai. 1987. The 5'-end sequence of the murine coronavirus genome: implications for multiple fusion sites in leader-primed transcription. Virology 156:321-330.

22. Siddell, S. G. 1983. Coronavirus JHM: coding assignments of subgenomic mRNAs. J. Gen. Virol. 64:113-125.

23. Soe, L. H., C.-K. Shieh, S. C. Baker, M.-F. Chang, and M. M. C. Lai. 1987. Sequence and translation of the murine coronavirus 5'-end genomic RNA reveals the N-terminal structure of the putative RNA polymerase. J. Virol. 61:3968-3976.

24. Spaan, W. J. M., H. Delius, M. Skinner, J. Armstrong, P. Rottier, S. Smeekens, B. A. M. van der Zeijst, and S. G. Siddell. 1983. Coronavirus mRNA synthesis involves fusion of non-contiguous sequences. EMBO J. 2:1839-1844.

25. Strauss, J. H. and E. G. Strauss. 1988. Replication of the RNAs of alphaviruses and flaviviruses. In "RNA Genetics." (E. Domingo, J.J. Holland, and P. Ahlquist, Eds.), Vol. I, pp. 71-90. CRC Press, Inc., Boca Raton, Florida.

26. Tabor, S., and C. C. Richardson. 1985. A bacteriophage T7 RNA polymerase/promoter system for controlled exclusive expression of specific genes. Proc. Natl. Acad. Sci. USA 82:1074-1078.

27. Wege, H., A. Muller, and V. ter Meulen. 1978. Genomic RNA of the murine coronavirus JHM. J. Gen. Virol. 41:217-227.

DETECTION OF MOUSE HEPATITIS VIRUS NONSTRUCTURAL PROTEINS USING

ANTISERA DIRECTED AGAINST BACTERIAL VIRAL FUSION PROTEINS

Philip W. Zoltick[1], Julian L. Leibowitz[2], James DeVries[2], Catherine J. Pachuk[1] and Susan R. Weiss[1]

[1]Department of Microbiology, University of Pennsylvania School of Medicine, Philadelphia, PA. 19104-6076 and [2]Department of Pathology and Laboratory Medicine, University of Texas Health Sciences Center, Houston, Texas 77225

ABSTRACT

Mouse hepatitis virus, strain A59 cDNAs were inserted into the procaryotic fusion vector pGE374. RecA/viral/LacZ tripartite fusion proteins were synthesized from these plasmids and purified from E. coli. Antisera were raised in rabbits against these fusion proteins. Viral nonstructural proteins were detected in infected murine fibroblasts and glial cells. The anti-gene B, ORF1 sera detect a 30K cytoplasmic protein while the anti-gene E, ORF2 sera detect a 9.6K protein. Sera raised against proteins encoded in cDNAs from 5' portions of gene A immunoprecipitate the 200-250K polypeptides synthesized in vitro from genome RNA. Antisera raised against proteins encoded in both 5' and 3' portions of gene A immunoprecipitate membrane associated polypeptides of 150K and >600K from MHV infected cells.

INTRODUCTION

Mouse hepatitis virus strain A59 contains three structural genes. These encode: N, the phosphorylated 60K basic nucleocapsid protein; E1, the transmembrane glycoprotein and E2, the peplomer protein which is responsible for cell fusion and is thought to play an important role in pathogenicity and antigenicity. The remaining four viral genes are thought to encode nonstructural proteins (1). The largest of these is the approximately 23 kb putative polymerase gene A (2), which may encode one or more polypeptides involved in viral RNA polymerase activity. Other smaller non-structural genes include gene B, which potentially encodes a 30K basic protein and possibly an additional glycoprotein (3), gene D which encodes a 14K protein in the case of MHV-JHM (4) or a 10K protein in the case of MHV-A59 (Weiss et al., unpublished) and gene E, which potentially encodes a 13K basic protein (ORF1) and a 9.6K hydrophobic protein (ORF2)(5,6).

It is possible that at least some of these proteins may be involved in RNA synthesis as there are at least six complementation groups of temperature sensitive mutants of MHV with RNA negative phenotypes (7). The sequences of the predicted gene E, ORF1 and gene B, ORF1 products suggest that these may be nucleic acid binding proteins.

The nonstructural proteins have been difficult to detect in the infected cell, probably due to their low abundance and a lack of specific antisera. Partial expression of gene A has been achieved by the cell-free translation of genome RNA. The 5' end of gene A is thought to encode p28 and p220, derived from a p250 precursor (8,9). These three polypeptides are presumed to be related to MHV polymerase. Of the predicted small, non-structural proteins the gene E, ORF2 product (10) and gene D product (11) have been detected in infected cells by the use of specific antisera. A 35K protein, the possible product of gene B, ORF1 has been observed in infected cells and in the products of cell free translation of mRNA 2 by the use of serum derived from an infected mouse (12).

We summarize here our use of procaryotic viral fusion vectors for the synthesis of fusion proteins which were used to raise antisera against the proteins encoded in MHV nonstructural genes A,B and E. We have validated the sera by reaction with in vitro translation products and then used the antisera to demonstrate the viral gene products in MHV-infected cells.

METHODS

Cells and viruses. The origin and growth of the 17Cl-1 and L-2 cell lines (13) as well as MHV-A59 (14) have been described previously. Mixed glial cell cultures, containing at least 90% astrocytes, were derived from newborn C57BL/6 mouse brains as described previously (15).

Protein labeling and subcellular fractionation. 17Cl-1 cells or glial cells were infected with MHV-A59 at an M.O.I. of 5-10 PFU/cell. Fourteen hours later (17Cl-1) and 24 hours later (glial) cells were labeled for one hour with ^{35}S-methionine and ^{35}S-cysteine as previously described (10,16). For subcellular fractionation, cells were divided into nuclear, membrane and cytoplasmic fractions by the procedures of Brayton et al., (17). Proteins were detected by radioimmunoprecipitation, immunoflorescence microscopy, immunoperoxidase staining or Western immunoblotting, all as described previously (10,20).

Recombinant DNA technology. Restriction enzymes as well as terminal deoxynucleotidyl transferase were used as suggested by the vendors. Viral cDNAs were cloned from MHV-A59 genome RNA using the procedures of Gubler and Hoffman (18) and mapped on the viral genome as previously described (2,19). DNA fragments were subcloned into pGem vectors as described previously (6,10,16).

Construction of fusion vectors. The prokaryotic expression vectors, pGE372 and pGE374 are derivatives of pBR322 that differ from each another at a synthetic DNA sequence between recA and lacZ elements and have been described in detail before (10,16). In both vectors, the 5' end of the E. coli recA structural gene (35 codons), as well as the recA promoter and ribosome binding site, are located upstream of the E. coli lacZ gene (1015 codons), which lacks its promoter and translation initiation site. The lacZ gene encodes a functional β-galactosidase. However, expression of the enzyme requires the recA transcription and translation initiation signals. In pGE372, the truncated recA and lacZ genes are in frame. In pGE374, the downstream lacZ sequence is out of frame with the recA sequence; these coding sequences are separated by a small synthetic DNA fragment which contains a Sma I site for insertion of DNA fragments.

Antisera production. The tripartite fusion proteins were usually recovered preparatively from the pellet following bacterial cell lysis in the presence of Triton X-100 and sonication (10,16). The fusion protein derived from gene E was recovered from a preparative polyacrylamide gel (10). Tripartite fusion proteins were used as immunogens directly and after denaturation with 1% SDS and 5% 2-mercaptoethanol (100°C for 5 minutes). Between 50 and 100 ug of protein was homogenized with complete Freund's adjuvant and injected subcutaneously in two NZW rabbits. Rabbits were subsequently boosted at approximately 4-week intervals by injection of antigen in incomplete Freund's adjuvant.

Antisera were initially evaluated by immunoblotting against bacterial extracts prepared from bacteria carrying the recombinant plasmids as well as pGE372, and pGE374. At least three immunizations were required before activity against the appropriate bands on the Western blots was observed. They were further evaluated for viral specificities as described below in Methods.

In vitro transcription and translation. The pGem recombinant vectors were linearized and transcripts were synthesized using the bacteriophage T7 or SP6 RNA polymerases as described by Krieg and Melton (21). Translation reactions (25ul) were in a rabbit reticulocyte lysates (Promega) and contained 1ug of the capped transcripts or purified genome RNA.

RESULTS

Anti-fusion protein antisera

For construction of viral/pGE374 fusion vectors, pGE374 DNA was linearized by digestion with Sma I, and tailed with deoxyguanosine triphosphate (22). Various fragments of DNA as diagrammed in Figure 1 were isolated from the MHV-A59 viral cDNAS, tailed with deoxycytosine triphosphate, annealed to Sma I digested, dG tailed pGE374, and used to transform MC1061. Colonies expressing a lacZ[+] phenotype were selected in the presence of XGal. The presence of viral sequences was verified by Southern blot hybridization (data not shown).

Colonies containing each of the viral inserts shown in Figure 1 were grown up in maxi-preps and RecA/viral/LacZ tripartite fusion proteins identified by immunblotting with anti-RecA serum as well as by their large size. Tripartite fusion proteins were isolated preparatively. Most of the tripartite fusion proteins were insoluble after bacterial cell lysis with Triton and sonication. These proteins were isolated directly from the bacterial pellets and used as a mixture of "native" and "denatured" proteins for immunization (see Methods). The remaining proteins, that were soluble after cell lysis, for example the gene E, ORF2 product tripartite protein, were purified by preparative SDS polyacrylamide gel electrophoresis and were used in denatured form for immunization. Inoculation of each protein into two rabbits and testing of the actitivy of the sera against the immunogens were carried out as described in Methods and as previously described (10,16,20).

Immunoprecipitation of in vitro translation products with antisera

Before testing the putative nonstructural protein antisera on infected cell lysates, the antisera were reacted with in vitro translation products representing portions of genes A,B and E. For testing of the gene A antisera, in vitro translation products of genome RNA were used. In vitro translation of the viral genome results in a group of large proteins of 200 to 250K among which are p220 and p250 described by Denison and Perlman (8,12). These correspond to the open reading frame initiated at the 5' end of the genome, the putative viral polymerase gene (9); the 250K of protein corresponds to the sequences found in approximately 7.5 kb at the 5' end of genome. These in vitro translated proteins were immunoprecipitated by the antisera directed against fusion proteins derived from clones 1410, 1533 but not those from 917, 1033 or from gene B (Figure 2A). Thus 1410 and 1533 antisera contain activity against the polypepetides encoded in the 5' end of genome as they should and the antisera derived from more 3' gene A clones do not. This suggests that antisera directed against proteins encoded in cDNAs 1410 and 1533 do contain activity against the polypeptides encoded in the 5' end of the polymerase gene and should be useful for the detection of polypeptides encoded in gene A in MHV infected cells. At present we do not observe cell free translation of more 3' regions of gene A so we do not have substrates with which to test these antisera.

The gene B and gene E antisera were validated similarly with in vitro translation products of RNAs generated by transcription from pGem constructs containing the appropriate ORFs. As we have published previously (6) we have inserted cDNAs containing gene E, ORF1 and ORF2 sequences either separately or in tandem into pGem vectors, transcribed RNAs from these vectors and used these in in vitro translation reactions to synthesize polypeptides

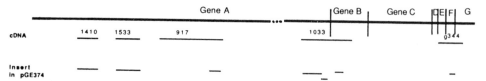

Figure 1. Schematic diagram of cDNA fragments used for synthesis of fusion proteins. cDNA clones are aligned on the viral genome map. Fragments of these clones used for insertion into the fusion vector are also diagrammed.

corresponding in size to the ORFs. We demonstrated a large amount of the 9.6K ORF2 product and only small amounts of the 13K ORF1 product. Using the 9.6K protein we demonstrated immuoprecipitation using the antisera directed against ORF2 but not using the antisera directed against ORF1. We were unable however to demonstrate activity by the gene E, ORF1 antiserum. Thus until now we have been unable to derive an anti-13K serum.

The ORF1 of gene B potentially encodes a 30K protein (3,22). An 820 base pair piece of DNA from clone 1033 containing the entire coding region of gene B, ORF2, was inserted into pGem. The resulting vector was linearized and then transcribed with T7 RNA polymerase. The resulting RNA was translated in vitro into a 30K polypeptide. This polypeptide was efficiently immunoprecipitated by antisera directed against gene B, ORF1, but not by antisera directed against sequences encoded in gene A.

Detection of MHV nonstructural proteins in infected cells

Now that we had demonstrated activity against the cell-free translation products of portions of genes A,B and E, we were ready to use the antisera to detect non-strucutral proteins in infected cells. We used the sera for gene A (1410, 1533, 917, 1033), gene B, ORF1 and gene E, ORF2) to immunoprecipitate radiolabeled proteins from infected cells. We used both murine

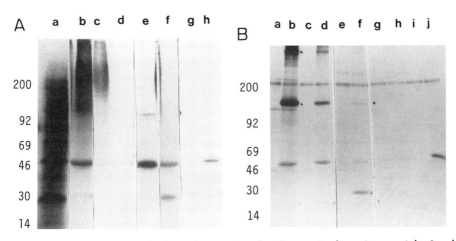

Figure 2. Immunoprecipitation of viral proteins by anti-fusion protein sera. Panel A. Purified viral genome was translated in vitro in a rabbit reticulocyte system. ^{3}H-leucine labeled proteins were either analyzed directly on SDS polacrylamide gels (lane a) or immunoprecipitated with antifusion protein sera prior to gel analysis. lane b, 1410 antiserum; lane c, 1533 antiserum; lane d, 917 antiserum; lane e, 1033 antiserum; lane f, anti-gene B, ORF1 serum; lane g, pre-immune rabbit serum; lane h, anti nucleocapsid monoclonal antibody. Panel B. ^{35}S-labeled protein from mock infected (lanes a,c,e,g,i) or infected (b,d,f,h,j) 17 Cl-1 cells was immunoprecipitated. Lanes a and b; 1410 antiserum; lanes c and d, 1033 antiserum; lanes f and g, gene B, ORF1 antiserum; lanes h and i, preimmune serum; lanes j and k, anti-nucleocapsid serum.

fibroblast cells (17Cl-1 and L-2) as well as primary murine glial cells derived from newborn mice. Infection of fibroblasts by MHV results in a lytic infection whereas infection of glial cells results in a persistent non-lytic infection. The antisera directed agaisnt fusion proteins derived from gene A cDNAs all immunoprecipitated a 150K band as well as a very large polypeptide that is in excess of 600K, as measured by migration of murine nebulin marker protein (estimated from 600-800K) (Figure 2B). This very large protein could be as large as 700K which might represent the entire length of gene A. We consider these two polypeptides as putative products of gene A. These proteins were found in glial cells as well as 17Cl-1 and L-2 fibroblasts and appeared with kinetics similar to those of the viral structural proteins.

The gene E, ORF2 antiserum detects a 9.6K protein in infected fibroblasts. This protein comigrates by SDS polyacrylamide gel electrophoresis with the product of in vitro translation of RNA containing gene E, ORF2 (6,10). The gene B, ORF1 antiserum detects a 30K protein in infected fibroblasts (Figure 2B) and in infected glial cells. This protein comigrates with the in vitro translation product of gene B, ORF1.

Subcellular localization of MHV nonstructural proteins

Since it had been reported that MHV polymerase activity was associated with membranes (17) we wanted to determine if the putative gene A products or the gene B 30K protein were membrane associated. Thus, we used radioimmunoprecipitation to examine the localization of radiolabeled proteins following subcellular fractionation of cells (17). Both the 150K and very large (>600K) proteins immunoprecipitated by the anti-gene A sera were found mostly in membranes. The 30K gene B, ORF1 product was found mostly in the cytoplasm as might be expected for a putative nucleic acid binding protein. As controls we used the strucutral proteins N and E1. As expected, N fractionated mostly with the cytoplasm and E1 mostly with membranes.

DISCUSSION

Anti fusion protein antisera

We have described here a method for generating fusion proteins to be used as immunogens to raise viral nonstructural protein antisera. The procaryotic fusion vector, pGE374 is an excellent expression vector. First the strategy of insertion of foreign DNA requires no detailed sequence information in order to determine if a coding sequence is present in the fusion DNA. If the DNA fragment used is longer than 110 bp there is less than a 1% chance that an open reading frame is a result of a random occurrence. We have used DNA inserts of from 250 bp to 2000 bp. Each of the inserts we have described here has resulted in approximately 5% lac Z positive colonies, which is close to the predicted value if there were one open reading frame in each fragment. Secondly, this vector has a high level recA promoter that can be induced to even higher levels with mitomycin C. Thirdly, the LacZ portion of the fusion protein can be assayed simply by a color reaction on bacterial colonies and the RecA portion may be assayed by Western blotting using a RecA antibody. The large size of the fusion protein also aids in its detection. Another useful feature of this system is that the insolubility of most of the fusion proteins allows a simple partial purification from the pellet of lysed bacteria. This also allows the use of both "native" and "denatured" forms of the protein to be used for immunizations. This makes it possible to use the antisera for the detection of both native and denatured forms of the proteins. We have found that the anti gene B, ORF1 serum is useful in Western blots and immunofluorescence as well as immunoprecipitation (20).

Detection of MHV nonstructural proteins

The MHV non-structural proteins have been very difficult to detect. The expected proteins have been predicted from RNA sequence analysis of cDNA clones for the small proteins encoded in genes B, D and E. In the cases of gene B, ORF1 (20), gene D (11) and gene E, ORF1 (6,10) the predicted proteins have been detected in the infected cells by the use of anti-fusion protein antisera. The gene B 30K and the gene E 9.6K proteins are detected both during lytic infection and during persistent infection in glial cells and appear with similar kinetics to that of MHV structural proteins.

Sequence analysis suggests that the gene B, ORF1 product and the gene D product are basic and may have nucleic acid binding potential while the gene E, ORF1 9.6K protein is quite hydrophobic and may be membrane associated. It is not clear whether the prediced 13K predicted gene E, ORF1 protein is expressed during infection. It has a suboptimal sequence around its initiation site for protein synthesis and is quite poorly translated in vitro compared to ORF2 which must be translated by internal initiation. Functions for these proteins are at present unknown. There are also to date no reports of expression of these in eukaryotic cells or description of mutants with lesions in these genes.

Sequence information is not yet available for the majority of MHV gene A. However, from the size of the gene (approximately 23kb) and by analogy with infectious bronchitis virus (IBV) genome RNA, it is thought that the gene will probably contain two large ORFs (23). If similar to IBV, the second ORF will be expressed via a frame shift mechanism. In vitro translation of genome has allowed the identification of p28, p220 and p250, likely translation products of gene A. However, there is at present no evidence that either p220 or p250 is synthesized in the infected cell or that any of these proteins is indeed part of a functional polymerase. We have preliminarily identified 150K and >600K polypeptides as putative products of gene A. We are at present comparing peptide maps of these polypeptides with those of the in vitro translation products of genome RNA and MHV structural proteins. The gene A antisera that we have generated hopefully will allow us to identify polypeptides encoded in gene A and to map these polypeptides along the length of the gene. We hope to be able to determine the fuunctions of the gene A polypeptides detected by these antisera by the use of the permeabilized cell system to study polymerase in vitro where the system may be more easily manipulated (24).

REFERENCES

1. Spaan, W.J.M., Cavanagh, D., Horzinek, M.C. 1988. Coronaviruses. Structure and genome expression. J. Gen. Virol. 69:2939-2952.
2. Pachuk, C.J., Bredenbeek, P.J., Zoltick, P.W., Spaan, W.J.M. and Weiss, S.R. (1988). Molecular cloning of the gene encoding the putative polymerase of mouse hepatitis coronavirus, strain A59. Virology 171:141-148.
3. Luytjes, W., Bredenbeek, P.J., Noten, A.F.S., Horzinek, M.C., Spaan, W.J.M. (1988).Sequence of mouse hepatitis virus mRNA 2: Indications for RNA recombination between coroanviruses and influenza C virus. Virology 166:415-422.
4. Skinner, M.A., Siddell, S.G. (1985).Coding sequence of coronavirus MHV-JHM mRNA4. J. Gen. Virol. 66:593-596.
5. Skinner, M.A., Ebner, D., Siddell, S.G. (1985). Coronavirus MHV-JHM mRNA 5 has a sequence arrangement which potentially allows translation of a second downstream open reading frame. J. Gen. Virol. 66:581-592.
6. Budzilowicz, C.J., Weiss, S.R. (1987). In vitro sythesis of two polypeptides from a nonstructural gene of coronvirus mouse hepatitis virus, strain A59. Virology 157:509-515.
7. Leibowitz, J.L., DeVries, J.R., Haspel, M.V. (1982). Genetic analysis of murine hepatitis virus. J. Virol. 42:1080-1087.
8. Denison, M.R., Perlman, S. (1986). Translation and processing of mouse hepatitis virus virion RNA in a cell free system. J. Virol. 60:12-18.
9. Soe, L., Shieh,C.K., Baker,S., Chang, M.F., Lai, M.M.C. (1987). Sequence and translation of murine coronavirus 5'end genomic RNA reveals the N-terminal structure of the putative RNA polymerase. J. Virol. 61:3968-3976.
10. Leibowitz, J.L., Perlman, S., Weinstock, G., DeVries, J.R., Budzilowicz, C.J., Weissmann, J.M., Weiss, S.R. (1988). Detection of a murine coronavirus nonstructural protein encoded in a downstream open reading frame. Virology 164:156-164.
11. Ebner, D., Siddell, S. (1986). Identification of the MHV-JHM mRNA 4 gene product using fusion protein antisera. In Advances in Experimental Medicine and Biology, Lai and Stohlman, eds. Plenum Press, N.Y. pp. 39-45.
12. Leibowitz, J.L., Weiss, S.R., Paavola, E., Bond, C.W. (1982). Cell-free translation of murine coronavirus RNA. J. Virol. 43:905-913.
13. Leibowitz, J.L., Wilhelmson, D.C., Bond, C.W. (1981). The virus specific intracellular RNA species of two murine coronaviruses: MHV-A59 and MHV-JHM. Virol. 114:39-51.
14. Sturman, L.S., Takemoto, K.K. (1972).Enhanced growth of a murine coronavirus in transformed mouse cells. Infect. Immunity 6:501-507.
15. Lavi, E., Suzumura, A., Hirayama, M., Silberburg, D.H., Weiss, S.R. (1987). Coroanvirus MHV-A59 causes a persistent productive infection in glial cell cultures. Microbiol Pathogenesis 3:79-86.
16. Zoltick, P.W., Leibowitz, J.L., DeVries, J.R., Weinstock, G., Weiss, S.R. A general method for the induction and screening of antisera directed against polypeptides encoded by cDNAs:Generation of antiserum specific for coronavirus MHV-A59 putative polyerase gene. Gene in press.
17. Brayton, P.R., Lai, M.M.C., Patton, C.D., Stohlman, S.A.(1982).Characterization of two RNA polymerase activities induced by mouse hepatitis virus. J. Virol. 42:847-853.

18. Gubler, U., Hoffman, B.J. (1983). A simple and very efficient method for generating cDNA libraries. Gene 25:263-269, 1983.
19. Budzilowicz, C.B., Wilczynski, S.P., Weiss, S.R. (1985).Three intergenic regions of mouse hepatitis virus strain A59 genome RNA contain a common nucleotide sequence that is homologous to the 3' end of the viral mRNA leader sequence. J. Virol. 53:834-840.
20. Zoltick, P.W., Leibowitz, J.L., Oleszak, E., Weiss, S.R. Mouse hepatitis virus gene B ORF1 is expressed in the cytoplasm of mouse fibroblasts and glial cells. Submitted to Virology.
21. Krieg, P.A., Melton,D.A.(1984). Functional messenger RNAs are produced by SP6 in vitro transcription of cloned cDNAs. Nucleic Acids Research,12:7075-7070.
22. Deng, G., and Wu, R., (1981). An improved procedure for utilizing terminal transferase to add homopolymers to the 3' terminus of DNA. Nuc. Acids. Res. 9:4173-4188.
23. Boursnell, M.E.G., Brown, T.D.K., Foulds, I.J., Green, P.H., Tomley, F.,. Binns, M.M. (1987). The complete sequence of the genome of avian infectious bronchitis virus. J. Gen. Virol. 68:57-77.
24. Leibowitz, J.L. DeVries, J.R.(1988). Synthesis of virus-specific RNA in permeabilized murine coronavirus infected cells. Virology 166:66-75.

NUCLEOTIDE SEQUENCE OF THE E2-PEPLOMER PROTEIN GENE AND PARTIAL NUCLEOTIDE
SEQUENCE OF THE UPSTREAM POLYMERASE GENE OF TRANSMISSIBLE GASTROENTERITIS
VIRUS (MILLER STRAIN)

Ronald D. Wesley

United States Department of Agriculture
Agricultural Research Service
National Animal Disease Center, Ames, Iowa, USA

ABSTRACT

The E2-peplomer protein gene of the virulent Miller strain of
transmissible gastroenteritis virus (TGEV) was sequenced from cDNA clones
and compared to the E2 gene sequence of the avirulent Purdue strain.
Sequence comparisons indicate that most amino acid differences occur in the
N-terminal half of the E2-peplomer which represents the most exposed region
of the protein. In addition, analysis of an incompletely sequenced open
reading frame (ORF) to the immediate 5'side of the E2 gene indicates
extensive sequence homology with the infectious bronchitis virus (IBV) F2
gene which is thought to encode a RNA polymerase.

INTRODUCTION

Transmissible gastroenteritis virus (TGEV) is an economically important
pathogenic coronavirus of swine. It is an enveloped RNA virus composed of 3
major structural proteins (E2, E1, and N), and a 23.6 kilobase (kb)
positive-stranded genome. At least 5 classes of neutralizing epitopes occur
on the E2-peplomer glycoprotein while complement-dependent neutralization
can be demonstrated only with E1 glycoprotein-specific monoclonal
antibodies. [1-4] Nucleotide sequencing studies have focused on the
avirulent Purdue 115 strain in which 8.3 kb at the 3' end of the genome have
been sequenced. [5-7] Base sequence comparisons of the Purdue and Miller
strains in the region between the E1 and E2 genes have shown that the Miller
TGEV genome contains an additional intergenic recognition sequence and a
larger ORF, perhaps, encoding a nonstructural protein. [8] In order to
further determine genetic differences between these 2 strains, the E2 gene
of the virulent Miller strain was sequenced. In addition, analysis of an
incomplete ORF upstream of the E2 gene indicates extensive sequence homology
with a presumed IBV polymerase gene. [9]

MATERIALS AND METHODS

Virus

A working stock of the virulent Miller strain of TGEV was prepared as
described previously. [10] For the isolation of genomic RNA, the virus was

first plaque-picked 3 times on swine testicular (ST) cells before virus purification and subsequent RNA isolation.[8] The plaque-picked virus remained lethal for neonatal piglets.

Cloning and DNA Sequencing

cDNA was prepared from TGEV genomic RNA and cloned into λgt11. First and second strand syntheses were carried out using calf thymus DNA oligodeoxynucleotides as primers and a cDNA synthesis kit (Amersham Corp., Arlington Heights, IL). EcoR1 linkers were added to blunt-ended, double-stranded cDNA. The cDNA was then ligated to EcoR1 cut λgt11 and packaged in vitro (Stratagene, La Jolla, CA).[32] Lambda phage containing viral inserts were identified by hybridization to ^{32}P-labeled cDNA prepared from genomic RNA.

To facilitate cDNA sequencing, viral inserts that hybridized to specific mRNAs were subcloned into the EcoR1 site of the multipurpose pBluescript phagemid vector (Stratagene, La Jolla, CA). Stepwise unidirectional deletions were constructed[11] and sequenced by the dideoxy chain-termination method.[12] Programs for computer analysis of the DNA sequence were purchased from DNASTAR (Madison, WI).

RESULTS

Figure 1 shows the location at the 3′end of the TGEV genome of the cDNA clones, pRP1 and pRP3, derived from the virulent Miller strain of TGEV that were used to obtain DNA sequences of the E2-peplomer gene and the 930 bases to the 5′side of the E2 gene. cDNA clone pRP1, 4256 base pairs (bp) in length, includes approximately 3/4 of the E2 gene sequence plus the 930 bases upstream. cDNA clone pRP3, 3232 bp in length, overlaps cDNA pRP1 by 72 bases, and contains the remaining 1/4 of the E2 gene sequence, the genetic region between the E2 and E1 genes and the entire E1 gene sequence except for the last 12 bases at the 3′end. For DNA sequencing of these clones overlapping unidirectional deletions were constructed by the exonuclease III/S1 nuclease method and double-stranded plasmid DNAs were sequenced by the dideoxynucleotide method.

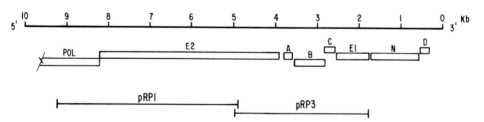

Fig. 1. Schematic diagram of the genomic organization of TGEV. The location at the 3′end of the genome of cDNA clones, pRP1 and pRP3, used for sequencing the gene encoding the E2-peplomer glycoprotein and the upstream POL ORF are shown. The relationship between the major structural protein genes E2, E1, and N and other large ORFs, A, B, C, D that might encode either non-structural or minor structural proteins are indicated. The POL ORF is part of a gene encoding a RNA polymerase.

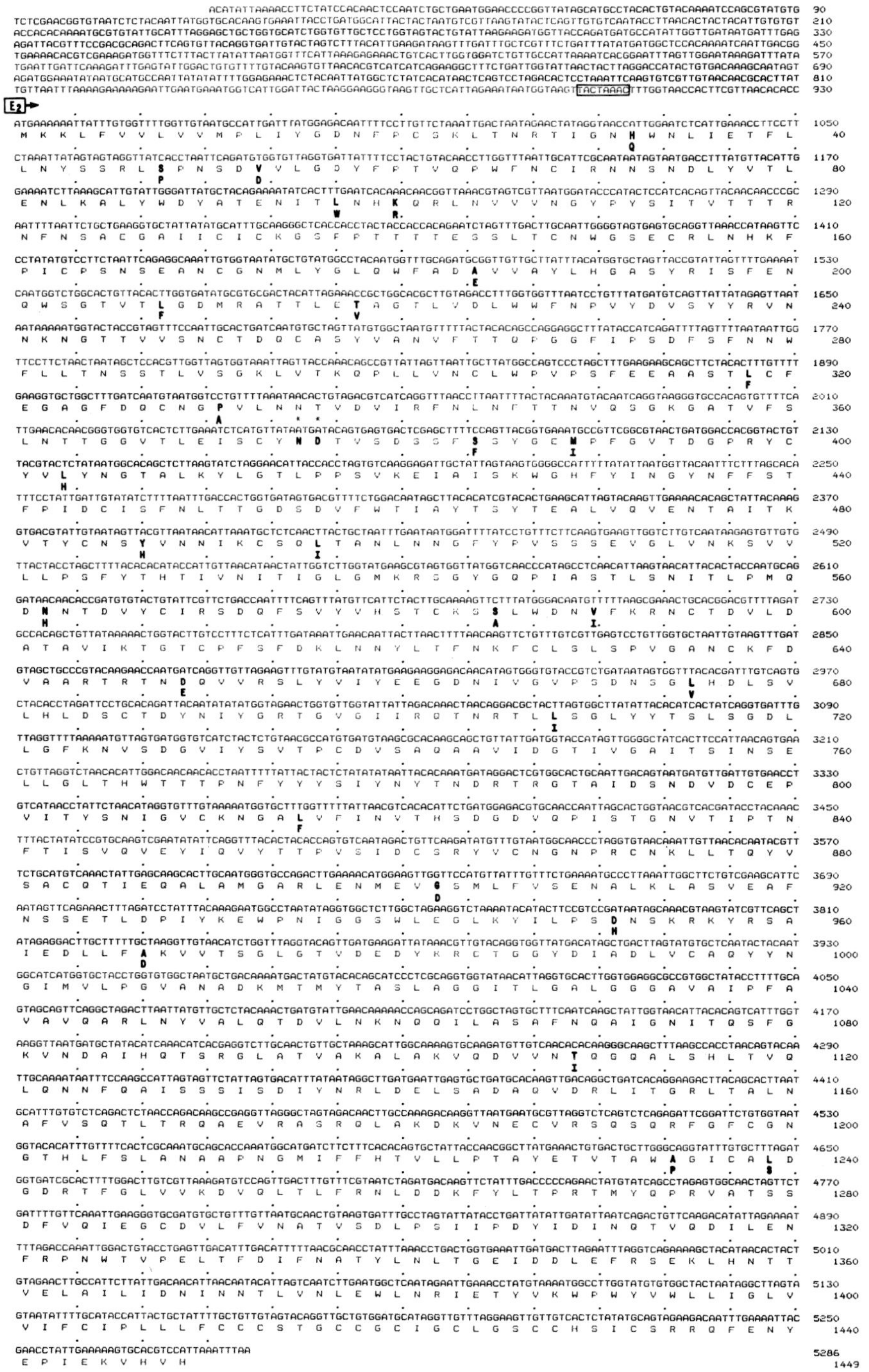

Fig. 2.   The nucleotide sequence and predicted amino acid sequence of the E2-peplomer protein of TGEV.   In addition, the base sequence (930 nucleotides) to the 5'side of the E2 gene is included.   Amino acid differences between the Miller and Purdue strains are shown in bold letters.   For the Miller strain, two extra amino acids are added at positions 375 and 376 that establish an additional potential glycosylation site.

The E2 gene sequence and the deduced amino acid sequence for TGEV, Miller strain, are shown in Figure 2 along with the 930 bases to the 5'side of the E2 gene. The nucleotide sequence was determined from both strands of the cDNA clones. The E2 gene primary translation product consists of 1449 amino acid residues, 2 residues longer than the E2 protein of the Purdue strain due to a 6 base insert at positions 2053-2058 (Fig. 2). There is 98% homology between the Miller strain and the Purdue strain E2 proteins at both the nucleotide and the amino acid levels. Between the 2 strains, there are 72 nucleotide differences in the E2 gene that resulted in the 30 amino acid changes shown as bold letters in Figure 2.

A single large ORF, overlapping only the initiation methionine of the E2 gene is found in the 930 bases to the 5'side of the E2 gene. Presumably, this is only a part of a much larger ORF. The amino acid translation product of this ORF is given in Figure 3 and compared with the IBV F2 ORF that is also located immediately 5' of the IBV E2 gene. Extensive sequence homology, 51% identity and 24% conservative amino acid changes, exists between the partial amino acid sequence determined for the TGEV ORF and the C-terminal 312 amino acid residues of the presumed IBV polymerase protein. Thus the base sequences immediately upstream from the E2 gene apparently code for a large RNA dependent-RNA polymerase in both IBV and TGEV.

DISCUSSION

The complete nucleotide sequence and the predicted amino acid sequence of the TGEV E2-peplomer gene (Miller strain) and a partial sequence of a presumed polymerase gene immediately to the 5'side of the E2 gene have been determined. The E2-peplomer gene of the virulent Miller strain shares 98% sequence homology at both the nucleotide and amino acid sequence levels with the E2 gene of the Purdue strain.[7] An additional 6 extra bases, positions 2053 to 2058 in the Miller strain E2 sequence, increase the length of the peplomer protein by 2 amino acids to 1449 residues and gives rise to a new potential glycosylation site. The amino acid differences between these strains do not occur randomly within the peplomer glycoprotein. Instead, over 75% of the amino acid changes occur in the N-terminal half of the peplomer which comprises the exposed club-shaped portion of the peplomer on top of a stalk. Only 7 amino acid differences occur in the C-terminal half of the peplomer which encompasses the stalk structure and the membrane anchoring domain. This feature of N-terminal amino acid variation in the peplomer glycoprotein has also been observed in mouse hepatitis virus (MHV) and IBV.[13,14] Further in the S1 protein of IBV which is the N-terminal cleavage product of the IBV peplomer protein, there are 2 regions of high amino acid variability; one of which has been shown to be associated with virus neutralization.[15,16] Similarly, most of the amino acid changes occur in the N-terminal half of the TGEV peplomer gene, however, no clustering of amino acid variation indicative of highly variable regions were apparent. The 30 amino acid changes in the E2 protein of the Miller and Purdue strains apparently are neutral substitutions since neutralizing monoclonal antibodies, representing 5 different noncompeting sites, were unable to distinguish between these 2 TGEV strains.

Coronaviruses have homologous recognition sequences that are involved in the initiation of transcription and the joining of a RNA leader sequence onto the 5'end of each subgenomic mRNA. The TGEV recognition sequence (A/T A/T)CTAAAC occurs 27 bases upstream from the E2 gene ATG start codon in both the Miller and Purdue strains. In the Purdue strain, a second (A/T A/T)CTAAAC sequence occurs 119 nucleotides into the E2 gene that might also function as an initiation site for a subgenomic mRNA. However, because of a C to T substitution at base 1056 (Fig. 2), the Miller strain E2 gene does not contain this second recognition sequence nor do any further

```
              10v        20v        30v        40v        50v        60v        70v        80v        90v       100v
MILLER  HIKTFYPQLQSAEWNPGYSMPTLYKIQRMCLERCNLYNYGAQVKLPDGITTNVVKYTQLCQYLNTTTLCVPHKMRVLHLGAAGASGVAPGSTVLRRWLPDD
IBVF2   SIKTCYPQLQSA-WTCGYNMPELYKVQNCVMEPCNIPNYGVGITLPSGILMNVAKYTQLCQYLSKTTICVPHNMRVMHFGAGSDKGVAPGSTVLKQWLPEG
              10^        20^        30^        40^        50^        60^        70^        80^        90^       190^
             110v       120v       130v       140v       150v       160v       170v       180v       190v
MILLER  AILVDNDLRDYVSDADFSVTGDCTSLYIEDKFDLLVSDLY--DGSTKSIDGENTSK--DGFFTYINGFIKEKLSLGGSVAIKITEFSWNKDLYELIQRFEY
        ::LVDND: DYVSDA: SV :DC..  .E:KFDL::SD:Y  ::S.:. :G  ::: D: F.Y:::F::::L:LGGS A:K:TE SW:. LY:: Q  ..
IBVF2   TLLVDNDIVDYVSDAHVSVLSDCNKYNTEHKFDLVISDMYTDNDSKRKHEGVIANNGNDDVFIYLSSFLRNNLALGGSFAVKVTETSWHEVLYDIAQDCAW
             110^       120^       130^       140^       150^       160^       170^       180^       190^       200^
        v         210v       220v       230v       240v       250v       260v       270v       280v       290v
MILLER  WTVFCTSVNTSSSEGFLIGINYLGPYCDKAIVDGNIMHANYIFWRNSTIMALSHNSVLDTPKFKCRCNNALIVNLKEKELNEMVIGLLRKGKLLIRNNGKL
IBVF2   WT:FCT:VN:SSSE:FLIG:NYLG:  .:K.  V.G:.:HANYIFWRN.. :. S  S::D.:KF. R :.: :VNLK..:  .::V:.L:: GKLL:R: G:
        WTMFCTAVNASSSEAFLIGVNYLGA-SEKVKVSGKTLHANYIFWRNCNYLQTSAYSIFDVAKFDLRLKATPVVNLKTEQKTDLVFNLIKCGKLLVRDVGNT
             210^       220^       230^       240^       250^       260^       270^       280^       290^       300^
        v         310v
MILLER  LNFGNHFVNTP
        :: FV T
IBVF2   SFTSDSFVCTM
             310^
```

Fig. 3. Comparison between predicted amino acid sequences of IBV F2 and TGEV. The IBV sequence represents the C-terminal 312 amino acid residues of the F2 ORF. The TGEV amino acid sequences is derived from the 930 bases immediately to the 5'side of the E2-peplomer gene. Identical amino acid residues are indicated. A colon indicates a conservative amino acid substitute. A dash indicates a deleted amino acid residue in order to achieve optional alignment.

(A/T A/T)CTAAAC sequences occur in the rest of the E2 gene. Interestingly, the sequence (A/T A/T)CTAAAT occurs 3 times within 150 nucleotides on either side of the E2 gene homologous recognition sequence and does not appear again in the rest of the E2 gene sequence.

MHV encodes a potential nonstructural protein (30-35 Kd) to the 5'side of the E2-peplomer gene that is the translation product of an additional subgenomic mRNA (RNA 2).[17,18] Analyses of TGEV subgenomic RNAs do not reveal a RNA larger than the E2 subgenomic mRNA but smaller than total genomic RNA.[6,8,19,20] In IBV replication, the E2 mRNA is the largest subgenomic mRNA. Large ORFs, upstream of the IBV E2 gene, are thought to encode potential polymerase genes F1 and F2, the latter overlapping the peplomer E2 gene sequence.[9] In this regard, the TGEV genome arrangement resembles more closely IBV than MHV. The evidence that a TGEV polymerase gene occurs to the immediate 5'side of the E2 gene is based on amino acid sequence homology at the C-terminus of the F2 polymerase enzyme of IBV (Fig. 3). Of the 310 amino acids deduced for the TGEV polymerase protein, 51% are identical to the C-terminus of IBV F2 and another 24% represent conservative amino acid changes.

ACKNOWLEDGMENT

The author wishes to thank David Michael for excellent technical assistance.

REFERENCES

1. B. Delmas, G. Gelfi, H. Laude, Antigenic structure of transmissible gastroenteritis virus. II. Domains in the peplomer glycoprotein, J. Gen. Virol. 67:1405-1418 (1986).

2. G. Jimenez, I. Correa, M. P. Melgosa, M. J. Bullido, and L. Enjuanes, Critical epitopes in transmissible gastroenteritis virus neutralization, J. Virol. 60:131-139 (1986).

3. R. D. Woods, R. D. Wesley, and P. A. Kapke, Neutralization of porcine transmissible gastroenteritis virus by complement-dependent monoclonal antibodies, Am. J. Vet. Res. 49:300-304 (1988).

4. R. D. Woods, R. D. Wesley, Unpublished result.

5. P. A. Kapke, and D. A. Brian, Sequence analysis of the porcine transmissible gastroenteritis coronavirus nucleocapsid protein gene, <u>Virol.</u> 151:41-49 (1986).

6. D. Rasschaert, J. Gelfi, and H. Lande, Enteric coronavirus TGEV: partial sequence of the genomic RNA, its organization and expression, <u>Biochimie.</u> 69:591-600 (1987).

7. D. Rasschaert, and H. Laude, The predicted primary structure of the peplomer protein E2 of the porcine coronavirus transmissible gastroenteritis virus, <u>J. Gen. Virol.</u> 68:1883-1890 (1987).

8. R. D. Wesley, A. K. Cheung, D. D. Michael, and R. D. Woods, Nucleotide sequence of coronavirus TGEV genomic RNA: evidence for 3 mRNA species between the peplomer and matrix protein genes, <u>Virus Res.</u> 13:87-101. (1989).

9. M. E. G. Boursnell, T. D. K. Brown, I. J. Foulds, P. F. Green, F. M. Tomley, and M. M. Binns, Completion of the sequence of the genome of the coronavirus avian infectious bronchitis virus, <u>J. Gen. Virol.</u> 68:57-77 (1987).

10. R. D. Wesley, R. D. Woods, I. Correa, L. Enjuanes, Lack of protection <u>in vivo</u> with neutralizing monoclonal antibodies to transmissible gastroenteritis virus, <u>Vet. Micro.</u> 18:197-208 (1988).

11. S. Henikoff, Unidirectional digestion with exonuclease III creates targeted breakpoints for DNA sequencing, <u>Gene</u> 28:351-359 (1984).

12. F. Sanger, S. Micklen, and A. R. Coulson, DNA sequencing with chain-terminating inhibitors, <u>Proc. Natl. Acad. Sci. USA</u>, 74:5463-5467 (1977).

13. W. Luytjes, L. S. Sturman, P. J. Bredenbeek, J. Charite, B. A. M. Van der Feijst, M. C. Horzinek, and W. J. M. Spaan, Primary structure of the glycoprotein E2 of coronavirus MHV-A59 and identification of the trypsin cleavage site, <u>Virology</u> 161:479-487 (1987).

14. J. G. Kusters, H. G. M. Niesters, J. A. Lenstra, M. C. Horzinek, and B. A. M. Van Der Feijst, Phylogeny of antigenic varients of avian coronavirus IBV, <u>Virology</u> 169:217-221 (1989).

15. H. G. M. Niesters, J. A. Lenstra, W. J. M. Spaan, A. J. Zijderveld, N. M. C. Bleumink-Pluym, F. Hong, G. J. M. van Scharrenburg, M. C. Horzinek, and B. A. M. van der Zeijst, The peplomer protein sequence of the M41 strain of coronavirus IBV and its comparison with Beaudett strains, <u>Virus Res.</u> 5:253-263 (1986).

16. D. Cavanagh, P. J. Davis, and A. P. A. Mockett, Amino acids within hypervariable region 1 of avian coronavirus IBV (Massachusetts serotype) spike glycoprotein are associated with neutralization epitopes, <u>Virus Res.</u> 11:141-150 (1988).

17. J. L. Leibowitz, S. R. Weiss, E. Paavola, and C. W. Bond, Cell-free translation of murine coronavirus RNA, <u>J. Virol.</u> 43:905-913 (1982).

18. S. Siddell, Coronavirus JHM: coding assignments of subgenomic mRNAs, <u>J. Gen. Virol.</u> 64:113-125 (1983).

19. S. Hu, J. Braszewski, T. Boone, and L. Souza, Cloning and expression of the surface glycoprotein gp195 of porcine transmissible gastroenteritis virus, in: "Modern Approaches to Vaccines," pp.219-223, Cold Spring Harbor Laboratory, New York (1984).

20. L. Jacobs, B. A. M. van der Zeijst, and M. C. Horzinek, Characterization and translation of transmissible gastroenteritis mRNAs, <u>J. Virol.</u> 57:1010-1015 (1986).

THE POLYMERASE GENE OF CORONA- AND TOROVIRUSES: EVIDENCE FOR AN

EVOLUTIONARY RELATIONSHIP

Peter J. Bredenbeek, Eric J. Snijder, Ans F.H. Noten, Johan
A. den Boon, Wim M.M. Schaaper[1], Marian C. Horzinek and
Willy J.M. Spaan

Institute of Virology, Department of Infectious Diseases and
Immunology, State University of Utrecht, P.O. Box 80.165
3508 TD, Utrecht, The Netherlands, [1]Central Veterinary
Institute, P.O. Box 65, 8200 AB Lelystad, The Netherlands

SUMMARY

In this paper we demonstrate that the organization of the polymerase
gene of toroviruses and coronaviruses is similar. The polymerase gene of
both virus families consists of at least two large ORFs (1a and 1b). Four
domains of conserved amino acid sequences have been identified in nearly
identical positions in the 3' ORF of the pol gene of toroviruses and
coronaviruses. The most 3' conserved domain which is still unique for these
viruses encodes a 33-kDA protein in MHV-A59, which is cleaved from a
precursor protein. Expression of ORF1b of the pol gene of both virus
families occurs by ribosomal frameshifting. A predicted stem-loop structure
and pseudoknot are conserved in the ORF1a/ORF1b overlap of toro- and
coronaviruses. On the basis of these results we postulate that toro- and
coronaviruses are ancestrally more related to each other than to other
families of positive stranded RNA viruses.

INTRODUCTION

Ancestral relationships between RNA viruses were first indicated by
similarities in genome organization and expression (1). The increasing
amount of sequence data on positive stranded RNA viruses has enabled
scientists to compare these viruses on the level of genetic information.
The presence of extensive sequence homologies and the similarities in
genome organization and expression have led to "supergroups" containing
more than one virus family which are thought to reflect ancestral
relationships among seemingly divergent viruses (see 2 and 3 for a review).
Among the positive stranded RNA viruses two superfamilies have been
recognized; the alphavirus like and picornavirus like families. Detailed
analysis of the nucleotide sequences has also revealed short stretches of
amino acid sequence similarity in most of the replicase proteins of
positive stranded plant and animal RNA viruses. This indicates that viruses
related in this way may have descended from a common ancestor (3). The two
most prominent amino acid motifs conserved in the replicase proteins are
the "GDD" or polymerase motif (4) and the "GKS/T" or nucleotide
triphosphate (NTP) binding motif (5, 6). Both motifs consist of several

stretches of conserved amino acids interspersed by variable numbers of non-conserved amino acids.

Coronaviruses have not been classified in either of the two superfamilies due to their different genome organization and expression. Infectious bronchitis virus (IBV) is still the only coronavirus of which the genome has been completely sequenced (7). The polymerase (pol) gene of IBV is about 20 kb in length and contains two large open reading frames (ORF) ORF1a and ORF1b (previously named F1 and F2) which potentially encode polypeptides of 441-kDa and 300-kDa, respectively. The second ORF is not expressed from a subgenomic mRNA but by ribosomal frameshifting (8, 9). Analysis of the predicted amino acid sequence of the IBV polymerase has revealed the presence of both amino acid motifs described above in ORF1b of the IBV pol gene (5, 10).

Two other groups of enveloped, positive stranded RNA viruses express their genetic information from a nested set of multiple subgenomic mRNAs; the arteriviruses (11; unpublished results) and the proposed family of Toroviridae (12). Equine arteritis virus, the prototype arterivirus, possesses an icosahedral nucleocapsid which contains a genomic RNA of approximately 13 kb. Initially, toroviruses were considered to be corona-virus-like, but analysis of the structure and replication of the family prototype Berne virus (BEV) has clearly distinguished them from corona-viruses. BEV contains an elongated tubular nucleocapsid which contains an RNA of approximately the same size as the coronavirus genome (13). In infected cells the genetic information of BEV is expressed by synthesis of four subgenomic mRNAs. These mRNAs are 3' co-terminal, but in contrast to the coronaviral mRNAs, no common leader sequence has been detected at their 5' end. From U.V. transcription mapping data it could be concluded that the synthesis of BEV mRNAs does not involve conventional cis-splicing (14)

In this paper we describe the analysis of the nucleotide sequence of a substantial part of the polymerase genes of both mouse hepatitis virus (MHV strain A59) and BEV. We present evidence demonstrating that in both toro- and coronaviruses expression of the polymerase gene involves ribosomal frameshifting and that both viruses are ancestrally related.

MATERIALS AND METHODS

cDNA synthesis, cloning and sequencing

cDNA was prepared from MHV-A59 genomic RNA and intracellular BEV poly(A)-selected RNA using oligo-(dT) and pentanucleotides as a primer. cDNA synthesis, cloning and sequencing was performed using standard procedures. Full details will be published elsewhere.

Computer analysis

Sequence data were analyzed using the computer programs of Staden (15) and Wisconsin (version 5, 1987). Comparison to the National Biomedical Research Foundation (NBRF) protein identification resource was made using the program FASTP (16).

Production of antisera

A peptide (CTRKEVFVGDSLVNVK) covering the 14 carboxyl terminal amino acids encoded by the MHV-A59 pol gene, linked to an amino-terminal cysteine residue to couple the peptide to keyhole limpet hemacyanin (KLH) was synthesized. Rabbits were injected intramuscularly and subcutaneously with 1 mg KLH coupled peptide suspended in 1 ml Freunds complete adjuvant. Sera were collected starting 6 weeks after immunization.

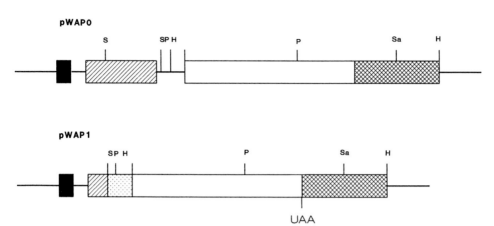

pWAP0

pWAP1

UAA

Figure 1. Construction of the plasmids pWAP0 and pWAP1. The position of the
T7 promoter is indicated as a black box. The nucleocapsid gene of BEV, the
MHV-A59 polymerase fragment and 30-kDa ns protein encoding fragment are
shown as a hatched, an open and a cross-hatched box, respectively. The
amino acids encoded by a part of the polylinker in pWAP1 are indicated by a
dashed box. S = SalI; P = PstI; H = HindIII and Sa = SacI. The position of
the stopcodon for the translation of the fusion protein in pWAP1 is shown.

Construction of pWAP1

To test the obtained sera for the presence of antibodies against the
MHV pol gene encoded product(s) the plasmid pWAP1 was constructed. An
HindIII fragment containing 1.85 kb of the 3' end of the MHV pol gene and
the complete first ORF of the unique region of mRNA2 was isolated from cDNA
clone 96 (17) and cloned downstream of the nucleocapsid gene of BEV in
pBSN1 (18). Plasmid DNA isolated from transformants was digested with PstI
to confirm the depicted orientation of the HindIII fragment (Fig. 1). The
internal Sal fragment was deleted by digestion of pWAP0 with SalI and
subsequent religation resulted in pWAP1, in which the MHV pol gene DNA
fragment was fused in frame to the N-terminal part of the BEV nucleocapsid
gene by making use of a number amino acids encoded by the polylinker of the
pBSN1 plasmid. Transcription of the BEV N/MHV pol hybrid gene is under the
control of the T7 promoter.

In vitro transcription and translation

Plasmid DNA of pWAP1 was linearized with SacI. Full details of the in
vitro transcription and translation will be described elsewhere (18).

Radioactive labeling of viral intracellular proteins

Monolayer cultures of Sac(-) cells were infected at a m.o.i. of 30
with MHV-A59 or mock infected using standard conditions. At 4 h after
infection (p.i.) the medium was replaced by methionine deficient MEM,
containing 50 μCi/ml [^{35}S]-methionine. At 8 h p.i. the medium was removed
and the cells were lysed (19).

Immunoprecipitation of proteins

Immunoprecipitations of the [^{35}S]-methionine labeled proteins were
essentially performed as described (19); 4 μl of in vitro translation
mixtures or 100 μl of the cell lysates were used. Immunoprecipitated
proteins were analyzed by electrophoresis on SDS- polyacrylamide gels.

RESULTS AND DISCUSSION

Nucleotide sequence analysis

The nucleotide sequence of 8.6 kb located in the 3' half of the
polymerase gene of MHV-A59 was determined. Analysis of the sequence data
revealed the 3' end of an ORF (ORF1a) overlapping with a large ORF (ORF1b)
covering the 3' half of the pol gene. ORF1b has a length of 8199
nucleotides and potentially encodes a protein of 309-kDa (2733 amino
acids). The first potential translation initiating codon is located at
position 405 in ORF1b and the ORF terminates just upstream of the junction
sequence AAAUCUAUAC. This region separates the gene encoding the 30-kDa
non-structural protein from the polymerase gene in MHV-A59 (17). ORF1a
overlaps ORF1b for 75 nucleotides.

Sequence analysis of the 3' half of the polymerase gene of BEV
revealed that the organization of this gene in toroviruses is very similar
to coronaviruses. An ORF of 6873 nucleotides (2291 amino acids) covering
the 3' half of the BEV pol gene was identified. This large ORF (ORF1b) has
a 12 nucleotide overlap with the 3' end of a preceding ORF.

Computer analysis of coronavirus and BEV polymerase genes

Dot matrix comparison of the predicted amino acid sequence of ORF1b of
MHV-A59 and IBV showed that almost the entire open reading frame is
extremely well conserved (Fig 2A). The positional identity in an alignment
of the amino acid sequence of ORF1b of MHV and IBV is 57%. Based on the
sequence analysis of a small part of the 3' end of the polymerase gene of
the feline coronavirus FIPV, which was found to be very similar to MHV-A59
as well as IBV (De Groot, unpublished results), we predict that the ORF1b
encoded product of coronaviruses is well conserved. No similarity could be
detected in the predicted amino acid sequence of the 5' end of ORF1a of the
IBV and MHV-A59 pol genes (20). However the putative carboxyl terminal
region of the ORF1a translation product of MHV-A59 and IBV is well

A   B

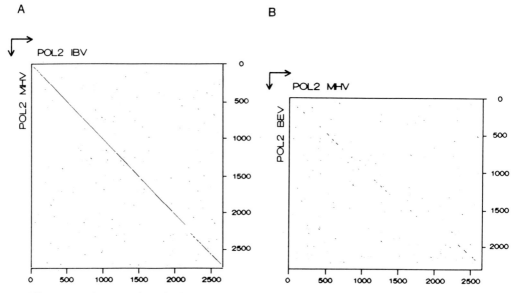

Figure 2. Proportional dot matrix comparisons. Numbers of the amino acid
residues are indicated at the axis. A) ORF1b of IBV-M42 and MHV-A59. B)
ORF1b of MHV-A59 and BEV.

conserved (data not shown). No similarity has been observed in the other MHV and IBV non-structural proteins while the structural proteins only showed significant similarity in relative small regions (reviewed by 21). These data suggest a selective pressure against mutations in the second ORF of the polymerase gene.

Remarkably, a proportional dot matrix comparison of the deduced amino acid sequences of BEV and MHV-A59 ORF1b showed a clustered but significant similarity (Fig. 2B). Identical results were obtained when the predicted amino acid sequences of IBV and BEV were compared. The overall identity between BEV and either MHV or IBV is approximately 19%. No similarity between the structural proteins of BEV and coronaviruses has been identified (18, unpublished results).

Detailed analysis of the regions in the pol products of toro- and coronaviruses which exhibit significant similarity revealed that they could be separated into four domains (Fig. 3). Three of these domains (domain 1-3 of Fig. 3) have also been described recently for ORF1b of IBV (10). Domain 1 contains the "GDD" motif. However, in contrast to the amino acid sequence GDD, which is thought to be the core of this motif, both coronaviruses and BEV contain the amino acid sequence SDD at this position. Although occasionally a M, C, V or L residue has been reported in the position of the G residue (4), no serine residue has been reported. immediately upstream of the two conserved aspartic acid residues. Domain 2 is characterized by a stretch of amino acids which contain a large number of conserved cysteine residues and a few conserved histidines. It is therefore tempting to speculate that this domain forms a metal binding "finger" structure of the cys-his type which could interact with nucleic acid (22) as pointed out by Gorbalenya et al. (10). However, the model proposed by Gorbalenya et al. (10) requires modification since some of the cysteine and histidine residues involved in their proposed "finger" structure are not conserved between MHV and IBV. Domain 3 represent the "GKS/T" motif or NTP binding motif (5, 10). The fourth conserved region is located at the carboxyl terminus of the product encoded by ORF1b and is still unique for toro- and coronaviruses since no significant similarity with any other amino acid sequence has been discovered.

Domains 1 and 3 have also been reported as present in the replicase proteins of viruses belonging to the alphavirus- and picornavirus-like superfamilies (3), but as indicated in fig. 3, the positional identity between toro-and coronaviruses is much higher as compared to viruses belonging to one of the two supergroups. In addition, the GDD motif (domain 1) is located downstream of the GKS/T motif (domain 3) in viruses belonging to the alphavirus- or picornavirus-like superfamily (3).

Analysis of the ORF1a/ORF1b overlapping sequence

It has been shown that the nucleotide sequence of the ORF1a/ORF1b overlapping region of the pol gene of IBV is capable of inducing ribosomal frameshifting in vitro and in vivo (8, 9). A predicted, stable stem-loop structure and RNA pseudoknot (Fig. 4A) were shown to be essential for accurate translational frameshifting in IBV (9). Comparison of the nucleotide sequence of the ORF1a/ORF1b overlap of MHV-A59 and IBV-M42 revealed a well conserved stretch of nucleotides. A nearly identical stem-loop structure and pseudoknot can be predicted for the MHV ORF1a/ORF1b overlapping region. The significance of these proposed secondary and tertiary RNA structures is emphasized by the presence of co-variation as indicated in figure 4A. Mutations in one part of the stem or in the nucleotide sequence of the predicted loop are compensated by complementary mutations in either the stem or in the downstream sequence involved in the potential pseudoknot (Fig. 4A). In both IBV and MHV the stop codon for the translation of ORF1a is located in this hairpin structure.

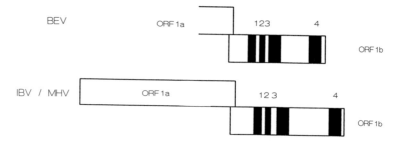

1)

```
BEV 514 CLIGVSK-Y-GLK--FSKFLKD-9-VF-GSDYTKCDRTFP-LSFR-37-LLNKPGGTSSGDA
IBV 585 VVIGTTKFYGGWDNMLRNLIQG-4-ILMGWDYPKCDRAMPNL-LR-41-IYVKPGGTSSGDA
MHV 594 VVIGTTKFYGGWDDMLRRLIKD-4-VLMGWDYPKCDRAMPNI-LR-41-YYVKPGGTSSGDA
         *                              *       *              ***
```

```
TTAHSNTFYN-51-FLNFLSDDSFIF-34-KGHIEEFCSAH-II-KTDGEYHFLP--SRGRLL 744 BEV
TTAYANSVFN-58-SLMILSDDGVVC-41-KGP-HEFCSQHTMLVEVDGDPKYLPYPDPSRIL 836 IBV
TTAFANSVFN-58-SMMILSDDGVVC-41-KGP-HEFCSQHTMLVKMDGDEVYLPYPDPSRIL 845 MHV
 * **         *   **  *         **        *
```

2)

```
BEV 845 ANFDKVCFCCPNPAVSVCEECYVPLPLCAYCYYVHVVISNHSKVEDKFKCFCGQDNIRELYI
IBV 929 LQSCGVCVVCNSQTILRCGNCIRKPFLCCKCCYDHVMHTDHKNVLSINPYICSQLGCGE-AD
MHV 938 LQSVGACVVCSSQTSLRCGSCIRKPLLCCKCAYDHVMSTDHKYVLSVSPYVCNSPGC-DVND
          *  *      *  *    * *  *    *      *           *
```

3)

```
V--LNNSICMYQCKNCVESDRLRI   928 BEV
VIKLYLGGMSYFCGNHKPKLSIPL  1013 IBV
VTKLYLGGMSYYCEDHKPQYSFKL  1022 MHV
    *  *
```

3)

```
BEV 1099 VMGPPGTGKTTFVYD--TYLSKA
IBV 1210 VQGPPGSGKSHFAIGLAVYFSSA
MHV 1218 VQGPPGTGKSHLAIGLAVYYCTA
         * *  ******
```

```
-53-THNTLPFIKSAVLIADEVSLI-15-VVLLGDPFQLSP-24-YLTACYRCPPQILSAFS-64-LGDVT-TI
-56-TINALPEVSCDILLVDEVSML-16-VVYVGDPAQLPA-28-FLAKCYRCPKEIVDTVS-75-LGLNVQTV
-56-TINALPELVTDIIVVDEVSML-16-YVYIGDPAQLPA-29-FLGTCYRCPKEIVDTVS-72-LGLQTQTV
    ** **   **           * ***  *            *** **               **
```

```
DSSQG-19-VNRVIVGCSRS 1367 BEV
DSSQG-19-INRFNVALTRA 1500 IBV
DSAQG-19-VNRFNVAITRA 1506 MHV
 **        *  **
```

4)

```
BEV 1921 HVFSGDFTEVGTDIGGVHHVVAL-29-
IBV 2274 HILYGEVDK--PQLGGLHTVIGM-38-
MHV 2322 HVVYGSFNQ--KIIGGLHLLIGL-38-
```

```
TLVDVCANQLYEKVK- 8-SKVIFVNIDFQDVQFMVFANGEDDIQTFYP-23-LKNYGQNPTFMP-3-NFAKYT
TVVDLLLLDDFLELLR-10-SKVVTVSIDYHSINFMTWFE-DGSIKTCYP-27-IPNYG-VGITLP-5-NVAKYT
TVIDLLLLDDFVDIVK- 7-SKVVNVNVDFKDFQFMLWCN-EEKVMTFYP-29-LWNYG-KPITLP-5-NVAKYT
```

```
QICTFI QDHVKVARNALVWHLGAAGVDGCSPGDIVL-32-NLIVSDIY-16-LALGGTIVFKTTESS-17-FF
QLCQYLSKTTICVPHNMRVMHFGAGSDKGVAPGSTVL-39-DLVISDMY-39-LALGGSFAVKVTETS-17-FC
QLCQYLSTTTLAVPANMRVLHLGAGSDKGVAPGSAVL-39-DLIISDMY-28-LALGGSVAIKITEFS-17-FC
```

```
TAGVNTSSSEVFVV 2209 BEV
TA-VNASSSEAFLI 2598 IBV
TN-VNASSSEGFLI 2641 MHV
```

Fig. 3. Localization (A) and amino acid sequences (B) of the conserved domains in ORF1b of the pol gene of BEV and the coronaviruses. The amino acids which are identical or conserved in these viruses are underlined. Domain 1; the "GDD" or polymerase motif, amino acids conserved according to (10) are indicated by asterisks. Domain 2; the cys-his motif, conserved cysteine and histidine residues are marked with asterisks. Domain 3; the "GKS/T" or helicase motif, asterisks indicate the amino acids conserved according to (5). Domain 4; the carboxyl terminal motif.

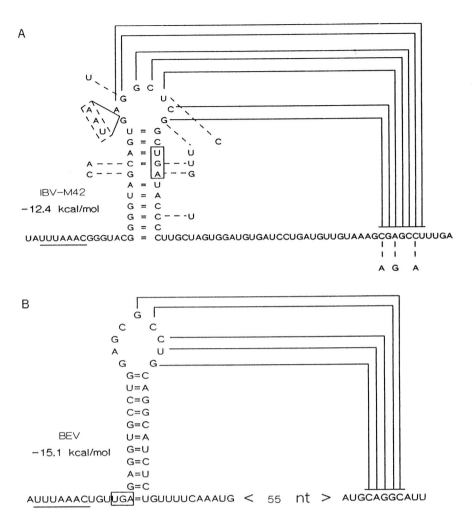

Figure 4. Predicted secondary and tertiary structure of RNA in the ORF1a/ORF1b overlap of IBV (A) and BEV (B). The conserved UUUAAAC sequence is underlined and the termination codon of the first ORFs are boxed. Solid lines illustrate the predicted pseudoknots. Differences between the nucleotide sequences involved in the predicted RNA structure of MHV and IBV are indicated in the IBV structure (A) with dashed lines (point mutations) and solid (insertions).

In addition to the underlined sequence UUUAAAC (Fig. 4) no nucleotide sequence similarity was observed between the ORF1a/ORF1b overlap of the pol genes of BEV and MHV or IBV. Nevertheless, a similar stem-loop structure and pseudoknot were predicted in the BEV ORF1a/ORF1b overlap (Fig. 4B). In comparison to the coronaviruses the distance between the stem-loop structure and the downstream region involved the pseudoknot may seem relatively large. However, this intervening sequence can be folded as a second separate stem-loop (data not shown), which reduces the distance and may stabilize the pseudoknot structure. The conserved sequence UUUAAAC probably functions as the actual site for ribosomal frameshifting in MHV and BEV since mutations in this sequence have been shown to influence ribosomal frameshifting in the IBV ORF1a/ORF1b overlap region (9). This

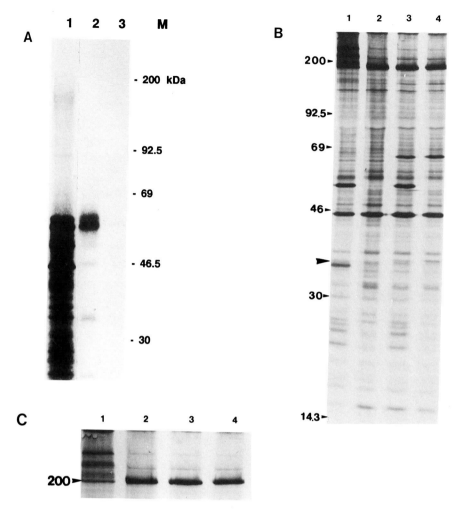

Figure 5. Identification of a 33-kDa protein encoded by the pol gene of MHV-A59. A) Lane 1, pWAP1 RNA in vitro translation products; pWAP1 translation products immunoprecipitated with antiserum (lane 2) and preserum (lane 3). B) Immunoprecipitation with the anti-peptide serum on lysates of MHV-A59 infected (lane 1) or mock infected (lane 2) Sac(-) cells. Lane 3 and 4 immunopprecipitations using preserum and lysates of infected and mock infected cells, respectively (exposure 7 days. C) Enlargement of the section containing proteins exceeding 200-kDa the autoradiograph shown in section B (exposure 3 days).

sequence has also been shown to function as a site for ribosomal frame-shifting in Rous sarcoma virus (23). Recently we have demonstrated that the ORF1a/ORF1b overlapping regions of both MHV and BEV are able to direct ribosomal frameshifting in vitro as well as in vivo (data not shown). The efficiency of this translational frameshifting was 40% and 25% for MHV and BEV, respectively.

As in retroviruses the BEV and coronaviral polymerase is probably produced as a fusion protein. Based on amino acid sequence analysis it is postulated that domain 1 of ORF1b (fig. 3), which is located downstream of the ribosomal frameshifting sequence, is the core domain of the replicase

Tabel 1. Predicted 3C protease-like cleavage sites in the carboxyl terminal region of ORF1b of the pol genes of IBV (10), MHV-A59 and BEV.

Virus	predicted cleavage site	position Q residue in the sequence
IBV	TCYPQLQ/SAWLCGY	2389
MHV	MTFYPLQ/AAADWKP	2434
BEV	NGEDDIQ/TFYPQKD	2021

of both corona- and toroviruses. It is tempting to speculate that the fusion protein is the functional polymerase, cleavage of this functional polyprotein will result in an inactive polymerase protein. This would explain the observed requirements for continuous de novo protein synthesis (24, 25).

A 33-kDa cleavage product from the putative MHV polymerase contains conserved domain 4.

To test the specificity of the antiserum raised against a peptide representing the carboxyl terminus encoded by ORF1b of MHV-A59, in vitro translation products of pWAP1 RNA were used in immunoprecipitations. Direct analysis of the in vitro translation products showed a large number of different sized proteins (Fig. 5A , lane 1). Most of these products probably result from premature termination of translation since only two proteins of the expected size (60-kDa and 62-kDa) were precipitated by the antiserum (Fig. 5A, lane 2). None of the translation products were recognized by the preimmune serum (Fig. 5A, lane 3). This antiserum was used to identify virus encoded protein(s) in infected cells and immuno-precipitated a 33-kDa protein from lysates of MHV-A59 infected cells (Fig. 5B, lane 1). This 33-kDa protein was not detected in mock infected cells (Fig. 5B, lane 2), or in similar immunoprecipitations using the preimmune serum (Fig. 5B, lane 3 and 4). Based on its size the 33-kDa protein should contain the complete fourth conserved domain. Enlargement and careful inspection of the upper region of the gel revealed several proteins with a high molecular weight which were only precipitated by the antisera from lysates of the infected cells (Fig. 5C). These observed products are likely to be precursors of the 33-kDa protein.

Recently Gorbalenya et al. (10) have described a putative protease domain in ORF1a of IBV which exhibits similarity to the well conserved 3C protease of picornaviruses. Based on the cleavage site of the picornavirus 3C proteases (26) potential cleavage sites in the pol products encoded by ORF1a and ORF1b of IBV were postulated. Inspection of the region in MHV ORF1b encoding the 33-kDa protein revealed that a potential 3C protease-like cleavage site present in a nearly identical position in MHV (tabel 1). If this cleavage site is used in MHV a 33-kDa carboxyl terminal protein is predicted from the sequence. In addition an other potential 3C protease-like cleavage site can be found in the amino acid sequence of this region in ORF1b of BEV (tabel 1). Usage of this cleavage site in BEV will result in 31-kDa protein containing the conserved domain 4.

CONCLUDING REMARKS

Recent studies on the molecular biology of corona- and toroviruses have revealed several unique similarities. Members of both virus families express their genetic information from a nested set of multiple subgenomic mRNAs. Sequence analysis and in vitro translation studies clearly demonstrate that they have an identical gene order: 5'POLYMERASE-PEPLOMER-MEMBRANE PROTEIN-NUCLEOCAPSID PROTEIN-3'. These similarities already indicate a possible evolutionary relationship between toro- and corona viruses. The data presented in this paper on the organization and expression of the pol gene and the significant level in the similarity in the products encoded by ORF1b suggest that these viruses are ancestrally more related to each other than to other families of positive stranded RNA viruses. If in the near future the toroviruses are classified as a new family of positive stranded RNA viruses the toro- and coronaviruses would then form a third superfamily of positive stranded RNA viruses.

ACKNOWLEDGMENTS

The help of Willem Luytjes during the initial stages of this work is greatly acknowledged. P. B. was supported by the Dutch Foundation for Chemical Research with financial aid from the Dutch Organization for the Advancement of Pure Research (project number 331-025). E. S. was supported by the Division for Health Research TNO in cooperation with the Foundation for Medical Research MEDIGON (project number 900-502-081).

REFERENCES

1. Strauss, J.H., and Strauss, E.G. (1983). Curr. Top. Microbiol. Immunol. 105, 1-98.
2. Goldbach, R., and Wellink, J. (1988). Intervirology 29, 260-267.
3. Strauss, J.H., and Strauss, E.G. (1988). Ann. Rev. Microbiol. 42, 657-683.
4. Argos, P. (1988). Nucl. Acids Res. 16, 9909-9916.
5. Hodgman, T.C. (1988). Nature 335, 22-23.
6. Gorbalenya, A.E., and Koonin, E.V., Donchenko, A.P., and Blinov, V.M. (1988). FEBS LETT. 235, 16-24.
7. Boursnell, M.E., Brown, T.D., Foulds, I.J., Green, P.F., Tomley, F.M., and Binns, M.M. (1987). J. Gen. Virol. 68, 57-77.
8. Brierley, I., Boursnell, M.E., Binns, M.M., Bilimoria, B., Blok, V.C., Brown, T.D. and Inglis, S.C. (1987). EMBO. J. 6, 3779-3785.
9. Brierley, I., Diggard, P. and Inglis, S.C. (1989). Cell 57, 537-547.
10. Gorbalenya, A.E., and Koonin, E.V., Donchenko, A.P., and Blinov, V.M. (1989). Nucl. Acids Res. 12, 4847-4861.
11. Van Berlo, M.F., Horzinek, M.C., Van der Zeijst, B.A.M. (1982). Virology 118, 345-352.
12. Horzinek, M.C. and Weiss, M. (1984). Zbl. Vet. Med. B. 31, 649-659.
13. Snijder, E.J., Ederveen, J., Spaan, W.J.M., Weiss, M. and Horzinek, M.C. (1988). J. Gen. Virol. 69, 2135-2144.
14. Snijder, E.J., Horzinek, M.C. and Spaan, W.J.M. J. Virol. in press.
15. Staden, R. (1986). Nucl. Acids Res. 14, 217-233.
16. Lipman, D.J. and Pearson, W.R. (1985). Science 227, 1435-1441.
17. Luytjes, W., Bredenbeek, P.J., Noten, A.F.H., Horzinek, M.C., and Spaan, W.J.M. (1988). Virology 166, 415-422.
18. Snijder, E.J., Den Boon, J.A., Spaan, W.J.M., Verjans, G.M.G.M. and Horzinek, M.C. J. Gen. Virol. in press.
19. De Groot, R.J., Ter Haar, R.J., Horzinek, M.C. and Van der Zeijst, B.A.M. (1987). J. Gen. Virol. 68, 995-1002.
20. Pachuk, C.J., Bredenbeek, P.J., Zoltick, P.W., Spaan, W.J.M., and Weiss, S.R. (1989). Virology 71, 141-148.
21. Spaan, W.J.M., Cavanagh, D., and Horzinek, M.C. (1988). J. Gen. Virol. 69, 2939-2952.
22. Klug, A. and Rhodes, D. (1987). TIBS 12, 464-468.
23. Jacks, T., Madhani, D.H., Masiarz, F.R., and Varmus H.E. (1988). Cell 55, 449-458.
24. Sawicki, S.G., and Sawicki, D.L. (1986). J. Virol. 57, 328-334.
25. Compton, S.R., Rogers, D.B., Holmes, K.V., Fertsch, D., Remenick, J., and McGowan, J.J. (1987). J. Virol. 61, 1814-1820.
26. Kräusslich, H.-G. and Wimmer, E. (1988). Ann. Rev. Biochem. 57, 701-754.

CHARACTERIZATION OF THE MHV-JHM NON-STRUCTURAL PROTEIN

ENCODED BY mRNA 2

Birgit Schwarz, Edward Routledge and Stuart Siddell

Institute of Virology
Versbacher Straße 7
D - 8700 Würzburg

INTRODUCTION

The genome of the murine coronavirus MHV-JHM is a positive-stranded RNA of approximately 30 Kb, which encodes 4 structural proteins (N, M, S and HE) and at least 4 non-structural proteins. The location of the major open reading frames (ORFs) in the genome is shown in Fig. 1. In the infected cell, expression of the viral proteins is mediated by a set of subgenomic mRNAs. In relation to the genome the mRNAs are 3' coterminal and extend to different positions in a 5' direction. The mRNAs 7, 6, 3 and 2-1 have been shown to encode the N, M, S and HE proteins respectively (Siddell, 1983; Pfleiderer et al., this volume). mRNA 4 encodes a 15,000 molecular weight (mol.wt.) non-structural protein (Ebner et al, 1988) and mRNA 5 has the potential to encode two non-structural proteins of 12,400 and 10,200 mol.wt. (Skinner et al., 1985). Earlier in vitro translation studies (Siddell, 1983), indicated that the MHV-JHM subgenomic mRNA 2 encodes a 30,000 mol.wt. non-structural protein, the expression of which was translationally regulated. Recent sequence analysis of the 5' proximal region of the closely related MHV-A59 mRNA 2 confirms the presence of a 261 aminoacid ORF at this position. Analysis of the predicted polypeptide sequence indicates a non-membrane protein which may possibly have nucleotide binding and phosphorylating properties (Luytjes et al., 1988).

In the experiments described here our aims were:

1. to construct and express a fusion protein containing sequences derived from the 5' proximal ORF of the MHV-JHM mRNA 2

2. to isolate monoclonal antibodies (MoABs) specific for the MHV-JHM mRNA 2 gene product

3. to identify the MHV-JHM mRNA 2 gene product in vitro and in vivo.

Coronaviruses and Their Diseases
Edited by D. Cavanagh and T.D.K. Brown
Plenum Press, New York, 1990

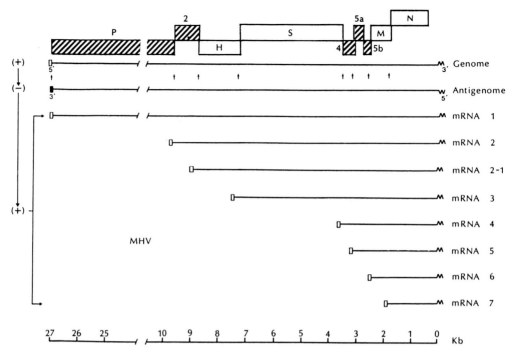

Fig. 1. A summary of the replication strategy of murine hepatitis virus, MHV-JHM. The organization of the major
open reading frames in the genome and their relationship to the subgenomic mRNAs is shown. The figure
includes data submitted for publication.

RESULTS

A cDNA clone encompassing the 5' proximal ORF of the MHV-
JHM mRNA 2 has been isolated and sequenced (Schwarz et al, in
preparation). This analysis reveals an ORF of 265 aminoacids
and the predicted polypeptide has 97 % similarity to the
corresponding MHV-A59 protein. A fusion protein vector, based
upon the pEX system (Stanley and Luzio, 1984) was constructed
to express sequences derived from the 5' proximal ORF of MHV-
JHM mRNA 2. Details of this construction will be given elsewhere. Essentially, the fusion protein consisted of a tripartite construct with amino acids 105 to 265 of the mRNA 2
ORF. The construct was introduced into E coli strain RR1
(pRK248cIts) where expression of the fusion protein is regulated by the temperature-sensitive λ phage repressor. Fig. 2
shows the proteins synthesized in induced (lanes 1 and 3) or
non-induced (lanes 2 and 4) bacteria which carry the ΔpEX
vector (lanes 1 and 2) (a modified pEX vector which expresses a
carboxyterminal truncated approx. 50,000 mol.wt. cro-ß-galacto-
sidase) or the fusion protein construct, ΔpEX-2, described
above (lanes 3 and 4). These results show that the fusion
protein (approx. 67,000 mol.wt) is expressed in both induced
and non-induced cells indicating the loss of the control,
pRK248cIts, plasmid.

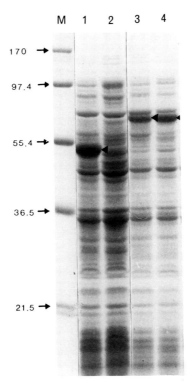

Fig. 2. Expression of the MHV-JHM mRNA 2 ORF fusion protein in
bacteria.

The fusion protein was purified by preparative SDS-polyacrylamide gel electrophoresis and electroelution and used to
immunize three months old Balb/c mice by a variety of routes
over a 14 week period. Three days after the final inoculation
spleen cells were fused to NSI plasmocytoma cells using
polethylene glycol. Hybridomas selected in HAT medium were
screened for fusion protein specific antibody production by
ELISA using lysates from induced bacteria carrying the ΔpEX or
the ΔpEX-2 as capture antigen. Ten specific cell lines could
be cloned and these were tested for their ability to recognize
MHV specific polypeptides _in vitro_ and _in vivo_.

PolyA+ RNA from MHV-JHM and MHV-A59 infected DBT cells was
isolated and translated in a rabbit reticulocyte lysate as previously described (Siddell, 1983) (Fig. 3, lane 2 and 3). The
in vitro translation products were immunoprecipitated using a
mixture of the fusion protein specific MoAbs (Fig. 3, lanes 5
and 6). The results clearly show that the fusion protein
specific antibodies immunoprecipitate an approximately 30,000
mol.wt. polypeptide from both the MHV-JHM and MHV-A59 trans-
lates. These polypeptides were not immunoprecipitated using
MoAbs directed against the MHV-N protein (data not shown).

319

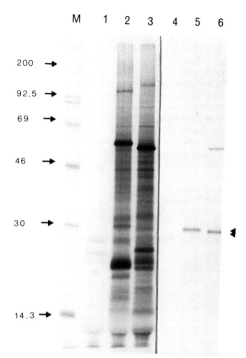

Fig. 3. Analysis of MHV _in vitro_ translation products with
MoAbs specific for the MHV-JHM mRNA 2 ORF fusion protein. The lanes 1 and 4 are H_2O controls.

To identify the MHV-JHM mRNA 2 gene product _in vivo_ we performed immunofluorescence, immunoprecipitation and Western
blotting. Indirect immunofluorescence was performed on acetone
fixed MHV-JHM infected and mock-infected DBT cells. Fig. 4
shows the staining of infected cells with the mixture of fusion
protein MoAbs (A) or an anti-spike protein MoAb (kindly provided by H. Wege) (C). In both cases a clear positive immune
reaction was evident, albeit less intensely for the fusion
protein MoAb. The immunostaining was restricted to the cytoplasm of syncytia, the characteristic cytopathic effect of MHV-
JHM infection. There was no staining in the nuclei of infected
cells nor in mock-infected cells (B).

The immunoprecipitation of ^{35}S methionine cell lysates
(Siddell et al., 1981) derived from MHV-JHM or MHV-A59 infected
DBT cells using either the fusion protein specific MoAb
mixture, an anti-S MoAb, or an anti ß-galactosidase MoAb is
shown in Fig. 5. The results show that, as expected, the anti S
MoAb immunoprecipitates a polypeptide of approximately 150-
160,000 mol.wt, the intracellular precursor of the spike

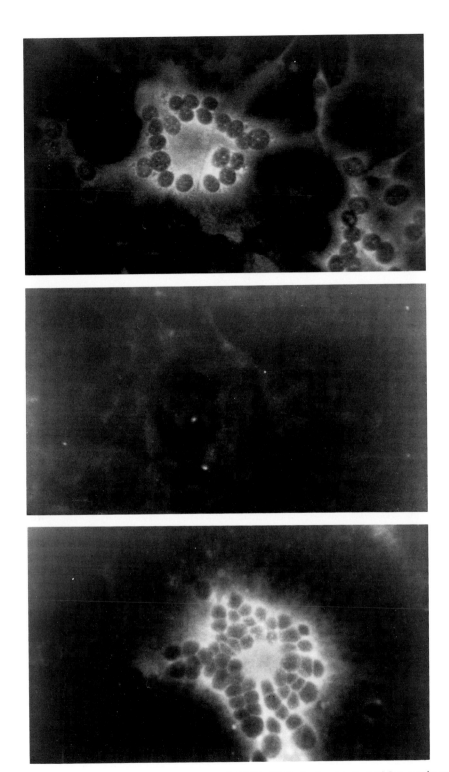

Fig. 4. Immunofluorescence of MHV-JHM infected cells using
        MoAbs specific for the mRNA 2 ORF fusion protein.

protein (Fig. 5, lanes 5 and 6). The fusion protein specific MoAbs again specifically immunoprecipitate an approximately 30,000 mol.wt. polypeptide from both JHM and A59 infected cells (Fig. 5 lanes 3 and 4). The anti ß-galactosidase MoAb did not show any immunoprecipitation (Fig. 5, lanes 7 and 8).

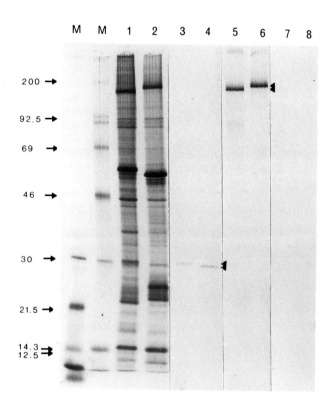

Fig. 5. Immunoprecipitation of polypeptides from MHV infected cells using MoAbs specific for the mRNA 2 ORF fusion protein.

Finally, the identity of the MHV-JHM mRNA 2 gene products was confirmed in vivo by immunoblotting. Cytoplasmic lysates were prepared from MHV-JHM and MHV-A59 infected DBT cells, electrophoresed on a 15 % SDS polyacrylamide gel and transferred to nitrocellulose. The 30,000 mol.wt. mRNA 2 gene product was then detected in both JHM and A59 infected cell lysates using the fusion protein specific MoAbs as shown in Fig. 6, lanes 1 and 2.

DISCUSSION

In this paper we have clearly demonstrated that the MHV-JHM mRNA 2 product is a 30,000 mol.wt. protein which has been previously identified as an _in vitro_ translation product (Siddell, 1983) and has been detected in small amounts in MHV-JHM infected cells (Siddell et al., 1981). The results also show that a homologous protein is synthesized in MHV-A59 infected cells. Furthermore, as predicted from the sequence analysis, the JHM and A59 proteins differ slightly in size (265 and 261 aminoacids, respectively) (this paper, Luytjes et al., 1988). The experiments we have reported also clearly demonstrate the

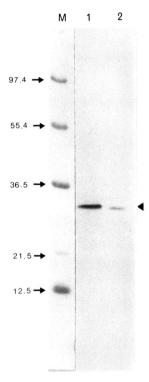

Fig. 6. Western blotting of cytoplasmic lysates from MHV infected cells using MoAbs specific for the mRNA 2 ORF fusion protein.

usefulness of the "fusion protein" strategy and the advantages of isolating fusion protein specific MoAbs, as compared to polyvalent sera. It should be noted that the mixture of fusion protein specific MoAbs is able to function in immunofluorescence, immunoprecipitation and immunoblotting. We believe that the MoAbs we have isolated may also be useful in elucidating the function of this protein, which at the moment is unknown.

ACKNOWLEDGMENT

We would like to acknowledge the technical help of Frau B. Schelle-Prinz. We thank Helga Kriesinger for typing the manuscript. This work was supported by the SFB 165 (B1).

REFERENCES

Ebner, D., Raabe, T., and Siddell, S.G., 1988, Identification of the coronavirus MHV-JHM mRNA4 product. J. gen. Virol. 69: 1041.

Luytjes, W., Bredenbeek, P.J., Noten, A.F.H., Horzinek, M.C., and Spaan, W.J.M., 1988, Virology 166:415.

Siddell, S.G., Wege, H., Barthel, A., and ter Meulen, V., 1981, Coronavirus JHM. Intracellular protein synthesis. J. gen. Virol. 53:145.

Siddell, S.G., 1983, Coronavirus JHM. Coding assignment of subgenomic mRNAs. J. gen. Virol. 64:113.

Skinner, M.A., Ebner, D., and Siddell, S.G., 1985, Coronavirus MHV-JHM mRNA5 has a sequence arrangement which potentially allows translation of a second, downstream open reading frame. J. gen. Virol. 66:581.

Stanley, K.K., and Luzio J.P., 1984, Construction of a new family of high efficiency bacterial expression vectors: identification of cDNA clones coding for human liver proteins, EMBO J. 3:1429.

Chapter 7

Transcription and Replication

BACKGROUND PAPER

TRANSCRIPTION AND REPLICATION OF CORONAVIRUS RNA: A 1989 UPDATE

Michael M.C. Lai

Department of Microbiology
University of Southern California School of Medicine
Los Angeles
CA 90033
USA

INTRODUCTION

The genomic RNA of coronaviruses has two unique features. Firstly, it is one of the largest stable RNAs known to exist in nature and is unquestionably the largest viral genomic RNA. The complete sequence of avian infectious bronchitis virus (IBV) RNA shows that its size is 27.6 kilobases (kb) (Boursnell *et al.*, 1987). Although the complete sequences of other coronavirus genomic RNAs are not yet available, preliminary data from several laboratories indicate that the genomic RNA of mouse hepatitis virus (MHV) is as long as 32 kb (Shieh and Lai, unpublished observations). The large size of these RNAs poses a theoretical quandary for the replication of coronavirus RNA, considering the high error frequency of RNA-dependent RNA synthesis observed in some systems (Holland *et al.*, 1982; Steinhauer and Holland, 1986). How does coronavirus RNA replicate faithfully despite the high error frequency of RNA synthesis? It is possible that a proof-reading mechanism operates to correct unavoidable mistakes which are expected to occur in almost every RNA molecule of this size. Secondly, coronavirus RNA contains a leader sequence (approximately 72 nucleotides) which is repeated at the 5'-end of every subgenomic mRNA species. This structural organization appears to be similar to that of most of eukaryotic mRNAs which contain leader sequences derived by RNA splicing. Yet the coronavirus RNA genome does not have consensus splicing signals and the virus replicates exclusively in the cytoplasm (Wilhelmson *et al.*, 1981; Brayton *et al.*, 1981), where there is no conventional RNA splicing machinery. Furthermore, UV transcriptional mapping studies suggest that coronavirus mRNA species are transcribed independently (Jacobs *et al.*, 1981), instead of being derived by cleavage of a precursor RNA. Thus, a new transcriptional mechanism must operate to transcribe coronavirus mRNAs.

LEADER-PRIMED TRANSCRIPTION OF SUBGENOMIC mRNAS

Several possible mechanisms could explain the generation of coronavirus subgenomic RNAs (Baric *et al.*, 1983). Over the last 4-5 years, a considerable body of evidence has been accumulated in support of a transcription mechanism unique to coronavirus, i.e. "leader-primed transcription" (Fig. 1.). This mechanism proposes that a leader RNA is transcribed first from the template RNA. It dissociates from the template as a free leader RNA species, which then binds to the template RNA again at various transcription initiation sites and serves as a primer for mRNA transcription.

The essence of this mechanism has been proven: (1) "Free" leader RNA species of 60-90 nucleotides have been detected in the cytoplasm of MHV-infected cells (Baric *et al.*, 1985, 1987). These RNAs are not associated with the template RNA. (2) A temperature-sensitive mutant has been isolated, which makes leader RNA, but no mRNAs at nonpermissive

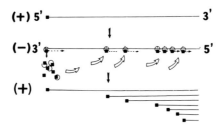

Fig. 1   Model of leader primed transcription. Solid squares represent leader RNA and open circles represent RNA polymerases.

temperature, suggesting that the synthesis of leader RNA and the synthesis of mRNAs are discontinuous and require different viral proteins (Baric *et al.*, 1985). (3) During mixed infection with two different MHV strains, the leader RNA of mRNAs can be freely exchanged between the coinfecting viruses as if the leader RNA exists as a separate transcription unit, independent of the rest of mRNAs (Makino *et al.*, 1986). (4) When two MHV strains which differ only in the sequence at the 3'-end of leader RNA were compared, it was found that the number of mRNA species transcribed by these two viruses was different (Makino and Lai, 1989) . For instance, a derivative of JHM strain which contains two UCUAA repeat sequences at the 3'-end of leader RNA transcribes an additional mRNA, 2b, while the same virus with three UCUAA repeats does not (Makino and Lai, 1989). This result gives the clearest evidence that the transcriptional initiation of coronavirus subgenomic mRNAs is controlled by leader RNA sequence. (5) Each mRNA species of MHV is heterogeneous, varying in the number of UCUAA repeats at the 3'-end of leader RNA (Makino *et al.*, 1988). Since this repeat sequence is present at both the 3'-end of leader RNA and the transcriptional initiation sites, this result suggests that these sequences are involved in leader RNA binding and that the leader RNA binding is imprecise. These studies indicate that coronavirus mRNA transcription is the result of interactions between the 3'-end of leader sequences and the transcription initiation sequences at the template RNA.

CONSENSUS SEQUENCES OF TRANSCRIPTIONAL INITIATION SITES AND LEADER RNA

A large number of various coronavirus genomic RNA sequences have already been obtained. Thus, it is now possible to derive a consensus sequence at the transcription initiation sites. Table 1 shows a compilation of the possible transcriptional initiation sites of various coronavirus strains. Since most of these sequences have not been confirmed by sequencing of mRNAs to be the actual transcriptional initiation sites, the designation of these sequences as transcriptional initiation sites was based on sequence homology and their localization at

Table 1. Consensus sequences at transcriptional initiation sites

Virus	Consensus sequence
MHV, BCV, HCV-229E	UCUAAAC
HCV-OC43	UCUAAAU
TGEV, FIPV	ACUAAAC
IBV	UUAACAA

intergenic regions. It is clear that these sequences are very well conserved, in contrast to the rest of the genomic sequences. The only exception is IBV, which has diverged extensively from other coronaviruses. When transcriptional initiation sites for different mRNAs on the same viral genome is compared, some minor divergence is noted in a few transcriptional initiation sites. These seven-nucleotide sequences appear to be the core of the leader-binding sites and is homologous between the 3'-end of the leader RNA and the intergenic sequences. It should be noted that leader-RNA binding probably involves sequences adjacent to these core sequences as well, as between the leader RNA and the transcriptional start sites (Shieh *et al.*, 1987). The degrees of this homology at different sites parallel, to a certain extent, the amounts of the different mRNA species transcribed, but this correlation is not absolute (Shieh *et al.*, 1987). It is also noted that the core sequence is devoid of any G residues. The minor heterogeneity observed at different transcriptional sites involves only A, C and U interchanges. The mutation of A to G within the core sequence in one of the mRNAs (mRNA 2b) of A59 strain of MHV completely eliminates the transcription within this region (Shieh *et al.*, 1989).

The remaining sequence of the leader RNA is less well conserved. However, the leader RNA appears to maintain the same basic conformation in all of the coronaviruses which have been sequenced so far (Fig. 2). The functional significance of these secondary structures is not clear at the present time.

THE STATE OF TEMPLATE RNA AND LEADER RNA IN INFECTED CELLS

The state of the template RNA for coronavirus transcription has been less well studied due to the small quantity of template (negative strand) RNA. The single report characterizing the size of the coronavirus template RNA indicated that it is a genomic-sized RNA (Lai *et al.*, 1982). There is currently a controversy concerning the kinetics of its synthesis: it is not known whether the negative-stranded RNA is synthesized only early in the infection (Brayton *et al.*, 1984) or throughout the infection (Sawicki *et al.*, 1986). Recently, it has been shown that TGEV may synthesize subgenomic template RNAs which have sizes equivalent to those of subgenomic mRNAs (D. Brian, this volume). This finding is hard to reconcile with the existing data. Clearly more studies on the negative-strand RNA are warranted.

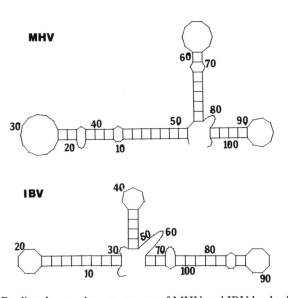

Fig. 2 Predicted secondary structures of MHV and IBV leader RNAs.

At least some of the leader RNAs exist as a free RNA species in the cytoplasm of infected cells. These RNAs range from 50 to 90 nucleotides in length (Baric *et al.*, 1985). It is not clear which leader RNA species is utilized for transcription. Leader RNAs have been shown to be associated with the nucleocapsid (N) protein of coronavirus (Baric *et al.*, 1988). Whether this association is a prerequisite to RNA transcription is not known. Biochemically it has not been demonstrated that these free leader RNAs could be chased into mature RNA species. Nor has the priming function of these leader RNAs been shown.

A MODEL OF LEADER-PRIMED TRANSCRIPTION

Given the current state of knowledge, a model of leader-primed transcription can be proposed (Fig. 3). The leader RNA is synthesized from the 3'-end of the template RNA. The transcriptional termination could occur at multiple sites between nucleotides 60 and 90 from the 5'-end, where there is a hairpin loop and a stretch of A-U-rich sequence (Shieh *et al.*, 1987). After termination, the leader RNA is dissociated from the template and is then associated with N protein and possibly also with RNA polymerase. This free leader RNA binds to the downstream transcriptional initiation sites via complementary sequences between the leader RNA and the intergenic regions on the template RNA. The binding sites include the UCUAAAC consensus sequence and possibly also neighboring sequences. The 3'-end single-stranded tail of the bound leader RNA is then removed by either an endonuclease or exonuclease activity associated with the polymerase. Alternatively, an endonuclease activity may recognize the mismatched nucleotide (e.g. at the initiation site of MHV mRNA 6) within the leader-binding sequence and cleave the leader RNA at a site upstream of the mismatched nucleotide. RNA transcription then takes place using the bound leader RNA as a primer. The endonuclease activity may be equivalent to a proof-reading activity for coronavirus RNA synthesis.

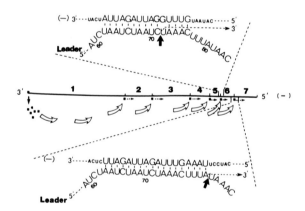

Fig. 3 <u>A detailed model of leader-primed trancription.</u>
Adapted from Lai (1986) with permission.

FREE LEADER RNA IN RNA REPLICATION

Coronavirus genomic size RNA in infected cells has two functions: it serves on the one hand as the mRNA for the polymerase proteins, and on the other as the genomic RNA destined to be packaged into virus particles. No clear structural difference could be detected between these two classes of RNAs. Thus, whether there is a switch from transcription to replication of RNA during coronavirus growth cycle is hard to evaluate. The only case where there is an obvious switch from RNA transcription to replication is with bovine coronavirus (BCV) (Keck *et al.*, 1988a). It is not clear whether transcription and replication utilize the same mechanism of RNA synthesis.

The understanding of the mechanism of coronavirus RNA replication has been aided by the studies of defective-interfering (DI) RNA. DI RNA has been generated from the JHM strain of MHV during high multiplicity passages of the virus (Makino *et al.*, 1984). It replicates at a very high efficiency, thus providing an opportunity to study the mechanism of RNA replication. Furthermore, DI RNAs are much smaller than the virion genomic RNA; for instance, the smallest DI RNA detected in MHV-infected cells is only 2.2 kb (Makino *et al.*, 1988) as compared to 32 kb for the entire virion genomic RNA. A complete cDNA clone of this DI RNA has been obtained and the *in vitro* transcribed RNA is capable of extremely efficient replication in the presence of a helper virus. Surprisingly, when the leader RNA in the DI RNA transfected cells was examined, it was found to contain the leader RNA from the helper virus, instead of its own leader RNA (Makino and Lai, this volume). This result suggests that a leader RNA supplied in trans is utilized in coronavirus DI RNA replication. Thus, the same mechanism of leader-primed RNA synthesis is likely to operate in the RNA replication step.

HIGH-FREQUENCY RNA RECOMBINATION SUGGESTS A DISCONTINUOUS MECHANISM OF RNA REPLICATION

Another interesting phenomenon which is relevant to coronavirus RNA replication is the high frequency of RNA recombination (Makino *et al.*, 1986). Recombination occurs both in tissue culture and in animals (Keck *et al.*, 1988b). Recombination frequency can be more than 10% under some conditions (Makino *et al.*, 1986). Such a high frequency of recombination resembles reassortment of segmented RNAs in influenza viruses, suggesting that segmented RNA intermediates may be generated during MHV RNA replication. RNA intermediates may account for RNA recombination by a copy-choice mechanism. Indeed, RNAs of discrete, non-message sizes have been detected in the cytoplasm of MHV-infected cells; these may correspond to transcriptional intermediates pausing at secondary structures in the template RNA (Baric *et al.*, 1987). These results suggest that coronavirus RNA replication proceeds by a discontinuous and non-processive mechanism, with transcriptional pauses occurring at sites of secondary structure. The occurrence of high-frequency RNA recombination may explain why the coronavirus RNA genome of enormous size (32 kb) can be maintained as a stable and infectious RNA.

ENZYMOLOGY OF RNA TRANSCRIPTION AND REPLICATION

Coronavirus RNA synthesis is mediated by virus-specific RNA-dependent RNA polymerase. The enzyme activity has been demonstrated in TGEV and MHV-infected cells; however, the protein responsible for the polymerase activity has not been identified. Based on the size of the possible gene products and analogy to other RNA viruses, it is assumed that the 5'-most gene (gene 1) encodes the polymerase proteins. This gene has been completely sequenced in IBV (Boursnell *et al.*, 1987). It is approximately 18 kb in length and has two open reading frames (ORFs) which overlap each other slightly. It has been shown that these two ORFs can be translated into a polyprotein by a ribosomal frame-shifting mechanism (Brierley *et al.*, 1987, 1989), resulting, presumably, in a polyprotein of M_r greater than 700,000. This polyprotein is most likely processed into multiple proteins (Brierley *et al.* this volume).

In the case of MHV, the sequencing of the gene encoding the polymerase protein has not been completed. This gene is approximately 23 kb long (Baker *et al.*, this volume). It has the capacity to encode a protein of M_r 800,000. Again, this polyprotein is most likely processed into multiple proteins. Indeed, it has already been shown that the N-terminus of this polyprotein is cleaved into a p28 protein (Denison and Perlman, 1986); Soe *et al.*, 1987); the cleavage is catalyzed by an autoproteolytic activity inherent in this polyprotein (Baker *et al.*, this volume). The proteins encoded by this gene very likely contain other activities in addition to the polymerase activity. For instance, the putative endonuclease required for processing the leader RNA, and other activities such as those required for the regulation of RNA transcription may also be present within this polyprotein.

The polymerases are likely to be associated with membranes (Dennis and Brian, 1982; Brayton *et al.*, 1982). Most likely, the transcription and replication complexes are in a membranous compartment, so that a high concentration of leader RNAs can be maintained locally and RNA recombination between coinfecting viruses can therefore occur at a high frequency.

PERSPECTIVES

Studies conducted so far have clearly established that coronaviruses utilize unique mechanisms for the transcription and replication of their RNAs. Many details of these mechanisms are, however, yet to be unveiled. Several areas of research in the future may be particularly useful in revealing additional insights into the mechanism of coronavirus RNA synthesis:

1. Establishment of An *In Vitro* Transcription and Replication System
Several in vitro systems capable of synthesizing either genomic or subgenomic RNAs have been reported (Dennis and Brian, 1982; Brayton *et al.*, 1982; Compton *et al.*, 1987; Leibowitz and DeVries, 1988). However, none of these are capable of utilizing exogenous RNAs as either template or primers. The ability of any *in vitro* system to transcribe or extend exogenous RNAs is a key to understanding the mechanism of RNA synthesis.

2. Temperature-Sensitive Mutants Defective in RNA Synthesis
An earlier report has grouped RNA (-) temperature-sensitive mutants into six complementation groups (Leibowitz *et al.*, 1982). However, no follow-up work has been reported. The characterization of phenotype and genotype of these mutants and genetic mapping of the temperature-sensitive lesions by complementation and recombination should yield valuable information on the possible gene products involved in coronavirus RNA synthesis.

3. Characterization of the Protein Products of the Gene Encoding the Putative Polymerase
This gene, ranging from 18 to 23 kb, very possibly encodes a polyprotein of M_r 700-800,000, which may subsequently be processed into multiple proteins. Its size is two to three times the size of the genomes of other positive-strand RNA viruses, such as flavi or picornaviruses. Thus, the primary gene product of this gene likely to undergo complex processing pathways, and possess multiple functions. The identification of these proteins and their functions will be an important contribution to the understanding of coronavirus RNA transcription and replication.

REFERENCES

Baric, R. S., Nelson, G. W., Fleming, J. O., Deans, R. J., Keck, J. G., Casteel, N., and Stohlman, S. A., 1988, Interactions between coronavirus nucleocapsid protein and viral RNAs: implications for viral transcription, J. Virol., 62:4280.

Baric, R. S., Shieh, C.-K., Stohlman, S. A., and Lai, M. M. C., 1987, Analysis of intracellular small RNAs of mouse hepatitis virus: evidence for discontinuous transcription, Virology, 156:342.

Baric, R. S., Stohlman, S. A., and Lai, M. M. C., 1983, Characterization of replicative intermediate RNA of mouse hepatitis virus: presence of leader RNA sequences on nascent chains, J. Virol., 48:633.

Baric, S. S., Stohlman, S. A., Razavi, M. K., and Lai, M. M. C., 1985, Characterization of leader related small RNAs in coronavirus-infected cells: further evidence for leader-primed mechanism of transcription, Virus Res., 3:19.

Boursnell, M. E. G., Brown, T. D. K., Foulds, I. J., Green, P. F., Tomley, F. M., and Binns, M. M., 1987, Completion of the sequence of the genome of the coronavirus avian infectious bronchitis virus, J. Gen. Virol., 68:57.

Brayton, P. R., Ganges, R. G., and Stohlman, S. A., 1981, Host cell nuclear function and murine hepatitis virus replication, J. Gen. Virol., 56:457.

Brayton, P. R., Lai, M. M. C., Patton, C. D., and Stohlman, S. A, 1982, Characterization of two RNA polymerase activities induced by mouse hepatitis virus, J. Virol., 42:847.

Brayton, P. R., Stohlman, S. A., and Lai, M. M. C., 1984, Further characterization of mouse hepatitis virus RNA-dependent RNA polymerase, Virology, 133:197.

Brierley, I., Boursnell, M. E. G., Binns, M. M., Bilimoria, B., Blok, V. C., Brown, T. D. K., and Inglis, S. C., 1987, An efficient ribosomal frame-shifting signal in the polymerase-encoding region of the coronavirus IBV, EMBO J., 6:3779.

Brierley, I., Digard, P., and Inglis, S. C., 1989, Characterization of an efficient coronavirus ribosomal frame-shifting signal: Requirement for an RNA pseudoknot, Cell, 57:537.

Compton, S. R., Rogers, D. B., Holmes, K. V., Fertsch, D., Remenick, J., and McGowan, J. J., 1987, In vitro replication of mouse hepatitis virus strain A59, J. Virol., 61:1814.

Denison, M. R., and Perlman, S., 1986, Translation and processing of mouse hepatitis virus virion RNA in a cell-free system, J. Virol., 60:12.

Dennis, D. E., and Brian, D. A., 1982, RNA-dependent RNA polymerase activity in coronavirus-infected cells, J. Virol., 42:153.

Holland, J., Spindler, K., Horodyski, F., Grabau, E., Nichol, S., and van de Pol, S., 1982, Rapid evolution of RNA genomes, Science, 215:1577.

Jacobs, L., Spaan, W.J.M., Horzinek, M.C. and van der Zeijst, B.A.M., 1981, The synthesis of the subgenomic mRNAs of mouse hepatitis virus is initiated independently: evidence from UV transcriptional mapping, J. Virol., 39:401.

Keck, J. G., Hogue, B. G., Brian, D. A., and Lai, M. M. C, 1988a, Temporal regulation of bovine coronavirus RNA synthesis, Virus Res., 9:343.

Keck, J. G., Matsushima, G. K., Makino, S., Fleming, J. O., Vannier, D. M., Stohlman, S. A., and Lai, M. M. C., 1988b, In vivo RNA-RNA recombination of coronavirus in mouse brain, J. Virol., 62:1810.

Lai, M. M. C., Patton, C. D., and Stohlman, S. A, 1982, Replication of mouse hepatitis virus: negative-stranded RNA and replicative form RNA are of genome length, J. Virol., 44:487.

Lai, M. M. C., 1986, Coronavirus leader-RNA-primed transcription: an alternative mechanism to RNA splicing, BioEssays, 5:257.

Leibowitz, J. L., DeVries, J. R., and Haspel, M. V., 1982, Genetic analysis of murine hepatitis virus strain JHM, J. Virol., 42:1080.

Leibowitz, J. L., and DeVries, J. R., 1988, Synthesis of virus-specific RNA in permeabilized murine coronavirus-infected cells, Virology 166:66.

Makino, S., Taguchi, F., and Fujiwara, K., 1984, Defective interfering particles of mouse hepatitis virus, Virology, 133:9.

Makino, S., Keck, J. G., Stohlman, S. A., and Lai, M. M. C., 1986, High-frequency RNA recombination of murine coronaviruses, J. Virol., 57:729.

Makino, S., Stohlman, S. A., and Lai, M. M. C., 1986, Leader sequences of murine coronavirus mRNAs can be freely reassorted: evidence for the role of free leader RNA in transcription, Proc. Natl. Acad. Sci. USA, 83:4204.

Makino, S., Shieh, C.-K., Soe, L.-H., Baker, S. C., and Lai, M. M. C., 1988, Primary structure and translation of a defective interfering RNA of murine coronavirus, Virology, 166:550.

Makino, S., Soe, L. H., Shieh, C.-K., and Lai, M. M. C., 1988, Discontinuous transcription generates heterogeneity at the leader fusion sites of coronavirus mRNAs, J. Virol., 62:3870.

Makino, S., and Lai, M. M. C., 1989, Evolution of the 5'-end of genomic RNA of murine coronaviruses during passages in vitro, Virology, 169:227.

Sawicki, S. G., and Sawicki, D. L., 1986, Coronavirus minus-straind RNA synthesis and effect of cycloheximide on coronavirus RNA synthesis, J. Virol., 57:328.

Shieh, C.-K., Soe, L. H., Makino, S., Chang, M.-F., Stohlman, S. A., and Lai, M. M. C., 1987, The 5'-end sequence of the murine coronavirus genome: implication for multiple fusion sites in leader-primed transcription, Virology, 156:321.

Shieh, C.-K., Lee, H.-J., Yokomori, K., La Monica, N., Makino, S., and Lai, M. M. C.,1989, Identification of a new transcriptional initiation site and the corresponding functional gene 2b in the murine coronavirus RNA genome, J. Virol., 63: 3729-3736.

Soe, L. H., Shieh, C.-K., Baker, S. C., Chang, M.-F., and Lai, M. M. C., 1987, Sequence and translation of the murine coronavirus 5'-end genomic RNA reveals the N-terminal structure of the putative RNA polymerase, J. Virol., 61: 3968-3976.

Steinhauer, D. A., and Holland, J. J, 1986, Direct method for quantitation of extreme polymerase error frequencies at selected single base sites in viral RNA, J. Virol., 57:219.

Wilhelmsen, K. C., Leibowitz, J. L., Bond, C. W., and Robb, J. A., 1981, The replication of murine coronavirus in enucleated cells, Virology, 110:225-230.

CORONAVIRUS SUBGENOMIC REPLICONS AS A MECHANISM FOR mRNA AMPLIFICATION

Phiroze B. Sethna, Shan-Ling Hung, and David A. Brian

Department of Microbiology
The University of Tennessee
Knoxville, Tennessee 37996-0845

INTRODUCTION

Assuming promoter sequences for synthesizing antigenome lie within the 3' noncoding region on the coronavirus genome (approximately 300 bases), and the promoter for synthesizing genome lie within the antileader sequence (approximately 80 bases) on the minus strand, we asked why do mRNAs not replicate? Coronavirus mRNAs have been shown to possess 3' and 5' noncoding regions in common with the genome (Brown et. al., 1984; Brown et. al., 1986; Lai et. al., 1984; Shieh et. al., 1987). If mRNA replication occurs, then we would predict the existence of (1) subgenomic (mRNA-length) minus strands, (2) subgenomic (mRNA-length) double-stranded replicative forms, and (3) subgenome mRNA replication rates that exceed that of the genome. We present evidence that suggests these three conditions are fulfilled for TGEV, and we, therefore, conclude that TGEV mRNAs undergo replication. We propose that this is a mechanism for mRNA amplification, a mechanism not yet described for any other RNA virus family having a nonsegmented genome.

MATERIAL AND METHODS

The Purdue strain of TGEV was plaque purified from infectious genomic RNA and a stock of virus made from passage 5 as previously described (Brian et. al., 1980; Kapke et. al., 1988) was used. Swine testicle cells in roller bottles were infected with a multiplicity of 10 and RNA was extracted as previously described (Kapke et. al., 1988) except that 10mM vanadyl ribonucleoside complex was added to the lysis buffer. RNA ($10\mu g$ per lane for cytoplasmic RNA and 20ng per lane for virion RNA) was electrophoresed in 1% agarose-formaldehyde gels essentially as described (Dennis and Brian, 1982) except that 20mM Mops buffer (pH7.0) was used. RNA was vacuum blotted onto Nytran membrane (Schleicher and Schuell) and bound by UV-crosslinking. Blots were hybridized with a synthetic oligodeoxynucleotide probe (probe 1; 5'-CAGCATGGAGGAAGACGAGCATCTCG-3') that is complementary to virus-sense RNA within the HP gene (Fig. 1), and that had been 5' end-labeled to a specific activity of 1.6 to 3.5×10^6 cpm per pmole by the forward reaction using $[\gamma-^{32}P]$ ATP (ICN). Probe 2 has a sequence that is complementary to probe 1 and it was likewise end-labeled. Membranes were prehybridized at 55°C for 2h in 5X SSC (1X SCC is 0.1%

Coronaviruses and Their Diseases
Edited by D. Cavanagh and T.D.K. Brown
Plenum Press, New York, 1990

335

Ficoll/0.1% polyvinyl pyrrolidine/0.1% bovine serum albumin/50 mM sodium phosphate, pH 7.0/1% SDS) that contained 100 μg sheared salmon sperm DNA and 50 μg tRNA per ml. Radiolabeled probes ($\approx$ 2x10^7 Cerenkov cpm per 120 cm^2 membrane) were denatured at 90°C for 5 min and added to the prehybridization solution, and hybridization was carried out at 55°C for 16h. The membrane was given three 10-min. washes in 2xSSC at 25°C and a fourth wash for 30 min at 55°C, air dried and exposed to Kodak XAR-5 film. Radioactive bands were excised for liquid scintillation counting in Scintiverse. The number of molecules of each mRNA species per cell was determined from the specific activity of the individual probe and from our measured yield of 10 μg of RNA per 1.6x10^6 cells.

For identification of double-stranded replicative forms, intracellular RNA extracted at 6 hpi was used. 60 μg of cytoplasmic RNA was dissolved in 40 μl 10mM Tris-HCl, pH 7.2/300mM NaCl/10mM MgCl$_2$/1mMEDTA containing 10 μg RNase A (Sigma) per ml, and incubated at 37°C for 30 min. Digestion was terminated by adding SDS to a final concentration of 2% and RNA was extracted with phenol-chloroform, and precipitated. RNA was analyzed by electrophoresis and blot hybridization as described above.

RESULTS

We and others have established the nucleotide sequence of the 3'-terminal 8.5 kilobases of the TGEV genome and have identified seven open reading frames (Fig. 1; Jacobs *et. al.*, 1987; Kapke and Brian, 1986; Kapke *et. al.*, 1988; Kapke *et. al.*, 1989; Laude *et. al.*, 1987; Rasschaert and Laude, 1987; Tung, 1987). mRNA transcripts have been identified for each of these ORFs by metabolic labeling (Dennis and Brian, 1982; Jacobs *et. al.*, 1986). To confirm that each transcript and genomic RNA can be identified by Northern blotting experiments, RNA blots were probed with a G+C-rich 26 mer complementary to a region within the HP gene (Fig. 1). Fig. 2 demonstrates that genomic RNA, and mRNAs for P, 7.7K, 27.7K, 9.2K, M, N and HP were each identifiable by this procedure, and yielded a pattern that is consistent with the 3' coterminal nested set structure of coronavirus mRNAs. Furthermore, by counting individual bands, an estimate of the number of molecules per cell for each species was made (Fig. 3A).

To determine whether subgenomic minus strands exist, probe 2 (which is complementary to probe 1) was used in Northern analyses (Fig. 2). A minus-strand counterpart (identified by α) for the genome and for each mRNA species was identified. Their numbers were likewise estimated (Fig

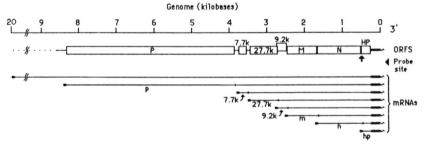

Fig. 1. Gene map for TGEV and site of the HP specific probes. The seven ORFs in the 3' end of the TGEV genome are drawn to scale. P=peplomer protein, M=matrix protein, N=nucleocapsid protein, HP=hydrophobic protein, and 7.7K, 27.7K, and 9.2K ORFs are potential nonstructural proteins. Corresponding mRNAs are respectively identified as p, m, n, hp, 7.7k, 27.7k, and 9.2k. Arrow identifies site from which the probe sequences came.

3B). Four observations suggested that probes designed to detect minus strands were not merely detecting abundant mRNA molecules nonspecifically. (1) Three of the eight minus-strand species (αhp, α27.7k, and α7.7k) did not migrate with the same mobility as did their presumed plus-strand counterparts. (2) A probe from within the N gene designed to detect minus strand, did so, and also detected the larger minus-strand species, but not αhp (data not shown). (3) The maximal abundance of minus-strand species occurred at 4 hpi., whereas that of plus strands occurred at 6 h.p.i. (Fig. 3). (4) Probes used to detect minus-strand species did not identify virion genomic RNA (Fig. 2, lane 20). We do not yet know the detailed structure of the molecules identified as high mol. wt. RNA and those identified by asterisks in Fig. 2.

To determine whether subgenomic double-strand replicative forms exist cytoplasmic RNA from infected cells at 6 h.p.i. was treated with pancreatic RNase A in 0.3M NaCl, and RNase resistant forms were denatured, electrophoresed, blotted and hybridized to probe 1 or probe 2 (Fig. 4A). Both plus and minus strands corresponding in size to mRNA species were found indicating that subgenomic replicative forms were present. Furthermore, within double-stranded forms, very few full-length (i.e., mRNA-length) plus strands were found, but full-length minus strand RNAs were abundant. We interpret this to mean that the replicative forms represented replicative intermediate structures on which a single minus-strand was serving as template for multiple plus strands (Fig. 4B). Plus strand molecules would have been degraded to protected species too small to be resolved in our electrophoretic system.

Both plus- and minus-strand subgenomic RNA species were, in general, synthesized at a rate inversely related to their length (Fig. 3, A and B). This can be seen by noting slopes throughout the first 6h for plus-strand

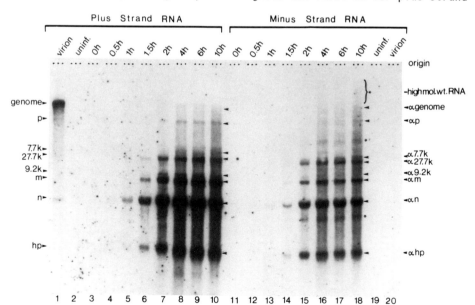

Fig. 2. Subgenomic plus- and minus-strand RNA species identified by hybridization. RNA from purified virions or from cytoplasm of uninfected or infected cells (hours postinfection are shown above the lanes) was electrophoresed, blotted, and hybridized with radiolabeled probe 1 to detect plus-strand RNA species (lanes 1-10) or with probe 2 to detect minus-strand RNA species (lanes 11-20). α indicates antisense (or minus strand) polarity; three dots at the top of each lane identify the well.

RNA synthesis, and throughout the first 4h for minus-strand RNA synthesis.

DISCUSSION

　　To our knowledge, this is the first demonstration of subgenomic minus-strand RNA for coronaviruses. The experimental approach used here may demonstrate subgenomic minus strands for other coronaviruses. We have shown them to exist for the bovine enteric coronavirus (M. Hofmann, P. Sethna, and D. Brian, unpublished data), for example, a close relative of the mouse hepatitis virus for which subgenomic minus strands were not demonstrable by other experimental methods (Lai *et. al.*, 1982).

　　The phenomenon of subgenomic mRNA replication does not rule out a mechanism like that of leader-primed transcription to explain the origin of subgenomic mRNAs. A mechanism such as leader-primed transcription must exist to explain the origin of mRNAs from a single, infectious coronavirus genome (Lai, 1986; Spaan *et. al.*, 1983). Once made, however, the individual subgenomic mRNA could serve as template for its replication. Conceivably, some mRNA species could enter the cells as part of the virion since they are known to be packaged (P. Sethna and D. Brian, unpublished data; Fig. 5).

　　Two biological consequences can be predicted from the replication of subgenomic mRNAs. First, replication may serve as an efficient mechanism to rapidly amplify mRNAs required for structural protein synthesis, thus freeing the full-length genome for genome replication and polymerase synthesis. Second, replicating mRNAs would most probably compete with genome for limiting factors required in RNA replication (such as the RNA polymerase) and in this way behave as genomes of defective interfering viruses. This may be a mechanism by which coronaviruses readily establish persistent infections in cell culture.

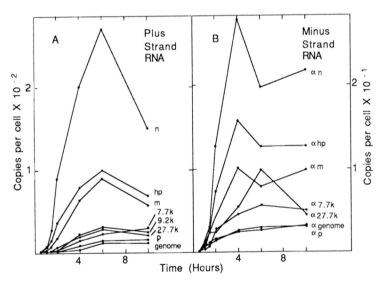

Fig. 3. Kinetics of plus strand (A) and minus-strand (B) RNA synthesis. Radiolabeled bands in Fig. 2 were excised and counted. Copy numbers were determined as described in Materials and Methods.

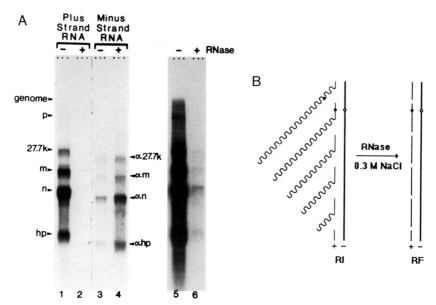

Fig. 4. (A) RNase-resistant species in replicative forms. Cytoplasmic RNA obtained from cells 6 hr postinfection was digested with RNase A in 0.3 M NaCl, electrophoresed in a denaturing gel, transferred and hybridized with probes from the HP gene sequence. Lane 1, 10 μg of untreated RNA, and lane 2, 30 μg of RNase-treated RNA, were hybridized with probe 1. Lane 3, 10 μg of untreated RNA, and lane 4, 30 μg of RNase-treated RNA, were hybridized with probe 2. Lanes 5 and 6 are extended exposures of lanes 1 and 2. (B) Models showing the relationship between the replicative intermediate (RI) and resulting double-stranded replicative form (RF) following RNase digestion for a replicative intermediate of 2.5 kilobases. Sites to which probes 1 (on the plus strand) and 2 (on the minus strand) would bind are depicted by a filled circle and an open circle, respectively.

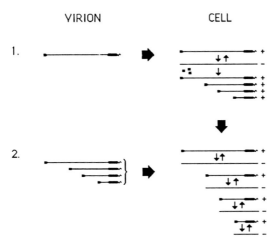

Fig. 5. Two schemes by which mRNAs potentially become available for replication. (1) mRNAs are derived by a mechanism such as leader-primed transcription. (2) mRNAs are carried into the cell by the infecting virion.

REFERENCES

Brian, D. A., D. E. Dennis, and J. S. Guy. 1980. Genome of porcine
    transmissible gastroenteritis coronavirus. J. Virol. 34:410-415.
Brown, T. D. K., M. E. G. Boursnell, and M. M. Binns. 1984. A leader
    sequence is present on mRNA A avian infections bronchitis virus. J.
    Gen. Virol. 65:1437-1442.
Brown, T. D. K., M. E. G. Boursnell, M. M. Binns, and F. M. Tomley. 1986.
    Cloning and sequencing of 5' terminal sequences from avian infectious
    bronchitis virus genomic RNA. J. Gen. Virol. 67:221-228.
Brown, T. D. K., M. E. G. Boursnell, M. M. Binns, and F. M. Tomley, 1986.
    Cloning and sequencing of 5' terminal sequences from avian infectious
    bronchitis virus genomic RNA. J. Gen. Virol. 67:221-228.
Dennis, D. E., and D. A. Brian. 1982. Coronavirus cell-associated RNA-
    dependent RNA polymerase activity in coronavirus-infected cells. J.
    Virol. 42:153-164.
Jacobs, L., B. A. M. Van Der Zeijst, and M. C. Horzinek. 1986.
    Characterization and translation of transmissible gastroenteritis
    virus mRNAs. J. Virol. 57:1010-1015.
Jacobs, L., R. DeGroot, B. A. M. Van Der Zeijst, M. C. Horzinek, and W.
    Spaan. 1987. Virus Res. 8:363-371.
Kapke, P. A., and D. A. Brian. 1986. Sequence analysis of the porcine
    transmissible gastroenteritis coronavirus nucleocapsid protein gene.
    Virology 151:41
Kapke, P. A., F. Y. T. Tung, and D. A. Brian. 1989. Nucleotide sequence
    between the peplomer and matrix protein genes of the porcine
    transmissible gastroenteritis coronavirus identifies three large open
    reading frames. Virus Genes. 2:293-294.
Kapke, P. A. K., F. Y. T. Tung, B. G. Hogue, D. A. Brian, R. D. Woods, and
    R. Wesley. 1988. The amino terminal signal peptide on the porcine
    transmissible gastroenteritis coronavirus matrix protein is not an
    absolute requirements for membrane translocation and glycosylation.
    Virology 165:367-376.
Lai, M. M. C. 1986. Coronavirus leader-RNA-primed transcription: an
    alternative mechanism to RNA splicing. Bio Essays 5:257-260.
Lai, M. M. C., R. S. Baric, P. R. Brayton, and S. A. Stohlman. 1984.
    Characterization of leader RNA sequences on the virion and mRNAs of
    mouse hepatitis virus, a cytoplasmic RNA virus. Proc. Natl. Acad.
    Sci. USA 81:3626-3630.
Lai, M. M. C., C. D. Patton, and S. A. Stohlman. 1982. Replication of
    mouse hepatitis virus: negative-stranded RNA and replicative form
    RNA are of genome length. J. Virol. 44:487-492.
Laude, H., D. Rasschaert, and J. C. Huet. 1987. Sequence and N-terminal
    processing of the transmembrane protein E1 of the coronavirus
    transmissible gastroenteritis virus. J. Gen. Virol. 68:1687-1693.
Rasschaert, D., and H. Laude. 1987. The predicted structure of the
    peplomer protein E2 of the porcine coronavirus transmissible
    gastroenteritis virus. J. Gen. Virol. 68:1883-1890.
Shieh, C. K., and L. H. Soe, S. Makino, M. F. Chang, S. A. Stohlman, and
    M. M. C. Lai. 1987. The 5'-end sequence of the murine coronavirus
    genome: implications for multiple fusion sites in leader-primed
    transcription. Virology 156:321-330.
Spaan, W., H. Delius, M. Skinner, J. Armstrong, P. Rottier, S. Smeekens,
    B. A. M. Van Der Zeijst, and S. G. Siddell. 1983. Coronavirus mRNA
    synthesis involves fusion of non-contiguous sequences. EMBO Journal
    2:1839-1844.

STUDIES OF CORONAVIRUS DI RNA REPLICATION USING *IN VITRO* CONSTRUCTED
DI cDNA CLONES

Shinji Makino and Michael M.C. Lai

Department of Microbiology, University of Southern California, School of Medicine
Los Angeles, CA 90033

ABSTRACT

Sequence analysis of an intracellular defective-interfering (DI) RNA, DIssE, of mouse hepatitis virus (MHV) revealed that it is composed of three noncontiguous genomic regions, representing the first 864 nucleotides of the 5'-end, an internal 748 nucleotides of the polymerase gene, and 601 nucleotides from the 3'-end of the parental MHV genome. DIssE had three base substitutions within the leader sequence and also a deletion of nine nucleotides located at the junction of the leader and the remaining genomic sequence. A system was developed for generating DI RNAs to study the mechanism of MHV RNA replication. A cDNA copy of DIssE RNA was placed downstream of T7 RNA polymerase promoter to generate DI RNAs capable of extremely efficient replication in the presence of a helper virus. We demonstrated that, in the DI RNA-transfected cells, the leader sequence of these DI RNAs was switched to that of the helper virus during one round of replication. This high-frequency leader sequence exchange was not observed if a nine-nucleotide stretch at the junction between the leader and the remaining DI sequence was deleted. This observation suggests that a free leader RNA is utilized for the replication of MHV RNA.

INTRODUCTION

Mouse hepatitis virus (MHV) contains a single-stranded infectious RNA genome of more than 32 kilobases (kb) (11; Shieh, C.-K. and Lai, M. M. C., unpublished data). It synthesizes in infected cells six major species of subgenomic mRNAs, which have a 3'-coterminal, nested-set structure (7, 12, 20) and contain an identical 5'-end leader sequence of 72-77 nucleotides (6, 9, 25). A considerable body of evidence suggests that MHV utilizes a leader-primed transcription mechanism, in which a leader RNA transcribed from the 3'-end of the genomic-sized negative-strand template RNA (10) is used as a primer for subgenomic mRNA transcription at downstream intergenic regions (5). As a result, the leader RNA can be freely exchanged between mRNAs of different co-infecting viruses (18). Furthermore, the leader sequence evolves very rapidly during virus passages in tissue culture; specifically, the number of pentanucleotide (UCUAA) repeat sequences at the 3'-end of the leader decreases upon serial passages (15). The change of leader sequences also resulted in the change of subgenomic mRNA species synthesized (15). Thus, the leader sequence of MHV is very important for MHV mRNA transcription. However, it is not clear whether the free leader RNA species is also involved in MHV RNA replication.

The JHM strain of MHV (MHV-JHM) has been shown to generate defective-interfering (DI) RNAs during high-multiplicity passages (14, 19). MHV DI RNAs are classified into two types. One is DI RNA of nearly genomic size, which is efficiently packaged into virus particles and replicates itself even in the absence of helper virus infection (16). Another group are smaller DI RNAs of the classical type. One of these RNAs, DIssE, which is the smallest DI RNA detected, has been analyzed in grerater detail (16). DIssE RNA synthesis requires a helper virus and are inefficiently packaged into virus particles (16). Thus, it may lack packaging signals. On the other hand, since it is efficiently replicated in DI-infected cells, DIssE RNA must contain the sequences essential for viral RNA replication. Since DI RNAs replicate more efficiently than the standard MHV RNA (16), DI RNAs provide an opportunity for the study of MHV RNA replication. In this study, we show that MHV DI RNA replication involves a high-frequency, site-specific leader sequence switching, suggesting that a leader RNA supplied *in trans* is also utilized for MHV RNA replication.

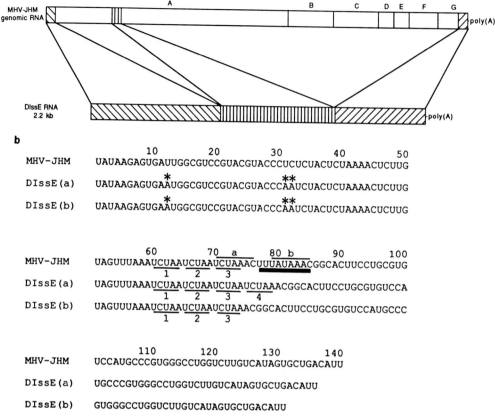

a

b

```
                    10        20        30        40        50
MHV-JHM    UAUAAGAGUGAUUGGCGUCCGUACGUACCCUCUCUACUCUAAAACUCUUG
                        *                   **
DIssE(a)   UAUAAGAGUGAAUGGCGUCCGUACGUACCCAAUCUACUCUAAAACUCUUG
                        *                   **
DIssE(b)   UAUAAGAGUGAAUGGCGUCCGUACGUACCCAAUCUACUCUAAAACUCUUG


                    60        70  a     80  b    90        100
MHV-JHM    UAGUUUAAAUCUAAUCUAAUCUAAACUUUAUAAACGGCACUUCCUGCGUG
                     1    2    3
DIssE(a)   UAGUUUAAAUCUAAUCUAAUCUAAUCUAAACGGCACUUCCUGCGUGUCCA
                     1    2    3    4
DIssE(b)   UAGUUUAAAUCUAAUCUAAUCUAAACGGCACUUCCUGCGUGUCCAUGCCC
                     1    2    3


                   110       120       130       140
MHV-JHM    UCCAUGCCCGUGGGCCUGGUCUUGUCAUAGUGCUGACAUU
DIssE(a)   UGCCCGUGGGCCUGGUCUUGUCAUAGUGCUGACAUU
DIssE(b)   GUGGGCCUGGUCUUGUCAUAGUGCUGACAUU
```

Figure 1. Diagram of the structure of DIssE RNA.
(a) A comparison between the sequence of DIssE RNA and that of standard MHV-JHM genomic RNA. A-G represent the seven genes of MHV (7).
(b) The 5'-end sequence of DIssE and MHV-JHM genomic RNA. The letters a and b represent the canonical seven-nucleotide sequence (22). A bold solid line represents the nine-nucleotide sequence which is deleted in DIssE but present in MHV-JHM. DIssE(a) and DIssE(b) represent the two species of DIssE RNA which have different number of UCUAA repeats. Sequence data were obtained from the primer extension analysis (data not shown). Three base substitutions are indicated by asteriks.

MATERIALS AND METHODS

Viruses and Cells. The plaque-cloned A59 strain of MHV (MHV-A59) was used as a helper virus. Mouse L2 cells and DBT cells were used for RNA transfection and propagation of viruses, respectively.

cDNA cloning of DIssE and DNA construction. cDNA cloning followed the general method of Gubler and Hoffman (4). Construction of various plasmids will be described elsewhere.

RNA transcription and transfection. Plasmid DNAs were linearized by Xba I digestion and transcribed with T7 RNA polymerase as previously described (24). RNA transfection was done as previously described (16).

Preparation of virus-specific intracellular RNA and agarose gel electrophoresis. Virus-specific RNAs in RNA-transfected cells or virus-infected cells were labeled with ^{32}P-orthophosphate as previously described (20). Virus-specific RNA was separated by electrophoresis on 1% agarose gels after denaturation with 1M glyoxal (21). Preparative gel electrophoresis in 1% agarose gels containing 6M urea was performed as previosly described (19).

RNA sequencing. Dideoxynucleotide chain termination methods adapted for RNA sequencing was used (26).

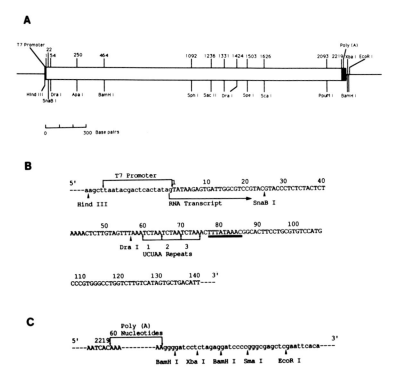

A

T7 Promoter ... Poly (A)

22
54 250 464 1092 1236 1331 1424 1503 1626 2093 2219/Xba I EcoR I

Hind III Dra I Apa I BamH I Sph I Sac II Dra I Spe I Sca I Ppu1 I BamH I
SnaB I

0   300 Base pairs

B

```
                      T7 Promoter
5'                     ┌─────────┐   10        20        30        40
----aagcttaatacgactcactatagTATAAGAGTGATTGGCGTCCGTACGTACCCTCTCTACTCT
    ▲                        └─────────────────┐        ▲
Hind III                     RNA Transcript     ──────→  SnaB I

        50        60        70        80        90        100
AAAACTCTTGTAGTTTAAATCTAATCTAATCTAAACTTTATAAACGGCACTTCCTGCGTGTCCATG
        ▲         ▲    ▲    ▲
      Dra I    1    2    3
              UCUAA Repeats

   110       120       130       140    3'
CCCGTGGGCCTGGTCTTGTCATAGTGCTGACATT----
```

C

```
              Poly (A)
              60 Nucleotides
5'    2219┌                                                      3'
----AATCACAAA---------AAgggggatcctctagaggatccccgggcgagctcgaattcaca----
              ▲      ▲      ▲     ▲      ▲
            BamH I  Xba I  BamH I  Sma I  EcoR I
```

Figure 2. Diagram of the structure of DE5-w3.
(A) Open box indicates DI cDNA sequence, and solid lines indicate vector sequences.
(B) Sequence of the 5'-end region of DI cDNA of DE5-w3. The nine-nucleotide sequence is underlined. The DI sequences are in capital letters while vector sequences are in lower cases.
(C) Sequence of the 3'-end region of DI cDNA of DE5-w3 and plasmid polylinker sites.

RESULTS

<u>cDNA cloning and sequencing of DIssE RNA.</u>   To understand the primary structure of DIssE RNA, cDNA clones were generated from gel-purified DIssE RNA using oligo(dT) as a primer. A diagram representing the structure of DIssE RNA and that of MHV-JHM genomic RNA are shown in Figure 1. Sequence analysis of DIssE cDNA clones revealed that DIssE RNA consists of three different regions of MHV-JHM genomic RNA. The first region represents 864 nucleotides from the 5'-end of the genomic RNA (24). The second region, 748 nucleotides in length, is a region within gene 1 that corresponds to the region at 3.3 to 4 kb from the 5'-end of genomic RNA (Baker et al., in press), and the third region contains a sequence of 601 nucleotides derived from the extreme 3'-end of the genomic RNA (23). The entire sequence of DIssE RNA is identical to that of the corresponding regions of MHV genomic RNA, with some exceptions in the leader sequence region, where 3 bases were substituted and nine nucleotides (UUUAUAAAC) were deleted in DIssE at the junction between the leader RNA and the remaining genomic sequences. Also the 5'-end of DIssE RNA was heterogeneous with respect to the number of UCUAA repeats within the leader sequence (Figure 1B).

<u>Construction of DI RNAs capable of efficient replication in the presence of helper virus.</u> To utilize DI RNAs for understanding the mechanism of MHV RNA synthesis and to assess the role of the 9 nucleotides at the junction between leader and the remaining genome sequence, we have constructed a complete DI cDNA clone (2.2 kb) which contains the complete leader sequence of MHV-JHM plus the 9 nucleotides. This DI sequence was placed downstream to the promoter for T7 RNA polymerase, so that one additional G residue is added to the 5'-end of the run-off RNA transcript (DE5-w3) (Figure 2). The 3'-end of this DI cDNA construct contains a poly (A) sequence, which is followed by a polylinker sequence (Figure 2). The plasmid was linearized by Xba I, and transcribed by T7 RNA polymerase in the presence of a cap analogue (m^{7}G(5')ppp(5')G). The RNA was transfected into monolayers of mouse L2 cells which had been infected with the A59 strain of MHV (MHV-A59), 1 hr prior to transfection. MHV-A59 can be distinguished from MHV-JHM in both leader and genomic sequences (6,22). Virus-specific RNAs were labeled with ^{32}P-orthophosphate in the presence of actinomycin D (20), and analyzed by agarose gel electrophoresis. As shown in Figure 3, DI RNA of 2.2 kb was detected as early as 6 hrs after transfection. When virus harvested from transfected cells (passage 1 virus) was used to infect

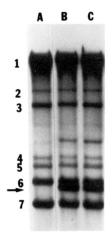

Figure 3. Intracellular RNA synthesis after transfection with DE5-w3 RNA and infection with MHV-A59. Lane A: mock-transfected and MHV-A59-infected cells, Lane B: DE5-w3-transfected and MHV-A59-infected cells, Lane C: passage 1 virus-infected cells. The arrow indicates the DI RNA.

L2 cells, the DI RNA was also detected in infected cells. This result indicates that this RNA could be packaged into virus particles. These data thus demonstrated that *in vitro* synthesized DE5-w3 RNA replicated efficiently in transfected cells in the presence of a heterologous helper virus, MHV-A59.

Change of 5'-end sequence of DI RNA in transfected cells. Since the leader sequences of mRNAs can be exchanged freely between different viruses during co-infection (18) and the leader sequence evolves rapidly during virus passages in tissue culture (15), we examined whether any alteration occurred at the 5'-end of DI RNA species in transfected cells. For this study, we have prepared several DI cDNA constructs which have different sequences within the leader sequence. The 5'-end structures of the transcripts are shown in Figure 4. The DI RNAs transcribed from these constructs were transfected into L2 cells as described above. The 5'-end sequence of gel-purified DI RNAs obtained from transfected cells were examined by RNA sequencing, using a primer complementary to nucleotides 172-188 from the 5' end of the genomic RNA. Results of RNA sequencing are shown in Figure 4. Surprisingly, all the DI RNA isolated from RNA-transfected-cells contained an A at position 35 and two repeats of the UCUAA sequence, which is identical to the leader sequence of MHV-A59 (6). All DI RNAs had a U at nucleotide 111, identical to parent MHV-JHM (22), whereas MHV-A59 had a C at this position, indicating that the leader sequence of DI RNA was replaced by the leader sequence of the helper virus MHV-A59.

To examine whether the sequence alteration was limited to the 5'-end of DI RNA or involved the entire DI genome, we examined the structure of DI RNA by T1-oligonucleotide fingerprinting. The fingerprinting analysis of the *in vitro* synthesized DE5-w3 RNA and the DI RNA isolated from the DE5-w3 RNA-transfected cells demonstrated that sequence alteration occurred only at the leader sequence and the rest of sequence did not undergo gross sequence alteration (data not shown). We therefore concluded that all of the DI RNAs switched the leader sequence with the helper virus.

A nine-nucleotide deletion eliminated the leader RNA switching. We have previously failed to detect leader RNA switching between a naturally occurring DI RNA and MHV-A59 (16). Since the naturally occurring DI RNA has a deletion of nine nucleotides at the junction between the leader and the remaining genomic sequence and has three nucleotide substitutions within leader sequence as compared to the standard MHV-JHM (22), we speculated that these sequence differences between the naturally occurring DI RNA and the *in vitro* constructed RNAs used here might have accounted for the difference in the leader RNA switching. Therefore we prepared three different DI cDNA constructs which contained a deletion of the nine nucleotides. As shown in Figure 5, the DI RNAs isolated from cells transfected with these DI RNA constructs retained the leader sequence of the input DI RNAs. Since the only difference between DE-1A and DE5-w4, and between DE-2c and DE107-w4 RNAs is the absence or presence of the nine nucleotides, we concluded that the presence of the nine nucleotides located at the junction between the leader and the remaining DI sequence is crucial for the leader sequence exchange with the helper virus during DI RNA replication.

344

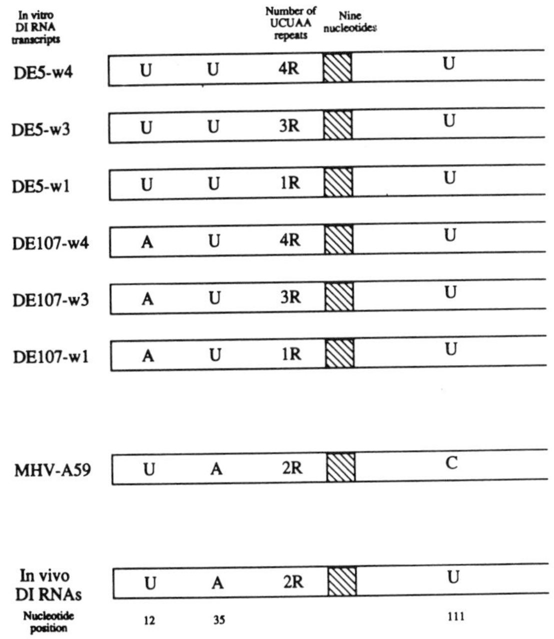

In vitro DI RNA transcripts			Number of UCUAA repeats	Nine nucleotides	
DE5-w4	U	U	4R	▨	U
DE5-w3	U	U	3R	▨	U
DE5-w1	U	U	1R	▨	U
DE107-w4	A	U	4R	▨	U
DE107-w3	A	U	3R	▨	U
DE107-w1	A	U	1R	▨	U
MHV-A59	U	A	2R	▨	C
In vivo DI RNAs	U	A	2R	▨	U
Nucleotide position	12	35			111

Figure 4. The schematic representation of the 5'-end sequences of DI RNAs synthesized *in vitro* and obtained from DI RNA-transfected cells.
Only the diverged nucleotides are indicated. 1R, 2R, 3R and 4R represent one, two, three and four repeats of UCUAA sequence, respectively. The nine-nucleotide sequences (UUUAUAAAC) are represented as cross-hatched boxes.

DISCUSSION

The sequence analysis of DIssE RNA revealed that it is composed of three discontiguous parts of the viral genome, including the 5'-end and 3'-end of genomic RNA. Our previous study has demonstrated that DIssE is replicated from its negative template in the presence of a helper virus (16). Therefore, the DIssE sequence likely contains essential recognition signals for MHV replication. The structure of DIssE RNA supports the likelihood that the recognition signals for the synthesis of negative-strand RNA and positive-strand RNA are localized at the 3'-end and 5'-end of genomic RNA, respectively.

We have also demonstrated that the leader sequence of DI RNAs switched to that of the helper virus during DI RNA replication. This leader sequence switching requires the presence of a nine-nucleotide sequence at the junction between leader RNA and the remaining genomic sequence. Since only one round of virus replication was required for the leader RNA switching and the majority of RNA in the DI RNA-transfected cells acquired the leader RNA of the helper virus, this leader RNA switching must have occurred very early in the DI replication process and at a very high frequency. This result is most consistent with the interpretation that a free leader RNA derived from the helper virus is involved in the replication of DI RNA. We have previously shown that leader RNA species can be freely exchanged between subgenomic mRNAs of two MHVs during mixed infection (18). These two studies suggest that both transcription and replication of MHV RNAs involve a free leader RNA species.

The MHV DI RNAs constructed here showed an extremely high efficiency of RNA replication. Considering the low efficiency of RNA transfection, this finding indicates that the DI RNA has a much higher efficiency of RNA replication than the mRNAs from helper viruses. This replication rate is even higher than that of comparable DI RNA of Sindbis virus, which requires several cycles of virus passages before DI RNAs could be detected (13). Thus, MHV DI RNA could be a potentially useful vector for expressing foreign genes in mammalian cells. It should be noted that in either DI RNA- transfected or passage 1 virus-infected cells, the helper virus RNA synthesis was not inhibited. This was probably due to the low efficiency of RNA transfection and lack of specific packaging signals in these DI RNAs. We have previously shown that DIssE RNA is packaged into virion particles nonspecifically and at a very low efficiency (16). Nevertheless, whatever small amount of RNA packaged apparently is enough to replicate into a major RNA species. The addition of a packaging signal to these DI cDNA constructs could further increase its utility as an expression vector.

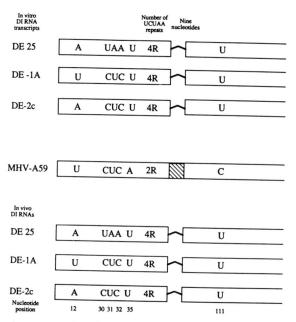

Figure 5. The schematic representation of the 5'-end sequences of DI RNAs containing a nine-nucleotide deletion.
2R and 4R represent the two and four repeats of UCUAA sequence, respectively. The nine-nucleotide sequence in MHV-A59 is represented by a cross-hatched box. The deletion of the nine-nucleotide is shown as a thin line. The nucleotide sequences which are not denoted in the diagram share the same sequence as that of DE5-w3 (see Figure 2B).

REFERENCES

1. Baric, R. S., Shieh, C.-K., Stohlman S.A., and Lai, M. M. C. (1987). Analysis of intracellular small RNAs of mouse hepatitis virus: Evidence for discontinuous transcription. Virology 156, 342-354.

2. Baric, R. S., Stohlman, S. A., and Lai, M. M. C. (1983). Characterization of replicative intermediate RNA of mouse hepatitis virus: Presence of leader RNA sequences on nascent chains. J. Virol. 48, 633-640.

3. Baric, R. S., Stohlman, S. A., Razavi, M. K., and Lai, M. M. C. (1985). Characterization of leader-related small RNAs in coronavirus-infected cells: Further evidence for leader-primed mechanism of transcription. Virus Res. 3, 19-33.

4. Gubler, U., and Hoffman, B. J. (1983). A simple and very efficient method for generating cDNA libraries. Gene 25, 263-269.

5. Lai, M. M. C. (1986). Coronavirus leader-RNA-primed transcription: an alternative mechanism to RNA splicing. BioEssays 5, 257-260.

6. Lai, M. M. C., Baric, R. S., Brayton, P. R., and Stohlman, S. A. (1984). Characterization of leader RNA sequences on the virion and mRNAs of mouse hepatitis virus, a cytoplasmic RNA virus. Proc. Natl. Acad. Sci. USA 81, 3626-3630.

7. Lai, M. M. C., Brayton, P. R., Armen, R. C., Patton, C. D., Pugh, C., and Stohlman, S. A. (1981). Mouse hepatitis virus A59: mRNA structure and genetic localization of the sequence divergence from hepatotropic strain MHV-3. J. Virol. 39, 823-834.

8. Lai, M. M. C., Makino, S., Soe, L. H., Shieh, C.-K., Keck, J. G., and Fleming, J. O. (1987). Coronavirus: A jumping RNA transcription. Cold Spring Harbor Symposia on Quantitative Biology, Vol. LII, 359-365.

9. Lai, M. M. C., Patton, C. D., Baric, R. S., and Stohlman, S. A. (1983). Presence of leader sequences in the mRNA of mouse hepatitis virus. J. Virol. 46, 1027-1033.

10. Lai, M. M. C., Patton, C. D., and Stohlman, S. A. (1982). Replication of mouse hepatitis virus: Negative-stranded RNA and replicative form RNA are of genome length. J. Virol. 44, 487-492.

11. Lai, M. M. C., and Stohlman, S. A. (1978). RNA of mouse hepatitis virus. J. Virol. 26, 236-242.

12. Leibowitz, J. L., Wilhelmsen, K. C., and Bond, C. W. (1981). The virus-specific intracellular RNA species of two murine coronavirus: MHV-A59 and MHV-JHM. Virology 114, 39-51.

13. Levis, R., Weiss, B. G., Tsiang, M., Huang, H. and Schlesinger, S. (1986). Deletion mapping of Sindbis virus DI RNAs derived from cDNAs defines the sequences essential for replication and packaging. Cell 44, 137-145.

14. Makino, S., Fujioka, N., and Fujiwara, K. (1985). Structure of the intracellular defective viral RNAs of defective interfering particles of mouse hepatitis virus. J. Virol. 54, 329-336.

15. Makino, S., and Lai, M. M. C. (1989). Evolution of the 5'-end of genomic RNA of murine coronaviruses during passages in vitro. Virology 169, 227-232.

16. Makino, S., Shieh, C.-K., Keck, J. G., and Lai, M. M. C. (1988). Defective-interfering particles of murine coronaviruses: Mechanism of synthesis of defective viral RNAs. Virology 163, 104-111.

17. Makino, S., Soe, L. H., Shieh, C.-K., and Lai, M. M. C. (1988). Discontinuous transcription generates heterogeneity at the leader fusion sites of coronavirus mRNAs. J. Virol. 62, 3870-3873.

18. Makino, S., Stohlman, S. A., and Lai, M. M. C. (1986). Leader sequences of murine coronavirus mRNAs can be freely reassorted: Evidence for the role of free leader RNA in transcription. Proc. Natl. Acad. Sci. USA 83, 4204-4208.

19. Makino, S., Taguchi, F., and Fujiwara, K. (1984). Defective interfering particles of mouse hepatitis virus. Virology 133, 9-17.

20. Makino, S., Taguchi, F., Hirano, N., and Fujiwara, K. (1984). Analysis of genomic and intracellular viral RNAs of small plaque mutants of mouse hepatitis virus, JHM strain. Virology 139, 138-151.

21. McMaster, G. K., and Carmichael, G. G. (1977). Analysis of single- and double-stranded nucleic acids on polyacrylamide and agarose gels by using glyoxal and acridine orange. Proc. Natl. Acad. Sci. USA 74, 4835-4838.

22. Shieh, C.-K., Soe, L. H., Makino, S., Chang, M.-F., Shohlman, S. A., and Lai, M. M. C. (1987). The 5'-end sequence of the murine coronavirus genome: Implications for multiple fusion sites in leader-primed transcription. Virology 156, 321-330.

23. Skinner, M. A., and Siddell, S. G. (1983). Coronavirus JHM: Nucleotide sequence of the mRNA that encodes nucleocapsid protein. Nucleic Acid Res. 15, 5045-5054.

24. Soe, L. H., Shieh, C.-K., Baker, S. C., Chang, M.-F., and Lai, M. M. C. (1987). Sequence and translation of the murine coronavirus 5'-end genomic RNA reveals the N-terminal structure of the putative RNA polymerase. J. Virol. 61, 3968-3976.

25. Spaan, W., Delius, H., Skinner, M., Armstrong, J., Rottier, P., Smeekens, S., van der Zeijst, B. A. M., and Siddell, S. G. (1983). Coronavirus mRNA synthesis involves fusion of non-contiguous sequences. EMBO J. 2, 1939-1944.

26. Zimmern, D., and Kaesburg, P. (1978). 3'-terminal nucleotide sequence of encephalomyocarditis virus RNA determined by reverse transcriptase and chain terminating inhibitors. Proc. Natl. Acad. Sci. USA 75, 4257-4261.

MURINE CORONAVIRUS TEMPERATURE SENSITIVE MUTANTS

Ralph S. Baric[1]*, Mary C. Schaad[1], Theodore Wei[2]
Kaisong Fu[1], Karen Lum[1], Carol Shieh[1] and
Stephen A. Stohlman[2]

[1]Department of Parasitology and Laboratory Practice
School of Public Health
University of North Carolina at Chapel Hill
Chapel Hill, North Carolina 27599

[2]Department of Neurology and Microbiology
University of Southern California
School of Medicine
Mckibben Annex 142
2025 Zonal Avenue
Los Angeles, California 90033

INTRODUCTION

Mouse hepatitis virus (MHV), a member of the Coronaviridae, contains a single-stranded, nonsegmented, plus-polarity RNA of 8.0×10^6 daltons molecular weight [1]. The ~32KB genomic RNA is organized into seven genetic regions each encoding one or more viral proteins [1,2]. In the virion, the RNA is enclosed in a helical nucleocapsid structure constructed from multiple copies of a 50-60KD phosphorylated nucleocapsid protein(N). The viral envelope is derived from modified host internal membranes and contains two virus-encoded glycoproteins designated M (gp23) and S(gp180/90) [1,3].

Upon entry into the host cell, the genomic RNA is translated into an RNA-dependent RNA polymerase which directs the synthesis of a full length negative-stranded RNA [4]. In turn, the negative-stranded RNA acts as template for the synthesis of seven virus specific mRNAs [4,5]. The most probable mechanism to explain the mechanism of MHV transcription involves the synthesis of a free leader RNA(s) which act in trans as a primer for mRNA synthesis [7,8,9,10,11]. Unfortunately, little data is available concerning the location and function of individual viral genes which participate in RNA synthesis. It is suspected that one or more viral proteins are encoded which regulate negative-strand synthesis, leader RNA synthesis, mRNA synthesis and genome replication.

Temperature sensitive (ts) mutants of animal viruses are useful for assigning particular physiologic, biochemical and pathogenic functions to individual viral genes. Complementation analysis of MHV ts mutants suggest that at least six RNA$^-$ and two RNA$^+$ complementation groups are encoded in the MHV genome [12,13]. The location and function of these complementation groups in viral transcription is not clear. In this article, we describe the isolation and characterization of several complementation groups of MHV-A59 which function in positive and/or

Coronaviruses and Their Diseases
Edited by D. Cavanagh and T.D.K. Brown
Plenum Press, New York, 1990

negative-strand synthesis. Utilizing genetic recombination techniques, these data indicate that the four RNA⁻ complementation groups used in this study map a linear array at the 5'end of the genome in the 21KB polymerase region, and also suggest that the RNA recombination frequency for the MHV-A59 genome may approach 25%.

METHODS
Virus and Cell Lines

The A59 strain of mouse hepatitis virus (MHV-A59) was used throughout the course of this study. Virus was propagated and cloned three times in the continuous murine astrocytoma cell line (DBT). Prior to use in these experiments, cloned MHV-A59 at passage level six at 39°C, was plaque purified 2X in DBT cells at 39°C.

Temperature Shift Experiments

Cultures of DBT cells were infected at a MOI of 2 with different ts mutants and maintained at 32°C. Following incubation at 32°C for 5.5 hrs, duplicate cultures were shifted to restrictive temperature by the addition of prewarmed media and virus progeny harvested at different times post-infection for analysis by plaque assay. In addition, intracellular RNA was extracted at 5.5, 7.5, 9.5, and 11.5 hrs post-infection and analyzed for the presence of viral mRNA with strand specific RNA probes representing the N gene sequence [13]. Alternatively, filters were probed with strand specific RNA probes which specifically hybridize genome or (-)-stranded RNA.

Recombination Test

Various combinations of ts mutants were mixed and inoculated onto cells at a multiplicity of infection of 10 each. Plates were rocked every 15 mins for 1 hr at room temperature and the inoculum removed. Individual wells were washed gently 2X with 2 mls of warm PBS and incubated at 32°C for 16 hrs in 2 mls of dMEM containing 10% antibiotic/antimycotic. Virus progeny were harvested and frozen at -70°C for future study. Each cross was titered at 32°C and 39.5°C by plaque assay and the recombination frequencies calculated as the percent of recombinant ts⁺ virus present in the progeny utilizing techniques previously reported for picornaviruses [15,16].

Recombination frequencies were standardized against a standard cross (LA7 x LA9) that was included in each experiment to obviate day to day variation. LA7 and LA9 were chosen as controls because LA7 maps 7 to 8KB from the 3'end of the genome in the gp180/90 envelope glycoprotein gene while LA9 maps in the polymerase gene at the 5'end of the genome [17,18,19,20]. The average recombination frequency for each cross was calculated from 5 to 10 individual crosses which had been standardized to the control cross. The ts mutants were arranged according to standard genetic practices.

RESULTS
Isolation and Characterization of MHV-A59 Ts Mutants

Mutants were screened for the ability to form plaques at the permissive, but not restrictive temperature, and only those isolates which showed a differential titer of at least 1 x 10⁻³ were retained for further study. Fourteen ts mutants were isolated from MHV-A59 infected cells that had been treated with 20ug/ml 5-azacytidine and an additional four mutants were isolated from 5-fluorouracil treated cultures. Two mutants were derived from cultures treated with either 350ug/ml of 5-fluorouracil (LA14, LA15) or with 450ug/ml of the drug (LA16, LA18). The

RNA phenotype of each mutant was analyzed at the nonpermissive temperature by the incorporation of ^{3}H-uridine into acid precipitable material from actinomycin D-treated virus-infected cells. Four of the ts mutants (LA7, LA12, LA13, NC5) were considered to be of RNA positive phenotype since levels of transcription at 39°C were at least 35% of the wildtype controls. The remaining 14 mutants were of the RNA⁻ phenotype since transcription at 32°C was less than 7% of the parental virus (Data not shown).

To determine the number of genetic functions represented in our panel of ts mutants, complementation analyses were performed. The complementation index for the ts mutants used in this study are summarized in Table 1. These data indicate that four RNA⁻ (A,B,C, and D) and one RNA⁺ (E) complementation groups are represented within this panel of ts mutants. These data are compatible with previous results obtained by other groups with MHV-A59, JHM, or MHV-3 ts mutants. All RNA⁻ mutants tested were incapable of transcribing mRNA, (-)-stranded RNA or genome at the restrictive temperature (Date not shown).

TABLE 1. COMPLEMENTATION GROUPS OF MHV-A59

GROUP A	-	LA3, LA6, LA16,
GROUP B	-	LA9, LA8, LA14,
GROUP C	-	LA10
GROUP D	-	LA18, NC4
GROUP E	-	LA7, LA12, NC5

Virus Growth Curves Following Temperature Shift

Temperature shift experiments immediately after the onset of positive strand RNA synthesis have elucidated the basic genetics of alphavirus transcription and replication. Duplicate cultures of cells were infected with different RNA⁻ or RNA⁺ ts mutants and incubated at 32°C for 5.5 hrs. One-half the cultures were shifted to restrictive temperature by the addition of prewarmed media, and virus progeny assayed at 7.5, 9.5, 11.5, and 16.0 hrs post-infection. Shift to restrictive temperature blocked the release of infectious virus from complementation groups A, C and D (RNA⁻ mutants). In contrast, the replication of the RNA⁻ group B mutant LA9 was unaffected by shift to restrictive temperature and continued to released infectious virus. The RNA⁺ group E mutant was also blocked in the ability to release infectious virus after shift to restrictive temperature (Data not shown).

Analysis of MHV RNA Synthesis following Temperature Shift

Previous studies demonstrated the presence of two classes of RNA⁻ mutants defective in either an early (Group B) or late function (Groups A,C,D,E) in virus replication. We next examined the ability of these mutants to transcribe mRNA following shift to restrictive temperature. Duplicate culture of cells were infected with ts mutants and maintained at 32°C for 5-6 hrs. One-half of the cultures were shifted to restrictive temperature by the addition of pre-warmed media, and intracellular RNA isolated at different times post-infection. The RNA was bound to nitrocellulose filters and hybridized with an N gene strand specific RNA probe which detects all viral positive-sensed mRNAs. As expected, the RNA⁺ complementation group synthesized viral RNA after shift to restrictive temperature. Consistent with the inability to shed infectious virus, RNA⁻ complementation groups A, C and D were defective in mRNA synthesis following shift to restrictive temperature. Conversely, the group E RNA$^+$ and group B RNA$^-$ complementation groups continued to transcribe RNA at restrictive temperature. Complementation groups A,C and D, but not B or E, were also defective in the synthesis of genomic RNA (Table 2).

In cultures radiolabeled with ^{32}P-orthophosphate, increasing amounts of viral mRNA were synthezied in group B-infected cells that were shifted to restrictive temperature at progressively later times post-infection (data not shown). These data indicate that the group B mutants were defective in an early event in virus transcription which effects the overall rates of positive strand synthesis later in infection.

TABLE 2. FUNCTIONAL ANALYSIS OF THE MHV-A59 COMPLEMENTATION GROUPS.

	GENOME	mRNA	(-) RNA	LEADER	FUNCTION
GROUP A	-	-	-	-	CORE
GROUP B	+	+	-	+	(-) RNA
GROUP C	-	-	?	+	mRNA
GROUP D	-	-	+	- ?	LEADER?
GROUP E	+	+	+	+	?

Complementation groups A,B and D were also examined for the ability to transcribe (-)-stranded RNA and leader RNA after shift to restrictive temperature. Infected cultures were maintained at permissive temperature for 5.5 hrs post-infection, and shifted to restrictive temperature. Intracellular RNA was extracted at 5.5, 7.5, 9.5 and 11.5 hrs post-infection and probed for the presence of (-)-stranded RNA with strand specific RNA probes. Complementation groups A and B were blocked in the ability to transcribe (-)-stranded RNA at restrictive temperature. Under identical conditions the group D mutants continued to transcribe (-)RNA following shift to restrictive temperature (Table 2). These data indicate that groups A and B are defective in (-)RNA synthesis at restrictive temperature while group D mutants were blocked at a later stage in the virus growth cycle. In cultures monitored for leader RNA synthesis following shift to restrictive temperature, complementation that groups A and D were probably defective in the synthesis of small leader RNAs while groups B,C and E were not (Table 2).

Recombination Mapping

Utilizing standard genetic recombination techniques, poliovirus and apthovirus ts mutants have been arranged into an additive, linear, genetic map with mutants at different locations differing in physiologic function [16,17,18]. To obtain a genetic recombination map, ts mutants from each complementation group were crossed with LA7 and LA9 and standardized to the standard cross (LA7 x LA9 - 4.45 $\pm$ 0.845). In addition, mutants from each group were crossed between mutants from other groups to provide unequivocal positioning. All the distances between complementation groups were within statistical limits and permit the construction of a genetic map (Figure 1). From the 5'end of the genome, the order of the complementation groups was: A, B, C, D, and E. Crosses between ts mutants in the same complementation group had characteristically low recombination frequencies. Not surprisingly, higher recombination frequencies were observed between mutants representing different complementation groups and were as high as 8.6% between group E (LA7) and group A (LA6) mutants. Group B and C mutants also had high recombination frequencies and support previous findings that these mutants map in the polymerase gene at the 5'end of the genome 18,19,20. It seems likely that the group D mutants also map at the 3'end of the polymerase gene since our data clearly indicate that this group is incapable of transcribing plus or minus-stranded RNA when maintained at restrictive temperature.

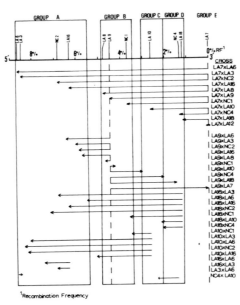

FIGURE 1. ESTABLISHING A GENETIC RECOMBINATION MAP OF THE MHV-A59 COMPLEMENTATION GROUPS

DISCUSSION

Little information is currently available concerning the number, location and function of the viral genes which participate in MHV transcription. Previous studies indicate that continous protein synthesis is a prerequisite for both positive and negative transcription and that MHV negative-strand synthesis is regulated temporally during infection [23]. Brayton et al [4,5] have described polymerase activities in MHV-infected cells which preferentially transcribe negative-stranded RNA, mRNA and genome. Temporal regulation of genome replication has been observed in BCV-infected cells [28]. Other groups have also demonstrated in vitro mRNA and/or genome transcription and shown that anti-N mABs block-in vitro transcription [24]. These data are supported by studies in our laboratory suggesting that N is tightly associated with the transcription complex and leader RNA. These data suggest that distinct functions are encoded in the MHV genome which regulate negative-strand synthesis, leader RNA synthesis, mRNA synthesis and genome replication.

The RNA⁻ mutants used in this study are incapable of transcribing any detectable levels of viral RNA at the restrictive temperature. However, temperature shift experiments after the onset of mRNA synthesis clearly revealed the presence of several classes of RNA⁻ mutants (Table 2). Preliminary data suggest that group A mutants are defective in leader RNA, mRNA, genome and negative-strand transcription at restrictive temperature and probably represent a core function required during each stage in RNA synthesis. One possibility is that the group A mutants

353

represent the protease encoded 5-6KB from the 5'end of the genome. Group C mutants synthesize leader RNA, but not mRNA at restrictive temperature, and probably encode a gene which functions during mRNA synthesis. Group D mutants transcribe negative-sensed RNA, but not leader RNA, mRNA or genome at restrictive temperature, and probably a function during leader RNA transcription. Complementation group B clearly encodes a genetic function which effects the rate of positive strand RNA synthesis following shift to restrictive temperature. Our data suggests that the group B allele functions during negative-strand synthesis. At least two additional RNA⁻ complementation groups have been demonstrated by other investigators in the field. The function of these groups is currently unclear.

T₁ fingerprint analysis of recombinant virus suggest that complementation groups A, B and C map in the polymerase gene at the 5'end of the genome and that the group E mutants map in the S envelope glycoprotein gene roughly 7-8KB from the 3'end of the genome [17,18,19,20]. Intratypic recombination frequencies between group A and E mutants approaches 8.6% or 17.2% assuming reciprocal crosses (Figure 2). Since LA7 maps ~23-24KB from the 5'end of the 32KB MHV genome and group A mutants probably do not map in the p28 protein encoded within the first 1.1KB at the 5'end of the genome, a 17.2% recombination frequency occurs over a ~22.5KB nucleotide domain or a 1% recombination frequency/1300 nucleotide pairs of RNA. Assuming an equivalent recombination frequency for the entire 32KB genome, these data predict that the recombination frequency for the MHV genome may approach 25%. Genetic recombination maps for poliovirus and apthoviruses predict a recombination frequency of 2.2% for the entire viral genome [15,16,17,29]. Thus, MHV high frequency recombination [37] approaches the reassortment frequency of segmented RNA viruses and suggests that segmented RNA intermediates may reassort during mixed MHV infection. We have previously demonstrated the presence of small RNA intermediates bound to or dissociated from the replicative intermediate RNA [9]. It remains to be determined if the small RNAs represent the functional intermediates of RNA transcription and recombination.

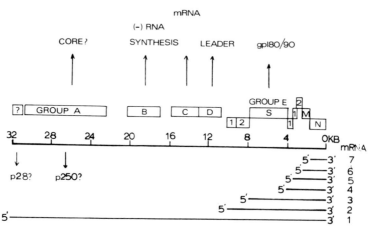

FIGURE 2. TENTATIVE MAP DOMAINS OF EACH MHV-A59 COMPLEMENTATION GROUP

Utilizing genetic recombination mapping techniques, we have formulated the first genetic map of the MHV-A59 ts mutants. The orientation of these complementation groups from the 5'end of the genome was A, B, C, D and E. Assuming a 1% recombination frequency/1300 nucleotide pairs of RNA, the nucleotide domains of each MHV-A59 complementation group can be calculated from the map domains illustrated in figure 1 (figure 2). Complementation groups A, B, C and D

definitively map in the polmerase region at the 5'end of the genome.
These data suggest that at least twelve genetic functions are encoded in
the MHV genome including four in the polymerase region, two each in
mRNAs2 and 5, and a single genetic function in mRNAs 3, 4, 6 and 7
(figure 2) [1,30,31,32,33]. The location of the two additional RNA⁻
complementation groups detected in other panels of ts mutants is unclear
but could reside in the polymerase region or internally in the viral
genome. By size analysis, the group A mutants map over a 7-8KB stretch
of RNA that could encode a protein of ~250-300KD molecular weight. In
vitro, the MHV genome is translated into a 250-300KD polyprotein which is
subsequently cleaved into a p28 and p220 protein [34,35]. The p28 protein
is encoded within the first 1.1KB from the 5'end of the genome [35,36].
These data suggest that the group A mutants do not map in the p28 protein
encoded at the 5'end of the genome and suggest that a fifth genetic
function is encoded in the polymerase region. We are currently
determining the genetic location and function of additional ts mutants of
MHV-A59.

ACKNOWLEDGEMENTS

The authors would like to express their appreciation to Phyllis
Driscoll and Gillian Harris for excellent technical and secretarial
assistance. This work was supported in part by a grant-in-aid from the
American Heart Association (AHA 871135) and a grant from the National
Institute of Health (AI 23946). This work was done during the tenure of
an Established Investigatorship of the American Heart Association (AHA
890193) (RSB).

REFERENCES

1. Spaan, W.J. et al (1988) J. Gen. Virol. 69:2939-2952
2. Siddell, S. (1983) J. Gen. Virol. 64:113-125
3. Sturman, L.S. et al (1980) J. Virol. 33:449-462
4. Brayton, P.R. et al (1982) J. Virol. 42:847-853
5. Brayton, P.R. et al (1984) Virol. 133:197-201
6. Lai, M.M.MC et al (1984) PNAS USA 81:3626-3630
7. Baric, R.S. et al (1983) J. Virol. 48:633-640
8. Makino, S. et al (1986a) PNAS USA 83:4204-4208
9. Baric, R.S. et al (1987) Virol. 156:342-354
10. Shieh, C-K., et al. (1987) Virology 156:321-330
11. Spaan, W.J. et al (1983) EMBO 2:1839-1844
12. Leibowitz, J. et al (1982) J. Virol. 42:1080-1087
13. Koolen, M.J. et al (1983) Viro. 125:393-402
14. Martin, J.P. et al (1988) J. Gen. Virol.
15. Mackenzie, J.S. et al (1975) J. Gen. Virol. 27:61-70
16. Lake, J.R. et al (1975) J. Gen. Virol. 27:355-367
17. Cooper, P.D. (1968) Virol. 35:584-596
18. Lai, M.M.C. et al (1985) J. Virol. 56:449-456
19. Keck, J.G. et al (1988b) J. Virol. 62:1810-1813
20. Keck, J.G. et al (1987) Virol. 156:331-341
21. Sawicki, D.L. and Sawicki, S.G. (1987) J. Virol. 25:19-27
22. Sawicki, S.G. and Sawicki, D.L. (1981) J. Virol. 115:161-172
23. Sawicki, S.G. and Sawicki, D.L. (1986) J. Virol. 57:328-334
24. Compton, S.R. et al (1987) J. Virol. 61: 1814-1820
25. Baric, R.S. et al (1988) J. Virol. 62: 4280-4287
26. Stohlman, S.A. et al (1988) J. Virol. 62:4288-4295
27. Baric, R.S. et al (1985)) Vir. Res. 3:19-33
28. Keck, J.G. et al (1988a) Vir. Res 9:343-356
29. Kirkkegaard, K. and Baltimore, D. (1986) Cell 47:433-443
30. Luytjes, W. et al (1988) Virol. In Press
31. Skinner, M.S. et al (1985) J. Gen. Virol 66:581-592

32. Skinner, M.A. et al (1985) J. Gen. Virol 66: 593-596
33. Amstrong, J. et al (1984) Nature (London) 308:731-752
34. Dennison, M.R. and S. Perlman (1987) Virol. 60:12-18
35. Dennison, M.R. and S. Perlman (1988) Virol. 157:565-568
36. Soe, L. et al (1987) J. Virol. 61:3968-3976
37. Fields, B.N. (1981) Corr. Top. Micro. Imm. 91:1-24

GENOMIC ORGANISATION OF A VIRULENT ISOLATE OF PORCINE TRANSMISSIBLE

GASTROENTERITIS VIRUS

P. Britton, K. W. Page, D. J. Pulford, D. J. Garwes,
K. Mawditt, F. Stewart, F. Parra*, C. Lopez Otin*,
J. Martin Alonso* and R. S. Carmenes*

AFRC Institute for Animal Health, Compton Laboratory
Compton, Newbury, Berkshire, RG16 0NN, U.K.
*Departamento de Biologia Funcional (Area de Bioquimica)
Universidad de Oviedo, Oviedo, Spain

INTRODUCTION

Transmissible gastroenteritis virus (TGEV) causes gastroenteritis in
pigs of all ages but has a high mortality in neonatal piglets. In piglets,
under two weeks of age, the first clinical sign is usually vomiting 18-24 h
after infection rapidly followed by a diarrhoea, resulting in loss of
weight and dehydration; death usually occurs after 2-5 days (1). Like all
the other coronaviruses TGEV proteins are expressed from a 'nested' set
of subgenomic mRNAs which have common 3' termini but different 5' extensions. The region of each mRNA responsible for the expression of a protein
appears to correspond to the 5'-terminal region that is absent on the
preceding smaller species. Mouse hepatitis virus (MHV) and infectious
bronchitis virus (IBV) mRNA species contain identical short non-coding
sequences at their 5' ends, specific to each virus, which appear to be
joined to the sequences encoding the viral genes by discontinuous transcription. A consensus sequence identified upstream of each gene/ORF may
act as a binding site for the RNA polymerase-leader complex (2, 3, 4, 5, 6).
It has been previously postulated that a heptameric sequence , ACTAAC (7)
or a hexameric sequence, CTAAAC (8, 9, 10) may be involved in the binding
of the TGEV RNA polymerase-leader complex. The TGEV virion contains three
major structural polypeptides; a surface glycoprotein (spike or peplomer
protein) with a monomeric M_r 200000, a glycosylated integral membrane
protein observed as a series of polypeptides of M_r 28000-31000 and a basic
phosphorylated protein (the nucleoprotein) of M_r 47000 associated with the
viral genomic RNA (11). TGEV infected cells, in addition to the genomic
RNA, have six species of subgenomic mRNA (12).

RESULTS AND DISCUSSION

Isolation of TGEV mRNA

TGEV strain FS772/70, a virulent British field isolate, was grown in
LLC-PK1 cells in the presence of [^{3}H]-uracil and actinomycin D (13).
Messenger RNA was isolated from the cells and purified on poly(U) Sepharose
as described previously (14). Analysis of the TGEV mRNA species isolated

Coronaviruses and Their Diseases
Edited by D. Cavanagh and T.D.K. Brown
Plenum Press, New York, 1990

357

from virus infected cells revealed six species whose products have now been determined by sequence and expression studies (14, 7, 15, 16, 17, 18).

cDNA cloning

A series of cDNA clones were obtained from TGEV mRNA species using either an oligo(dT)-tailed vector-primer, a specific restriction endo-nuclease fragment as a primer (7) or a specific oligonucleotide primer (15, 16). The clones shown in Fig. 1 overlapped each other and covered 10.5 kb of the TGEV genome from the 3' end. Clone pTS15-1 was generated using an oligo(dT)-tailed vector primer (7). Clone pF4F-36 was generated using a specific restriction endonuclease fragment derived from clone pTS15-1 (15). The rest of the clones were generated using a specific oligonucleotide primer whose sequence was derived from clone pF4F-36 and was complementary to a sequence between the integral membrane protein and nucleoprotein genes (15, 16). The clones were mapped using restriction endonuclease mapping and northern blot analysis to TGEV mRNA species.

DNA sequencing

The cDNA clones were sequenced, as described previously (7, 15, 16), by the dideoxy method, using restriction endonuclease fragments from the various cDNA clones in M13. Parts of the clones containing ORFs 1-3 were sequenced using specific oligonucleotides as primers (16). Most of clone pTG47 was sequenced using specific oligonucleotides as primers (unpublished results).

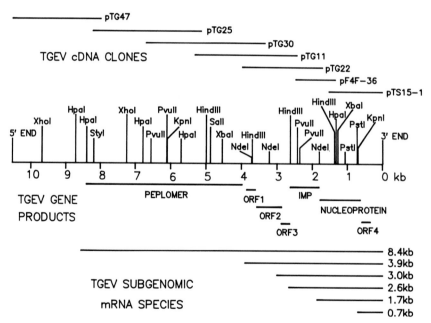

Fig. 1.   Shows the positions of the cDNA clones used to determine the nucleotide sequence and the identification of the various TGEV genes. The restriction sites shown were used in the mapping of the various clones and are not always unique sites.

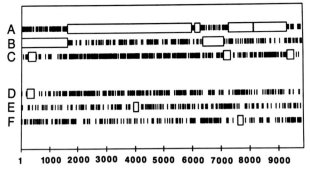

Fig. 2. Diagram showing the positions of potential open reading frames
along the TGEV genome sequenced. The letters denote the six
reading frames on both strands: A, B and C represent ORFs on the
positive sense and D, E and F ORFs on the negative sense strands.
Gene sequences of 170 bp and greater are shown and are represented
as open boxes. The vertical lines denote stope codons.

Analysis of the TGEV genome

Fig. 2 shows the translation of all six reading frames, using the
computer program SIXFRAMES, 9866 nucleotides from the 3'. end of the TGEV
(FS772/70) genome. Potential open reading frames were identified by the
initiation codon, ATG, and the presence of one of the three stop codons at
a determined distance.

Four potential open reading frames were identified from Fig. 2 in
frame A of the positive strand. The largest open reading frame (ORF)
corresponding to a polypeptide of M_r 159811 is the peplomer gene. The
identity of this gene product was initially determined by its homology to
other coronavirus peplomer proteins. The confirmation that the open reading
frame was the peplomer gene resulted from the construction of the gene from
the various cDNA clones (unpublished result) and by its expression in
recombinant vaccinia viruses (18). The next ORF, ORF-1, has a capacity to
express a polypeptide of M_r 6600 (16). The potential gene is slightly
smaller than the one identified from the avirulent Purdue strain of TGEV
(10), X2a, corresponding to a polypeptide of M_r 7700. The next two ORFs on
frame A encode polypeptides of M_r 29459 and M_r 43483 and are the integral
membrane protein and nucleoprotein genes. These were initially identified
by homology to other coronavirus proteins. The identity of the nucleoprotein gene was confirmed by antibodies raised against a β-galactosidase
chimaera which reacted against nucleoprotein produced in TGEV infected
cells (14) and by the expression of the nucleoprotein gene in Saccharomyces
cerevisiae (7) and by recombinant vaccinia virus (18). The identity of
the integral membrane protein gene was confirmed by antibodies raised
against a β-galactosidase chimaera reacting with the integral membrane
protein from TGEV infected cells (15) and by the expression of the integral
membrane protein gene by recombinant vaccinia virus and recombinant baculovirus (18).

Analysis of frame B revealed two potential ORFs. The first was a
contiguous ORF from the 5' end of the cDNA with no initiation codon and
will be dealt with later in the article. The second ORF, ORF-2, encodes a
potential polypeptide of M_r 27600. This potential gene is much larger than
the one identified from the avirulent Purdue strain of TGEV (10), X2b,
corresponding to a polypeptide of M_r 18800.

Analysis of frame C revealed the presence of three potential ORFs. The first was within the contiguous ORF identified at the 5' end of the cDNA. The other two ORFs, ORF-3 and ORF-4, encode potential polypeptides of M_r 9200 and M_r 9068. ORF-3 is very similar to the ORF, X1, identified from the avirulent Purdue strain of TGEV (10). ORF-4 is very similar to the ORF identified from the avirulent Purdue strain of TGEV (8, 10), termed X3.

Antibodies were raised against a synthetic oligopeptide, 12B/86 (17), whose sequence was taken from the derived amino acid sequence from the FS772/70 ORF-4 cDNA sequence (7). The antibodies reacted to a polypeptide of M_r 14000 in TGEV infected cells when analysed by SDS polyacrylamide gel electrophoresis. The difference between the predicted and observed molecular weights of this polypeptide may arise from the very hydrophobic nature of the polypeptide (35% leucine residues). Comparison of ORF-4 gene product from FS772/70 with Purdue has identified an amino acid substitution at residue 30, introducing a potential N-glycosylation site (7), which may account for the difference observed between the expected and the experimentally determined M_r. The cellular location of the polypeptide was shown to be the cell nucleus using 12B/86 antibodies against TGEV infected and uninfected cells fixed with acetone. At 10 h post-infection the cells underwent a marked cytopathology and the presence of ORF-4 was less obvious due to degradation of the nucleus (17). There is some evidence of a "leucine zipper" motif (19), at leucine residues 21, 28 and 35 of ORF-4, which is a characteristic property of some DNA-binding proteins indicating a possible reason for the location of ORF-4 in the cell nucleus.

The amino acid sequences of ORFs 1-3 show no homology to any other coronavirus proteins, proteins in the PIR protein database, or deduced amino acid sequences from the DNA sequences in the EMBL (20) and GENBANK (21) nucleic acid sequence database using the TFASTA (22) computer program (16). A potential gene, with homology to the TGEV ORF-4 gene product, encoding a polypeptide of M_r 11000 has been identified 3' to the nucleoprotein in feline infectious peritonitis virus (FIPV) (23). ORF-4 does not have any homology to any other coronavirus proteins, proteins in the PIR database, or the deduced amino acid sequences from the nucleotide sequence databases. The presence of this gene in TGEV and FIPV, the homology of other genes and cross-reactivity of their antibodies, indicate that the two viruses may have evolved from a common ancestral virus. The gene in FIPV has an insert increasing the size of the potential product and is followed by yet another potential gene that is absent from TGEV (23). It will be interesting to know if FIPV has the equivalents of the TGEV ORFs 1-3.

Consensus sequence

A heptameric sequence, ACTAAAC, has been observed at the start of each of the three structural protein genes and most of the other ORFs. Analysis of the 9866 nucleotide sequence with this heptameric sequence by the FITCONSENSUS program (24) is shown in Table 1. The only gene that does not have the complete consensus sequence is ORF-3 which has the hexameric sequence CTAAAC. It is interesting to note that the ORF-3 mRNA species is the least abundant message (12), possibly resulting from the difference in the consensus sequence. This may allow some control over the level of synthesis and translation of the gene product. ORFs 1-2 are carried at the 5' end of the 3.9 kb mRNA (16) and whether both or just one is translated has yet to be determined. ORF-3 is present on the 5' end of the 3.0 kb mRNA (16). No 3.7 kb mRNA species, which would correspond to the theoretical size of a mRNA with just the ORF-2 at the 5' end, was detected in TGEV infected cells using specific cDNA probes from within the gene sequence (16). The mRNA species containing the other TGEV genes at their 5' ends are shown in Fig. 1.

Table 1. Computer search for the heptameric sequence ACTAAAC
using FITCONSENSUS (24)

Score	Position	Sequence	TGEV mRNA/gene
85.71	19	ACTAAgC	
85.71	214	AaTAAAC	
100	1611	ACTAAAC	PEPLOMER
85.71	2433	ACTAcAC	
85.71	2529	ACcAAAC	
85.71	3502	ACTtAAC	
85.71	4203	ACTAcAC	
100	6072	ACTAAAC	ORF-1/ORF-2
85.71	6293	AgTAAAC	
85.71	6326	ACaAAAC	
85.71	6522	ACaAAAC	
85.71	7059	tCTAAAC	ORF-3
100	7349	ACTAAAC	IMP
85.71	8086	ACTcAAC	
100	8147	ACTAAAC	NUC
85.71	9114	ACTgAAC	
100	9304	ACTAAAC	ORF-4
85.71	9472	ACTAAAa	

Codon usage

An amino acid codon usage table was constructed using the three
structural protein genes and ORFs 1-4. These are shown in Table 2. There
is a distinctive bias for some of the codons, for example the codon GGT
for glycine is used three times more than two of the other glycine codons

Table 2. Codon usage table determined from the TGEV
structural protein genes and from ORFs 1-4

F TTT	94.	S TCT	55.	Y TAT	67.	C TGT	43.
F TTC	33.	S TCC	21.	Y TAC	49.	C TGC	25.
L TTA	75.	S TCA	39.	* TAA	5.	* TGA	1.
L TTG	54.	S TCG	4.	* TAG	1.	W TGG	42.
L CTT	66.	P CCT	39.	H CAT	26.	R CGT	21.
L CTC	16.	P CCC	9.	H CAC	14.	R CGC	10.
L CTA	36.	P CCA	27.	Q CAA	60.	R CGA	4.
L CTG	9.	P CCG	5.	Q CAG	26.	R CGG	4.
I ATT	84.	T ACT	72.	N AAT	120.	S AGT	63.
I ATC	17.	T ACC	24.	N AAC	56.	S AGC	22.
I ATA	58.	T ACA	74.	K AAA	68.	R AGA	44.
M ATG	40.	T ACG	18.	K AAG	40.	R AGG	24.
V GTT	89.	A GCT	68.	D GAT	82.	G GGT	90.
V GTC	32.	A GCC	24.	D GAC	45.	G GGC	32.
V GTA	48.	A GCA	63.	E GAA	75.	G GGA	31.
V GTG	48.	A GCG	7.	E GAG	17.	G GGG	7.

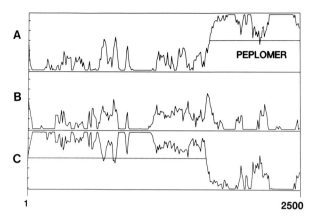

Fig. 3. Diagram showing the potential gene 5' to the peplomer gene using codon usage determined from the three TGEV strucutral protein genes and ORFs 1-4 as shown in Table 2. Note the reading frames are different to those shown in Fig. 2 resulting from the output of different programs.

whereas GGG is rarely used. In fact, G or C in the third position appears to be the least favourable choice. Analysis of the codon usage for individual TGEV genes has shown that the codons GCG (ala), TCG (ser), CGA (arg), CTG (leu) and ATC (ile) are very rarely used suggesting that ORFs 1-3 encode genetic information and have not evolved by random incorporation of nucleotides. A TGEV codon usage table was used to analyse the contiguous ORF identified at the 5' end of the 9866 nucleotide sequence. The codons within this predicted ORF are consistent with those seen for TGEV genes indicating that this ORF is a TGEV gene (Fig. 3).

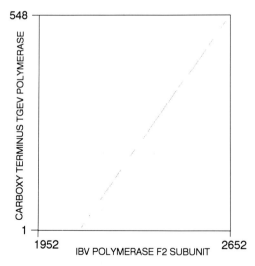

Fig. 4. Dot matrix analysis of the 548 amino acid sequence derived from the potential gene 5' to the peplomer gene against the last 700 amino acids at the carboxyl terminus of the F2 subunit from the IBV RNA-dependent-RNA polymerase. The analysis was carried out using the DIAGON program (25) using a span length of 15.

362

Comparison of the deduced amino acid sequence of this ORF with the last 700 amino acids of the F2 subunit of IBV RNA-dependent-RNA polymerase revealed high level homology (Fig. 4). Homologies between the TGEV and IBV structural proteins have been low (7, 15) indicating that the viruses diverged a long time ago and have evolved relatively different protein sequences. This is in contrast to coronaviruses of the same serological subgroup like TGEV and FIPV or MHV and BCV which show very good homologies. The homology between the contiguous 5' ORF and the carboxyl terminus of the IBV F2 subunit indicates that the TGEV ORF is the carboxyl terminus of the TGEV RNA polymerase and that the polymerase molecules may not have diverged from each other as seen with other coronavirus proteins. Whether the TGEV polymerase consists of two subunits, as seen with IBV (26), has yet to be determined.

ACKNOWLEDGEMENTS

This research was supported by the Biomolecular Engineering Programme of the Commission of the European Communities Contract No. BAP-0235-UK(HI) for Compton and Contract No. BAP-0219-E(A) for Spain. We would like to thank Dr. M. E. G. Boursnell of this Institute for the computer programme SIXFRAMES.

REFERENCES

1. D. J. Garwes, Coronaviruses in Animals, in: "Virus infection of the gastrointestinal tract," D. A. J. Tyrrell and A. Z. Kapikian, eds., Marcel Dekker Inc., New York (1982).
2. W. J. M. Spaan, H. Delius, M. Skinner, J. Armstrong, P. Rottier, S. Smeekens, B. A. M. van der Zeijst and S. G. Siddell, Coronavirus mRNA synthesis involves fusion of non-contiguous sequences. EMBO J., 2: 1839-1844 (1983).
3. T. D. K. Brown, M. E. G. Boursnell and M. M. Binns, A leader sequence is present on mRNA A of avian infectious bronchitis virus. J. Gen. Virol., 65:1437-1442 (1984).
4. M. M. C. Lai, R. S. Baric, P. R. Brayton and S. A. Stohlman, Characterization of leader RNA sequences on the virion and mRNAs of mouse hepatitis virus, a cytoplasmic RNA virus. Proc. Nat. Acad. Sci., 81:3626-3630 (1984).
5. C. J. Budzilowicz, S. P. Wilczynski and S. R. Weiss, Three intergenic regions of coronavirus mouse hepatitis virus strain A59 genome RNA contain a common nucleotide sequence that is homologous to the 3' end of the viral mRNA leader sequence. J. Virol., 53:834-840 (1985).
6. C-K. Shieh, L. H. Soe, S. Makino, M-F. Chang, S. A. Stohlman and M. M. C. Lai, The 5'-end sequence of the murine coronavirus genome: implications for multiple fusion sites in leader-primed transcription. Virology, 156:321-330 (1987).
7. P. Britton, R. S. Carmenes, K. W. Page, D. J. Garwes and F. Parra, Sequence of the nucleoprotein from a virulent British field isolate of transmissible gastroenteritis virus and its expression in Saccharomyces cerevisiae. Mol. Microbiol., 2:89-99 (1988).
8. P. A. Kapke and D. A. Brian, Sequence analysis of the porcine transmissible gastroenteritis coronavirus nucleocapsid protein gene. Virology, 151:41-49 (1986).
9. D. Rasschaert, B. Delmas, B. Charley, J. Grossclaude, J. Gelfi and H. Laude, Surface glycoproteins of transmissible gastroenteritis virus: functions and gene sequence. Adv. Exp. Med. Biol., 218:109-116 (1987).
10. D. Rasschaert, J. Gelfi and H. Laude, Enteric coronavirus TGEV: partial sequence of the genomic RNA, its organisation and expression. Biochimie, 69:591-600 (1987).

11. D. J. Garwes and D. H. Pocock, The polypeptide structure of transmissible gastroenteritis virus. J. Gen. Virol., 29:25-34 (1975).

12. P. Britton, D. J. Garwes, G. C. Millson, K. Page, L. Bountiff, F. Stewart and J. Walmsley, Towards a genetically-engineered vaccine against porcine transmissible gastroenteritis virus. In: "Biomolecular Engineering in the European Community. Final Report," E. Magnien, ed., Martinus Nijhoff, The Netherlands (1986).

13. D. J. Garwes, L. Bountiff, G. C. Millson and C. J. Elleman, Defective replication of porcine transmissible gastroenteritis virus in a continuous cell line. Adv. Exp. Med. Biol., 173:79-93 (1984).

14. P. Britton, D. J. Garwes, K. Page and J. Walmsley, Expression of porcine transmissible gastroenteritis virus genes in E. coli as β-galactosidase chimaeric proteins. Adv. Exp. Med. Biol., 218:55-64 (1987).

15. P. Britton, R. S. Carmenes, K. W. Page and D. J. Garwes, The integral membrane protein from a virulent isolate of transmissible gastroenteritis virus: Molecular characterization, sequence and expression in Escherichia coli, Mol. Microbiol., 2:297-505 (1988).

16. P. Britton, C. Lopez Otin, J. M. Martin Alonso and F. Parra, Sequence of the coding regions from the 3.0 kb and 3.9 kb mRNA subgenomic species from a virulent isolate of transmissible gastroenteritis virus, Arch. Virol., 105:(in press) (1989).

17. D. J. Garwes, F. Stewart and P. Britton, The polypeptide of M_r 14000 of porcine transmissible gastroenteritis virus: Gene assignment and intracellular location, J. Gen. Virol., 70:(in press) (1989).

18. D. J. Pulford, P. Britton, K. W. Page and D. J. Garwes, Expression of transmissible gastroenteritis virus structural genes by virus vectors, (This book).

19. W. H. Landschulz, P. F. Johnson and S. L. McKnight, The leucine zipper: A hypothetical structure common to a new class of DNA binding proteins, Science, 240:1759-1764 (1988).

20. G. H. Hamm and G. N. Cameron, The EMBL data library, Nucl. Acids Res., 14:5-10 (1986).

21. H. S. Bilofsky, C. Burks, J. W. Fickett, W. B. Goad, F. I. Lewitter, W. P. Rindone, C. D. Swindell and C-S. Tung, The Genbank genetic sequence database, Nucl. Acids Res., 13:1-4 (1986).

22. W. R. Pearson and D. J. Lipman, Improved tools for biological sequence comparison, Proc. Nat. Acad. Sci., 85:2444-2448 (1988).

23. R. J. De Groot, A. C. Adeweg, M. C. Horzinek and W. J. M. Spaan, Sequence analysis of the 3' end of the feline coronavirus FIPV 79-1146 genome: Comparison with the genome of porcine coronavirus TGEV reveals large insertions, Virology, 167:370-376 (1988).

24. J. Devereux, P. Haeberli and O. Smithies, A comprehensive set of sequence analysis programs for the VAX, Nucl. Acids Res., 12:387-395 (1984).

25. R. Staden, An interactive graphics program for comparing and aligning nucleic acid and amino acid sequences, Nucl. Acids Res., 10:2951-2961 (1982).

26. M. E. G. Boursnell, T. D. K. Brown, I. J. Foulds, P. F. Green, F. M. Tomley and M. M. Binns, Completion of the sequence of the genome of the coronavirus avian infectious bronchitis virus, J. Gen. Virol., 68:57-77 (1987).

Chapter 8

Aspects of Coronavirus Variation and Evolution

BACKGROUND PAPER

ASPECTS OF CORONAVIRUS EVOLUTION

D. Cavanagh and T.D.K. Brown

AFRC Institute for Animal Health
Houghton Laboratory, Huntingdon
Cambridgeshire PE17 2DA, UK

Department of Pathology
University of Cambridge
Tennis Court Road
Cambridge CB2 2QQ, UK

The word "evolution" usually evokes thoughts of events which occurred in the distant past, but it is self-evidently an ongoing process. The application of intense selective pressure, for example by the wide-spread use of vaccination, and also the transport of infected animals over large distances may have contributed to what may be considered "short-term" evolution. Papers relevant to putative coronavirus evolution in both recent and distant time-scales are presented in this volume.

A major contribution to our understanding of the evolution of this genus was the demonstration, both *in vitro* and *in vivo*, of high frequency recombination between strains of murine hepatitis virus (MHV) (1,3,5). Recombination has been shown to occur at many positions throughout the genome and may be related to the propensity of the replicase to fall off its template and then to continue RNA replication on the homologous or heterologous template (copy choice mechanism) during a mixed infection. A more unexpected finding has been the discovery that the HE glycoprotein possessed by some coronaviruses has homology with the HEF 1 subunit of the influenza virus C glycoprotein (4; chapter 2, this volume). This implies that at some time a coronavirus and an influenza virus (or their respective progenitors) have undergone non-homologous recombination.

Given the experimental evidence for recombination of MHV strains and the revelation regarding the HE glycoprotein it will not be surprising to find that some coronavirus isolates from the field are, in fact, recombinants. Indeed sequencing of the S and M genes of infectious bronchitis virus (IBV) strains has provided circumstantial evidence for this having occurred (2; Cavanagh *et al.*, this chapter).

Another observation which may be related to the tendency of the replicase to fall off its template is the highly variable length of the S protein among strains of MHV (7; papers in this chapter). MHV strains with different passage histories both *in vitro* and in *vivo* can differ by as many as 150 amino acids in the length of the S1 subunit. Moreover, such variants which have been selected with monoclonal antibodies differ in neurovirulence from the parental population.

An example of the economic consequences of a coronavirus "evolutionary" event, which may have occurred in the recent past, is that of the emergence of porcine respiratory coronavirus (PRCV) (chapter 9, this volume). First isolated in 1984, in Western Europe (6), this virus is closely related to porcine transmissible gastroenteritis virus (TGEV). Unlike the latter, however, the primary replication site is not the gut but the respiratory tract.

It is to be hoped that in the near future it will be made clear to what extent possession of HE affects host cell range and pathogenicity. Further elucidation of the functional domains of the S protein will help to explain the differences in neurovirulence exhibited by monoclonal antibody selected variants. The elucidation of the molecular basis for the different tissue tropisms of TGEV and PRCV is eagerly awaited. Also required is further evidence for recombination among IBV strains since, if confirmed, this factor must be taken into account when attempting to clarify the epizootiology of this widespread, economically important virus. One thing is clear that, through one mechanism or another, an important feature of the coronaviruses is the inconstant nature of the genome.

REFERENCES

1. Keck, J.G. *et al.*, 1988, *In vivo* RNA-RNA recombination of coronavirus in mouse brain, J. Virol., 62: 1810.
2. Kuster, J.G. *et al.*, 1989, Phylogeny of antigenic variants of avian coronavirus IBV, Virology, 169:, 217.
3. Lai, M.M.C. *et al.*, Recombination between nonsegmented RNA genomes of murine coronaviruses, J. Virol., 56: 449.
4. Luytjes, W. *et al.*, Sequence of mouse hepatitis virus A59 mRNA 2: indications for RNA recombination between coronaviruses and influenza C virus, Virology, 166: 415.
5. Makino, S. *et al.*, High frequency RNA recombination of murine coronaviruses, J. Virol., 57: 729.
6. Pensaert, M. *et al.*, Isolation of a porcine respiratory, non-enteric coronavirus related to transmisible gastroenteritis, Vet. Quart., 8: 257.
7. Taguchi, F. *et al.*, Characterisation of variant virus selected in rat brains after infection by coronavirus mouse hepatitis virus JHM, J. Virol., 54: 429.

MOLECULAR BASIS OF THE VARIATION EXHIBITED BY AVIAN INFECTIOUS

BRONCHITIS CORONAVIRUS (IBV)

D. Cavanagh, P. Davis, J. Cook and D. Li

AFRC Institute for Animal Health, Houghton Laboratory
Houghton, Huntingdon, Cambridgeshire, PE17 2DA, UK

ABSTRACT

IBV serotype-specific, virus neutralising (VN) antibody is induced
by the S1 subunit of the spike (S) glycoprotein. A Portuguese isolate
(Port/322/85) is considered to be an in vivo recombinant. VN tests
showed that it belongs to the Massachussetts (Mass) serotype. Corresp-
ondingly, the sequence of S1 and S2 was extremely similar to that of
older Mass isolates. However, the matrix (M) glycoprotein and upstream
gene sequences were atypical of these Mass strains and more closely
resembled other serotypes isolated in Europe. The recombination event
had occurred within the sequence between the M and S genes (corresponding
to mRNA 3) or near the 3' terminus of the S2 gene.

INTRODUCTION

It has been known for decades that IBV exhibits extensive antigenic
variation. On the basis of VN tests isolates have been assigned to
serotypes, the number of which continues to increase[1,2]. Serotype-
specific VN antibody is induced by S1, the amino-(N)-terminal half of the
spike (S) glycoprotein[3-6]. Moreover, amino acid differences between
isolates are concentrated within the N-terminal 25% of S1 residues[6-8] and
some epitopes for VN antibody are situated in this region[6] (Fig.1).

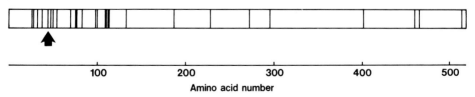

Fig.1. Amino acid variation within S1 of 8 Mass serotype strains (from
reference 6). Vertical lines indicate where at least one of seven Mass
strains differed in sequence from the M41 strain. The arrow shows the
position of an amino acid substitution in a mutant of M41 which resisted
neutralization by a monoclonal antibody.[6]

In this communication we present evidence that a strain of the Massachusetts serotype is actually a recombinant.

METHODS

Isolate Portugal/322/85 was received in 1985 and was serotyped by virus neutralization (VN) tests in chicken tracheal organ cultures[1]. IBV RNA was produced and sequenced essentially as described previously[9].

RESULTS

Strains of the Mass serotype have always been a major cause of severe outbreaks of IB and the most widely used vaccines are of the Mass serotype. Our analysis of a number of vaccine and field strains, all of the Mass serotype but isolated over a four decade period, showed that S1 had been strongly conserved (S2 was not sequenced)[6] (Fig.1). Taken as a group, the 7 strains analysed varied from the M41 strain, at only 6% of amino acids. The 3c ORF and M gene of the vaccinal strains had also been highly conserved[9].

Isolate Port/322/85 was neutralised by antisera to several Mass strains including M41 and H120 and was considered to be of the Mass serotype. Sequencing of S1 gave data which correlated with the serological analysis. Thus the S1 protein of Port/322/85 shared 94.9% homology with that of M41 (Fig.2). Several of the amino acids possessed by Port/322/85 and different from M41 were identical to those in the vaccine strain H120, the field strain HVI-140 (Fig.2) and the other Mass strains previously sequenced[6]. However, the 3c ORF and M gene sequence of Port/322/85 was not at all like that of these other Mass strains (Fig.3). Rather, it more closely resembled the sequences of UK/6/82 and UK/200/83[9], both in terms of deletions and the possession of specific nucleotides. We then sequenced the S2 part of the S gene. There was 97.4% amino acid homology with S2 of M41 (we determined 87% of the S2 sequence of Port/322/85). We were not able to determine the carboxy-(C-)-terminal amino acids because of the complete failure of the oligonucleotide used to prime the reverse transcription of this part of the gene. The oligonucleotide was complementary to IBV-M41 sequence a few nucleotides downstream from the C-terminus of S2, in the 3a ORF.

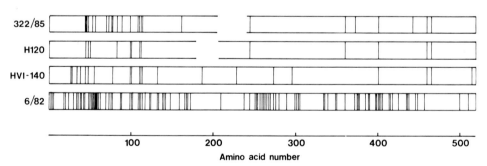

Fig.2. Comparison of the S1 amino acid sequence of Mass serotype strains Port/322/85, H120 and HVI-140 and the non-Mass strain UK/6/82 with that of the M41 strain. Each vertical line represents an amino acid difference.

```
(a)
M41        UGGUAGAAAACUUAACAAUCCGGAAUUAGAAGCAGUUAUUGUCAACGAGUUUCCUAAGAACGGUUGGAAUAAUAAAAAUCCAGCAAAUUUUCAAG
MM/Bronch                                                   U
H52/H120                      U                             U
Ibvax                        U                       G      U
322/85         A             A      G     A G                      C    A        AC ********************
UK/200/83  C   A             A      G G   A G                           A        AC ********************
UK/6/82    C   A             A      G     A G   .          A       A    A        AU********************
(b)
M41        AUGUCCAACGAGACAAAAUUGUACUCUUGACUUUGAACAGUCAGUUGAGCUUUUUAAAGAGUAUAAU
MM/Bronch
H52/H120              A
Ibvax                A
322/85     *********AU          A      UAC C G   AGU  C .    .. C  G  U
UK/200/83  ****** UGACAGA              UAC       AG   C     C    G  A
UK/6/82        GAU   ACC  C            GUAC      AG   C          G  A
(c)
M41        UUAUUUAUAACUGCAUUCUUGUUGUUCUUAACCAUAAUACUUCAGUAUGGCUAUGCAACAAGAAGUAAG
MM/Bronch                                                             .....
H52/H120                                               U
Ibvax                                                  U
322/85     C  .  CG      G   C U     C       C        .     G  C  G  CCG
UK/200/83           C  C  C       UC U  U   C U        A  C    U  G  CCGU
UK/6/82    C     G       C                  C         A  C    U  G AC

(d)
M41,MM,Bronch,   MSNETNCTLDFEQSVELFKEYNLFITAFLLFLTIILQYGYATRSK
H52, H120,Ibvax
322/85     ***M     TQ VA. . D    V        L        R
UK/200/83  **MTE    T  A Q                 L        R
UK/6/82    D T     GT  A Q      V          L        N
```

Fig.3. M gene sequences. Only those nucleotides which differ from those
of M41 are shown; unidentified nucleotides are marked with a dot (.).
(a) sequences of the 3' end of the 3c ORF; (b) sequence coding for the
exposed part of M; (c) sequence for the first membrane-embedded part of
M. Nucleotides absent from some sequences are indicated by asterisks[*];
(d) comparison of the amino acid sequences of the M protein corresponding
to nucleotide sequences in (b) and (c).

The striking similarity of the S1 genes of Port/322/85 and M41 and
equally striking dissimilarity of their 3c ORF and M sequences indicates
that Port/322/85 is a recombinant. The recombinantion event would have
occurred either within the gene 3 ORFs or, given the failure of the
above-mentioned oligonucleotide, near the C-terminus of S2.

DISCUSSION

The results presented herein and the recent findings of Kusters et
al.[8] strongly support the view that some IBV isolates are naturally
occurring recombinants. Given the high frequency of recombination which
occurred during experimental mixed infections with murine hepatitis virus
strains[10] it seems likely that many IBV strains are recombinant at one or
more loci.

Strains of the Mass serotype continue to be isolated, 50 years after
the first Mass isolate was made. Given the widespread use of Mass serotype vaccines - some countries, including the UK, permit only live vaccines of this serotype - it might be assumed that a Mass isolate is a
re-isolate of a vaccine strain. Sequencing of S1 can indicate if a
Mass isolate is a vaccine strain, a mutant of a vaccine or a nonvaccine
related Mass field strain (which from the data reported herein, some

isolates clearly are). However, given the phenomenon of recombination, such data can be no more than a tentative indication of the identity of an isolate. Sequencing of the M gene improves the situation but this still leaves unexamined more than 20 000 nucleotides, among which there may have been point mutations, deletions, insertions and/or recombination events!

ACKNOWLEDGEMENT

We wish to thank Miss Carolyn Payne and Mrs Marjorie Ellis for technical assistance.

REFERENCES

1. Cook, J.K.A. The classification of new serotypes of infectious bronchitis virus isolated from poultry flocks in Britain between 1981 and 1983. Avian Path. 13: 733 (1984).
2. Cook, J.K.A. and Huggins, M.B. Newly isolated serotypes of infectious bronchitis virus: their role in disease. Avian Path. 15: 129 (1986).
3. Cavanagh, D., Darbyshire, J.H., Davis, P. and Peters, R.W. Induction of humoral neutralising and haemagglutination-inhibiting antibody by the spike protein of avian infectious bronchitis virus. Avian Path. 13: 573 (1984).
4. Mockett, A.P., Cavanagh, D and Brown, T.D.K. Monoclonal antibodies to the S1 spike and membrane proteins of avian infectious bronchitis coronavirus strain Massachusetts M41. J. gen. Virol. 65: 2281 (1984).
5. Cavanagh, D., Davis, P.J., Darbyshire, J.H. and Peters, R.W. Coronavirus IBV: Virus retaining spike glycopolypeptide S2 but not S1 is unable to induce virus-neutralizing or haemagglutination-inhibiting antibody, or induce chicken tracheal protection. J. gen. Virol. 67: 1435 (1986).
6. Cavanagh, D., Davis, P.J. and Mockett, A.P.A. Amino acids within hypervariable region 1 of avian coronavirus IBV (Massachusetts serotype) spike glycoprotein are associated with neutralization epitopes. Virus Res. 11: 141 (1988).
7. Binns, M.M. Boursnell, M.E.G., Tomley, F.M. and Brown, T.D.K. Comparison of the spike precursor sequences of coronavirus IBV strains M41 and 6/82 with that of IBV Beaudette. J. gen. Virol. 67: 2825 (1986).
8. Kusters, J.G., Niesters, H.G.M., Lenstra, J.A., Horzinek, M.C. and van der Zeijst B.A.M. Phylogeny of antigenic variants of avian coronavirus IBV. Virology, 169: 217 (1989).
9. Cavanagh, D., and Davis, P.J. Evolution of avian coronavirus IBV: sequence of the matrix glycoprotein gene and intergenic region of several serotypes. J.gen.Virol. 69: 621 (1988).
10. Keck, J.G., Matsushima, G.K., Makino, S., Fleming, J.O., Vannier, D.M., Stohlman, S.A. and Lai, M.M.C. In vivo RNA-RNA recombination of coronaviruses in mouse brain. J. Virol. 62: 1810 (1988).

SEQUENCE COMPARISONS OF THE 3' END OF THE GENOMES OF

FIVE STRAINS OF AVIAN INFECTIOUS BRONCHITIS VIRUS

Ellen W. Collisson[1], Anna K. Williams[1], Ray
Vonder Haar[2], Wang Li[1], and Loyd W. Sneed[1]

[1]Department of Veterinary Microbiology
[2]Department of Biology
Texas A&M University
College Station, TX

INTRODUCTION

Avian infectious bronchitis virus (IBV) causes an acute, highly contagious respiratory disease of chickens characterized by tracheal rales, coughing and sneezing[1]. The disease was first described in 1931 by Schalk and Hawn[1] and since that time, many strains have been defined[2,3]. These strains vary widely in virulence and tissue tropism. A number of serologically distinguishable strains of infectious bronchitis virus have been isolated from poultry in the U.S.A. Of the strains included in this study, Beaudette, Conn. and Ark DPI 75 are vaccine strains, Gray and AustT are known to be nephropathogenic causing limited respiratory disease, and infections with Ark99, Mass41 and a Japanese strain (KB8523) are generally thought to result in severe respiratory disease in the absence of nephritis and nephrosis[4].

In this study, the 3' end of the Ark99 and Gray strains were compared with the published data for Mass41 and Beaudette[5] and a Japanese strain, KB8523[6]. An insert in the 3' noncoding region of the genome described in the Beaudette and Japanese strains, but absent in the Mass41 strain, was also found in the Ark99 and Gray strains.

MATERIALS AND METHODS

Viral Preparation

The Gray and Ark99 strains of IBV were purified in our lab by three terminal dilution cycles in embryonating chick embryos (ECE) and were propagated by allantoic sac inoculation into 11-day old specific pathogen free (SPAFAS) ECE. Virus was precipitated with polyethylene-glycol and banded on a 30-50% glycerol/potassium tartrate gradient. After concentrating by ultracentrifugation, virus was reconstituted and the virions were disrupted with Proteinase K and SDS. The RNA was extracted in phenol/chloroform/isoamyl and ethanol precipitated[7].

Cloning of The Gray and Ark99 Strains

First strand cDNA synthesis was carried out by reverse transcriptase using an oligo dT primer and second strand synthesis with DNA Pol1 and RNase H[8]. The double stranded cDNA was tailed with deoxy C's using

Table 1.   Percent similarity among the four strains
            having the insert in the 3' non-coding
            region not present in the Mass41 strain.

	Beau	KB8523	Ark99	Gray
Beau	100	67.4	91.9	92.9
KB8523	67.4	100	69.4	69.9
Ark99	91.9	69.4	100	94.6
Gray	92.9	69.9	94.6	100

Table 2. Percent similarities among the 3' non-coding regions
         of the genomes of five strains of IBV.

	Mass41	Beau	KB8523	Ark99	Gray
Mass41	100	99.1	97.1	93.3	96.9
Beau	99.1	100	98.1	94.0	97.7
KB8523	97.1	98.1	100	93.2	95.1
Ark99	93.3	94.0	93.2	100	96.1
Gray	96.9	97.7	95.1	96.1	100

terminal deoxy transferase and annealed with oligo dG tails in the Pst1
site of the pUC9 plasmid[9]. Clones containing 1-2Kb of IBV cDNA were
selected after transformation of E. coli JM109 cells. Dideoxy sequencing of
plasmid cDNA[10] and of single-stranded cDNA following subcloning into M13[11]
was performed, and the resulting sequences of Ark99 and Gray were compared
with each other and with the published data for the Mass41 and Beaudette
strains[5] and the Japanese strain, KB8523[6], using the University of
Wisconsin Genetics Computor Group programs.

Results

     The 3' ends of the genomes of the Gray and Ark99 strains of IBV were
cloned and sequenced. The 1712 bases of the cDNA for Gray included the
entire nucleocapsid gene and 346 bases of the 3' non-coding region.
Approximately 170 bases were missing from the 3' end of the Gray clone as
determined by comparing the sequence with the other strains (Fig.1). Other
Gray cDNA clones are currently being sequenced to complete this data. The
cDNA of the Ark99 clone was 1255 bases in length and apparently included
all of the 3' non-coding region but according to the data from the other
four strains, Ark99 was missing 485 bases of the 5' end of the nucleocapsid
structural gene (fig.1). Therefore, comparisons with the Ark99 strain were
based on the 3' 742 bases of the nucleocapsid coding region (247 amino

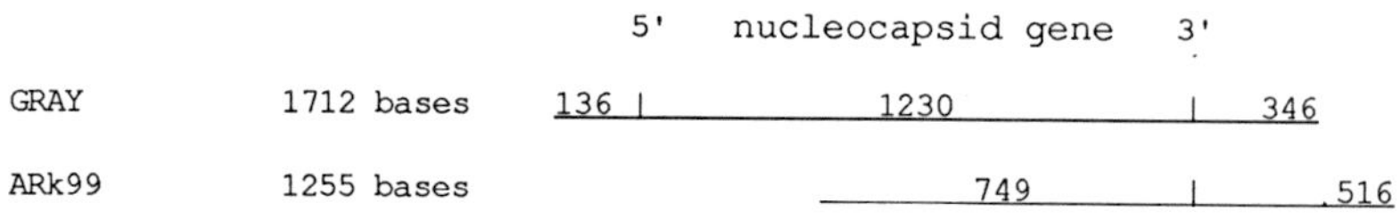

```
              5'    nucleocapsid gene    3'

GRAY      1712 bases    136 |_____1230_____|__346

ARk99     1255 bases           _____749_____|___.516
```

Fig.1. cDNA clones of the 3' ends of Gray and Ark99

374

acids) present in this clone.The complete open reading frame for the nucleocapsid gene of Gray, as with Beau, Mass41 and KB8523 contained 1227 bases, contain Kozac's consensus sequence at the AUG start codon and coded for a basic protein of 409 amino acids. The available amino acid sequencing data of the nucleocapsid proteins of Gray and Ark99 were compared to each other and with the amino acid sequences for the nucleocapsid proteins of Beaudette, Mass41 and KB8523. The similarities of the amino acid sequences of the nucleocapsid proteins of these 5 strains of IBV ranged from 90.7 to 96.3 with the Gray strain showing the least overall similarity to the other strains. There is an area of divergence in the Gray nucleocapsid protein sequence from residues 230-250 when compared to the other strains as can be seen in Fig.2 which shows the alignment comparison of the amino acids of the Gray and Beaudette strains. However, the significance of this apparent divergence is unknown.

The nucleotide sequences of the 3' non-coding regions of Gray and Ark99 were compared with each other and with the published data for Mass41, Beaudette and a Japanese strain KB8523. In the 3' end of the genome, 4 bases downstream from the stop codon for the nucleocapsid gene, there is a region that ranges from 184 to 187 bases in length that is present in the KB8523, Beaudette, Gray and Ark99 strains and is missing in the Mass41 strain. This region was from 67.4 to 94.6% similar among the strains containing this sequence with the Japanese strain being the most divergent (Table 1).

```
  1 MASGKAAGKTDAPAPVIKLGGPKPPKVGSSGNASWFQAIKAKKLNTPPPK 50
    ||||||  ||||||||||||||| ||||||||||||||||||||| | ||
  1 MASGKATGKTDAPAPVIKLGGPRPPKVGSSGNASWFQAIKAKKLNSPQPK 50

 51 FEGSGVPDNENIKPSQQHGYCRRQARFKPGKGGRKPVPDAWYFYYTGTGP 100
    |||||||||||| |||||| |||||||||||| |||||||||||||||||
 51 FEGSGVPDNENFKTSQQHGYWRRQARFKPGKGRRKPVPDAWYFYYTGTGP 100

101 AADLNWGDTQDGIVWVAAKGADTKSRSNQVTRDPDKFDQYPLRFSDGGPD 150
    ||||||||| |||||||||||| |||||| ||||||||||||||||||||
101 AADLNWGDSQDGIVWVAAKGADVKSRSNQGTRDPDKFDQYPLRFSDGGPD 150

151 GNFRWDFIPLNRGRSGRSTAASSAAASRAPSREGSRGRRSDSGDDLIARA 200
    |||||||||||||||||||||||| |||| |||||||||||| |||||||
151 GNFRWDFIPLNRGRSGRSTAASSAASSRPPSREGSRGRRSGSEDDLIARA 200

201 AKIIQDQQKKGSRITKAKADEMAHRRYCKRTIPPNYRVDQVFGPRTKGKE 250
    |||||||||||||||||||||||||     |   ||  | | |||||
201 AKIIQDQQKKGSRITKAKADEMVIAGIASALFHLVIRLIKFLVPGTKGKE 250

251 GNFGDDKMNEEGIKDGRVTAMLNLVPSSHACLFGSRVTPKLQLDGLHLRF 300
    |||||||||||||||||||||||||||||||||||||||||| ||||| |
251 GNFGDDKMNEEGIKDGRVTAMLNLVPSSHACLFGSRVTPKLQPDGLHLKF 300

301 EFTTVVPCDDPQFDNYVKICDQCVDGVGTRPKDDEPKPKSRSSSRPATRG 350
    |||||| |||||||||||||||||||||||||||||||||||||||||||
301 EFTTVVPRDDPQFDNYVKICDQCVDGVGTRPKDDEPKPKSRSSSRPATRT 350

351 NSPAPRQQRPKKEKKLKKQDDEADKACTSDEERNNAQLEFYDEPKVINWG 400
    ||||||| ||||| |||||| ||| ||| ||||||||||| |||||||||
351 SSPAPRQQRLKKEKRPKKQDDEVDKALTSDEERNNAQLEFDDEPKVINWG 400

401 DAALGENEL* 410
    | ||||||||
401 DSALGENEL* 410
```

Fig.2. Optimal alignment of the amino acid
       sequences of Beaudette and Gray from
       the UWGCG GAP program.

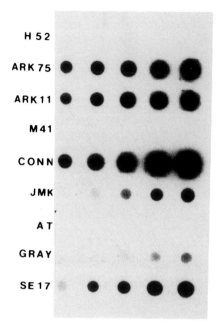

H 52

ARK 75

ARK 11

M 41

CONN

JMK

A T

GRAY

SE 17

Fig.3. Northern blot analysis of 9
strains of IBV using 3'non-
coding region "insert"-
specific 40bp probe.

    In order to determine the occurence of this 184bp region in various
strains of IBV, a 40 base oligonucleotide was synthesized to the middle
portion of the Ark insert and hybridized[12] to genomic RNA of several IBV
strains (fig.3). In addition to the Ark99 and Gray strains, the Conn, JMK
and SE17 strains had the 184 base insert; whereas the Mass41, Aust T and
the Hol152 strains were missing this region. The remaining noncoding region
was from 93.2 to 99.1% similar among the strains (Table 2) with the Ark99
strain showing somewhat less homology. The putative secondary structure of
the non-coding 3' ends indicated that the Mass41 without the "insert" had
two branches with hairpin loops and the other strains showed 4 hairpin
loops with Beaudette, 5 with Gray, and 6 with the KB8523 and Ark99 strains.

Ark99
GGAT TCAGCTTT AGG   TGA GAAT G AAC T TTGA G**TAA**||**AGTT** CAA TAG TAAG AGT TA AGG GAGA TAGG

Gray
                  AGG TGAGAATG AACT C TGA G**TAA**||**AGT T**CAA TA GTAAGAGT TAAGGA

Beaudette
                      GAGAATGA ACT TTGAG **TAA**||**AAT T**CA AT AGTAAG AG

Mass41
                  TAG GAGA GAAT GAA CTT TGA G **TAA**|**AAT** TCAAT AGT AAG AGT TAAG GAA GAT

K8523
                      GAA AA TGAA C TTTGA TTAA||**AGTT**T ATTGA AAGT T AAG GA

Fig.4. Sequences flanking the 3' non-coding region "insert." Underlined
sequences represent mirrored sequences and the bold letters
represent common sequences adjacent to the "insert."

376

However, these structures were computed only with the 3' non-coding region, and therefore the impact of the rest of the genome is not known. Also, the completion of the sequencing of the 3' end of Gray may result in an altered secondary structure for this strain. The significance of the differences resulting from the "insert" sequences on the function of this end of the genome is not known. This extemely AT rich "insert" appears to be in the same location in several strains of IBV (fig.4.) and mirrored sequences flanking this region also appear as loops in the secondary structures of the strain in which this sequence is absent. The sequence 5' of this 184bp insert is consistently TAA and the sequence 3' is either AATT or AGTT in the strains analyzed to date. Boursnell et al.[5] found the sequence AGTTTA to be repeated 6 times downstream of the "insert" in the 3' noncoding region of the Mass41 and Beau strains and the sequence TTTAGTTTAA repeated 3 times. Seven repeats of AGTTTA were found in the corresponding region of KB8523 and 5 in Ark99, and the latter sequence was repeated twice in the KB8523 and Ark99 strains. This portion of the 3'non-coding region of Gray was not represented in this data. The function(s) of the these mirrored and repeated sequences is unknown, but it is possible that they are important in producing a secondary structure facilitating more efficient polymerase and/or leader sequence binding and hence, more efficient transcription.

REFERENCES

1. A. F. Schalk, and M. C. Hawn, An apparantly new respiratory disease of baby chicks, JAVMA.78:418-422 (1931).

2. J. H. Darbyshire, J. G. Rowell, J. K. A. Cook, and R. W. Peters,Taxonomic studies on strains of avian infectious bronchitis virus using neutralization tests in tracheal organ cultures, Arch.Virol. 61:227-238 (1979).

3. S. R. Hopkins, Serologic comparisons of strains of infectious bronchitis using plaque-purified isolates, Avian Dis. 18:231-239 (1974).

4. R. B. Cumming, The etiology of uremia of chickens, Aust.Vet.J. 39:145-147 (1963).

5. M. Boursnell, M. Binns, I. Foulds, and T. Brown, Sequences of the nucleocapsid genes from two strains of avian infectious bronchitis virus, J.Gen.Virol. 66:573-580 (1985).

6. S. Shizuyo, S. Seiji, T. Okabe, M. Nakai, and N. Sasaki, Cloning and sequencing of genes encoding structural proteins of avian infectious bronchitis virus, Virology 165: 589-595 (1988).

7. L. Wang, M. C. Kemp, P. Roy, and E. Collisson, Tissue tropism and target cells of Bluetongue virus in the chicken embryo. J.Virol. 62:887-893 (1988).

8. U. Gubler and B. J. Hoffman, A simple and very efficient method for generating cDNA libraries, Gene 25:263-269 (1983).

9. S. L. Berger and A. R. Kimmel, Guide to Molecular Cloning Techniques; in Meth. in Enzym. 152 (1987).

10. E. Y. Chen and P. H. Seeburg, Supercoil sequencing: A fast and simple method for sequencing plasmid DNA, DNA 4(2):165-170 (1985).

11. F. Sanger, S. Nicklen, A. R. Coulson, DNA sequencing with chain-terminating inhibitors. PNAS USA 74:5463-5467 (1977).

12. L. Sneed, G. Butcher, L. Wang, M. Kemp, and E. Collisson, Protein and RNA comparisons of several strains of IBV. Southern Conference on Avian Disease. (March 1987)

SELECTION OF VARIANTS OF AVIAN INFECTIOUS BRONCHITIS VIRUS

SHOWING TROPISM FOR DIFFERENT ORGANS

Koichi Otsuki, Kohei Matsuo, Nobuyuki Maeda,
Takeshi Sanekata, Misao Tsubokura

Department of Veterinary Microbiology, Faculty of
Agriculture, Tottori University, Tottori 680, Japan

ABSTRACT

Avian infectious bronchitis virus strain Kagoshima-34 isolated from the
kidneys of a chicken that died of nephrosis/nephritis lost its nephropathogenicity during intratracheal passage in SPF chickens. The resultant virus
acquired stronger respirotropism but reduced tropism for kidneys. On the
other hand strain Tottori-2 isolated from the trachea of a chicken suffering
from severe respiratory disease did not lose its respirotropism after serial
intravenous passage in SPF chickens.

The serological properties of the passaged virus were investigated by
virus neutralisation test. The antibody titres of both strains of virus
fluctuated with progressive passage. The serological properties of the
virus isolated from respiratory organs were not necessarily the same as
those of the isolates made from the kidneys.

INTRODUCTION

Avian infectious bronchitis virus (IBV) grows not only in respiratory
organs of chickens but also in the kidneys[1,2,5]. IBVs causing respiratory
disease have strong respirotropism and those causing nephrosis/nephritis
have nephrotropism[5]. We had already shown experimentally that IBV changed
its serological properties after serial passages in cultured mammalian
cells[3]. It is well known that most strains of IBV lose their virulence
for chickens following repeated passage in vitro or in ovo. It is
possible that IBV changes its properties including its organ tropism with
ease. We have tried to induce IBV to alter its organ tropism.

MATERIALS AND METHODS

Virus. Two Japanese isolates were tested in this investigation. Strain
Kagoshima-34, isolated from the kidneys of a chicken that died of nephrosis/
nephritis and strain Tottori-2, isolated from the trachea of a chicken
showing severe respiratory signs[5]. Neither virus caused any CPE in
cultivated chick kidney (CK) cells, but both strains caused curling or
dwarfing of hen's embryos.

Virus titration. Virus was titrated as described previously[5].

Virus neutralisation test. Immune sera were prepared according to the
method described previously[4]. Virus neutralisation test was carried out

in 8-day-old hen's eggs by the constant-serum varying-virus method[5].

In vivo passage of IBVs.

Intravenous passage. With both strains, virus at a titre of $10^{6.5}$ EID_{50} was injected into the ulvar cutaneous vein of two 6-week-old SPF chickens. The chickens were killed 4 days postinoculation (p.i.). Kidneys and such respiratory organs as trachea and lungs were taken aseptically, homogenised respectively with sterile sand and suspended to approximately 10% in Eagle's MEM. After clarification, portions of the supernatant of the kidneys were injected into the ulvar cutaneous vein of another two SPF chickens. Both IBV strains were passaged in this way ten times.

Intratracheal passage. With both strains, virus at a titre of $10^{6.5}$ EID_{50} was inoculated intratracheally into two 6-week-old SPF chickens. Trachea, lungs and kidneys were taken 3 or 4 days p.i., the former two tissues were pooled and homogenised. After clarification supernatant of the respiratory suspension was inoculated intratracheally another two SPF chickens. IBV was passaged ten times in the same manner.

Experimental infection with IBV. For each strain, 12 10-week-old SPF chickens were inoculated with $10^{6.0}$ EID_{50} of virus intratracheally. Two chickens were killed at 1, 2, 3, 5, 7 and 10 days p.i.. Trachea, lungs and kidneys were taken aseptically and the former two tissues were pooled and virus recovery attempted as described previously[5].

RESULTS

Organ tropism of passaged IBV

Initially, we tried to passage both strains of IBV by intratracheal inoculation. Strain Kagoshima-34 was passed ten times via the respiratory tract of SPF chickens. As shown in Table 1, this virus altered its organ tropism during passage. After 10 passages the virus caused only mild respiratory disease and macroscopical lesions in respiratory organs. Neither diarrhoea nor macroscopical lesions were observed in the kidneys, although considerable amounts of virus were still recovered from that tissue.

Table 1. Pathogenicity of strain Kagoshima-34 passaged in the respiratory organs

Passage number	Virus titre recovered from		Respiratory signs	Diarrhoea	Macroscopical change in	
	R.O.*	Kidneys			R.O.	Kidneys
1	2.3**	1.2	+ +	+ +	+ +	+ +
2	4.5	3.3	+ +	+ +	+ +	+ +
3	5.5	2.8	+ +	+ +	+ +	- -
4	5.5	2.8	- -	- -	+ +	- -
5	5.5	2.7	- -	- -	- -	- -
6	4.1	3.5	- -	- -	- -	- +
7	5.0	4.0	- -	- -	- -	- +
8	3.3	4.0	- -	- -	- -	- -
9	5.5	3.0	+ +	- -	- -	- +
10	4.4	4.0	+ +	- -	+ +	- -

For Tables 1 and 2   *: respiratory organ   +: positive
                    **: $\log_{10}/0.2$ g   -: negative

Virus passaged in respiratory organs grew lesser in kidneys than did its parent virus, but grew better in respiratory organs than its parent virus (Fig. 1).
Strain Tottori-2 passaged in the same manner did not change its organ tropism but grew better than the parent virus in any target organs.

Next, we tried to pass both strains by intravenous injection. Strain Tottori-2 hardly survived ten passages in kidneys. There was no obvious difference in pathogenicity between passaged and parent virus (Table 2). Virus recovery of passaged virus was similar to that of its parent. On the other hand, strain Kagoshima-34 could not be passed more than five times in kidneys.

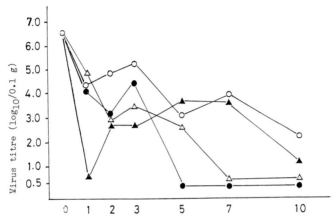

Fig. 1. Virus growth in chickens infected with strain Kagoshima-34. Comparison of the virus passed ten times in respiratory organs with the parent strain.
o———o virus passaged from respiratory organs; •———• parent virus virus passaged from kidneys; △———△ from respiratory organs; ▲———▲ parent virus from kidneys.

Table 2. Pathogenicity of strain Tottori-2 passaged in the kidneys of chickens

Passage number	Virus titre recovered from		Respiratory signs	Diarrhoea	Macroscopical change in	
	R.O.*	Kidneys			R.O.	Kidneys
1	3.9**	3.0	– –	+ +	– –	– –
2	1.1	0.3	– –	– –	– –	– –
3	1.7	2.0	– –	– –	– –	– –
4	1.8	1.4	– –	+ –	– –	– –
5	1.6	1.8	– –	– –	– –	– –
6	5.2	2.8	– –	+ –	– –	– –
7	1.3	1.3	– –	+ +	– –	– –
8	1.8	3.0	– –	– –	– –	– –
9	1.0	2.7	– –	+ +	– –	– –
10	1.0	0.0	– –	– –	– –	– –

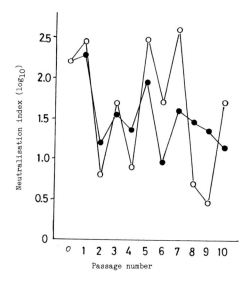

Fig. 2. Antigenicity of strain Tottori-2 passaged in respiratory
organs. o———o virus recovered from respiratory organs;
•———• virus recovered from kidneys.

Antigenicity of passaged IBV

The antigenicity of IBV passaged in respiratory organs was tested by
virus neutralisation test using virus recovered from the respiratory organs
and kidneys respectively and hyperimmune sera against the parent virus.
Fig. 2 shows that the antigenicity of Tottori-2 isolated from respiratory
organs is not necessarily the same as that from kidneys even if they were
recovered from the same chicken. The neutralising index of those viruses
fluctuated with progressive passage, this was particularly so with virus
recovered from the respiratory organs. Similar results were obtained with
Kagoshima-34 (Fig. 3).

Resistance of passaged IBV to exposure to chemical and physical agents

Resistance of both strains of IBV passaged 3, 6, 8 and 10 times in
respiratory organs of kidneys to exposure to pH 3.0 (4°C, 30 min), 5%
chloroform (4°C, 20 min), 20% ethyl ether (4°C, 18 h) and heating (56°C, 15
min) was examined. All viruses were sensitive to all agents except to
exposure to pH 3.0. These results are the same as those for the parent
viruses.

DISCUSSION

IBV causing nephrosis/nephritis in chickens grows not only in the
kidneys but also in the respiratory organs[1,2,5]. In this investigation,
strain Kagoshima-34 isolated from the kidneys of a chicken that died of

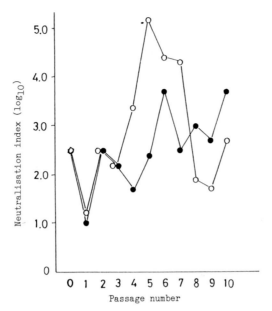

Fig. 3.   Antigenicity of strain Kagoshima-34 passaged in respiratory
organs.   ○────○ Virus recovered from respiratory organs;
●────● Virus recovered from kidneys.

nephrosis/nephritis lost its nephropathogenicity following passage in respiratory organs of chickens but still caused respiratory disease.   Strain Tottori-2 did not acquire obvious nephrotropism in spite of serial passages in kidneys.   These results suggest that the target organ for IBV is not initially kidneys, but respiratory tissues.

With both virus strains, the antigenicity of the IBV recovered from kidneys was different from that recovered from the respiratory organs, even if both viruses were recovered from the same chicken.   Antigenic alteration seemed to occur during passage regardless of whether virus was grown in respiratory organs or kidneys.   In this investigation, it appears that alteration of organ tropism of IBV occurred unrelated to changes in antigenicity.

As we reported previously[3], an IBV strain seems to consist of various subpopulations.   Thus it is possible that a subpopulation having respirotropism does not necessarily have nephrotropism.   Both IBV strains tested here consist of considerably varied subpopulations and the antigenicity of these subpopulation varies.

Taguchi et al.[6] selected acute encephalitis-causing virus clone from mouse hepatitis virus JHM strain by intracerebral inoculation.   They reported that the molecular size of a variant virus was larger than that of its parent virus.

Recently in Japan the incidence of nephrosis/nephritis caused by IBV is increasing even though several kinds of live IB vaccines have been widely used.   It is possible that such vaccines caused selection of strongly nephrotropic IBV in the field, although we did not succeed in selecting nephrotropic virus clones from respiratory disease-causing IBV strains.

ACKNOWLEDGEMENTS

   We are grateful to Dr Jane K. A. Cook for her advice in the preparation of this manuscript.

REFERENCES

1. D.J. Alexander and R.E. Gough.   Isolation of avian infectious bronchitis virus from experimentally infected chickens. Res. Vet. Sci., 23:344 (1977).
2. R.C. Jones.   Nephrosis in laying chickens caused by Massachusetts-type infectious bronchitis virus. Vet. Rec., 95:319 (1974).
3. K. Otsuki, Y. Tagawa and M. Tsubokura.   Antigenic variation of avian infectious bronchitis virus during replication in BHK-21 cells. Arch. Virol., 73:75 (1982).
4. K. Otsuki, K. Noro, H. Yamamoto and M. Tsubokura.   Studies on avian infectious bronchitis virus (IBV). II. Replication of IBV in several cultured cells. Arch. Virol., 60:115 (1979).
5. K. Otsuki, T. Nakamura, N. Kubota, Y. Kawaoka and M. Tsubokura. Comparison of two strains of avian infectious bronchitis virus for their interferon induction, viral growth and development of virus -neutralizing antibody in experimentally infected chickens. Vet. Microbiol., 15:31 (1987).
6. F. Taguchi, S.G. Siddel, H. Wege and V. Meulen.   Characterization of a variant virus selected in rat brain after infection by coronavirus mouse hepatitis virus JHM. J. Virol., 54:429 (1985).

MONOCLONAL ANTIBODY-SELECTED VARIANTS OF MHV-4 CONTAIN

SUBSTITUTIONS AND DELETIONS IN THE E2 SPIKE GLYCOPROTEIN

Thomas M. Gallagher and Michael J. Buchmeier

Department of Neuropharmacology
Scripps Clinic and Research Foundation
La Jolla, CA

ABSTRACT

Selection and analysis of MHV-4 (strain JHM) variants resistant to E2-specific neutralizing MAbs was performed. Two types of variation in the E2 spike glycoprotein were found. From minimally passaged stocks of MHV-4, putative point mutants were obtained. These mutants were resistant only to the MAb used to select them. In contrast, multiply passaged stocks were found to harbor variants uniformly resistant to two selecting MAbs. Northern and Western blot analysis of the viral RNAs and proteins synthesized by these doubly-resistant variants showed that they contained large deletions in both mRNA 3 and its E2 translation product, localized to a 15 kilodalton region within the amino terminal 90B post-translational fragment. The selective advantage of this second class of variants lacking sequences within E2 90B was a result of their reduced cytopathology, thereby allowing cultures to support virus production for prolonged periods.

INTRODUCTION

Variants of neurotropic murine coronaviruses have received much attention in the past decade because they serve as useful tools for the correlation of viral genotype and virus-induced disease. Methods for variant generation and selection have included chemical mutagenesis followed by isolation of temperature sensitive virus (1) or multiple passaging in vivo and purification of resulting small plaque virus (2). In contrast to the fatal encephalitis caused by MHV-4 infection of murine brain, infection with these variants typically results in a non-fatal demyelinating disease.

MHV-4 variants have also been selected for their ability to escape the effects of neutralizing MAbs (3-5). In most cases neutralizing MAbs directed against the 180 kilodalton spike glycoprotein E2 have been used as selecting agents. A neuroattenuation phenotype has often been observed among the

Coronaviruses and Their Diseases
Edited by D. Cavanagh and T.D.K. Brown
Plenum Press, New York, 1990

resulting neutralization-resistant mutants (3-5) indicating
that at least one determinant of neurovirulence resides on
E2.

In our laboratory, variants uniformly resistant to
neutralization by two E2-specific MAbs 4B11.6 and 5A13.5
have been isolated from stocks of MHV-4 passaged in Sac-
culture (3). Although these variants were shown to be
neuroattenuated (3) the precise nature of the genetic lesion
in E2 correlating with this attenuation was not determined.
Because one source of heterogeneity among strains and
variants of MHV involves extensive deletion and insertion of
sequences within the E2 gene (6-8) we sought to determine
whether any of these neutralization-resistance mutations
were deletions. We found that these original variants were
indeed deletion mutants lacking sequences from the middle of
E2 post-translational fragment 90B.

METHODS

Cells and Virus

All cell lines were grown as monolayer cultures in DMEM
supplemented with either calf or fetal calf serum.
Infections were performed as described by Sturman et al. (9)
and progeny virus infectivity was determined by plaque assay
on DBT cells.

Selection of MAb-Resistant Variants

The properties of the MAbs used in this study have been
described previously (10). Selection of MAb-resistant
mutants followed those described (3) except that in most
cases resistant virus populations rather than individual
plaque isolates were selected for subsequent analysis.

Analysis of Viral RNA and Protein

Electrophoretic analysis of phenol-extracted RNA from
infected Sac- cells was performed on denaturing agarose
gels. Following transfer of separated RNAs to
nitrocellulose, Northern blot hybridization with a [^{32}P]
RNA complementary to nucleotides 636 to 840 of MHV-A59 RNA 7
was utilized to visualize all seven MHV-4 mRNAs.

For detection of the E2 proteins of MHV-4 and variants,
[^{35}S] methionine labeled infected cell proteins were
immune precipitated with antiserum directed against E2 and
subjected to SDS-polyacrylamide gel electrophoresis.
Further analysis by Western blotting was performed according
to standard methods (11) using antibodies raised against
peptides represented in the known MHV-A59 E2 sequence (6) as
detection agents.

RESULTS

Original Neuroattenuated and Neutralization-Resistant
Variants Contain Deletions in E2

Electrophoretic analysis of the viral RNAs induced by
infection with MHV-4 and two representative variants

revealed a difference in the sizes of the largest three of
the seven 3' coterminal viral mRNAs (Figure 1, Panel A).
Such shifts indicated the presence of deletions within mRNA
3, the gene encoding E2. The increased mobility of variant
mRNA 3 species (8.3 kb) suggested that about 400 nucleotides
were deleted in each of the variants. These deletions were
similarly reflected in the E2 protein. Radiolabeling of E2
in the presence of the glycosylation inhibitor tunicamycin
followed by immune precipitation and electrophoresis
revealed that the variant polypeptides lacked about 150
amino acids relative to MHV-4 (Figure 1, Panel B).

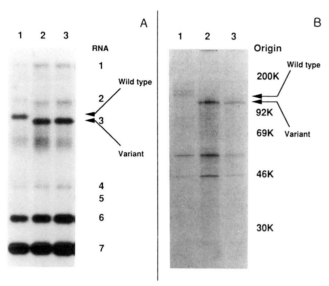

Fig. 1. Electrophoretic profiles of viral RNAs (A) and E2
        polypeptides (B) from infected Sac- cells. Infected
        cell RNAs were denatured with formamide and electro-
        phoresed on formaldehyde-agarose gels prior to detec-
        tion by hybridization with [^{32}P] complementary RNA
        7 transcripts. Infected cell proteins were radio-
        labeled with [^{35}S] methionine in the presence of
        tunicamycin (1 ug per ml) then immune precipitated
        with antiserum against E2 and electrophoresed on
        Laemmli slab gels. Lanes represent RNAs and proteins
        from wild type MHV-4 (1), V4B11.3 deletion mutant (2)
        and V5A13.1 deletion mutant (3) infection.

     Antipeptide antibodies directed against selected
portions of the E2 polypeptide were used on Western blot
analyses to localize these deletions to one of the two
post-translational products of E2. To this end, virus was
partially purified and concentrated by sedimentation through
sucrose gradients and prepared for Western blotting.
Immunoblotting of the immobilized protein showed that
antiserum against peptide A, which corresponds to residues
near the middle of the MHV-A59 90B fragment, recognized E2
90B from MHV-4 but not the variants V4B11.3 and V5A13.1
(Figure 2, Panel A). Specific binding to a previously
unidentified band at 75 K (p75) was also observed, as was
non-specific binding to nucleocapsid. Antipeptide B serum,
directed against the carboxyl terminus of E2 cleavage

produce 90B, reacted with distinct 90 K proteins from MHV-4 and the variants (Figure 2, Panel B). The different increases in electrophoretic mobility of the variant 90B chains was indicative of varying extents of deletion. Serum reactive to the sequence present on the amino terminus of E2 cleavage product 90A (peptide C) bound to two bands at 90 K and 270 K. The co-electrophoresis of MHV-4 and variant 90A-specific proteins, which represent monomers (90 K) and trimers (270 K), indicated that no large deletions were present in this fragment. Together these results indicate that the major deletions in the neuroattenuated variants V4B11.3 and V5A13.1 are localized to the middle of the E2 cleavage product 90B.

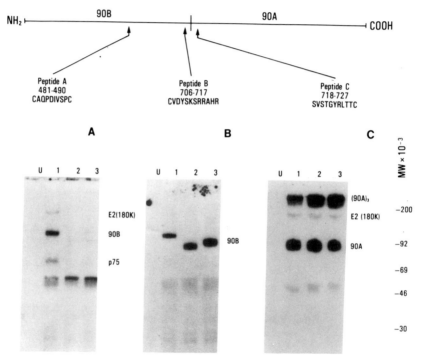

Fig. 2. <u>Western blot analysis of MHV-4 and deletion variant virion proteins</u>. Virions were purified from infected Sac- cells and electrophoresed on SDS-polyacrylamide gels prior to transfer to nitrocellulose. Proteins were then incubated in the presence of rabbit anti-peptide antibodies A, B and C, directed against the indicated portions of the MHV-A59 E2 protein. Bound antibodies were detected with [125I] protein A. U; uninfected control, 1; MHV-4, 2; V4B11.3, 3; V5A13.1.

Isolation of Deletion Mutants Requires Multiple Passaging of Virus Stocks in Cell Culture

To assess the frequency with which deletions in E2 arise in MHV-4 stocks we isolated pure MHV-4 from a single well-isolated plaque on a DBT cell lawn and prepared passage 2 virus by two short 12 hour growth cycles in Sac- culture. The resulting stock was then subjected to neutralization by

each of three E2-specific MAbs 4B11.6, 5A13.5 and 5B19.2.
In all three neutralizations, resistant virus capable for
forming plaques on DBT cells was observed. However, only
small plaque virus (less than 0.1 cm diameter) escaped the
initial round of neutralization by MAbs 4B11.6 and 5B19.2;
amplification of these small plaque variants under selecting
MAbs resulted in restoration of normal (0.5 cm diameter)
plaque size. Thus disabling mutations conferring
neutralization resistance are followed by additional
compensating mutation(s) in the viral genome. All of the
large plaque variants were neurovirulent in Balb/c mouse
brain (data not shown).

Table 1. Frequencies of MAb-Resistant Variants in Low and
High Passage MHV-4 Stocks[a]

MHV-4 Passage	Selecting MAb	Percent Resistance
2	4B11.6	0.0027
	5A13.5	0.0027
	4B11.6 + 5A13.5	<0.00045
10	4B11.6	12
	5A13.5	20
	4B11.6 + 5A13.5	13

[a]MHV-4 stocks of known titer were subjected to MAb ascites
fluids (1:20) and plated onto DBT cells. Plaque development
was for 3 days in the presence of 1:50 dilutions of MAb.

All three of these variants from MHV-4 passage 2
synthesized viral RNAs and proteins electrophoretically
identical to MHV-4-specific RNAs and proteins (data not
shown) indicating that large deletions were not present in
the variant genomes. Evidence that two of these variants
likely harbored point mutations was suggested by their
10^{-4} to 10^{-5} selection frequency (Table 1) which is the
expected frequency of point mutation in RNA virus
populations (12). In addition, each of the three variants
displayed resistance only to the MAb used to select them
(Table 2). Resistance to both MAbs 4B11.6 and 5A13.5 was
not observed, indicating that deletion mutants possessing
this double-resistance character were below the limits of
detection.

These results were in marked contrast to those observed
upon selection of MAb-resistant variants from MHV-4 passaged
ten times in Sac- cells. In these passaged stocks the
frequency of virus resistant to either of two MAbs (4B11.6
and 5A13.5) was as high as 20% (Table 1). In addition,
variants selected by MAbs 4B11.6 were resistant to MAb
5A13.5, and vice versa (Table 2). Western blot analyses
using antipeptide antibodies (not shown) revealed that these
doubly-resistant populations contained large deletions in
90B whose size and location were similar to those seen in
the original neuroattenuated mutants. Thus serial passage
of MHV-4 in Sac- culture resulted in the selective
amplification of deletion mutants.

Table 2. Neutralization Resistance Patterns for Selected
          Variants[a]

Virus	Origin of Variant	Neutralizing MAb		
		4B11.6	5A13.5	5B19.2
MHV-4 (P2)		+	+	+
V4B11	MHV-4 (P2)	−	+	+
V5A13	"	+	−	+
V5B19	"	+	+	−
V4B11	MHV-4 (P10)	−	−	+
V5A13	"	−	−	+

[a]Virus samples were treated as described in Table 1. A (+)
indicates >99% neutralization while a (−) represents <30%
neutralization relative to untreated controls.

A Selective Advantage for Deletion Mutants Exists Only in Cell Lines Susceptible to Virus-Induced Cytopathic Effects

We found that high multiplicity MHV-4 infection of a
number of cultured cell lines, including DBT, Sac-, C1300
and Neuro 2A, resulted in extensive cell-cell fusion after
about 8 hours. Destruction of cell monolayers was complete
by 16 hours post-infection. In contrast, 4 out of 4
independently isolated deletion mutants exhibited a delayed
induction of fusion in these cell lines. Although
cytopathic, these deletion mutants typically induced fusion
4 to 6 hours later than MHV-4. That this reduced
cytotoxicity permitted cells to support virus replication
for prolonged periods was shown by pulse labeling of
infected cultures with [^{3}H] uridine in the presence of
actinomycin D, an inhibitor of host but not coronavirus
transcription (13). The relative amount of radiolabel
incorporation into acid insoluble material showed that Sac-
cells supported equivalent amounts of wild type and variant
RNA for the first 10 hours of infection. However between 10
and 16 hours post-infection, variant RNA accumulated whereas
wild type RNA synthesis rapidly declined (Figure 3, Panel
A). This profile of viral RNA synthesis correlated well
with the onset of cytopathic effects. In addition the fact
that 5 to 10 times more variant-specific RNA was produced
throughout the time course was consistent with the 10-fold
higher yields of infectious variant progeny typically
obtained from Sac- cultures (Table 3).

Two continuous neuronal cell cultures derived from
central nervous system olfactory bulb, OBL 21 and OBL 21A,
supported MHV-4 replication without suffering from any
virus-induced cytopathic effect. With the OBL 21A line a
slight preference for MHV-4 replication relative to the
deletion mutant was observed (Figure 3, Panel B). MHV-4
progeny yields were slightly higher in the OBL 21A line
(Table 3). Thus in the fusion-negative OBL 21A line, where
no selective advantage for diminished viral cytotoxicity
exists, wild type virus with its full-length E2 was
favored. In this regard the OBL 21A line mimicked in vivo

infection in murine brain, which consistently produced more wild type virus (Table 3).

Table 3.   Yields of Wild Type and Deletion Mutant Viruses in Selected Neuronal and Non-neuronal Cultures and in Murine Brain[a]

Host	Fusion	Virus Yields MHV-4	V4B11.3	V5A13.1
DBT	+	2.2[b]	208	188
Sac−	+	320	3000	2800
C1300	+	192	1280	800
Neuro 2A	+	148	1760	1480
OBL 21	−	1.6	0.6	1.2
OBL 21A	−	2.2	1.3	1.0
Balb/c brain		57[c]	14	2

[a]Inoculation multiplicities were 0.01 PFU per cell for cultures and 100 PFU per mouse for intracerebral injections.
[b]Progeny PFU x 10^{-4} per ml at 24 hours post-infection.
[c]Progeny PFU x 10^{-3} per gram at 4 days post-infection.

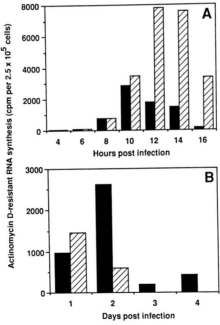

Fig. 3.   Time courses of viral RNA synthesis in Sac− (A) and OBL 21A (B) cell lines.   Monolayers were infected with MHV-4 (solid bars) or deletion mutant V5A13 (hatched bars) at 2 PFU per cell.   RNA synthesis was monitored at the indicated times after infection by 0.5 hour (Sac− cells) or 2 hour (OBL 21A cells) [^{3}H] uridine labeling periods in the presence of actinomycin D (5 ug per ml).   Acid insoluble radioactivity was counted immediately after labeling.

DISCUSSION

Point mutations represent the expected outcome of MAb-selection on RNA virus populations. Thus the result of MAb selection on minimally passaged stocks of MHV-4 is typical. We have no evidence that mutants selected from these stocks contain any gross alteration in E2 structure. In fact, nucleotide sequence analysis which is currently in progress has identified single base substitutions in both V4B11 and V5B19. We anticipate that complete variant sequences will not only clearly identify neutralization epitopes on E2 but also point to sites important in receptor binding and/or fusion, as both V4B11 and V5B19 initially displayed a small plaque phenotype in culture.

Viable deletion mutants are unexpected among RNA viruses, although defective interfering (DI) deletion mutants are common among all virus populations (14). Like DI genome generation, viable deletion mutant MHV-4 formation required multiple passaging in culture. Previously described "copy-choice" mechanisms (15,16) provide the most attractive explanation for generation of these mutants. Copy-choice involves transfer of RNA polymerase and nascent genome to alternate site(s) on a template followed by replication reinitiation and elongation. Non-homologous transfers would result in deletion or insertion mutants.

Viable deletion mutants of MHV-4 are rare but are selectively amplified in some cell cultures. In fact, MAbs are not required for selection of deletions in Sac- cells. Continual passaging eventually results in relatively pure stocks of virus with a smaller E2. This is because infected Sac- cells can survive beyond 12 hours post-infection to support the low-cytotoxicity mutants but not the more potent MHV-4. Thus far our comparative analyses of MHV-4 and deletion mutant E2 synthesis, processing and transport have revealed no differences at early stages of infection. Therefore we believe that E2 lacking a region within the middle of 90B is less fusogenic in culture than MHV-4 E2.

What is the in vivo function of these dispensable sequences in E2? There does not appear to be any absolute in vitro or in vivo requirement for this part of E2 90B -- we have yet to find a cell line or murine host that will support the growth of MHV-4 but not the mutants. However these variants do not induce the fatal encephalitis seen with MHV-4. Whether or not this is due to a lack of infection of essential brain cells by the deletion mutants is currently under investigation.

ACKNOWLEDGMENTS

This is Publication Number 5970-IMM from the Department of Neuropharmacology, Scripps Clinic and Research Foundation, La Jolla, CA 92037. This work was supported in part by USPHS grants AI-25913 and NS-12428. TMG was supported by NIH training grant 5-T32-AG-00080.

REFERENCES

1. M.V. Haspel, P.W. Lampert, and M.B.A. Oldstone, Temperature-sensitive mutants of mouse hepatitis produce a high
   incidence of demyelination. Proc. Natl. Acad. Sci. USA
   75:4033 (1978).
2. S. Stohlman, P. Brayton, J. Fleming, L. Weiner, and M.
   Lai, Murine coronaviruses: isolation and
   characterization of two plaque morphology variants of
   JHM neurotropic strain. J. Gen. Virol. 63:265 (1982).
3. R.G. Dalziel, P.W. Lampert, P.J. Talbot, and M.J.
   Buchmeier, Site-specific alteration of murine hepatitis
   virus type 4 peplomer glycoprotein E2 results in reduced
   neurovirulence. J. Virol. 59:463 (1986).
4. J.O. Fleming, M.D. Trousdale, F.A.K. El-Zaatari, S.A.
   Stohlman, and L.P. Weiner, Pathogenicity of antigenic
   variants of murine coronavirus JHM selected with
   monoclonal antibodies. J. Virol. 58:869 (1986).
5. H. Wege, J. Winter, and R. Meyermann, The peplomer
   protein E2 of coronavirus JHM as a determinant of
   neurovirulence: Definition of critical epitopes by
   variant analysis. J. Gen. Virol. 69:87 (1988).
6. W. Luytjes, L.S. Sturman, P.J. Bredenbeek, J. Charite,
   B.A.M. van der Zeijst, M.C. Horzinek, and W.J.M. Spaan,
   Primary structure of the glycoprotein E2 of coronavirus
   MHV-A59 and identification of the trypsin cleavage
   site. Virology 161:479 (1987).
7. V.L. Morris, C. Tieszer, J. Mackinnon, and D. Percy,
   Characterization of coronavirus JHM variants isolated
   from Wistar Furth rats with a viral-induced
   demyelinating disease. Virology 169:127 (1989).
8. F. Taguchi and J.O. Fleming, Comparison of six different
   murine coronavirus JHM variants by monoclonal antibodies
   against the E2 glycoprotein. Virology 169:233 (1989).
9. L.S. Sturman, K.V. Holmes, and J. Behnke, Isolation of
   coronavirus envelope glycoproteins and interaction with
   the viral nucleocapsid. J. Virol. 33:449 (1980).
10. P.J. Talbot, A.A. Salmi, R.L. Knobler, and M.J.
    Buchmeier, Topographical mapping of epitopes on the
    glycoproteins of murine hepatitis virus-4 (strain JHM):
    Correlation with biological activities. Virology
    132:250 (1984).
11. W.N. Burnette, Western blotting: electrophoretic
    transfer of proteins from sodium dodecyl sulfate-poly-
    acrylamide gels to unmodified nitrocellulose and
    radiographic detection with antibody to radioiodinated
    protein A. Anal. Biochem. 112:195 (1981).
12. D.A. Steinhauer and J.J. Holland, Rapid evolution of RNA
    viruses. Ann. Rev. Microbiol. 41:409 (1987).
13. J.A. Robb and C.W. Bond, Coronaviridae, in:
    "Comprehensive Virology," H. Frankel-Conrat and R.R.
    Wagner, eds., Plenum Publishing Corp., New York (1979).
14. A.J. Huang and D. Baltimore, Defective interfering
    animal viruses. Comp. Virol. 10:73 (1977).
15. M.M.C. Lai, S. Makino, L.H. Soe, C.-K. Shieh, J.G. Keck,
    and J.O. Fleming, Coronaviruses: A jumping RNA
    transcription. Cold Spring Harbor Symp. Quant. Biol.
    LII:359 (1987).
16. R.A. Lazzarini, J.D. Keene, and M. Schubert, The origins
    of defective interfering particles of the negative
    strand RNA viruses. Cell 26:145 (1981).

RNA SEQUENCE ANALYSIS OF THE E2 GENES OF WILDTYPE AND
NEUROATTENUATED MUTANTS OF MHV-4 REVEALS A HYPERVARIABLE
DOMAIN

Suezanne E. Parker and Michael J. Buchmeier

Department of Neuropharmacology
Scripps Clinic and Research Foundation
La Jolla, CA

INTRODUCTION

Murine hepatitis virus 4 (MHV-4) is a neurotropic
coronavirus (1-4). Infection of the CNS in susceptible mice
strains results in a fatal encephalitis with destruction of
neurons accompanied by demyelination. The few mice that
survive the acute infection develop a chronic demyelinating
disease characterized by episodes of demyelination followed
by remyelination (2,5). The extensive white matter disease
is believed to arise as the consequence of viral infection
and destruction of oligodendrocytes (2,3,6).

There is substantial evidence indicating that the MHV-4
E2 glycoprotein plays a crucial role in determining the
neurovirulence of an MHV-4 infection. E2, the major
constituent of the viral spike or peplomer (7,8), is
initially synthesized as a 180 kDa peripheral membrane
glycoprotein and is subsequently cleaved into two
non-identical 90 kDa subunits compromising the amino
terminal (S_1 or 90B) and the carboxy terminal (S_2 or
90A) regions of the protein (9). The E2 glycoprotein
mediates the attachment of the virion to susceptible cells,
is responsible for cell to cell fusion after infection and
is the major target on the virus for neutralizing antibodies
(9-12). Passive transfer of neutralizing MAbs to E2 alters
the course of MHV-4 induced disease from a fatal
encephalitis to a chronic demyelinating disease (13).
Furthermore, variants of MHV-4 selected for their ability to
escape neutralization by anti-E2 MAbs are neuroattenuated
and induce chronic demyelination (14-16).

The selection of neuroattenuated variants by antibodies
specific for E2 provides some of the strongest evidence that
E2 plays a pivotal role in the outcome of a CNS infection.
To localize the genetic alteration(s) in E2 responsible for
neuroattenuation we have sequenced the viral RNA encoding
the E2 gene of MHV-4 and of the neuroattenuated variants.
The carboxy terminal half of E2 was found to be highly
conserved whereas in contrast, the amino terminal half is

Coronaviruses and Their Diseases
Edited by D. Cavanagh and T.D.K. Brown
Plenum Press, New York, 1990

very polymorphic and contains deletions of up to 159 amino acids in the antibody resistant variants.

METHODS

The parental strain of MHV-4 was originally obtained from L.P. Weiner and propagated on Sac- cells as previously described (7). Neuroattenuated variants V5A13.5(86) and V4B11.3(86) were isolated from a 1986 plaque purified stock of MHV-4 by their ability to resist neutralization by MAb 5A13.5 (epitope E2B) and 4B11.6 (epitope E2C) respectively, as previously described (14). V5A13(88) was recently isolated from a 1988 plaque purified stock of MHV-4 (17). JHM-X, a variant of MHV-JHM which has been shown to have a smaller E2 gene as well as a truncated E2 glycoprotein compared to wildtype (18) was kindly provided for sequence analysis by Dr. M.M.C. Lai.

The sequence of the viral RNA was determined by the dideoxy primer extension method using radiolabeled synthetic oligonucleotides 20 bases in length as primers (19,20). Viral RNA was isolated from infected cells by guanidine isothiocyanate extraction (21). Sequence data was compiled and analyzed using the University of Wisconsin Genetics Computer Group sequence analysis software package (22).

RESULTS AND DISCUSSION

Direct RNA sequence analysis of the E2 gene of the neuro-attenuated variants of MHV-4 and the JHM-X revealed that the variants had large deletions ranging in size from 426 to 477 nucleotides in the 5' coding region of the E2 gene. As a consequence of the nucleotide deletions, the E2 glycoproteins of the variants have large deletions ranging from 142 amino acids in the case of V5A13.1(86) to 159 amino acids in the case of V4B11.3(86). Table 1 lists the size and location of the deletions. As a consequence of the deletion in the E2 glycoprotein of V5A13.1(86), there is a lysine to asparagine substitution at amino acid 433 at the 5' boundary of the deletion (Fig. 1). The deletions in E2 all map to a localized region in the amino terminal half of the protein (Fig. 1) thus defining the location of major epitopes determining both neutralization and neurovirulence.

Table 1. Location of Deletions in E2

Virus	Nucleotide Deletion	Amino Acid Deletion
MHV-JHM	423 (1,359-1,781)	141 (454-594)
JHM-X	458 (1,336-1,794)	153 (446-598)
V5A13.1(86)	426 (1,298-1,723)	142 (434-575)
V5A13(88)	447 (1,307-1,753)	149 (436-585)
V4B11.3(86)	477 (1,285-1,761)	159 (429-586)

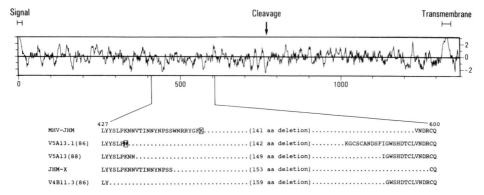

Fig. 1. Hydropathicity plot of the MHV-4 E2 glycoprotein
according to the analysis of Kyte and Doolittle (40)
and localization of the deletions in the amino
terminal domain of MHV-4 E2.   The vertical scale is
the average hydropathicity (+2 to -2) index for each
residue over a window of 9 amino acids.   Hydrophobic
sequences appear above the midline and hydrophilic
sequences appear below the midline.   Below is an
alignment of comparable amino acid sequences from
MHV-JHM (29), JHM-X, and MHV-4 variants V8A13.1(86),
V4B11.3(86) and V5A13(88). The numbering is relative
to the MHV-4 E2 amino acid sequence.   Dots indicate
deletions and boxed amino acids indicate sequence
changes from MHV-4 E2.   The signal sequence,
putative cleavage site and transmembrane domains of
E2 are indicated.

     Selection by MAbs of viral escape mutants with large
deletions is uncommon.   Most often it has been shown that
MAb selected variants have point mutations which affect
antibody binding to a given epitope (23-28).   The E2 glycoprotein may be unique in that it can accommodate large
deletions while retaining functions necessary for virus
growth both in vitro and in vivo.

     A comparison of the amino acid sequence of E2 for our
parental strain of MHV-4 (see Fig. 2 for the complete
sequence of E2 for MHV-4) with that of MHV-JHM (29), and of
MHV-A59 (30) reveals that the carboxy terminal region is
highly conserved whereas the amino terminal region of E2 is
very heterogeneous with respect to size.   Of importance is
the finding that the E2 glycoprotein of MHV-4 contains an
additional 141 amino acids (aa 454-594) as compared to
MHV-JHM (Fig. 2).   This clearly demonstrates that MHV-4 and
MHV-JHM which were previously considered to be synonymous,
are in fact distinct viruses.   Given the near sequence
identity of E2 for the two viruses, MHV-JHM may actually be
a deletion variant of MHV-4.   The E2 glycoprotein of MHV-4
also contains an additional 52 amino acids (501-552)
compared to MHV-A59.   This heterogeneity in E2 maps to the
same region of the protein which is deleted in the variants
of MHV-4 (Fig. 2).   Heterogeneity in terms of size of E2 has
also been reported to occur as a result of the in vitro and
in vivo passage of MHV where variants with both a smaller E2

(31) as well as variants with a larger E2 than the parental strain have been described (32,33). As the sequence data becomes available for these variants it will be of interest to determine if these differences represent deletions or insertions of the polymorphic sequences that we have described.

```
                                                                              TAATCTAAAC
1
M  L  F  V  F  I  L  L  L  P  S  C  L  G  Y  I  G  D  F  R  C  I  Q  T  V  N  Y  N  G  N  N  A  S  A  P  S  I  S  T  E     40
ATGCTGTTCGTCTTTATTTTACTATTACCCTCCTTGTTTAGGGTATATTGGTGATTTTAGATGTATCCAGACCGTGAATTATAACGGCAATAATGCTTCTGCGCCTAGCATTAGCACCGAA   120
  o o o o o o o o R o o o o o o
A  V  D  V  S  K  G  L  G  T  Y  Y  Y  V  L  D  R  V  Y  L  N  A  T  L  L  L  L  T  G  Y  Y  P  V  D  G  S  N  Y  R  N  L  A     80
GCAGTCGATGTTTCCAAAGGTCTGGGCACTTACTATGTTTTAGATCGTGTTTACTTAAATGCCACGTTATTGCTTACTGGTTATTATCCTGTGGACGGTTCCAATTATCGGAATCTCGCG   240

L  T  G  T  N  T  L  S  L  T  W  F  K  P  P  F  L  S  E  F  N  D  G  I  F  A  K  V  Q  N  L  K  T  N  T  P  T  G  A  T     120
CTTACAGGCACTAATACCTTAAGCCTTACGTGGTTTAAACCACCCTTTCTAAGTGAGTTTAATGATGGTATATTGCTAAGGTCCAGAACCTCAAGACAAATACGCCAACAGGTGCAACC   360

S  Y  F  P  T  I  V  I  G  S  L  F  G  N  T  S  Y  T  V  V  L  E  P  Y  N  N  I  I  M  A  S  V  C  T  Y  T  I  C  Q  L     160
TCATATTTTCCCACTATAGTTATAGGTAGTTTGTTTGGTAACACTTCCTATACCGTAGTTTTAGAGCCATATAATAATATTATAATGGCTTCTGTTTGTACATATACCATTTGTCAATTA   480

P  Y  T  P  C  K  P  N  T  N  G  N  R  V  I  G  F  W  H  T  D  V  K  P  P  I  C  L  L  K  R  N  F  T  F  N  V  N  A  P     200
CCTTACACACCCTGTAAGCCTAATACCAATGGTAATCGTGTTATTGGATTTTGGCACACAGATGTCAAACCGCCGATTTGTCTTTTAAAGCGTAATTTTACGTTTAATGTTAATGCCCCT   600

W  L  Y  F  H  F  Y  Q  Q  G  G  T  F  Y  A  Y  Y  A  D  K  P  S  A  T  T  F  L  F  S  V  Y  I  G  D  I  L  T  Q  Y  F     240
TGGCTTTATTTCCATTTTTATCAGCAGGTGGTACTTTTTATGCGTACTATGCGGATAAACCTTCCGCTACTACGTTTTTGTTTAGTGTGTATATTGGCGACATTTTAACACAGTATTTT   720
                                                                       A
V  L  P  F  I  C  T  P  T  A  G  S  T  L  L  P  L  Y  W  V  T  P  L  L  K  R  Q  Y  L  F  N  F  N  E  K  G  V  I  T  S     280
GTGTTACCTTTTATTTGTACTCCAACAGCTGGTAGCACTTTACTGCCGCTCTATTGGGTTACACCTTTACTTAAGCGCCAATATTTGTTTAATTTTAATGAAAAGGGTGTCATTACTAGT   840

A  V  D  C  A  S  S  Y  I  S  E  I  K  C  K  T  Q  S  L  L  P  S  T  G  V  Y  D  L  S  G  Y  T  V  Q  P  V  G  V  V  Y     320
GCTGTTGATTGCGCCAGCAGCTACATTAGTGAAATAAAATGTAAGACCCAAAGTCTCTTACCGAGTACTGGTGTCTATGATCTATCCGGTTACACGGTCCAACCTGTTGGAGTTGTGTAC   960

R  R  V  P  N  L  P  D  C  K  I  E  E  W  L  T  A  K  S  V  P  S  P  L  N  W  E  R  R  T  F  Q  N  C  N  F  N  L  S  S     360
CGGCGTGTTCCTAACCTACCTGATTGTAAAATAGAGGAATGGCTCACTGCTAAATCTGTGCCGTCACCTCTCAATTGGGAGCGTAGGACTTTCCAAAATTGTAATTTTAATTTAAGCAGC   1080

L  L  R  Y  V  Q  A  E  S  L  S  C  N  N  I  D  A  S  K  V  Y  G  M  C  F  G  S  V  S  V  D  K  F  A  I  P  R  S  R  Q     400
CTGCTACGTTATGTCCAGGCTGAGTCTTTGTCGTGTAATAATATTGATGCGTCCAAAGTGTATGGTATGTGCTTTGGTAGTGTCTCAGTTGATAAGTTTGCTATCCCCCGAAGCCGTCAA   1200
                                                                  V4B|86|        V5A|86|  V5A|88|
I  D  L  Q  I  G  N  S  G  F  L  Q  T  A  N  Y  K  I  D  T  A  A  T  S  C  Q  L  Y  Y  S  L  P  K  N  N  V  T  I  N  N     440
ATTGATTTACAAATTGGCAACTCCGGATTTTTGCAAACGGCTAATTATAAGATTGATACCGCTGCCACATCAGTCAGCTGTATTACAGTCTTCCTAGAATAATGTTACCATAAATAAC   1320
      JHMX                       K  JHM
Y  N  P  S  S  W  N  R  R  Y  G  F  N  D  A  G  V  F  G  K  S  K  H  D  V  A  Y  A  Q  Q  C  F  T  V  R  P  S  Y  C  F     480
TATAACCCCTCGTCTTTGGAATAGGAGGTATGTTTTAATGATGTCTGGTGGTGTGTTTGGCAAAAGTAAACATGATGTTGCCTACGCCCAGCAATGTTTTACTGTGCGACCTAGCTATTGTCCG   1440
                               A59
C  A  Q  P  D  I  V  S  A  C  T  S  Q  T  K  P  M  S  A  Y  C  P  T  G  T  I  H  R  E  C  S  L  W  N  G  P  H  L  R  S     520
TGTGCACAACCGGACATAGTTAGCGCTTGCACTAGTCAGACCAAACCCATGTCTGCTTATTGCCCCCACAGGCACAATTCATCGTGAGTGTTCTCTTTGGAATGGGCCCCATTTGCGCTCG   1560
                                                          A59
A  R  V  G  S  G  T  Y  T  C  E  C  T  C  K  P  N  P  F  D  T  Y  D  L  R  C  G  Q  I  K  T  I  V  N  V  G  D  H  C  E     560
GCACGTGTAGGTTCCGGCACGTACACGTGTGAGTGCACTTGTAAACCCAATCCATTTGATACGTATGATCTCCGCTGTGGGCAAATTAAAACTATTGTTAATGTGGGCGATCATTGTGAA   1680
        V5A|86|                        V5A |88|  V4B|86|              JHM    JHMX
G  L  G  V  L  E  D  K  C  G  N  S  D  P  H  K  G  C  S  C  A  N  D  S  F  I  G  W  S  H  D  T  C  L  V  N  D  R  C  Q     600
GGTCTGGGTGTTTTAGAAGATAAATGTGGCAATAGCGATCCACATAAGGGCTGTTCTTGTGCCAATGATTCTTTTATCGGATGGTCACATGACACTTGTTTAGTAAATGATCGCTGCCAA   1800

I  F  A  N  I  L  L  N  G  I  N  S  G  T  T  C  S  T  D  L  Q  L  P  N  T  E  V  A  T  G  V  C  V  R  Y  D  L  Y  G  I     640
ATTTTTGCTAACATATTGTTAAATGGCATTAATAGTGGGACTACGTGTTCCACAGATTTACAATTGCCTAATACTGAAGTGGCCACTGGCGTTTGCGTCAGATATGACCTCTATGGTATT   1920

T  G  Q  G  V  F  K  E  V  K  A  D  Y  Y  N  S  W  Q  A  L  L  Y  D  V  N  G  N  L  N  G  F  R  D  L  T  T  N  K  T  Y     680
ACTGGTCAAGGTGTTTTTAAAGAGGTCAAGGCTGACTATTATAATAGCTGGCAGGCCCTATTATATGATGTTAATGGTAACTTAAACGGGTTCCGTGACCTTACCACTAACAAGACTTAT   2040

T  I  R  S  C  Y  S  G  R  V  S  A  A  Y  H  K  E  A  P  E  P  A  L  L  Y  R  N  I  N  C  S  Y  V  F  T  N  N  I  S  R     720
ACGATAAGGAGCTGTTATAGTGGCCGTGTTTCTGCTGCATATCATAAAGAAGCACCCGAACCGGCTCTGCTCTATCGTAATATAAATTGTAGTTATGTTTTTACTAATAATATTTCCCGT   2160
                                                                    N
E  E  N  P  L  N  Y  F  D  S  Y  L  G  C  V  V  N  A  D  N  R  T  D  E  A  L  P  N  C  D  L  R  M  G  A  G  L  C  V  D     760
GAGGAAAACCCCCTTAACTATTTTGATAGTTATTTGGGTTGTGTTGTTAATGCTGATAACCGCACGGATGAGGCGCTTCCTAATTGCGATCTCCGTATGGGTGCTGGACTATGCGTAGAT   2280

Y  S  K  S  R  R  A  R  R  S  V  S  T  G  Y  R  L  T  T  F  E  P  Y  M  P  M  L  V  N  D  S  V  Q  S  V  G  G  L  Y  E     800
TATTCAAAGTCACGCAGAGCCCGCCGATCAGTTTCTTACTGGCTATCGATTAACCACATTCGAGCCATACATGCCGATGTTAGTCAATGATAGCGTTCAATCCGTAGGTGGATTATATGAG   2400

M  Q  I  P  T  N  F  T  I  G  H  H  E  E  F  I  Q  I  R  A  P  K  V  T  I  D  C  A  A  F  V  C  G  D  N  A  A  C  R  Q     840
ATGCAAATACCAACCAATTTTACTATTGGTCATCATGAGGAATTCATCCAGATAAGGGCTCCCAAGGTGACTATAGATTGTGCTGCATTTGTTTGTGGTGATAACGCTGCATGCAGACAG   2520

Q  L  V  E  Y  G  S  F  C  D  N  V  N  A  I  L  N  E  V  N  N  L  L  D  N  M  Q  L  Q  V  A  S  A  L  M  Q  G  V  T  I     880
CAGTTGGTTGAGTATGGCTCTTTTTGTGATAATGTTAATGCCATTCTTAATGAGGTTAATAACCTCTTGGATAATATGCAATTACAAGTTGCTAGTGCATTAATGCAGGGTGTTACTATA   2640

S  S  R  L  P  D  G  I  S  G  P  I  D  D  I  N  F  S  P  L  L  G  C  I  G  S  T  C  A  E  D  G  N  G  P  S  A  I  R  G     920
AGTTCGAGGCTGCCAGATGGCATCTCCGGCCCTATAGATGACATTAATTTTCAGTCCTCTACTTGGATGCATAGGTTCAACATGTGCTGAAGACGGCAATGGACCTAGTGCGATACGGGGG   2760
```

Recombination between heterologous strains of coronaviruses has been reported to occur at a relatively high
frequency (34-36) and is believed to occur as a consequence
of the discontinuous mechanism of "leader primed transcription" that has been described for MHV replication. Presumably, during MHV replication RNA transcription frequently
pauses at sites of secondary structure on the template RNA
releasing the transcriptional complex and the nascent RNA
strand which subsequently rejoins the template and reinitiates transcription (37). Deletions of genomic RNA
could occur by the same mechanism whereby the transcriptional complex reinitiates at a distant site on the template
RNA from where the initial disassociation event occurred.
Because E2 can accommodate large deletions, the progeny
virions resulting from a recombination in the E2 may require
site specific recombination without the accompanying loss of
genetic information.

```
R  S  A  I  E  D  L  L  F  D  K  V  K  L  S  D  V  G  F  V  E  A  Y  N [N] C  T  G  G  Q  E  V  R  D  L  L  C  V  Q  S    960
CGTTCAGCTATAGAGGATTTATTATTTGACAAGGTCAAACTATCTGACGTTGGCTTTGTCGAGGCTTATAACAATTGCACTGGTGGTCAAGAAGTTCGCGACCTCCTTTGCGTACAGTCT  2880

F  N  G  I  K  V  L  P  P  V  L  S  E  S  Q  I  S  G  Y  T  A  G  A  T  A  A  A  M  F  P  P  W  T  A  A  A  G  V  P  F   1000
TTTAATGGCATCAAAGTATTACCTCCCGTGTTGTCTGAGAGTCAAATCTCTGGCTACACAGCGGGTGCTACTGCGGCAGCTATGTTCCCACCTTGGACTGCAGCTGCTGGTGTGCCATTC  3000

S  L  N  V  Q  Y  R  I  N  G  L  G  V  T  M  N  V  L  S  E  N  Q  K  M  I  A  S  A  F  N  N  A  L  G  A  I  Q  E  G  F   1040
AGTTTAAATGTTCAATATAGGATTAATGGTTTAGGTGTCACTATGAATGTTCTTAGTGAGAACCAAAAGATGATTGCTAGTGCTTTTAACAACGCGCTCGGTGCTATTCAGGAAGGGTTC  3120

D  A  T  N  S  A  L  G  K  I  Q  S  V  V  N  A  N  A  E  A  L  N  N  L  L  N  Q  L  S  N  R  F  G  A  I  S  A  S  L  Q   1080
GATGCAACCAATTCTGCTCTAGGTAAGATCCAGTCCGTTGTTAATGCAAACGCTGAAGCACTTAATAATTTATTAAACCAACTTTCTAATAGGTTTGGTGCTATTAGTGCTTCTTTACAA  3240

E  I  L  T  R  L  D  A  V  E  A  K  A  Q  I  D  R  L  I  N  G  R  L  T  A  L  N  A  Y  I  S  K  Q  L  S  D  S  T  L  I   1120
GAAATTCTCAACGCGGCTTGACGCTGTAGAAGCAAAGGCCCAGATAGATCGTCTTATTAATGGCAGGTTAACTGCACTTAATGCGTATATATCCAAGCAACTCAGTGATAGTACGCTTATT  3360

K  F  S  A  A  Q  A  I  E  K  V  N  E  C  V  K  S  Q  T  T  R  I  N  F  C  G  N  G  N  H  I  L  S  L  V  Q  N  A  P  Y   1160
AAATTTAGTGCTGCTCAGGCCATCGAAAAGGTCAATGAGTGCGTTAAGAGCCAAACTACGCGCATTAATTTCTGTGGCAATGGTAATCACATATTATCACTTGTCCAGAATGCGCCTTAT  3480

                                                                          A
G  L  C  F  I  H  F  S  Y  V  P  T  S  F  K  T  A [N] V  S  P  G  L  C  I  S  G  D  R  G  L  A  P  K  A  G  Y  F  V  Q   1200
GGCTTATGTTTTATTCATTTCAGCTACGTGCCAACATCCTTTAAAACGGCAAATGTGAGTCCTGGACTATGCATTTCTGGTGATAGAGGATTGGCACCTAAAGCTGGATATTTTGTTCAA  3600

D  N  G  E  W  K  F  T  G  S  N  Y  Y  Y  P  E  P  I  T  D  K  N  S  V  V  M  I  S  C  A  V [N] Y  T  K  A  P  E  V  F   1240
GATAATGGAGAGTGGAAGTTCACAGGCAGTAATTATTACTACCCTGAACCCATTACAGATAAAAATAGTGTTGTCATGATCAGTTGCGCTGTGAATTACACAAAAGCGCCTGAAGTTTTC  3720

L [N] N  S  I  P  N  L  P  D  F  K  E  E  L  D  K  W  F  K [N] Q  T  S  I  A  P  D  L  S  L  D  F  E  K  L [N] V  T  F   1280
TTGAACAACTCAATACCAAATCTACCCGACTTTAAGGAGGAGTTAGATAAATGGTTTAAGAATCAGACGTCTATTGCGCCTGATTTATCCCTCGATTTCGAGAAGTTAAATGTTACTTTC  3840

L  D  L  T  Y  E  M  N  R  I  Q  D  A  I  K  K  L [N] E  S  Y  I  N  L  K  E  V  G  T  Y  E  M  Y  V  K  W  P  W  Y  V   1320
CTGGACCTGACTTATGAGATGAACAGGATTCAGGATGCAATTAAGAAGTTAAATGAGAGCTACATCAACCTCAAGGAAGTTGGCACATATGAAATGTATGTGAAATGGCCTTGGTATGTT  3960

W  L  L  I  G  L  A  G  V  A  V  C  V  L  L  F  F  I  C  C  C  T  G  C  G  S  C  C  F  R  K  C  G  S  C  C  D  E  Y  G   1360
TGGTTGCTAATTGGTTTAGCTGGTGTGACCGTTTGTGTGTTATTATTCTTTATATGTTGCTGCACAGGTTGCGGCTCATGTTGTTTTTAGAAAATGCGGAAGTTGTTGTGATGAGTATGGA  4080
●  ●  ●  ●  ●  ●  ●  ●  ●  ●  ●  ●  ●  ●  ●  ●  ●  ●  ●  ●  ●  ●  ●  ●  ●  ●  ●  ●  ●  ●  ●  ●
G  H  Q  D  S  I  V  I  H [N] I  S  A  H  E  D  *    1376
GGACACCAGGACAGTATTGTGATACATAATATTTCAGCCCATGAGGATTGACTATCACA  4139
```

Fig. 2. Nucleotide and predicted amino acid sequence of the
         MHV-4 E2 gene. The numbering starts at the ATG codon.
         Open circles indicate the N-terminal signal sequence
         (calculated according to the algorithm of Von Heijne
         [38], as described by Fazakerley and Ross [39]) and
         closed circles indicate the hydrophobic carboxy-
         terminal transmembrane domain. Potential glyco-
         sylation sites are indicated by boxed asparagine
         residues. The intergenic homology sequence
         TAATCTAAAC is boxed. The putative proteolytic
         cleavage site between the amino terminal and carboxy
         terminal domain is indicated by an arrowhead. The
         MHV-JHM amino acid sequence (29) is indicated where
         differences occur. Brackets denote the boundaries
         of the deletion for the indicated viruses.

By direct RNA sequence analysis of the E2 gene of wild-type MHV-4 and of neuroattenuated variants we have demonstrated that the E2 glycoprotein of MHV is very heterogeneous with respect to deletions in a localized region of the amino terminal half of the protein. Sequences localized within this polymorphic region of the protein are important in determining the neurovirulence of an MHV-4 infection of the CNS. Studies are currently underway to further assess the role of this domain in an in vivo infection.

ACKNOWLEDGMENTS

The authors thank Maria Salvato and Elaine Shimomaye for advice on RNA sequencing, Joseph O'Neill for technical assistance and Gay Schilling for manuscript preparation. This work was supported by NIH grants AI-25913 and NS-12428. SEP was the recipient of a National Multiple Sclerosis Society Fellowship. This is Publication Number 5971-IMM from the Department of Neuropharmacology, Research Institute of Scripps Clinic, La Jolla, CA 92037.

REFERENCES

1. L.P. Weiner, Pathogenesis of demyelination induced by a mouse hepatitis virus (JHM virus), Arch. Neurol. 28:298 (1973).
2. P.W. Lampert, J.K. Sims, and A.J. Kniazeff, Mechanism of demyelination in JHM virus encephalomyelitis, Electron microscopic studies, Acta. Neuropathol. 24:76 (1973).
3. M.V. Haspel, P.W. Lampert, and M.B.A. Oldstone, Temperature sensitive mutants of mouse hepatitis virus produce a high incidence of demyelination, Proc. Natl. Acad. Sci. USA 75:4033 (1978).
4. H. Wege, S. Siddel, and V. ter Meulen, The biology and pathogenesis of coronaviruses, Curr. Top. Microbiol. Immunol. 99:165 (1982).
5. R.L. Knobler, P.N. Tunison, P.W. Lampert, and M.B.A. Oldstone, Selected mutants of mouse hepatitis virus type 4 (JHM strain) induce different CNS diseases, Am. J. Pathol. 109:157 (1982).
6. M.E. Dubois-Dalcq, E.W. Doller, M.V. Haspel, and K.V. Holmes, Cell tropism and expression of mouse hepatitis virus (MHV) in mouse spinal cord cultures, Virology 119:317 (1982).
7. L.S. Sturman, K.V. Holmes, and J. Behnke, Isolation of coronavirus envelope glycoproteins and interaction with the viral nucleocapsid, J. Virol. 33:449 (1980).
8. S. Siddel, H. Wege, and V. ter Meulen, The structure and replication of coronaviruses, Curr. Top. Microbiol. Immunol. 99:131 (1982).
9. L.S. Sturman, C.S. Ricard, and K.V. Holmes, Proteolytic cleavage of the E2 glycoprotein of murine coronavirus: Activation of cell-fusing activity of virions by trypsin and separation of two different 90K cleavage fragments, J. Virol. 56:904 (1985).
10. A.R. Collins, R.L. Knobler, H. Powell, and M.J. Buchmeier, Monoclonal antibodies to murine hepatitis virus-4 (strain JHM) define the viral glycoprotein responsible for attachment and cell-cell fusion, Virology 119:358 (1982).

11. P.J. Talbot, A.A. Salmi, R.L. Knobler, and M.J. Buchmeier, Topographical mapping of epitopes on the glycoproteins of murine hepatitis virus-4 (strain JHM): Correlation with biological activities, _Virology_ 132:250 (1984).

12. H. Wege, R. Dorries, and H. Wege, Hybridoma antibodies to the murine coronavirus JHM: Characterization of epitopes on the peplomer protein (E2), _J. Gen. Virol._ 65:1931 (1984).

13. M.J. Buchmeier, H.A. Lewicki, P.J. Talbot, and R.L. Knobler, Murine hepatitis virus-4 (strain JHM)-induced neurological disease is modulated _in vivo_ by monoclonal antibody, _Virology_ 132:261 (1984).

14. R.G. Dalziel, P.W. Lampert, P.J. Talbot, and M.J. Buchmeier, Site-specific alteration of murine hepatitis virus type 4 peplomer glycoprotein E2 results in reduced neurovirulence, _J. Virol._ 59:463 (1986).

15. J.O. Fleming, M.D. Trousdale, F.A.K. El-Zaatari, S.A. Stohlman, and L.P. Weiner, Pathogenicity of antigenic variants of murine coronavirus JHM selected with monoclonal antibodies, _J. Virol._ 58:869 (1986).

16. H. Wege, J. Winter, and R. Meyermann, The peplomer protein E2 of coronavirus JHM as a determinant of neurovirulence: Definition of critical epitopes by variant analysis, _J. Gen. Virol._ 69:87 (1988).

17. T.M. Gallagher, S.E. Parker, and M.J. Buchmeier, Neutralization resistant variants of a neurotropic coronavirus are generated by deletions within the amino terminal portion of the E2 spike glycoprotein, _J. Virol._ submitted (1989).

18. F. Taguchi and J.O. Fleming, Comparison of six different murine coronavirus JHM variants by monoclonal antibodies against the E2 glycoprotein, _Virology_ 169:233 (1989).

19. P.H. Hamlyn, M.J. Gait, and C. Milstein, Complete sequence of an immunoglobulin mRNA using specific priming and the dideoxynucleotide method of RNA sequencing, _Nuc. Acids Res._ 9:4485 (1981).

20. F. Sanger, S. Nicklen, and A.R. Coulson, DNA sequencing with chain terminating inhibitors, _Proc. Natl. Acad. Sci. USA_ 74:5463 (1977).

21. J.M. Chirgwin, A.E. Przybyla, R.J. MacDonald, and W.J. Rutter, Isolation of biologically active ribonucleic acid from sources enriched in ribonuclease, _Biochemistry_ 18:5294 (1979).

22. J. Devereux, P. Haberli, and O. Smithies, A comprehensive set of sequence analysis programs for the VAX, _Nuc. Acids Res._ 12:387 (1984).

23. D.M.A. Evans, P.D. Minor, G.S. Schild, and J.V. Almond, Critical role of an eight-amino acid of VP_1 in neutralization of poliovirus type 3, _Nature_ 304:459 (1983).

24. I. Seif, P. Coulon, S.E. Rollin, and A. Flamand, Rabies virulence: Effect on pathogenicity and sequence characterization of rabies virus mutations effecting antigenic site III of the glycoprotein, _J. Virol._ 53:926 (1985).

25. J.W. Yewdell, A.J. Caton, and W. Gerhard, Selection of influenza A virus adsorptive mutant by growth in the presence of a mixture of monoclonal anti-hemagglutinin antibodies, _J. Virol._ 57:623 (1986).

26. R. Bassel-Duby, D.R. Spriggs, K.L. Tyler, and B.N. Fields, Identification of attenuating mutations on the reovirus type 3^1 double-stranded RNA segment with a rapid sequencing technique, J. Virol. 60:64 (1986).
27. S.D. Thompson and A. Portner, Localization of functional sites on the hemagglutinin-neuraminidase glycoprotein of Sendai virus by sequence analysis of antigenic and temperature-sensitive mutants, Virology 160:1 (1987).
28. L. Luo, Y. Li, R.M. Snyder, and R.R. Wagner, Point mutations in glycoprotein gene of vesicular stomatitis virus (New Jersey serotype) selects resistance to neutralization by epitope-specific monoclonal antibodies, Virology 163:341 (1988).
29. I. Schmidt, M. Skinner, and S. Siddel, Nucleotide sequence of the gene encoding the surface projection glycoprotein of coronavirus MHV-JHM, J. Gen. Virol. 68:47 (1987).
30. W. Luytjes, L.S. Sturman, P.J. Bredenbeek, J. Charite, B.A.M. van der Zeijst, M.C. Horzinek, and W.J.M. Spaan, Primary structure of the glycoprotein E2 of coronavirus MHV-A59 and identification of the trypsin cleavage site, Virology 161:479 (1987).
31. V.L. Morris, C. Tieszer, J. Mackinnon, and D. Percy, Characterization of coronavirus JHM variants isolated from Wistar Furth rats with a viral induced demyelinating disease, Virology 169:127 (1989).
32. F. Taguchi, S.G. Siddel, H. Wege, and V. ter Meulen, Characterization of a variant virus selected in rat brains after infection by coronavirus mouse hepatitis virus JHM, J. Virol. 54:429 (1985).
33. F. Taguchi, P.T. Massa, and V. ter Meulen, Characterization of a variant virus isolated from neural cell culture after infection of mouse coronavirus JHMV, Virology 155:267 (1986).
34. M.M.C. Lai, R.S. Baric, S. Makino, J.G. Keck, J. Egberg, J.L. Leibowitz, and S.A. Stohlman, Recombination between nonsegmented RNA genomes of murine coronaviruses, J. Virol. 56:449 (1985).
35. S. Makino, J.G. Keck, S.A. Stohlman, and M.M.C. Lai, High frequency of RNA recombination of murine coronaviruses, J. Virol. 57:729 (1986).
36. J.G. Keck, G.K. Matsushima, S. Makino, J.O. Fleming, D.M. Vannier, S.A. Stohlman, and M.M.C. Lai, In vivo RNA-RNA recombination of coronavirus in mouse brain, J. Virol. 62:1810 (1988).
37. R.S. Baric, C.-K. Chien, S.A. Stohlman, and M.M.C. Lai, Analysis of intracellular small RNAs of mouse hepatitis virus: Evidence for discontinuous transcription, Virology 156:342 (1987).
38. G. von Heijne, A new method for predicting signal sequence cleavage sites, Nuc. Acids Res. 14:4683 (1986).
39. J.K. Fazakerley and A.M. Ross, Computer analysis suggests a role for signal sequences in processing polyproteins of enveloped RNA viruses and as a mechanism of viral fusion, Virus Genes 2:219 (1989).
40. J. Kyte and R.F. Doolittle, A simple method for displaying the hydropathic character of a protein, J. Mol. Biol. 157:105 (1982).

CHARACTERIZATION OF ATTENUATED MUTANTS OF MHV3 : IMPORTANCE OF THE E2

PROTEIN IN ORGAN TROPISM AND INFECTION OF ISOLATED LIVER CELLS

J.P. MARTIN, W. CHEN, G. OBERT, F. KOEHREN

Laboratoire de Virologie de la Faculté de Médecine et Unité
INSERM 74
3, rue Koeberlé 67000 STRASBOURG

INTRODUCTION

MHV3 is an hepatotropic coronavirus. The injection of this virus
into susceptible.BALB/c mice causes a mortal fulminating hepatitis. Several viral genes have been implicated as determinants of MHV virulence,
including the nucleocapsid (5), E2 (4, 6) and polymerase genes (7). The
E2 glycoprotein plays a central role in determining cellular tropism and
MHV virulence. It is responsible for the attachment of the virus to the
cell and point mutations in the E2 gene could thus modify virus pathogenicity and the target organ. The selection of antibody "escape mutants"
has been used by several laboratories to confirm the importance of E2 as
a viral determinant of virulence (8). In the case of the MHV3 strain, no
results have so far been reported. We have selected MHV3 variants by virtue of their resistance to neutralization by monoclonal antibodies. Two
of the mutants selected were less pathogenic than the parental strain.
This difference in the biological effect may be associated with a modification in organ tropism and failure to recognize viral receptors on
certain hepatic cells.

METHODS

Cells and Virus

MHV3 was a clonal isolate produced in L929 cell cultures. Viral suspensions were assayed on L2 cells (9) for titration and for ELISA assays
the virus was concentrated on a cushion of 50 % sucrose,   bothbefore and
after being purified through a 20-40 % sucrose gradient.

Preparation of the Hepatic Cells

Kupffer cells and endothelial cells. This technique has already been
described (11). Briefly, mouse livers were perfused in situ with 0.05 %
collagenase and then incubated for 30 min in a rotary water bath shaker
with 0.05 % collagenase. The sinusoidal cells were collected by density
gradient centrifugation with metrizamide. The endothelial cells and Kupffer cells were separated by centrifugal elutriation. The cells were
cultured in 96-well microtiter plates at a concentration of 3 x 10^5

Coronaviruses and Their Diseases
Edited by D. Cavanagh and T.D.K. Brown
Plenum Press, New York, 1990

cells/well in Dulbecco's modified Eagle's medium supplemented with 20 % fetal bovine serum.

Ito cells (fat-storing cells) (FSC). The FSC were prepared according to the procedure previously described (3). In brief, Kupffer cells or endothelial cells were isolated and cultured. On account of their high rate of multiplication, the FSC, which contaminated the culture by 3-5 %, reached around 50 % after 15 days. They were then purified by negative selection based on their inability to form rosettes with IgG-coated sheep erythrocytes. Following this, the FSC were cultured in 96-well microtiter plates at a concentration of 2 x 10^4 cells/well in Dulbecco's modified Eagle's medium supplemented with 10 % fetal bovine serum.

Hepatocytes. Mouse hepatocytes were isolated according to Berry (1) and Seglen (10), partially modified by Braunwald (unpublished data). Briefly, after perfusion in situ via the portal vein with Hank's balanced salt solution followed by 0.05 % collagenase in Williams' E medium, the cellular suspension was filtered through nylon wool. After centrifugation and triple washing, the hepatocytes were diluted in Williams' E medium containing 4 ug/ml insulin and 20 % inactivated fetal bovine serum and seeded in 35 mm Petri dishes at a concentration of 1.2 x 10^6 cells/dish.

Isolation of Mutants

L2 cells in 96-well plates were infected with 300 PFU of MHV3 per well in the presence of specific monoclonal antibodies. The cells producing virus surviving neutralization were harvested by freeze-thawing and a second selection with antibody was performed. Each mutant was cloned twice by limited dilution and 100 PFU were injected intraperitonally into BALB/c mice.

ELISA Assays

The virus was adsorbed for 2hrs at 4°C on intact cells and washed by immersion in PBS. The plates were then examined for specific binding of the monoclonal antibody using a streptavidin-biotinyled alkaline phosphase preformed complex. The optical density was measured as being 405 nm.

RESULTS

Selection and Characterization of Mutants Resistant to Monoclonal Antibodies

Mutants were selected from the MHV3 strain with 15 neutralizing monoclonal antibodies which recognized the E2 protein by radio-immuno-precipitation (not shown). The number of mutants isolated with each monoclonal antibody was variable though the largest number was generally obtained with monoclonal antibodies which did not inhibit cell fusion. 283 mutants were isolated and after amplification of each virus in the presence of the specific monoclonal antibody, 100 PFU of each mutant were inoculated by intraperitoneal injection into five sensitive BALB/c mice. Only two mutants, 51.6 and Cl 12, revealed a modified pathogenic effect. The resistance of these two mutants to the selective monoclonal antibody was checked by indirect immunofluorescence in infected cells and immunoprecipitation coupled with PAGE. 51.6 and Cl 12 were obtained with two different monoclonal antibodies (A51 and A37 respectively). These antibodies were able to neutralize MHV3 at high dilutions (> 10,000), slightly inhibited cellular fusion and did not protect the sensitive mice against MHV3 injection. No difference in the size of the mRNA coding for

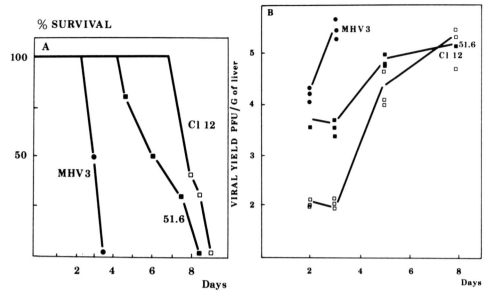

Fig 1A.   Survival of mice after I.P. injection of 100 PFU of wt MHV3 or
          mutants.

Fig 1B.   Virus titer in liver homogenates at different times after
          injection of wt MHV3 or mutants.

the E2 protein was detected by agarose gel electrophoresis nor in the
si e of the E2 protein studied by immunoprecipitation.

Biological Activity of the Resistant Mutants

   Mortality. Twenty   sensitive BALB/c mice free of coronavirus antibodies were injected intraperitoneally with 100 PFU of each mutant and
wild type virus. A 50 % mortality rate was reached after 3 days p.i. and

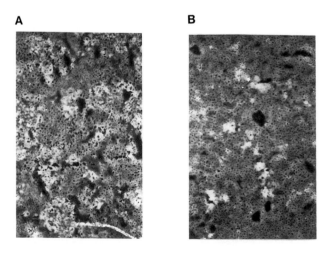

Fig 2.   Viral antigens in liver sections detected by indirect
         immunofluorescence. A : Wt MHV3, B : Cl 12

after 6 days p.i. with the 51.6 mutant or 8 days p.i. with Cl 12 (Fig 1A). The two mutants were thus not avirulent though their lethal affect was retarded to the same extent.

Detection of viral antigens. Viral antigens were examined in frozen liver samples taken at different times after infection. At 3 days p.i. with wt virus, the liver appeared invaded with viral antigens and the necrotic foci were very large. At 8 days p.i., with the mutants, the necrotic foci were small and were slow to enlarge even slightly (Figs 2A et B).

Viral titer in the liver. In the liver homogenates wild type virus was detectable at 48h p.i. (Fig 1B). Multiplication was intensive between 48h and 72h with wt virus. With Cl 12, viral replication occurred mainly

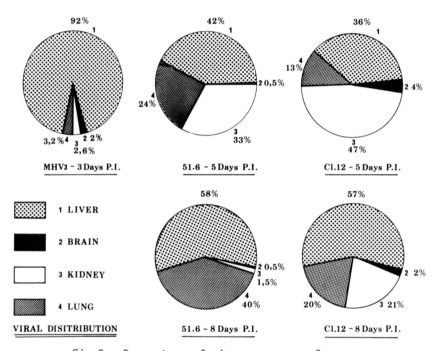

Fig 3 . Percentage of virus per gram of organ.

between 4 days and 5 days p.i., then it slowed down until the 8th day. The 51.6 mutant behaved in an intermediate manner. It is remarkable that the final titer at 3 days p.i. with wt virus and 8 days p.i. with mutants was very similar.

Organ Tropism

The determination of the amounts of virus in the liver, brain, lung and kidney showed that at 3 days p.i. 90 % of the wt virus was concentrated in the liver (Fig 3). With the mutants only about 40 % was found in the liver at 5 days p.i. Prior to the death of the mice, (8 days p.i.) less than 60 % was present in the liver. At that time the major part of mutant 51.6 was localized in the lung and mutant Cl 12 was equally distributed between the lung and the kidney. The brain seemed only slightly infected.

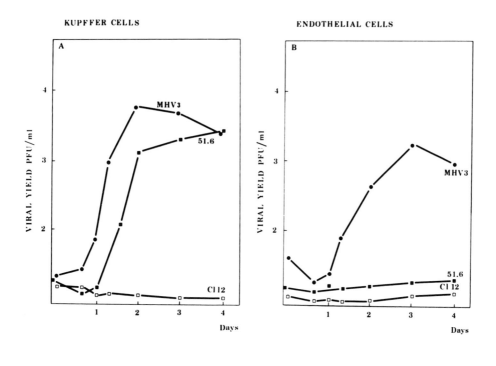

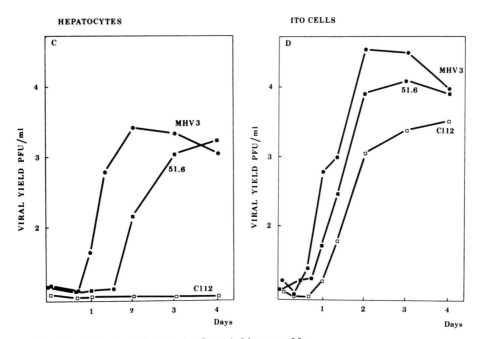

Fig 4. Viral yield in isolated liver cells

A : Kupffer cells, B : Endothelial cells, C : Hepatocytes,
D : Ito cells.

Table 1. Summarize table of the permissivity of isolated hepatic cells and optical densities in ELISA assays of virus binding to whole cells.

	PERMISSIVITY OF CELLS				ELISA ON WHOLE CELLS		
	KC	EC	HC	IC	L2	KC	EC
MHV3	+	+	+	+	1.130	0.603	0.440
51.6	+	-	+	+	1.082	0.538	0.121
CL.12	-	-	-	+	1.058	0.085	0.041

The mutants appeared to be somewhat less hepatotropic. To understand why the mutants multiplied less rapidly in the liver, we isolated liver cells and infected them in vitro.

In Vitro Multiplication

Titer in the hepatic cells. Viral yields were measured in the hepatic cells, the sinusoidal cells (Kupffer cells, endothelial cells, Ito cells) and hepatocytes (Figs 4A, B, C, D). The maximum yield was usually obtained after 48h p.i. with wt virus except in the endothelial cells (72h p.i.) and the 51.6 mutant multiplied in all but not in the endothelial cells. In cells permissive for this mutant, the titer was similar to the wt virus, but multiplication was delayed by about 24 hours. Cl 12 multiplied only in the Ito cells, all other cell types being non-permissive. Table 1 shows the importance of the endothelial cells in retarding mortality and in modifying organ tropism, since the endothelial cells alone were non-permissive for the two mutants.

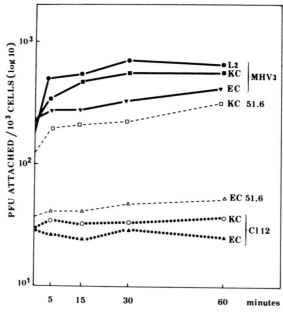

Fig 5. Adsorption of wt MHV3 and mutants on isolated sinusoidal cells

Virus adsorption to the hepatic cells. Sinusoidal cells were isolated and cultur and 24h later virus was adsorbed for 2h at + 4°C on the non-fixed cells. An other monoclonal antibody against the E2 protein was added and subsequently detected by ELISA assays. The data were compared with those for L2 cells which are permissive for the 3 viruses (Table 1). Measurement of the optical density revealed that: (i) adsorption of mutants on KC and EC was very poor, (ii) the efficiency of adsorption on L2 cells was similar in all cases, (iii) for a virus, adsorption was different between KC, EC and L2 cells. The results showed that the non-permissive cells were unable to bind virus.

Adsorption assay by PFU determination. Adsorption was measured at different times after virus-cell contact at 4°C (Fig 5). The apparent interactions between Cl 12 and the KC and EC respectively were very poor and remained at the same level throughout the entire assay. Identical results were obtained with 51.6 and EC. On the other hand, adsorption onto KC was close to the level observed with wt virus.

CONCLUSIONS

In this study we have analyzed the behaviour of two MHV3 mutants which resist neutralization by monoclonal antibodies directed against the E2 protein. Although the mutants were not avirulent, a considerable delay in mortality was observed in BALB/c mice. This delay seemed to correspond to a modification in the organ tropism of the mutants since the liver, which is the main target organ for MHV3, was no longer a major replication site for the mutants which, to the contrary appeared to accumulate in the lungs and kidneys. Our results suggest that liver endothelial cells play a major role in virus diffusion within this organ since the fact that the mutants were attenuated corresponded to a loss in permissivity for the mutants of in vitro cultur endothelial cells. Moreover, the endothelial cells' lack of susceptibility could be explained by the failure of these cells to recognize and adsorb mutant virus. The viral receptors on liver cells are identified in this study as being the key components of MHV3 hepatotropism. The finding that the two mutants isolated behaved differently towards different liver cell types suggests that several cell receptors may be involved in MHV3 recognition. Furthermore, the apparent number of viral receptors seems to vary according to the cell type examined. A given number of mouse L2 cells adsorbs twice the amount of virus particles in comparison with a similar number of sinusoidal cells. Our results bear out the findings for the MHV-A59 virus (2) that MHV3 cell receptors play a major role in tissue tropism and in the pathogenesis of this virus.

Acknowledgements

We are grateful to Michèle Valle for excellent technical assistance, Robert Drillien for helpful comments and Véronique Risch for excellent help with the manuscript.

REFERENCES

1. Berry, M.N., Friend, D.S., 1969, High-yield preparation of isolated rat liver parenchymal cells. J. Cell. Biol., 43:506-520.

2. Boyle, J.F., Weismiller, D.G., Holmes, K.W., 1987, Genetic resistance to mouse hepatitis virus correlates with absence of virus-binding activity on target tissues. J. Virol., 61:185-189.

3. Chen, W., Gendrault, J.L., Steffan, A.M., Jeandidier, E., and Kirn, A., 1989, Isolation, culture and main characteristics of mouse fat-storing cells : Interaction with viruses. Hepatology, 9:352-362.

4. Dalziel, R.G., Lampert, P.W., Talbot, P.J. and Buchmeier, M.J., 1986, Site-specific alteration of murine hepatitis virus type 4. Peplomer glycoprotein E_2 results in reduced neurovirulence. J. Virol., 59:463-471.

5. Fleming, J.O., Stohlman, S.A., Harmon, R.C., Lai, M.M.C., Frelinger, J.A., and Weiner, L.P., 1983, Antigenic relationships of murine coronaviruses : analysis using monoclonal antibodies to JHM (MHV-4) virus. Virology, 131:296-307.
6. Fleming, J.O., Trousdale, M.D., El-Zaatari, F.A.K., Stohlman, S.A., and Weiner, L.P., 1986, Pathogenicity of antigenic variants of murine coronavirus JHM selected with monoclonal antibodies. J. Virol., 58:869-875.

7. Lai, M.M.C., Brayton, P.R., Armen, R.C., Patton, C.D. Pugh, C., and Stohlman, S.A., 1981, Mouse hepatitis virus MHV A59 : mRNA structure and genetic localization of the sequence divergence from hepatotropic strain MHV3. J. Virol., 39:823-834.

8. Leibowitz, J.L., De Vries, J.R., Rodriguez, M., 1986, Increased hepatotropism of mutants of MHV, strain JHM, selected with monoclonal antibodies, in Coronavirus, Lai M.M.C., Stohlman, S.A., Eds. Plenum Press, New-York, London.

9. Martin, J.P., Koehren, F., Rannou, J.J. and Kirn, A., 1988, Temperature-sensitive mutants of mouse hepatitis virus type 3 (MHV3) : isolation, biochemical and genetic characterization. Arch. Virol., 100:147-160.

10. Seglen, P.O., 1976, Preparation of isolated rat liver cells. Methods Cell. Biol., 13:29-81.

11. Steffan, A.M., GENDRAULT, J.L., Mac Cuskey, R.S., Mac Cuskey, P.A., Kirn A., 1986, Phagocytosis, an unrecognized property of murine endothelial liver cells. Hepatology, 6:830-836.

MURINE HEPATITIS VIRUS JHM VARIANTS ISOLATED FROM WISTAR FURTH RATS WITH

VIRAL-INDUCED NEUROLOGICAL DISEASE

V.L. Morris,[1] G.A.R. Wilson,[1] C.E. McKenzie,[1] G. Tieszer,[1] N. La Monica,[2] L. Banner,[2], D. Percy,[3] M.M.C. Lai,[2] S. Dales[1]

[1]Cytobiology Group, Dept. Microbiology & Immunology, Univ. of Western Ontario, London, ON, Canada N6A 5C1, [2]Depts. Microbiology & Neurology, Univ. of S. California, Sch. of Med., Los Angeles, CA 90033, [3]Dept. Pathology, Ont. Vet. College, Univ. of Guelph, Guelph, ON, Canada N1G 2W1

INTRODUCTION

Murine Hepatitis Virus (MHV) can produce neurological disease in murine species.(1) Intracerebral (ic) inoculation of 2-day old Wistar Furth rats with the JHM virus (JHMV) strain of MHV generally produces an acute encephalitis which kill the rats within one week of inoculation.(2,3) Grey matter lesions generally predominate in the central nervous system (CNS) of these rats. Wistar Furth rats which are inoculated at 10 days of age with JHMV generally develop a chronic demyelinating disease characterized by hind leg paralysis or paresis.(2,3,4) These symptoms generally do not develop until 2-4 weeks post inoculation.(2,4) The rats that live for 3 weeks post inoculation or longer generally have predominately white matter lesions.(2,3,4)

Wild type JHMV produces 7 mRNAs in mouse fibroblast (L-2) cells which have molecular weights of approximately 0.8, 1.1, 1.4, 1.6, 3, 4, 5.8 x 10^6 Da.(5,6,7,8) By convention, the highest molecular weight RNA, which is of genomic size, is designated mRNA 1, and the lowest molecular weight mRNA is called mRNA 7.(9,10) The mRNAs form a 3'-coterminal nested set extending for different lengths in a 5' direction. (5,9,11,12,13,14,15) The coding sequence utilized during infection is located at the 5' end of each mRNA not present in smaller mRNA species.(8,16) The E2 glycoprotein is a heterodimer with a molecular weight of 180 kDa.(17) This molecule forms the projecting peplomers of the virus and its functions likely include attachment to cells, induction of cell to cell fusion, and elicitation of neutralizing antibodies.(18,19,20,21)

MHV has a high rate of recombination.(22) Recombinant virus arises at a high frequency in mouse CNS tissue that is infected with a mixture of ts mutants of A59 and JHMV.(23) We have shown that a truncated E2 glycoprotein mRNA is present in the CNS of Wistar Furth rats with a JHMV-induced demyelinating disease.(4) Further work has shown that JHMV E2 glycoprotein can be detected in individual cells of JHMV infected CNS tissue; however, the ratio of detectable E2 antigen to nucleocapsid antigen in the total CNS tissue of infected rats is reduced by more than 13 fold compared with the same ratio in JHMV-infected tissue culture cells.(2) We have now isolated and are examining JHMV variants from the CNS of Wistar Furth rats with a JHMV-induced demyelinating disease. We have found that differences in mRNAs produced by the viral variants and wild type JHMV were accompanied by differences in the biological properties of these viruses.

RESULTS AND DISCUSSION

CHARACTERIZATION OF VIRAL VARIANTS

We isolated viral variants from the brain and spinal cord of a 10 day-old Wistar Furth rat pup (designated AT11f) that was inoculated ic with a cloned isolate of the murine hepatitis virus (MHV) strain JHMV. This pup was severely runted and developed hind leg paresis by 14 days post inoculation when it was sacrificed. Virus was recovered independently from the brain and spinal cord and designated AT11f brain virus and AT11f cord virus, respectively. We thus were able to compare two virus isolates recovered from a single inoculated rat pup. A littermate of AT11f (called AT11e) was also inoculated with the same stock of JHMV at 10 days of age. At 13 days post inoculation, rat AT11e had symptoms similar to those of AT11f and was killed. Virus was isolated from the brain of rat AT11e and was designated AT11e brain virus. Results obtained with AT11f brain virus were generally similar to those obtained with AT11e brain virus.

All of the viral variants and wild-type JHMV formed massive syncytia in mouse fibroblast L-2 cells.(24) However, AT11f brain virus, AT11e brain virus, and wild-type JHMV virus-infected oligodendroglioma cells (G26-24) resembled uninfected G26-24 cultures except individual cells "rounded up" and lifted off from the monolayer.(24) These infected cultures only rarely contained viral-induced syncytia. In contrast, AT11f cord virus formed massive syncytia equally well in mouse L-2 and G26-24 cells.(24) The wild type JHMV and all of the viral variants are capable of forming syncytia which cover 60-80% of the monolayer in a neuroblastoma cell line (C1300). We have also examined C6 cells which are of Wistar Furth rat astrocytoma origin and RN2-2 which are of BD1X rat Schwannoma cell origin.(25) Neither wild type JHMV nor any of the variant viruses produced any significant numbers of syncytia in these cells. Starting with a single stock of AT11f cord virus, the ratio of the titer in G26-24 cells to the titer in L-2 cells was 0.472 (Table 1). However, the same ration for AT11f brain virus was 0.008, for AT11e brain virus was 0.011, and for wild-type JHMV was 0.010 (Table 1). Therefore, the ratio of the viral titer in G26-24 cells to the titer in L-2 cells was approximately 50-fold higher for AT11f cord virus than for the brain virus variants and wild-type JHMV (Table 1). We also find that the AT11f cord virus variant grows better in C6 cells than do the wild-type JHMV, the AT11f brain virus, or the AT11e brain virus (Table 1). The ratio of the virus titer in C6 cells to the titer in L-2 cells was more than a hundred fold greater for AT11f cord virus than the same ratio was for wild-type JHMV or the brain virus variants (Table 1). The ratio for AT11f cord virus was maintained even when residual virus remaining after adsorbtion and penetration was removed by washing 3 times with a 0.05% Tween 20 solution or treatment with JHMV antibody. It has been previously shown that the C6 cells are restrictive to JHMV replication by preventing the early penetrating stage of the viral replicative cycle.(26) Therefore the alterations in AT11f cord virus allows this variant to at least partially overcome this restriction. The wild type JHMV appears to grow marginally (5-10 fold) better in C1300 (mouse neuroblastoma cell line) than do the viral variants. There is no significant difference in the ability of the viral variants to grow in a Schwannoma (RN2-2) cell line. Our data with the wild-type JHMV are in good agreement with previously published results.(25)

Primary cultures of oligodendrocytes and astrocytes were established from the cerebral cortices of neonatal Wistar Furth rats (27) and challenged with wild type JHMV and variant AT11f cord virus. Infection of Wistar Furth oligodendrocytes resulted in a productive infection with AT11f cord virus producing at least 10 fold more virus than wild type JHMV at 24

Table 1. Titers of Viral Variants and Wild-Type JHM.

Virus[a]	Cell Line[b]	Titer (PFU/ml)	Titer in cell line/ titer in L-2 cells
AT11f cord[c]	G26-24	8.5×10^6	0.472×10^0
AT11f cord[c]	L-2	1.8×10^7	
AT11f brain[c]	G26-24	7.0×10^4	0.8×10^{-2}
AT11f brain[c]	L-2	9.0×10^6	
AT11e brain[c]	G26-24	8.5×10^4	0.11×10^{-1}
AT11e brain[c]	L-2	7.5×10^6	
JHM[c]	G26-24	4.9×10^5	0.1×10^{-1}
JHM[c]	L-2	4.9×10^7	
AT11f cord	C-6	2.5×10^4	0.17×10^{-2}
AT11f cord	L-2	1.5×10^7	
AT11f brain	C-6	6×10^1	0.6×10^{-5}
AT11f brain	L-2	1×10^7	
AT11e brain	C-6	1.2×10^2	0.15×10^{-4}
AT11e brain	L-2	8×10^6	
JHM	C6	4×10^1	0.7×10^{-5}
JHM	L-2	5.5×10^6	
AT11f cord	RN2-2	3×10^2	0.6×10^{-4}
AT11f cord	L-2	5×10^6	
AT11f brain	RN2-2	2.2×10^3	0.22×10^{-3}
AT11f brain	L-2	1×10^7	
AT11e brain	RN2-2	1×10^3	0.13×10^{-3}
AT11e brain	L-2	8×10^6	
AT11f cord	C1300	9.5×10^5	0.6×10^{-1}
AT11f cord	L-2	1.5×10^7	
AT11f brain	C1300	2.3×10^5	0.23×10^{-1}
AT11f brain	L-2	1.0×10^7	
AT11e brain	C1300	6.5×10^5	0.81×10^{-1}
AT11e brain	L-2	8×10^6	
JHM	C1300	1.8×10^6	0.33×10^0
JHM	L-2	5.5×10^6	

a) For each virus and infected cell line the identical virus preparation was used to infect L-2 cells.
b) L-2 cells are a mouse fibroblast cell line. G26-24 cells are a C57B1/6 mouse oligodendroglioma cell line. C6 cells are a Wistar Furth rat astrocytoma cell line. RN2-2 cells are a BD1X Schwannoma cell line. C1300 cells are an A/J mouse neuroblastoma cell line.
c) Data was taken from Table 1 of (24).

hours post inoculation. AT11f cord virus infection also continued to be more productive at later times when compared with wild type JHMV, but neither AT11f cord virus nor wild type JHMV had any observable increase in the amount or extent of cell-to-cell fusion in these cultures. Inoculation of Wistar Furth astrocytes with either wild-type JHMV or AT11f cord virus, failed to produce any infection, even at the earliest time points assayed, consistent with previous studies reporting an unambiguous tropism of JHMV for rat oligodendrocytes.(27) Therefore, while AT11f cord virus resembled wild type JHMV with respect to tropism for oligodendrocytes, AT11f cord virus infects oligodendrocytes more productively than the wild type JHMV.

Wistar Furth rat littermates inoculated with AT11f cord virus and AT11f brain virus had different courses of disease. When seventeen 10-day old pups were inoculated with AT11f cord virus, a more chronic demyelinating disease typified by hind leg paralysis developed; these rats died in an average time of 20 days.(24) In nineteen 10-day old injected rats, AT11f brain virus produced a rapid encephalitis which killed the rats in an average time of 9 days.(24) When twelve 2 day old Wistar Furth rats were inoculated with AT11f cord virus, the rats died in an average time of 10.8 days. When thirteen rats from the same litters were inoculated with AT11f brain virus, the rats died in an average time of 5.5 days. None of the uninoculated control rats showed any symptoms. Histopathological examination indicated that, in general, the white matter lesions were more extensive in the spinal cord and brain stem region (metencephalon and mesencephalon) in rats inoculated at 10 days with AT11f cord virus when compared with rats inoculated at 10 days with the brain virus variants.(24)

COMPARISON OF mRNA AND PROTEINS SYNTHESIZED BY JHMV VARIANTS

We examined the mRNAs produced in L-2 or G26-24 cells infected with wild type JHMV or the viral variants. Northern transfer analysis indicated that viral mRNAs 4, 5, 6 (E1 envelope glycoprotein), and 7 (nucleocapsid) comigrated for all the viral variants and JHMV wild-type viruses.(24) However, a truncated mRNA 3 with a molecular weight of 2.85×10^6 Da was produced in AT11f cord virus infected cells; wild type JHMV and the other viral variants produced a mRNA 3 of 3×10^6 Da. In addition, AT11f brain and AT11e brain virus each produced two novel mRNA species (3.3 and 3.6×10^6 Da). These mRNA species are distinct from the 4.0×10^6 Da mRNA species seen with the wild-type JHMV.(24) In addition, a uniform deletion of approximately 1.5×10^5 Da exists in the E2 glycoprotein and higher molecular weight mRNAs produced in AT11f cord virus infected cells when compared with cells infected by the brain virus variants.(24)

We next examined the E2 protein synthesized by variant viruses and wild type JHMV. The E2 glycoprotein produced by AT11f cord virus had an apparent molecular weight of 165 kDa while the E2 glycoprotein made by the brain virus variants and wild type JHMV had an apparent molecular weight of 180 kDa.(24) To make sure that these differences were not simply due to differences in glycosylation, we compared the sizes of the E2 polypeptides synthesized in the presence of tunicamycin. The differences in the sizes of the E2 glycoprotein were still apparent even when the viruses were grown in the presence of tunicamycin.(24) Thus the E2 glycoprotein mRNA produced by the AT11f cord virus contains a deletion in its coding region. Sequencing studies indicated that a 441 base deletion occurred 1324 bases from the 5' end of the E2 coding region of the viral genome. This result is in good agreement with the 390 base deletion we had estimated from the Northern transfer analysis (24). This general location in the E2 coding region appears to be a common site for recombinations and deletions (unpublished results Dr. M. Lai, Univ. Southern California, California, USA). The viral variants' production of novel mRNA species with molecular weights lower than the 4×10^6 Da mRNA 2 species suggests that there may also be deletions in the coding region of mRNA 2 in these viruses. This possibility is under current investigation.

The deletion in the E2 glycoprotein of AT11f cord virus is thus associated with an increased ability of the virus to infect some cells of neural origin (G26-24 and C6 cells lines and primary oligodendrocyte cells). The increased ability of AT11f cord virus to replicate in C6 cells is apparently due to the ability of the virus to overcome a block in the penetration of the cells. This deletion in the E2 glycoprotein is also accompanied by the ability of the AT11f cord virus to cause a demyelinating disease in Wistar Furth rats with an increased white matter involvement. These results fit with the functions of the E2 glycoprotein which include attachment of virus to cells, induction of cell to cell fusion, and elicitation of neutralizing antibodies.(18,19,20,21) Future work will explore the possible role of deletions or alterations in mRNA 2 in the propensity of the AT11f and AT11e brain viruses to cause an acute encephalitis in rats.

ACKNOWLEDGEMENTS

G.A.R.W. was supported by a studentship from the MS Society of Canada. This work was supported by a grant from the MRC of Canada awarded to V.L.M., grants from the MS Society of Canada and the MRC of Canada awarded to S.D., and a NSERC grant awarded to D.P.

REFERENCES

1. F. S. Cheever, J. B. Daniels, A. M. Pappenheimer, and O. T. Bailey, A murine virus (JHM) causing disseminated encephalomyelitis with extensive destruction of myelin: I. Isolation and biological properties of the virus, J. Exp. Med. 90:195 (1949).
2. D. Parham, A. Tereba, P. J. Talbot, D. P. Jackson, and V. L. Morris, Analysis of JHM central nervous system infections in rats, Arch. Neurol. 43:702 (1986).
3. O. Sorensen, D. Percy, and S. Dales, In vivo and in vitro models of demyelinating diseases. III. JHM virus infection of rats, Arch. Neurol. 37:478 (1980).
4. D. P. Jackson, D. H. Percy, and V. L. Morris, Characterization of murine hepatitis virus (JHM) RNA from rats with experimental encephalomyelitis, Virol. 137:297 (1984).
5. S. Cheley, R. Anderson, M. J. Cupples, E. C. Chan, and V. L. Morris, Intracellular murine hepatitis virus-specific RNAs contain common sequences, Virol. 112:596 (1981).
6. S. Cheley, V. L. Morris, M. J. Cupples, and R. Anderson, RNA and polypeptide homology among murine coronaviruses, Virol. 115:310 (1981).
7. I. Schmidt, M. Skinner, and S. Siddell, Nucleotide sequence of the gene encoding the surface projection glycoprotein of coronavirus MHV-JHM, J. Gen. Virol. 68:47 (1987).
8. S. Siddell, H. Wege, and V. ter Meulen, The biology of coronaviruses, J. Gen. Virol. 64:761 (1983).
9. W. J. Spaan, P. J. Rottier, M. C. Horzinek, and B. A. van der Zeijst, Isolation and identification of virus-specific mRNAs in cells infected with mouse hepatitis virus (MHV-A59), Virol. 108:424 (1981).
10. H. Wege, S. Siddell, M. Sturm, and V. ter Meulen, Coronavirus JHM: Characterization of intracellular viral RNA, J. Gen. Virol. 54:213 (1981).
11. M. M. Lai, and S. A. Stohlman, Comparative analysis of RNA genomes of mouse hepatitis viruses, J. Virol. 38:661 (1981).
12. J. L. Leibowitz, K. C. Wilhelmsen, and C. W. Bond, The virus specific intracellular species of two murine coronaviruses: MHV-A59 and MHV-JHM, Virol. 114:39 (1981).
13. D. F. Stern, and S. I. T. Kennedy, Coronavirus multiplication strategy. I. Identification and characterization of virus-specific RNA, J. Virol. 34:665 (1980).

14. D. F. Stern, and S. I. T. Kennedy, Coronavirus multiplication strategy. II. Mapping the avian infectious bronchitis virus intracellular RNA species to the genome. J. Virol. 36:440 (1980).

15. S. R. Weiss, and J. L. Leibowitz, Characterization of murine coronavirus RNA by hybridization with virus-specific cDNA probes, J. Gen. Virol. 64:127 (1983).

16. J. L. Leibowitz, S. R. Weiss, E. Paavola, and C. W. Bond, Cell-free translation of murine coronavirus RNA, J. Virol. 43:905 (1982).

17. L. S. Sturman, C. S. Ricard, and K. V. Holmes, Proteolytic cleavage of the E2 glycoprotein of murine coronavirus: activation of cell-fusing activity of virions by trypsin and separation of two different 90K cleavage fragments, J. Virol. 56:904 (1985).

18. A. R. Collins, R. L. Knobler, H. Powell, and M. J. Buchmeier, Monoclonal antibodies to murine hepatitis virus-4 (strain JHM) define the viral glycoprotein responsible for attachment and cell-cell fusion, Virol. 119:358 (1982).

19. J. O. Fleming, S. A. Stohlman, R. C. Harmon, M. M. Lai, J. A. Frelinger, and L. P. Weiner, Antigenic relationships of murine coronaviruses: analysis using monoclonal antibodies to JHM (MHV-4) virus, Virol. 131:296 (1983).

20. L. S. Sturman, and K. V. Holmes, Proteolytic cleavage of peplomeric glycoprotein E2 of MHV yields two 90K subunits and activates cell fusion, Adv. Exp. Med. Biol. 173:25 (1984).

21. S. G. Siddell, H. Wege, and V. ter Meulen, The structure and replication of Coronaviruses, Curr. Topics in Microbiol. and Immunol. 99:131 (1982).

22. M. M. Lai, R. S. Baric, S. Makino, J. G. Keck, J. Egbert, J. L. Leibowitz, and S. A. Stohlman, Recombination between nonsegmented RNA genomes of murine coronaviruses, J. Virol. 56:449 (1985).

23. J. G. Keck, G. K. Matsushima, S. Makino, J. O. Fleming, D. M. Vannier, S. A. Stohlman, and M. M. Lai, In vivo RNA-RNA recombination of coronavirus in mouse brain, J. Virol. 62:1810 (1988).

24. V. L. Morris, C. Tieszer, J. MacKinnon, and D. Percy, Characterization of coronavirus JHM variants isolated from Wistar Furth rats with a viral-induced demyelinating disease, Virol. 169:127 (1989).

25. A. Lucas, W. Flintoff, R. Anderson, D. Percy, M. Coulter, and S. Dales, In vivo and in vitro models of demyelinating diseases: tropism of the JHM strain of murine hepatitis virus for cells of glial origin, Cell 12:553 (1977).

26. S. Van Dinter, and W.F. Flintoff, Rat glial C6 cells are defective in murine coronavirus internalization, J. Gen. Virol. 68:1677 (1987).

27. S. Beushausen, and S. Dales, In vivo and in vitro models of demyelinating disease. XI. Tropism and differentiation regulate the infectious process of coronavirus in primary explants of the rat CNS, Virol. 141:89 (1985).

Chapter 9

Porcine Respiratory Coronavirus

BACKGROUND PAPER

THE APPEARANCE OF THE PORCINE RESPIRATORY CORONAVIRUS HAS

CREATED NEW PROBLEMS AND PERSPECTIVES

M. Pensaert

Laboratory of Virology-Immunology
Faculty of Veterinary Medicine
State University of Gent
Casinoplein 24
9000 Gent
Belgium

In 1984, the appearance of a new porcine coronavirus related to TGEV was suspected based on an unexpected but widespread prevalence of antibodies to TGEV found in the swine population of several European countries. Most remarkable was the observation that this widespread occurrence of TGEV antibodies was seen in the absence of previous outbreaks or epizootics of diarrhea and also the fact that such findings were made in countries, e.g. Denmark, which had never experienced TGEV infection previously. The ease with which the virus spread, not only within a country, but also across national borders, pointed towards long distance virus transmission, almost certainly by the aerogenic route.

The virus involved was isolated in 1986 from the respiratory tract of swine and was found to be a coronavirus very closely related to the well-characterised TGEV. It was called porcine respiratory coronavirus (PRCV). Soon after its isolation, comparative antigenic studies between PRCV and TGEV were performed with the use of monoclonal antibodies which had been prepared against different epitopes of the Purdue strain of TGEV. It was found that in the TLM strain of PRCV three peplomer S epitopes, present in TGEV, are lacking or have been modified. Monoclonal antibodies directed against these epitopes have no virus-neutralizing capacity. Therefore, infection with TGEV or PRCV in swine induces neutralizing antibodies which are similar in titre and differentiation cannot be made by the sero-neutralisation test. An examination for the presence or absence of the differentiating epitopes on TGEV strains and PRCV strains showed that 6 virulent field TGEV strains, and 8 different TGEV attenuated strains (used as vaccine) bound the differentiating monoclonal antibodies while none of the 4 PRCV field strains did so. These studies permitted the conclusion that PRCV was not an attenuated TGEV which had "escaped" and been able to circulate in the swine population. This possibility had to be considered since it has been published that some TGEV strains, concomitantly with artificial attenuation, gradually acquire a tropism for the respiratory tract.

The slight difference found in epitope structure provided a means for serological differentiation between pigs which have been infected with TGEV and those which have been infected with PRCV. There is a definite need for such differentiation particularly in countries which export swine to countries which require that the imported animals are free from a previous infection with the enteropathogenic virulent TGEV. A differentiating ELISA test has been developed for this purpose but more data will be reported in this chapter on the molecular aspects of PRCV compared to TGEV and their possible use in differentiation.

Coronaviruses and Their Diseases
Edited by D. Cavanagh and T.D.K. Brown
Plenum Press, New York, 1990

The slight difference in molecular structure and particularly in the external glycoprotein composition has markedly altered the virus-host interactions of PRCV compared to that of TGEV. With TGEV, the pathogenesis in neonatal pigs is straightforward. After oral uptake of the virus, a massive replication occurs in the absorptive cells on the small intestinal villi with cell degeneration, desquamation and watery diarrhoea as a consequence. With PRCV, however, oronasal inoculation in neonatal pigs leads to virus replication to very high titers (up to $10^{8.3}$ TCID$_{50}$ per gram lung tissue) in the respiratory tract. Replication occurs in nasal, tracheal, bronchial, bronchiolar and alveolar epithelial cells and also in alveolar macrophages. Tonsillary tissue also supports virus replication.

One of the key points from a pathogenetic point of view is whether PRCV had kept its tropism for the intestine or not. Upon aerosol inoculation of 1 week old colostrum-deprived pigs, virus replication can be found in the small intestine, but the intestinal infection evolves totally differently from that of an enteric virus. Replication starts in the ileum and gradually spreads towards the duodenum. Immunofluorescence remains limited to a few cells located at crypt or villus sites. It is not clear which type of cell is involved and research is under way to identify it. Infected cells are found only on some villi and their number remains limited to one or a small group. They are often difficult to find. It can be assumed that they are not common villous enterocytes since one might then expect them all to be of equal sensitivity for the virus. In that case, the infection would be expected to run a normal progressive course with more cells infected at the peak of virus replication. That the intestine is not very sensitive to PRCV virus can be concluded from the finding that virus titres in the intestine remain low (maximally $10^{3.7}$ TCID$_{50}$). Also, more than 10^3 TCID$_{50}$ of PRCV are needed to consistently start the intestinal infection by direct virus inoculation in the lumen of the small intestine. PRCV certainly does not behave as an enteric virus since virus transmission does not occur through faeces. The amount of virus excreted via the faeces is probably insufficient to initiate an intestinal infection in a contact animal. A respiratory infection is needed so that sufficiently high quantities of virus can be ingested to initiate the intestinal infection.

An important practical question is whether PRCV infection, as it occurs in the field, induces an immunity to TGEV. In the field, PRCV regularly persists on farms and pigs usually become infected between the ages of 5 and 8 weeks. At that time, the respiratory infection occurs in the presence of relatively low titres of maternal antibodies in the blood. Whether or not intestinal replication also occurs in pigs infected at that age and in the presence of passive serum antibodies is not known. This aspect may be important from an immunological point of view as will be explained elsewhere in this chapter.

The PRCV-TGEV tandem opens perspectives for future research on virus-cell interactions and immunity mechanisms:

1. It is remarkable that a slight change in molecular arrangement in the E2 peplomer protein creates a virus which exhibits a totally different cell tropism. A prototype highly enteropathogenic TGEV has turned into a respiratory virus which has lost tropism for common villous enterocytes. Apparently the altered molecular site must be crucial for determining virus-cell interactions.

2. The tandem may present an ideal model for studying mucosal immunity and to test the concept of a common mucosal immune system in pigs. A PRCV infection with immunological stimulation in the respiratory tract can be used to find out if an immunological effect occurs against TGEV in the intestine. Vice versa, an intestinal infection with TGEV can be employed to examine a possible immunological reaction in the respiratory tract against PRCV.

3. It is known that an enteric viral infection in sows leads to a stimulation of the gut-mammary link with appearance of IgA in the milk (lactogenic immunity). However, TGEV neutralizing IgA is also found in the milk after an (exclusively?) respiratory infection with PRCV as will be reported further. It will be interesting to find out if IgA in the milk also can be obtained via a respiratory-tract-mammary gland link and if lactogenic immunity can be afforded in the intestine by this respiratory-induced IgA.

420

INDUCTION OF MILK IGA ANTIBODIES BY PORCINE RESPIRATORY CORONAVIRUS

INFECTION

P. Callebaut, E. Cox, M. Pensaert and K. Van Deun

Laboratory of Virology, Faculty of Veterinary Medicine
State University of Gent.
Casinoplein 24, 9000 Gent, Belgium

ABSTRACT

An ELISA was developed to examine the prevalence of TGEV-specific immunoglobulin (Ig)A in the milk of sows, infected in the field with PRCV or with TGEV. It was shown that previous PRCV-infections can induce the secretion of IgA antibodies in the milk. However, only 9 out of 28 PRCV-infected sows had IgA in their milk whereas 11 TGEV-infected sows all secreted IgA. On farms where a reinfection with PRCV occurred, the number of IgA-secreting sows increased from 2 to 11 on a total of 13 sows. This showed that the presence of IgA antibodies in the milk may depend upon the occurrence of reinfection with PRCV. As demonstrated by density gradient analysis, the milk IgA induced by PRCV was 11S secretory IgA and had the capacity to neutralize TGEV.

INTRODUCTION

In sow milk the most abundant class of immunoglobulin (Ig) is IgA[1]. It is mainly produced in the mammary tissue[2]. However, with transmissible gastroenteritis (TGE) as a model, it has been shown that the antigenic stimulation of the IgA secreting cells in the mammary gland occurs at a distant mucosal site, i.e. the gut associated lymphoid tissues[3]. IgA lymfocytes, stimulated in the gut, subsequently migrate to the mammary gland where they become localized and synthesize IgA antibodies which are secreted in the milk. This mechanism is referred to as the gut-mammary immunologic link. It is considered to be the basis of passive "lactogenic" immunity against enteric infections in suckling piglets, nursing immune sows.

It has been shown that following an infection with respiratory syncytial virus IgA antibodies are secreted in the milk of women[4]. This gives evidence that IgA secretion in the mammary gland may be induced at a mucosal site other than the gut, such as the respiratory tract.

As the porcine respiratory coronavirus (PRCV) primarily replicates in epithelial cells of the respiratory tract[5], the question arises if a PRCV-infection provokes the secretion of IgA antibodies in the milk of sows. In the present communication an ELISA is described for the detection of IgA antibodies against TGEV/PRCV in sow milk, together with the results of a comparative study of the prevalence of these antibodies in PRCV- and TGEV-

Coronaviruses and Their Diseases
Edited by D. Cavanagh and T.D.K. Brown
Plenum Press, New York, 1990

infected sows. In order to determine some of the properties of the IgA antibodies, milk immunoglobulins were separated by density gradient centrifugation.

MATERIALS AND METHODS

Specimens

On each of 6 farms between 5 and 8 sows were selected. Milk samples, to be examined for the presence of IgA antibody, were taken at different time intervals between 1 and 4 weeks after farrowing. Serum pairs were collected at the time of farrowing and 4 weeks later.

On 2 of these farms, designated TGEV-A and -B, a TGE outbreak had occurred 2,5 months and 2,5 years, respectively, prior to the time of sampling. The diagnosis of the TGEV-infection had been made by IF staining on gut sections of killed animals at the time of the outbreak. The selection for the present study of individual sows, which had been infected with TGEV on these farms, was based on the demonstration of the presence of differen-tial serum antibodies against TGEV by the competitive inhibition ELISA.

On 4 farms, designated PRCV-A, -B, -C and -D, an infection with PRCV had occurred prior to the time of sampling. The diagnosis of the PRCV-infection and the selection of individual PRCV-infected sows on these farms was made by demonstrating in serum samples the presence of TGEV neutralizing antibodies and the absence of differential TGEV-antibodies. On farm PRCV-D, the selected sows were experimentally reinfected by oronasal inoculation with 10^6 TCID50 of the Belgian PRCV-isolate TLM 83^6 at 7 days after far-rowing.

Control Specimens

Control TGEV-antibody negative milk samples, used to test the specifi-city of the IgA ELISA, were collected on 2 farms from 6 and 16 sows, respectively, between 1 and 4 weeks after farrowing.

Collection and Preparation of Milk

Milk was obtained manually following IM injection of 30 IU of oxytocin. Whole milk was centrifuged at 10 000 x g for 30 min. at 4° C. The middle fraction was collected and used for the titration fo antibody by VN and IgA ELISA. From samples, to be separated by density gradient centrifugation, casein was removed by pelleting at 85 000 x g for 1 h at 4° C.

Virus Neutralization (VN) Test

VN tests with heat inactivated (30 min. at 56° C) serum and milk speci-mens were performed as described previously[7], using the Purdue strain of TGEV as the antigen.

Competitive Inhibition ELISA

The competitive inhibition ELISA for the detection of differential serum antibodies against TGEV, permitting the differentiation of pigs infected with TGEV or PRCV, was performed as described elsewhere[8].

Separation of Milk Immunoglobulins

Milk immunoglobulins were separated by sucrose density gradient centri-fugation, performed as described by Vaerman[9] with minor modifications.

Briefly, 0,4 ml milk was layered on top of a 12 to 32,5 % (wt/wt) sucrose gradient in phosphate-buffered saline (PBS), pH 7,2, and centrifuged in a Beckman SW 41 Ti rotor at 200 000 x g for 17 h at 4° C. After centrifugation 0,5 ml fractions were collected and the location of protein peaks was determined by reading the absorbence of the fractions at 280 nm. The fractions were screened by IgA ELISA and tested for the presence of IgA, IgM and IgG by double micro-immunodiffusion utilizing antisera against the Fc fragments of porcine IgA, IgM and IgG (Nordic, Tilburg, The Netherlands). Four fractions, containing predominantly IgA, and 4 fractions with predominantly IgG were pooled, dialyzed overnight against PBS and tested for antibody titer by VN and IgA ELISA. Titers were corrected for the 5 x dilution factor of the immunoglobulins.

TGEV-specific IgA ELISA

The ELISA was performed in polystyrene microtiter plates (Nunc-Immuno plate Maxisorp F96), using 100 μl volumes of reagents per well. Optimal dilutions of reagents were determined by checkerboard titrations. Plates were coated with a 1/10 000 dilution in 0,05 M carbonate buffer, pH 9,6 of a mixture of equal volumes of 2 TGEV-specific monoclonal antibody (MAb) ascites fluids, kindly provided by Dr. L. Enjuanes, Madrid, Spain. The two MAb used have been designated 1DB12 and 6AC3; their preparation and characteristics have been described elsewhere[10]. Following overnight incubation at 37° C, the plates were washed three times with water containing 0,01 % Tween 80. A 1/50 dilution of viral antigen in PBS containing 0,01 % Tween80 and 10 % fetal calf serum (FCS) was added to alternating rows of wells. Diluent without viral antigen was added to the remaining rows, to be used as blanks. The viral antigen was the Purdue strain of TGEV, grown in the swine testicle ST cell line and prepared as described previously[8]. The plates were incubated for 5 h at 37° C and washed 4 times. Two-fold serial dilutions of milk samples (starting at 1/5) or sucrose gradient fractions (at a 1/5 dilution) were added each to wells with and without viral antigen and incubated overnight at room temperature. The plates were washed 4 times and a goat anti-swine IgA (Fc)-horseradish peroxidase conjugate, diluted 1/2 500, was added to each well for 1 h at 37° C. The conjugate was prepared according to the method of Wilson and Nakane[11], using immunoglobulins, purified from antiserum (Nordic) by conventional methods. Test samples and conjugate were diluted in 0,5 M NaCl, pH 7,2, containing 0,05 % Tween 80 and 10 % FCS. The plates were washed six times and substrate solution was added, containing 1mg/ml 5-aminosalicylic acid-0,005 % H_2O_2 in 0,01 M sodium phosphate, 1 mM Na2EDTA, pH 6,0. After overnight incubation at 4° C, the absorbence at 450 nm was read with a Multiskan (Flow Labs). A sample dilution was scored positive if the absorbence in the well with viral antigen, after subtraction of the absorbence in the blank well, was $\geq$ 0,050. The IgA antibody titer was determined as the reciprocal of the highest positive dilution. One IgA antibody-positive milk sample was included in each plate as a control to establish reproducibility.

RESULTS

Antibody Responses in Serum

In the serum, taken at the time of farrowing, all the 39 sows from the 6 farms had VN antibody. The geometric mean titer (GMT) was 122 (24-4096). On the farms TGEV-A and TGEV-B the GMT of the VN antibodies increased from 82 at the time of farrowing to 259 four weeks later. As shown in Table 1, 4-fold or higher titer rises were found in the paired sera from some of these sows. Using competitive inhibition ELISA, no significant titer rises of the differential TGEV-antibodies were found; the GMT was 19 (5-160) and 29 (5-160) at the time of farrowing and 4 weeks later, respectively.

Table 1. VN-antibody responses in serum and milk and IgA antibody responses in milk of sows, previously infected with TGEV or PRCV

Sow group**	Sow	VN titer				IgA ELISA titer in milk	
		Serum		Milk			
		0 wpp*	4 wpp*	1 wpp*	4 wpp*	1 wpp*	4 wpp*
TGEV-A	1	32	256	8	48	160	160
	2	64	384	16	48	40	160
	3	192	384	12	16	160	160
	4	1536	256	48	48	640	1280
	5	64	96	3	6	80	40
TGEV-B	1	24	192	12	192	320	1280
	2	24	512	24	96	320	5120
	3	64	192	8	32	80	160
	4	192	768	16	32	40	40
	5	64	96	48	256	320	640
	6	64	256	48	192	640	320
PRCV-A	1	192	192	6	6	<5	<5
	2	4096	1024	32	32	<5	<5
	3	24	256	32	12	640	.2560
	4	96	1536	8	256	<5	160
	5	48	512	12	48	10	160
PRCV-D	1	96	3072	2	24	<5	80
	2	24	512	2	384	<5	320
	3	24	512	<2	64	<5	320
	4	48	768	6	96	<5	320
	5	96	512	4	96	<5	80
	6	64	256	4	96	<5	640
	7	64	1536	3	96	<5	80
	8	768	3072	6	64	<5	320

*wpp = weeks post partum; **TGEV-A = infected with TGEV, 2,5 months previously; TGEV-B = infected with TGEV, 2,5 years previously; PRCV-A = infected previously with PRCV; PRCV-D = infected previously with PRCV and experimentally inoculated with PRCV at 1 wpp.

On farms PRCV-A and -D the GMT of the VN-antibodies increased between the time of farrowing and the end of the lactation period from 98 to 728. Eleven out of the 13 sows showed significant titer rises in the paired sera (Table 1). No VN-titer rises were found in the serum pairs from the sows at farms PRCV-B and -C: the GMT was 198 (48-1024) and 213 (32-1536) at the time of farrowing and 4 weeks later, respectively. All sera, collected on farms PRCV-A to D were negative (titer <5) in the competitive inhibition ELISA.

VN-antibody Responses in the Milk

The VN-antibody responses in the milk of TGEV- or PRCV-infected sows at different time intervals between 1 and 4 weeks after farrowing are shown in Table 2. The sows from farms TGEV-A and -B had VN-antibodies in all milk samples collected throughout the lactation period. Titers were minimal between 1 and 2 weeks after farrowing and increased towards the end of the lactation period. As indicated in Table 1, some sows showed a 4-fold or higher VN-titer rise between 1 and 4 weeks after farrowing.

Table 2. Prevalence and titers of VN- and IgA ELISA antibodies in the milk
of sows, previously infected with TGEV or PRCV

Sow group** (no.)	Time of milk collection (wpp)*	Geometric mean VN titer (range)	IgA ELISA positive	
			No.	Geometric mean titer (range)
TGEV-A	1	16(3–48)	5	240(80–1280)
(n = 5)	2	15(3–48)	5	140(40–1280)
	3	14(4–32)	5	240(80–640)
	4	26(6–48)	5	200(40–1280)
TGEV-B	1	27(6–96)	6	127(20–320)
(n = 6)	2	21(8–48)	6	201(40–640)
	3	63(8–256)	6	284(40–5120)
	4	99(32–768)	6	452(40–5120)
PRCV-A	1	22(12–128)	2	56(5–640)
(n = 5)	2	12(6–32)	2	113(5–1280)
	3	14(3–48)	3	80(20–640)
	4	38(6–256)	3	402(160–2560)
PRCV-B	1–2	19(6–128)	2	80(40–160)
(n = 7)	3–4	19(6–384)	2	80(20–320)
PRCV-C	1–2	63(12–256)	5	40(5–320)
(n = 8)	3–4	23(6–96)	5	40(5–320)
PRCV-D	1	3(2–6)***	0	<5
(n = 8)	3	79(4–384)	8	160(40–640)
	4	87(24–384)	8	207(80–640)

*wpp = weeks post partum; ** TGEV-A = infected with TGEV, 2,5 months
previously; TGEV-B = infected with TGEV, 2,5 years previously; PRCV-A, -B,
-C = infected previously with PRCV on 3 different farms; PRCV-D = infected
previously with PRCV and experimentally inoculated with PRCV at 1 wpp;
*** one negative sow not included.

On the farms with a previous PRCV-infection, all sows except one had
VN milk antibodies throughout the lactation period. The latter sow (group
PRCV-D) was negative 1 week after farrowing (not included in Table 2). In
groups PRCV-A and PRCV-D VN-titers increased at the end of the lactation.
As indicated in Table 1, 10 out of the 13 sows showed 4-fold or higher titer
rises or became positive between 1 and 4 weeks after farrowing. No VN-antibody titer rises were observed in the groups PRCV-B and -C.

IgA Antibody Responses in the Milk

Twenty two control milk specimens, containing no VN antibody (titer <2),
were negative in the IgA ELISA (titer <5).

The antibody responses in the milk of TGEV- or PRCV-infected sows as
determined by IgA ELISA are shown in Table 2. All sows from farms TGEV-A
and -B had IgA antibodies in the milk throughout the lactation. Titers
increased at the end of the lactation period. As indicated in Table 1, some
sows in both groups showed a 4-fold or higher titer rise between 1 and 4
weeks after farrowing.

Table 3. VN- and IgA ELISA antibody titers in milk and in isolated milk IgA
and IgG from sows, previously infected with PRCV or TGEV

Sow group*	Sow no.	Milk**		IgA		IgG	
		VN titer	IgA ELISA titer	VN titer	IgA ELISA titer	VN titer	IgA ELISA titer
TGEV-A	1	48	160	60	50	<10	<25
	2	48	160	15	200	<10	<25
TGEV-B	3	256	640	240	400	30	25
	4	192	320	120	200	40	<25
PRCV-A	5	32	2560	30	3200	15	50
	6	256	160	160	100	320	<25
	7	32	<5	15	<25	80	<25
PRCV-B	8	384	320	480	400	20	<25
	9	12	<5	<10	<25	20	<25
PRCV-C	10	96	320	80	400	10	<25
	11	32	320	30	200	<10	<25
	12	128	<5	40	<25	120	<25
PRCV-D	13	384	320	480	200	40	<25
	14	96	640	40	400	<10	<25

*groups as in Table 2; **all milk specimens were collected 4 weeks post partum.

As shown in Table 2, 9 out of the 28 sows were positive in the IgA
ELISA 1 week after farrowing on the farms with a previous PRCV infection.
The GMT was 50 (5-640). In group PRCV-A, 1 sow became positive 3 weeks
after farrowing, whereas two other sows showed 4-fold or higher titer rises
between 1 and 4 weeks after farrowing (Table 1). Two sows remained
negative. In group PRCV-D, the 8 sows became positive 3 weeks after farrowing. The GMT in the 2 groups PRCV-A and -D reached a maximum value of
248 (80-2560) at 4 weeks after farrowing. In the groups PRCV-B and -C, no
IgA antibody titer rises were observed. Eight sows from the latter 2 groups
were negative during the whole lactation period.

Density Gradient Separation of Milk Immunoglobulins

The results of the separation of immunoglobulins in milk specimens from
the different groups of TGEV- and PRCV-infected sows, collected 4 weeks
after farrowing, are indicated in Table 3. The IgA ELISA- and VN-activity
in milk from 4 TGEV-infected sows was the highest in the isolated IgA. The
IgA containing gradient fractions were located in a position between 7S IgG
and 19S IgM (not shown). Six out of 7 PRCV-infected sows, containing IgA
ELISA reactivity in their milk, gave an identical result. In 1 sow the VN-
activity was equally distributed between the isolated IgA and IgG. Three
milk samples from PRCV-infected sows, containing VN antibodies but without
IgA ELISA reactivity, had the highest VN-titer in the isolated IgG.

DISCUSSION

From the present results it is clear that previous PRCV-infections can
induce the secretion of IgA antibodies in the milk of sows. These antibodies can be demonstrated using an ELISA for the detection of TGEV-specific

IgA. The specificity of the test is indicated by the results on control specimens from non-immune sows. Evidence of its isotype-specificity is obtained from the findings with density gradient separated specimens from TGEV- and PRCV-infected sows. Milk samples scored positive by ELISA contain TGEV-specific IgA, as proven by the presence of VN-activity in the isolated IgA. Furthermore, the ELISA reactivity is associated with the isolated IgA. The weak ELISA reactivity found in the isolated IgG from 2 specimens is thought to be due to contamination with IgA resulting from slight over-lapping of the IgG and IgA peaks. Milk samples scored negative by ELISA probably do not contain TGEV-specific IgA, since the VN-activity of these samples is mainly associated with the isolated IgG.

The results obtained by density gradient separation further indicate that the IgA secreted by TGEV- and PRCV-infected sows have indistinguishable characteristics. It is considered 11S secretory IgA on the basis of its position in the gradient[9]. Furthermore, the isolated IgA has the capacity to neutralize TGEV. As demonstrated in Table 3, there is no correlation between the VN- and IgA ELISA titer of the IgA, isolated from different sows. This indicates that the proportion of total TGEV-specific IgA, neutralizing the virus, varies depending upon individual differences.

The finding that TGEV-infected sows secrete IgA antibodies in the milk confirms previous reports by others[12]. The results obtained with PRCV-infected sows, showing that not all of them secrete IgA in the milk, cannot be fully explained. As demonstrated by the significant VN-titer rises in the serum of the PRCV-D sows following experimental inoculation with PRCV, a previous infection with PRCV and the presence of serum antibodies do not prevent reinfection with PRCV. Similar VN-titer rises in the serum, without a concomittant rise or appearance of differential TGEV-antibodies, were found in 3 out of 5 remaining sow groups. This demonstrates that in these groups a natural PRCV (re)infection has occurred during the lactation period and that PRCV reinfection may be a frequent event. Reinfection results in the rise or appearance of VN- and IgA-antibodies in the milk. This indicates that in PRCV-infected sows the occurrence of reinfections may determine the prevalence of IgA in the milk.

The mechanism accounting for the presence of IgA antibodies in the milk following PRCV-infection is not known. On the one hand, PRCV replicates to high titers in the respiratory tract and is likely to stimulate IgA-positive lymfocytes in the bronchi associated lymphoid tissue. Therefore, the secretion of IgA in the milk may be an indication for migration of the stimulated cells from the lung to the mammary gland. On the other hand it cannot be excluded that some of the PRCV-antigen reaches the gut associated lymphoid tissue, by ingestion and/or by limited replication in the gut. The secretion of IgA in the milk would involve then the gut-mammary link, known to be operative in the pig[3].

It has been established already that milk IgA, produced following an enteric TGEV-infection, provides protection of suckling piglets against that infection[3]. It is not clear if sows, previously infected with PRCV, protect their suckling piglets against TGEV-infection. So far, contra-dictory results have been reported[13, 14, 15]. As no attention was paid to the IgA content of the sow's milk in these studies, the protective properties against TGE of the milk IgA induced by a previous PRCV infection remain unknown.

Further work is in progress to clarify these points as it may open new ways for vaccination against TGEV.

ACKNOWLEDGEMENTS

This work was supported by the Institute for the Encouragement of Scientific Research in Industry and Agriculture (IWONL), Brussels, Belgium. The technical assistance of K. De Rudder is gratefully appreciated.

REFERENCES

1. J. Curtis and F.J. Bourne, Immunoglobulin quantitation in sow serum, colostrum and milk and the serum of young pigs, Biochim. Biophys. Acta 236: 319 (1971).
2. F.J. Bourne and J. Curtis, The transfer of immunoglobulins IgG, IgA and IgM from serum to colostrum and milk in the sow, Immunology 24: 157 (1973).
3. E.H. Bohl, R.K.P. Gupta, M.V.F. Olquin,and L.J. Saif, Antibody responses in serum, colostrum and milk of swine after infection or vaccination with transmissible gastroenteritis virus, Infect. Immun. 6: 289 (1972).
4. N. Nandapalan, C. Taylor, R. Scott,and G.L. Toms, Mammary immunity in mothers of infants with respiratory syncytial virus infection, J. Med. Virol. 22: 277 (1987).
5. E. Cox, J. Hooyberghs, and M.B. Pensaert, Sites of replication of a porcine respiratory coronavirus related to transmissible gastro- enteritis virus in pigs, Res. Vet. Sci. (in press).
6. M. Pensaert, P. Callebaut, and J. Vergote, Isolation of a porcine respir- atory, non-enteric coronavirus related to transmissble gastroenteritis, Vet. Q. 8: 257 (1986).
7. M.T. Voets, M. Pensaert, and P.R. Rondhuis, Vaccination of pregnant sows against transmissible gastroenteritis using 2 attenuated virus strains and different inoculation routes, Vet. Q. 2: 211 (1980).
8. P. Callebaut, M.B. Pensaert, and J. Hooyberghs, A competitive inhibition ELISA for the differentiation of serum antibodies from pigs infected with transmissible gastroenteritis virus (TGEV) or with the TGEV-re- lated porcine respiratory coronavirus, Vet. Microbiol. 20: 9 (1989).
9. J.P. Vaerman, "Studies on IgA immunoglobulins in man and animals", Thesis, Louvain (1970).
10. G. Jiménez, J. Correa, M.P. Melgosa, M.J. Bullido, and L. Enjuanes, Critical epitopes in transmissible gastroenteritis virus neutralization, J. Virol. 60: 131 (1986).
11. B. Wilson and P.K. Nakane, Recent developments in the periodate method of conjugating horseradish peroxidase (HRPO) to antibodies, in: "Immunofluorescence and related staining techniques", W. Knapp, K. Holubar and G. Wick, eds., Elsevier/North Holland Biomedical Press, Amsterdam/New York (1978).
12. L.J. Saif, E.H. Bohl, and R.K.P. Gupta, Isolation of porcine immuno- globulins and determination of the immunoglobulin classes of trans- missible gastroenteritis viral antibodies, Infect. Immun. 6:600 (1972).
13. J. Hooyberghs, M.B. Pensaert, and P. Callebaut, Transmissible gastro- enteritis: outbreaks in swine herds previously infected with a TGEV- like porcine respiratory coronavirus, Proc. Int. Pig Vet. Soc. Congress 10: 200 (1988).
14. J.M. Aynaud, P. Have, E. Bottreau, S. Bernard,and J. Szymanski, Natural infection of the sows with the porcine respiratory coronavirus (PRCV) induces protective lactogenic immunity against transmissible gastro- enteritis (TGE), in: "Résumés réunion mixte des Sociétés Française et Britannique d'Immunologie", Paris (1988).
15. D.J. Paton and I. Brown, Evaluation of porcine respiratory coronavirus induced cross-protection against transmissible gastroenteritis in suckling pigs, Abstr. Congress European Soc. Vet. VIrol. 1: 46 (1989).

SITES OF REPLICATION OF A PORCINE RESPIRATORY CORONAVIRUS IN 5-WEEK-

OLD PIGS WITH OR WITHOUT MATERNAL ANTIBODIES

E. Cox, M. Pensaert, J. Hooyberghs and K. Van Deun

Laboratory of Virology
Faculty of Veterinary Medicine
State University of Gent
Casinoplein 24
9000 Gent
Belgium

ABSTRACT

On farms, where the porcine respiratory coronavirus (PRCV) is enzootic, pigs usually become infected between 5 and 10 weeks of age while losing their maternal antibodies. It was examined whether PRCV replicates in the small intestine in such pigs. This point is important since intestinal replication with PRCV might induce immunity against TGEV not only by stimulating mucosal intestinal immunity, but also by the induction of a lactogenic IgA response at later age via the gut-mammary link.

Five week old pigs with and without maternal antibodies were inoculated by aerosol or directly into the intestinal lumen. In aerosol inoculated pigs, virus replication was observed to high titres in the respiratory tract. Replication occurred in epithelial cells of nasal mucosa, trachea, bronchi bronchioli and alveoli and in alveolar macrophages. Small amounts of virus produced in the respiratory tract were ingested, but no intestinal replication of PRCV was demonstrated. Differences were not observed in virus titre and sites of replication in seronegative pigs compared to those in pigs with maternal antibodies. Upon inoculation of 10^5 or 10^7 TCID$_{50}$ directly into the lumen of the cranial jejunum, no intestinal replication could be demonstrated.

INTRODUCTION

In 1984, a porcine respiratory coronavirus (PRCV) appeared in the swine population of Belgium (1). This virus was antigenically closely related to the enteropathogenic coronavirus, transmissible gastroenteritis virus (TGEV) (2). Upon infection with PRCV, pigs develop TGEV-neutralizing antibodies. PRCV has spread to such an extent that nearly 100 % of the Belgian swine farms are now infected (3). Similar spread has been observed in other European countries (4,5,6).

Presently, the virus is enzootic in the Belgian swine population. Regular episodes of infection and reinfection occur on breeding farms. On these farms, pigs usually become infected between 5 and 10 weeks of age while losing their maternal antibodies (3). The aim of the present study was to examine if PRCV replicates in the intestine of such pigs. This point is important since intestinal replication of PRCV may result in the induction of immunity against TGEV by stimulating IgA secreting lymphocytes in the gut-associated-lymphoid-tissue (GALT). In this way, a PRCV infection may not only induce an intestinal mucosal immunity against TGEV, but also an anti-TGEV lactogenic IgA response at a later age via the gut-mammary-link (7) , as observed following TGEV infection (8).

Coronaviruses and Their Diseases
Edited by D. Cavanagh and T.D.K. Brown
Plenum Press, New York, 1990

MATERIALS AND METHODS

Virus stock

The TLM 83 isolate of PRCV was used in this study (l). The stock for the experimental infection represented the first passage in ST cells of a 20 percent suspension of lung tissue from an experimentally inoculated pig. The infectivity titer of this stock was $10^{6.7}$ ($TCID_{50}$) per ml.

Inoculation by Aerosol of 5-week-old Pigs with or without Maternal Antibodies

Three colostrum-deprived pigs and three conventionally reared pigs with maternal PRCV antibodies were used in this experiment. Serum was sampled at inoculation. The pigs were inoculated by aerosol with $10^{7.0}$ $TCID_{50}$ TLM 83 in 8 ml phosphate buffered saline (PBS) at the age of 5 weeks. The virus suspension was nebulized using the "Wright" nebuliser (particle size <8 µm) during 40 minutes for each pig individually. Rectal swabs were collected daily for viral isolation (VI). One seronegative and one seropositive pig were killed at 3, 4 and 5 days post inoculation (PI) respectively. Immediately after bleeding the pigs, the following tissues were collected for VI and immunofluorescence (IF): nasal mucosa, trachea, lungs (apical, cardiac, diaphragmatic lobes), tonsils, small intestine, spleen and lymph nodes (mesenteric, bronchial). The small intestine was divided in 7 segments of equal length: duodenum, jejunum 1 to 5 and ileum. A piece of approximatively 1.5 cm long was removed for IF. VI was performed on the remaining parts. Caecal, rectal contents and stomach tissue were collected for VI only.

Furthermore, a post mortem lung washing was performed by injecting 50 ml of PBS containing 50 percent (v/v) Alsever's solution through a polyethylene catheter in the left bronchus. The fluid was immediately aspirated whereafter the cells were sedimented by centrifugation (10 minutes at 300 g). Next, the erythrocytes were lysed with NH_4Cl. Sedimented cells were resuspended in 5 ml Eagle's minimum essential medium, whereafter smears were prepared for IF.

Some additional samples were collected for VI in the seronegative pigs only i.e. plasma daily between the time of inoculation and euthanasia; small intestinal contents, liver, plasma and inguinal and cervical lymph nodes at euthanasia.In seropositive piglets, the following samples were also collected for VI at euthanasia: oesophagal swabs and contents of stomach and of the 7 small intestinal segments.

Intraintestinal Inoculation of 4- to 5-week-old Pigs with or without Maternal Antibodies

Three conventionally reared pigs without seroneutralizing antibodies were housed together in isolation. They were inoculated with PRCV directly into the lumen of the cranial jejunum after laparotomy at the age of 4 weeks. The inoculation dose was 10^5 $TCID_{50}$ TLM 83 in 5 ml PBS. They were followed serologically during 4 weeks. Rectal and tonsillar swabs were collected for VI daily until 2 weeks PI, whereafter they were collected 3 times a week until 4 weeks PI.

A catheter was implanted after laparotomy in the ileum of a 5-week-old pig with maternal TGEV antibodies in order to allow frequent sampling of intestinal content at the site of virus replication. PRCV was inoculated in a dose of 10^7 $TCID_{50}$ TLM 83 in 5 ml PBS into the lumen of the cranial jejunum at the time of surgery. Serum was sampled at inoculation and 3 weeks later. Ileal contents were collected for VI at 4 hours interval during the first 3 days PI and subsequently 2 times a day until 1 week PI.

Viral Isolation, Viral Titration, Immunofluorescence and TGEV sero-neutralization test

VI isolation was performed according to standard procedures. The supernatant of a 20 percent suspension in PBS of each sample was inoculated on swine testicle (ST) cells in Flow tubes. Quantitative titrations of infectious virus were performed by inoculating 10-fold dilutions of the supernatants on ST cells in microtiter plates. The IF-test was performed using as hyperimmune serum a specific antiserum to TGEV. The SN-test was performed in SK6 cells using the Purdue-114 strain of TGEV.

RESULTS

Sites of Replication of PRCV upon Aerosol Inoculation of 5-week-old Pigs with or without Maternal Antibodies

No virus was isolated from rectal swabs sampled daily. Virus was isolated from one plasma sample of the seronegative pig 1665 taken one day PI.

Results of virus titration and of IF of tissues of 3 pigs without and 3 with maternal antibodies inoculated by aerosol and euthanatized 3, 4 and 5 days PI are presented in Table 1. Virus was isolated from nasal mucosa, trachea, lungs, tonsils and bronchial lymph nodes of all 6 pigs. The highest titres were detected in lung tissue (up to $10^{6.3}$ in seronegative and up to $10^{7.3}$ TCID$_{50}$ per g tissue in pigs with maternal antibodies). Titres decreased in seronegative pigs in most respiratory tract tissues and in bronchial lymph nodes from 3 up to 5 days PI. Fluorescence was observed in all the pigs in the epithelial cells of nasal mucosa, trachea and lungs. IF in lungs was seen in epithelial cells of alveoli, bronchioli and rarely of bronchi. Furthermore, fluorescence was observed in alveolar macrophages in the lung washing fluids in all pigs.

Table 1. Results of virus titration and immunofluorescence of tissues from pigs with and without maternal antibodies inoculated by aerosol with TLM 83 at the age of 5 weeks

	Virus titre ($\log_{10}$ TCID$_{50}$/g in pig number)						IF[a]
	1665[n]	1845[ma]	1666[n]	1847[ma]	1667[n]	1846[ma]	all pigs
Day killed p.i.	3	3	4	4	5	5	3, 4, 5
Tissue							
Respiratory tract							
Nasal mucosa	4.5	5.7	4.5	5.5	4.7	5.0	+
Trachea	4.5	5.0	4.3	4.3	3.9	4.0	+
Lung	6.3	7.3	6.0	6.5	4.0	6.7	+
Tonsil	2.1	4.5	1.8	3.3	1.3	4.5	-
Bronchial lymph nodes	3.7	4.5	2.2	3.3	1.8	4.5	-
Digestive tract							
Oesophagal swab	nt[b]	2.7	nt	2.7	nt	1.8	
Stomach	neg.[c]	2.2	1.4	neg.	neg.	neg.	nt
Duodenum	1.5	neg.	1.3	neg.	neg.	neg.	-
Jejunum 1	neg.	neg.	1.3	neg.	neg.	neg.	-
Jejunum 2-5	neg.	neg.	neg.	neg.	neg.	neg.	-
Ileum	neg.	neg.	neg.	neg.	neg.	neg.	-
Caecal contents	neg.	neg.	neg.	neg.	neg.	neg.	-
Mesenteric lymph nodes	neg.	neg.	1.7	neg.	neg.	neg.	-
Other							
Liver	neg.	nt	neg.	nt	neg.	nt	nt
Peripheral lymph nodes[d]	neg.	nt	neg.	nt	neg.	nt	nt
Spleen	neg.	nt	neg.	nt	neg.	nt	nt
Plasma	neg.	nt	neg.	nt	neg.	nt	

a: -, no fluorescence; +, 5% or less of epithelial cells fluorescing. b: nt, not tested.
c: neg, no virus isolated. d: inguinal and cervical lymph nodes. n: no maternal antibody. ma: maternal antibody titre of 48

Virus was isolated from the stomach, gastric content, the mesenterial lymph nodes and the cranial small intestine in some pigs and from oesophagal swabs in all the seropositive pigs. Fluorescence was not seen in any of the pigs in the small intestine or mesenterial lymph nodes.

Intraintestinal Inoculation of 4- to 5-week-old Pigs with or without Maternal Antibodies

A TGEV-SN-titer of 6 appeared 4 weeks PI in 1 of 3 seronegative pigs which had been inoculated into the lumen of the cranial jejunum. No virus was isolated from rectal swabs of this pig taken between 1 to 7 days PI. The other 2 pigs remained seronegative. Upon the intraintestinal inoculation, virus was not isolated from any sample of ileal content collected during the 1st week PI in the pig with the ileal catheter. The neutralizing-titer in the serum of the latter pig was 8 at inoculation and 3, 3 weeks later.

DISCUSSION AND CONCLUSION

No significant differences were observed in virus titres and immuno-fluorescence in respiratory tract tissue between the 5-week-old pigs with or without maternal antibodies. These results show that low maternal antibody titres do not decrease virus production at the respiratory tract surface. A similar observation was made upon infection with bovine respiratory syncytial virus of calves with or without maternal antibodies (9). In this latter study, it was suggested that the results could be attributed to the presence of only a weak diffusion of serum antibodies into lung alveoli.

Previous pathogenesis experiments have been performed in which 1-week-old piglets were inoculated with PRCV by aerosol (10). The virus was observed to replicate at high titres in the respiratory tract (up to $10^{8.3}$ TCID$_{50}$ TLM 83 per g lung tissue). Replication occurred in epithelial cells of the nasal mucosa, trachea, bronchi, bronchioli and alveoli and in alveolar macrophages. Replication was also observed in tonsillary tissue. In the present study, replication of PRCV in tonsils could not be demonstrated by fluorescence. Virus titres and fluorescence observed in lung tissue of the 5-week-old pigs were generally lower than those in the 1-week-old piglets.

Upon aerosol inoculation, virus was isolated inconsistently and at low titres from the cranial digestive tract in pigs with or without maternal antibodies. Since no fluorescence was found in the cranial small intestine, this was considered to be ingested virus.

In 1-week-old piglets, PRCV was observed to replicate in the small intestine upon aerosol inoculation (10). The intestinal replication of PRCV started in the ileum and spread within a few days to the duodenum. Intestinal replication remained limited to few unidentified cells. In the present study, virus could not be isolated either from mid and caudal small intestine or from contents of this part of the small intestine.

It was previously shown that the susceptibility of the small intestine of 1-week-old piglets to infection with PRCV is very low. More than 10^3 TCID$_{50}$ of TLM 83 must be inoculated into the lumen of the cranial jejunum in order to induce an intestinal infection consistently (11). Results of the present study show that the small intestine in older pigs is fully resistant to PRCV infection since inoculation of 10^5 to 10^7 TCID$_{50}$ into the lumen of the cranial jejunum induced no intestinal replication. The very weak and late serological reaction observed in one seronegative pig may have been due to gastrointestinal antigen uptake (12).

The results of the present study show that no intestinal replication occurs upon aerosol inoculation with PRCV of older pigs. Therefore, TGEV- specific IgA which was observed in the milk of sows previously infected with PRCV (Callebaut et al., this volume) is most likely induced by stimulating lymphocytes present in the bronchus-associated-lymphoid-tissue. The occurrence of TGEV-IgA in milk following respiratory PRCV infection suggest the presence of a common mucosal immune system and a lung-mammary link in swine.

ACKNOWLEDGEMENTS

These studies were supported by the Institute for the Encouragement of Research in Industry and Agriculture (IWONL), Brussels, Belgium. Dr. J.A. Decuypere (Laboratory of Nutrition and Hygiene, RUG) is thanked for his advice concerning the ileal catheterization. The excellent technical assistance of Mrs. L. Sys and Mr. K. De Rudder is gratefully acknowledged.

REFERENCES

1. M. Pensaert, P. Callebaut, and J. Vergote, Isolation of a porcine respiratory, non-enteric coronavirus related to transmissible gastroenteritis, Vet. Quarterly, 8: 257 (1986).
2. P. Callebaut, I. Correa, M. Pensaert, G. Jiminez, and L. Enjuanes, Antigenic differentiation between transmissible gastroenteritis virus of swine and a related porcine respiratory coronavirus, J. Gen. Virol., 69: 1725 (1988).
3. M. Pensaert, and E. Cox, A porcine respiratory coronavirus related to transmissible gastroenteritis virus, Agri-Practice, 10: 17 (1989).
4. I. Brown, and S. Cartwright, New porcine coronavirus ? Vet. Rec., 119 : 282 (1986).
5. A. Jestin, Y. Le Forban, P. Vannier, F. Madec, and J. Gourreau, Un nouveau coronavirus porcin. Etudes séro-épidémiologiques retrospectives dans les élevages de Bretagne, Rec. de Med. Vet., 163: 567 (1987).
6. A.P. van Nieuwstadt, and J.M.A. Pol, Isolation of a TGE virus-related respiratory coronavirus causing fatal pneumonia in pigs, Vet. Rec., 124: 43 (1989).
7. F.J. Bourne, The mammary gland and neonatal immunity, Vet. Sci. Commun., 1: 141 (1977).
8. E.H. Bohl, R.K.P. Gupta, M.V.F. Olquin, and L.J. Saif, Antibody responses in serum, colostrum and milk of swine after infection or vaccination with transmissible gastroenteritis virus, Infect. Immun., 6: 289 (1972).
9. T.G. Kimman, F. Westenbrink, B.E.C. Schreuder, and P.J. Straver, Local and systemic antibody response to bovine respiratory syncytial virus infection and reinfection in calves with or without maternal antibodies, J. Clin. Microbiol.25: 1097 (1989).
10. E. Cox, J. Hooyberghs, and M.B. Pensaert, Sites of replication of a porcine respiratory coronavirus related to transmissible gastroenteritis virus in pigs, Res. Vet. Sci., (in press).
11. E. Cox, M.B. Pensaert, P. Callebaut, and K. Van Deun, Intestinal replication of a porcine respiratory coronavirus antigenically closely related to the enteric transmissible gastroenteritis virus, Vet. Microbiol., (in press).
12. P. Brandtzaag, K. Baklien, K. Bjerke, T.O. Rognum, H. Scott, and K. Valnes, Nature and properties of the human gastrointestinal immune system, In: Immunology of the Gastrointestinal tract, Miller K. and Nicklin S. eds. Florida, CRC Press pp. 1 (1987).

INFECTION WITH A NEW PORCINE RESPIRATORY CORONAVIRUS IN
DENMARK: SEROLOGIC DIFFERENTIATION FROM TRANSMISSIBLE GASTRO-
ENTERITIS VIRUS USING MONOCLONAL ANTIBODIES

Per Have

State Veterinary Institute for Virus Research
Lindholm
DK-4771 Kalvehave, Denmark

ABSTRACT

In 1984 neutralizing antibodies against transmissible
gastroenteritis virus (TGEV) were detected in pig herds in a
small geographical area in the southern part of Denmark. No
clinical symptoms were observed and accumulating epidemiological evidence gradually pointed towards a respiratory infection. In 1986 a TGE-like virus, tentatively named porcine
respiratory coronavirus (PRCV), was isolated from the lungs of
swine. The virus was partially characterized using monoclonal
antibodies against TGEV and this showed that some (mainly non-
neutralizing) epitopes of the peplomer glycoprotein E2 were
absent in PRCV, whereas the major neutralizing domains were
conserved. These findings allowed the design of competitive
antibody immunoassays either discriminating or not discriminating the immune responses against the two viruses. However,
the discriminating epitopes studied so far have shown minor
immunodominance and some steric interference from non-
discriminating epitopes.

INTRODUCTION

Until 1984 transmissible gastroenteritis (TGE) had never
been diagnosed in Denmark either virologically or serologically, nor had firm clinical evidence of TGE been observed. The
absence of the infection was confirmed by periodic serological
surveys. During the spring of 1984 seropositive animals were
identified in a few herds in the southern part of Jutland. Comprehensive serological examinations of in-contact herds revealed a number of seropositive herds. No clinical disease
could be associated with seroconversion in any of these herds.
Initially a voluntary eradication programme based on serological examinations was undertaken. However, in the beginning of
1986 the infection spread massively to other parts of the country and PRCV can now be considered enzootic in Denmark with a
prevalence of seropositive animals of 75 - 80 %. Similar infections have been described in several other European countries.[1-4] Despite intensive efforts, the putative TGE-like

Coronaviruses and Their Diseases
Edited by D. Cavanagh and T.D.K. Brown
Plenum Press, New York, 1990

435

virus was not isolated until June 1986, thus confirming the
contagious nature of the seroreactions. Conventional crossneutralization did not reveal significant differences between
PRCV and TGEV. Therefore, studies employing anti-TGEV monoclonal antibodies were undertaken to characterize PRCV in more
detail with the aim of identifying possible antigenic differences that might be used as markers in differential diagnosis.

METHODS

Virus Strains

The following TGEV strains were used: FS 216 (kindly provided by Dr. S. Cartwright, Central Veterinary Laboratory, Weybridge), Purdue (kindly provided by Professor M. Pensaert,
Faculty of Veterinary Medicine, Ghent) and Riems (kindly
provided by Professor W. Bathke, Friedrich Loeffler Institute,
Insel Riems). PRCV strain DK 1/86 was isolated from the lungs
of a pig that died of pneumonia (courtesy of Dr. L. Rønsholt,
State Veterinary Institute for Virus Research, Lindholm). All
virus strains were grown in primary porcine kidney cells in
roller bottles. Virus titrations were performed in microplates
using primary porcine thyroid cells.

Monoclonal Antibodies

Eight monoclonal antibodies against the peplomer protein
E2 and 4 monoclonal antibodies against the transmembrane
protein E1 of Purdue strain of TGEV[5] were kindly provided by
Dr. H. Laude, INRA, Jouy-En-Josas. Two neutralizing monoclonal
antibodies against TGEV were kindly provided by Dr. N. Juntti,
Biomedicum, Uppsala. The latter monoclonals were subsequently
shown to correspond to domain A of the peplomer protein according to the classification of Delmas et al.[6] (data not shown).

Immunofluorescence Test

Reactivity of monoclonal antibodies against each virus
strain was tested on acetone-fixed monolayers of primary porcine kidney cells on multiwell slides. FITC-conjugated rabbit
anti-mouse IgG (DAKO) was used at a dilution of 1/50 in PBS.

Blocking ELISA

The Purdue strain of TGEV was grown in primary porcine
kidney cells in roller bottles. After 48 h the supernatant was
clarified by low-speed centrifugation followed by pelleting of
virus in a Beckman JA 14 rotor for 4 h. The pellet was resuspended in 1/100 of the original vol. in PBS and stored at
-80°C. Microplates were coated overnight at 4°C with a predetermined dilution of virus, washed and stored ready for use at
-20°C. Appropriate dilutions of test sera in PBS-0.1% Tween 20
(PBST) were incubated overnight at 4°C. The test was completed
by incubation with a predetermined dilution of monoclonal antibody (E4 or 44-4) in PBST containing 10 % normal bovine serum
followed by incubation with peroxidase-conjugated rabbit anti
mouse IgG (DAKO) diluted 1/800 in the same buffer.

Test Sera

The following porcine sera have been included in the present study: 748 TGEV antibody negative sera from another country (sampled 1988), 440 randomly selected Danish sera (sampled 1987), 32 sera from pigs experimentally infected with Riems strain of TGEV, 35 sera sampled in France during 1979-85 and 141 sera sampled in France in 1987-88 (both sets kindly provided by Dr. P. Vannier, Ploufragan).

RESULTS

Indirect Immunofluorescence

The reactivity of monoclonal antibodies with strains of TGEV and PRCV is shown in Table 1. Of the monoclonal antibodies directed against the peplomer protein E2 only 4 fail to react with PRCV. These are 40 (domain D) and 6.179, 67.9 and 44.4 (outside domain A-D). Monoclonal antibodies 6.179 and 67.9 seem to be very strain specific in that they only react with the Purdue strain which was used to generate these antibodies. Two monoclonal antibodies (9.34 and 49.22) against the transmembrane protein E1 showed no reaction with PRCV and 1 monoclonal antibody (25.22) showed a very weak reaction with PRCV. The results are in concordance with those published by Laude et al.[7] From these results only monoclonal antibodies 40 and 44.4 against E2 could be considered possible candidates as specific markers of TGEV antibodies in competition assays. The monoclonal antibodies 49.22, 25.22 and 9.34 against E1 could not be used as markers since they did not react with all strains of TGEV.[7]

ELISA

Initially, all monoclonal antibodies against E2 were titrated in ELISA. Subsequently, each monoclonal antibody was tested in blocking assays against TGEV and PRCV reference sera

TABLE 1. Reactivity of monoclonal antibodies (MAB) with strains of TGEV and PRCV.

Protein	MAB	FS216	Purdue	PRCV	Riems
		VIRUS			
E2	11	20480	1280	5120	20480
	25	40960	20480	40960	40960
	40	5120	5120	<20	5120
	48	20480	5120	20480	10240
	51	40960	40960	81920	40960
	6.179	<20	320	<20	<20
	67.9	<20	80	<20	<20
	44.4	20480	81920	<20	81920
	E3	20480	5120	320	2560
	E4	81920	81920	81920	81920
E1	3.60	5120	5120	5120	1280
	25.22	320	1280	20	5120
	9.34	320	320	<20	1280
	49.22	5120	5120	<20	320

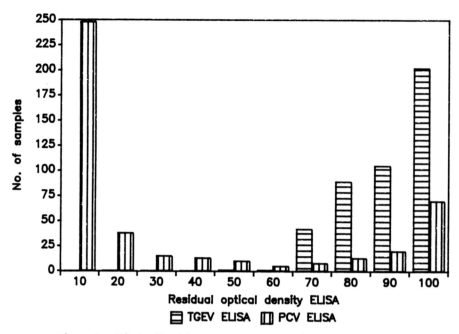

Fig. 1. Distribution of 440 porcine sera in E4
ELISA (termed PCV) and in 44.4 ELISA
(termed TGEV).

to evaluate its usefulness as marker antibody. Monoclonal antibodies E4 and 44.4 proved to be especially useful as markers of
common and TGEV-specific antibodies, respectively (data not
shown).

The specificity of E4 ELISA has been evaluated using 748
TGEV and PRCV antibody negative sera. These showed on the average 0 % inhibition with a standard deviation of ±11 %. One
hundred PRCV antibody positive sera were used to compare the
sensitivity of E4 ELISA (50 % cut-off level) with virus neutralization test using TGEV. The two tests showed a high correlation (r=0.88) and E4 ELISA was on the average 2-fold more
sensitive than neutralization test.

The specificity of 44.4 ELISA (TGEV-specific) was evaluated using 440 randomly sampled Danish sera of which most were
PRCV antibody positive but assumed to be free of TGEV antibodies. The results (see Fig. 1) showed that up to 40 % inhibition may be encountered by PRCV antisera in 44.4 ELISA
(single determinations). Regression analysis of these data
showed that PRCV antibodies do interfere with the 44.4 epitope
(average of 20 % inhibition for PRCV positive sera, slope 0.2).

The sensitivity of 44.4 ELISA was studied using sera from
4 experimentally TGEV-infected pigs. These results showed that
the TGEV-specific response was delayed up to 1 week and
remained 2-4 fold lower than that of the E4 response even
though this study used a cut-off level for 44.4 ELISA of 25 %
inhibition.

The 44.4 ELISA has been further evaluated (cut-off level
25 %) using sera from various sources. Thus, the 100 PRCV

antibody positive sera used to evaluate E4 ELISA were all
negative in 44.4 ELISA. Of 130 French sera sampled in 1987 and
suspected to be PRCV positive, 127 were positive in E4 ELISA
and only 1 was positive in 44.4 ELISA. In contrast, of 35 sera
sampled in France during 1979-85 34 were positive in E4 ELISA
and 30 were positive in 44.4 ELISA which is to be expected if
these sera were sampled before the introduction of PRCV.
Furthermore, 11 sows vaccinated against TGEV were all strongly
positive in both tests.

DISCUSSION

    The E4 ELISA has been shown to be a sensitive and specific
test for antibodies against TGEV and PRCV. The 44.4 ELISA has
proven useful for serologic differentiation between TGEV and
PRCV infections. However, the specificity of this test is
limited due to some interference from PRCV antibodies. This
requires the cut-off level to be adjusted accordingly, leading
to decreased sensitivity which is furthermore influenced by the
apparent low avidity of antibodies against the 44.4 epitope and
incomplete immune response against this epitope (data not
shown). A similar test has been described by Callebaut et al.[8]
which supports these findings and conclusions. Thus, the 44.4
test is useful for differentiating TGEV and PRCV infections but
indiscriminate use in individual pigs is not warranted at
present.

REFERENCES

1. M. Pensaert, P. Callebaut & J. Vergote, Isolation of a
   porcine respiratory, non-enteric coronavirus related to
   transmissible gastroenteritis. Vet. Quart. 8(3): 257
   (1986).
2. I. Brown & S. F. Cartwright, New porcine coronavirus? Vet.
   Rec. 119: 282 (1986).
3. A. Jestin, Y. Leforban, P. Vannier, F. Madec & J.-M.
   Gourreau, Un nouveau coronavirus porcin. Rec.Méd.Vét.
   163(5): 567 (1987).
4. A. P. van Nieuwstadt & J. M. A. Pol, Isolation of a TGE
   virus-related respiratory coronavirus causing fatal
   pneumonia in pigs. Vet.Rec. 124: 43 (1989).
5. H. Laude, J.-M. Chapsal, J. Gelfi, S. Labiau & J.
   Grosclaude, Antigenic structure of transmissible
   gastroenteritis virus. I. Properties of monoclonal
   antibodies directed against virion proteins. J.gen.Vir.
   67: 119 (1986).
6. B. Delmas, J. Gelfi & H. Laude, Antigenic structure of
   transmissible gastroenteritis virus. II. Domains in the
   peplomer glycoprotein. J.gen.Vir. 67: 1405 (1986).
7. H. Laude, J. Gelfi, D. Rasschaert & B. Delmas,
   Caractérisation antigénique du coronavirus respiratoire
   porcin a l'aide d'anticorps monoclonaux dirigés contre le
   virus de la gastro-entérite transmissible. Journées Rech.
   Porcine en France 20: 89 (1988).
8. P. Callebaut, M. B. Pensaert & J. Hooyberghs, A competitive
   inhibition ELISA for the differentiation of serum
   antibodies from pigs infected with transmissible
   gastroenteritis virus (TGEV) or with the TGEV-related
   porcine respiratory coronavirus. Vet.Microbiol. 20: 9
   (1989).

MOLECULAR ASPECTS OF THE RELATIONSHIP OF TRANSMISSIBLE GASTROENTERITIS

VIRUS (TGEV) WITH PORCINE RESPIRATORY CORONAVIRUS (PRCV)

P. Britton, D. J. Garwes, K. Page and F. Stewart

AFRC Institute for Animal Health, Compton Laboratory
Compton, Newbury, Berkshire, RG16 ONN, U.K.

INTRODUCTION

Transmissible gastroenteritis, caused by a coronavirus (TGEV), has been recognised as a viral disease since 1946 when the virus was first isolated by Doyle and Hutchings (1). TGEV has been shown to cause diarrhoea in pigs of all ages but has a high mortality, often 100%, in neonatal piglets. The TGEV virion, like all coronaviruses, contains an envelope, whose lipids are derived from the host cell endoplasmic reticulum, a single-stranded RNA genome, of positive polarity, and three structural proteins. The virion proteins are: a surface glycoprotein (peplomer) of M_r 200000, a glycosylated integral membrane protein observed as a series of polypeptides of M_r 28000-31000 and a basic phosphorylated protein (nucleoprotein) of M_r 47000 associated with the viral genomic RNA (2). Like all the coronaviruses the TGEV proteins are expressed from a series of subgenomic mRNA species, six in the case of TGEV (3), which have common 3' ends but different 5' extensions. The region of each mRNA responsible for the expression of a protein appears to correspond to the 5'-terminal region, often referred to as the 'unique' region, that is absent from the preceding smaller species. The TGEV genome encompassing the structural protein genes has been cloned and sequenced from a virulent British isolate, FS772/70 (4, 5, 6, 7, 8 and unpublished results), and from the avirulent Purdue strain (9, 10, 11, 12, 13, 14). This has led to the identification of five other potential genes, one of which appears to be the polymerase gene (8), another that appears to be located in the host cell nucleus and not in TGEV virions (8, 15) and three others whose products have yet to be identified in TGEV infected cells.

A virus antigenically related to TGEV has recently appeared, and spread rapidly, throughout the pig population in several European countries between 1984 and 1986. The virus does not cause diarrhoea and has been shown to replicate in the respiratory tract with little or no clinical signs (16). The causative agent, isolated in Belgium (16) and in Britain (17), was identified as a coronavirus that produced a serological response that could not be distinguished from TGEV-infected pigs by available diagnostic tests. The respiratory form of TGEV has been named porcine respiratory coronavirus (PRCV) and shown not to replicate in the enteric tract upon oronasal inoculation. This is in contrast to TGEV which preferentially grows in the enterocytes covering the tips of the villi in the small intestine, causing diarrhoea and dehydration. TGEV has also been

shown to be present in lung tissue by immune fluorescence and virus
isolation (18). PRCV is fully neutralised by antisera prepared against
TGEV and the majority of monoclonal antibodies (mAbs) raised against any
of the TGEV virion proteins do cross react with PRCV. However, mAbs raised
against antigenic determinants of the peplomer protein from either the
virulent British isolate FS772/70 (19) or the avirulent Purdue strain (20)
of TGEV, have been identified that do not recognise PRCV. None of the
mAbs that reacted with TGEV but not PRCV had any neutralising effect on
TGEV indicating that the difference between the peplomer molecules,
recognised by these mAbs, is probably in a part of the molecule not
involved in virus neutralisation. PRCV is not related to two other pig
coronaviruses, porcine epidemic diarrhoea virus (PEDV) and porcine haemagglutinating encephalomyelitis virus (HEV), neither of which belong to
the TGEV subgroup (21).

Here we report the characterisation of polypeptides synthesised by a
British isolate of PRCV in infected cells and describe differences in the
subgenomic mRNA species of the two viruses.

METHODS

Virus production and RNA isolation

The 86/137004 isolate, Burkle strain, of PRCV and the FS772/70 strain
of TGEV were grown and plaque assayed in secondary adult pig thyroid (APT/2)
cell cultures (2). Viral subgenomic mRNA was isolated from infected
LLC-PK1 cells as described previously (4). Monolayer cultures of APT/2
cells, 850 cm^2, in plastic roller bottles were infected with TGEV or PRCV
(m.o.i. = 5 pfu/cell) for 2 h at 37°C, transferred to methionine-free
medium for a further 2 h and metabolically labelled with [^{35}S]-methionine
at 100 µCi/ml for a further 14 h. Cultures were frozen and thawed and
the virions purified by sucrose gradient centrifugation (2).

Analysis of [^{35}S]-methionine labelled viral polypeptides

LLC-PK1 cells were infected with TGEV or PRCV, at a m.o.i. of 5-10
pfu/cell, and incubated at 37°C for 2 h. The inoculum was replaced with
methionine free Eagles MEM medium and the cells incubated for a further
2 h as described previously (19). The infected cells were then incubated
in the same medium containing 250 µCi of [^{35}S]-methionine and lysed (19).
Protein samples were denatured by heating at 100°C for 2 mins in PAGE
sample buffer and analysed on 12-20% polyacrylamide gels.

Messenger RNA analysis

Specific restriction fragments from TGEV cDNA clones were separated
on agarose gels, purified by Geneclean^{TM}, and labelled with [α^{32}P-dATP]
(5). TGEV and PRCV subgenomic mRNA species were denatured with 6M glyoxal,
electrophoresed into 1% agarose gels, northern blotted onto Biodyne
membrane and hybridised to ^{32}P-labelled TGEV cDNA fragments (5). The
probes were hybridised and washed as described previously (7).

RESULTS

Viral polypeptides

TGEV and PRCV, grown in APT/2 cells in the presence of [^{35}S]-methionine,
were purified by sucrose gradient centrifugation and Figure 1 shows that
the two viruses have a similar overall structure, with the three major

442

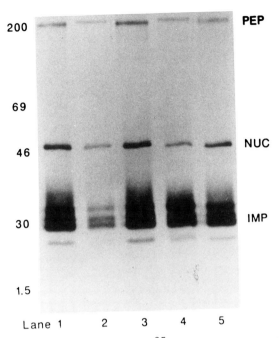

Fig. 1. Polypeptides purified from [^{35}S]-methionine labelled virions of TGEV (Tracks 2 and 4) and PRCV (Tracks 1, 3 and 5). PEP: peplomer; NUC: nucleoprotein; IMP: integral membrane protein; analysed by PAGE.

polypeptide species, the peplomer, nucleoprotein and integral membrane protein. LLC-PK1 cells, uninfected or infected with either TGEV or PRCV and incubated between 1-5 h, 5-10 h and 10-15 h post infection in the presence of [^{35}S]-methionine, were lysed and analysed by PAGE. Figure 2 shows that by 5 h after infection the TGEV nucleoprotein is detectable but the equivalent protein is not detectable in PRCV infected cells until between 5-10 h post infection. There is a marked suppression of host cell protein synthesis in the TGEV-infected cells between 5-10 h after infection bu this is not apparent in the PRCV cultures. The major polypeptide species discernible in the infected cel lysates with both viruses are the peplomer, nucleoprotein, the truncated form of the nucleoprotein (M_r 42000), the integral membrane protein and polypeptides of M_r 17000 and 14000. It can be seen from Figs. 1 and 2 that the PRCV peplomer protein (M_r 190000) is slightly smaller than the TGEV peplomer and that the PRCV nucleoprotein (M_r 48000) is slightly larger than the TGEV protein. The truncated form of the PRCV nucleoprotein (M_r 43000) is also slightly larger than the TGEV product. There is no detectable difference in the size of the PRCV integral membrane protein. The polypeptide of M_r 14000, TGEV ORF-4 gene product (5, 8, 15), is also present in PRCV infected cells and migrates identically to the TGEV product. A polypeptide of M_r 17000, observed in TGEV infected cells but not assigned to any TGEV gene (15), is also present in PRCV infected cells and migrates identically to the polypeptide observed in TGEV infected cells.

Viral mRNA analysis

Subgenomic mRNA from cells infected with either TGEV or two different isolates of PRCV were blotted onto membranes and probed with ^{32}P-labelled TGEV cDNA. This revealed the series of mRNA species shown in Figure 3.

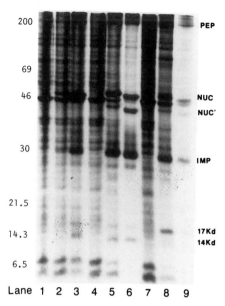

Fig. 2.   Polypeptides from uninfected or virus infected cells labelled with [^{35}S]-methionine during 1-5 h (Tracks 1-3), 5-10 h (Tracks 4-6) and 10-15 h (Tracks 7-9) post infection. Uninfected cells (Tracks 1, 4 and 7); PRCV-infected (Tracks 2, 5 and 8); TGEV-infected (Tracks 3, 6 and 9).

The overall number of mRNA species was six for both viruses. The sizes of the TGEV species were 8.4, 3.9, 3.0, 2.6, 1.7 and 0.7 kb (3, 4, 5, 6, 7, 8). The pattern of mRNA from PRCV-infected cells was very similar, with

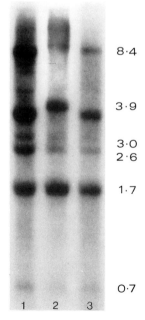

Fig. 3.   Autoradiograph of northern blotted TGEV mRNA (Track 2) and from two strains of PRCV (Track 1; 86/137004, Track 3; 86/135308) probed with ^{32}P-labelled TGEV cDNA derived from several genes.

identical sizes for the 3.0, 2.6, 1.7 and 0.7 kb species but the PRCV
equivalent to the TGEV 3.9 kb mRNA migrated faster than that of TGEV,
relating to a size of 3.6-3.7 kb. The peplomer mRNA (8.4 kb TGEV) from
PRCV also migrated faster than the TGEV equivalent.

DISCUSSION

     Comparison of the virion proteins between British isolates of TGEV
an PRCV shows very little difference in their molecular weights. The
differences seen, a slightly smaller peplomer and slightly larger nucleoprotein in the case of PRCV, are of the same magnitude as those seen
between TGEV and other members of the same serological group, namely feline
infectious peritonitis virus (FIP) and canine coronavirus (CCV). The
difference observed in the size of the peplomer polypeptides may be due to
variations in the extent of glycosylation. the variations in the size of
the nucleoprotein cannot be attributed to glycans as this protein is not
glycosylated. It is interesting to note that the truncated form of
nucleoprotein is also larger in the case of PRCV. The polypeptide of
M_r 14000, product of the TGEV ORF-4 gene, is also present in PRCV infected
cells.

     TGEV has been shown to produce six subgenomic mRNA species and one,
3.9 kb, has two potential open reading frames at its 5' 'unique' region.
The four smallest mRNA species from TGEV and PRCV appear to have the same
size but the two larger species, 8.4 and 3.9 kb, appear to be smaller in
PRCV. The mRNA equivalent to the TGEV 3.9 kb mRNA is 3.6-3.7 kb in PRCV
infected cells. Comparison of the cDNA sequences, from TGEV and PRCV,
corresponding to the 5' ends of this mRNA shows that there are deletions
within this region of PRCV. Sequence data indicates that the smaller size
of the mRNA in PRCV is probably due to a new consensus sequence, ACTAAAC,
preceding the ORF-2 gene (unpublished result). This sequence appears to
be involved in the synthesis of TGEV mRNA species and precedes the TGEV
ORF-1 gene on the 3.9 kb mRNA species.

ACKNOWLEDGEMENTS

     This research was supported by the Biomolecular Engineering Programme
of the Commission of the European Communities Contract No. (BAP-0235-UK(HI)).
We would like to thank Dr. S. F. Cartwright for supplying the British
isolates of PRCV.

REFERENCES

 1. L. P. Doyle and L. M. Hutchings, A transmissible gastroenteritis in
       pigs, J. Am. Vet. Med. Assoc., 108:257-259 (1946).
 2. D. J. Garwes and D. H. Pocock, The polypeptide structure of trans-
       missible gastroenteritis virus, J. Gen. Virol., 29:25-34 (1975).
 3. P. Britton, D. J. Garwes, G. C. Millson, K. Page, L. Bountiff, F.
       Stewart and J. Walmsley, Towards a genetically-engineered vaccine
       against porcine transmissible gastroenteritis virus. In:
       "Biomolecular Engineering in the European Community. Final Report,"
       E. Magnien, ed., Martinus Nijhoff, The Netherlands (1986).
 4. P. Britton, D. J. Garwes, K. Page and J. Walmsley, Expression of
       porcine transmissible gastroenteritis virus genes in E. coli as β-
       galactosidase chimaeric proteins. Adv. Exp. Med. Biol., 218:55-64
       (1987).
 5. P. Britton, R. S. Carmenes, K. W. Page, D. J. Garwes and F. Parra,
       Sequence of the nucleoprotein from a virulent British field isolate

of transmissible gastroenteritis virus and its expression in
Saccharomyces cerevisiae, Mol. Microbiol., 2:89-99 (1988).

6. P. Britton, R. S. Carmenes, K. W. Page and D. J. Garwes, The integral
   membrane protein from a virulent isolate of transmissible gastroenteritis virus: Molecular characterization, sequence and expression
   in Escherichia coli, Mol. Microbiol., 2: 497-505 (1988).

7. P. Britton, C. Lopez Otin, J. Martin Alonso and F. Parra, Sequence of
   the coding regions from the 3.0 kb and 3.9 kb mRNA subgenomic species
   from a virulent isolate of transmssible gastroenteritis virus, Arch.
   Virol., 105:(in press) (1989).

8. P. Britton, K. W. Page, D. J. Pulford, D. J. Garwes, K. Mawditt, F.
   Stewart, F. Parra, C. Lopez Otin, J. Martin Alonso and R. S. Carmenes,
   Genomic organisation of a virulent isolate of porcine transmissible
   gastroenteritis virus, (This book).

9. P. A. Kapke and D. A. Brian, Sequence analysis of the porcine transmissible gastroenteritis coronavirus nucleocapsid protein gene,
   Virology, 151:41-49 (1986).

10. P. A. Kapke, F. Y. C. Tung, D. A. Brian, R. D. Woods and R. Wesley,
    Nucleotide sequence of the porcine transmissible gastroenteritis
    coronavirus matrix protein, Adv. Exp. Med. Biol., 218: 117-122 (1987).

11. H. Laude, D. Rasschaert and J. C. Huert, Sequence and N-terminal
    processing of the transmembrane protein E1 of the coronavirus
    transmissible gastroenteritis virus, J. Gen. Virol., 68:1687-1693
    (1987).

12. D. Rasschaert, B. Delmas, B. Charley, J. Grossclaude, J. Gelfi and
    H. Laude, Surface glycoproteins of transmissible gastroenteritis
    virus: functions and gene sequence, Adv. Exp. Med. Biol., 218:109-116
    (1987).

13. D. Rasschaert and H. Laude, The predicted structure of the peplomer
    protein E2 of the porcine coronavirus transmissible gastroenteritis
    virus, J. Gen. Virol., 68:1883-1890 (1987).

14. D. Rasschaert, J. Gelfi and H. Laude, Enteric coronavirus TGEV: partial
    sequence of the genomic RNA, its organisation and expression.
    Biochimie, 69:591-600 (1987).

15. D. J. Garwes, F. Stewart and P. Britton, The polypeptide of M_r 14000
    of porcine transmissible gastroenteritis virus: Gene assignment and
    intracellular location, J. Gen. Virol., 70:(In press) (1989).

16. M. B. Pensaert, P. E. Callebaut and J. Vergote, Isolation of a porcine
    respiratory non-enteric coronavirus related to transmissible gastro-
    enteritis. Vet. Q., 8:257-260 (1986).

17. I. Brown and S. Cartwright, New porcine coronavirus? Vet. Rec.,
    119:282-283 (1986).

18. N. R. Underdahl, C. A. Mebus, E. L. Stair, M. B. Rhodes, L. D. McGill
    and M. J. Twiehaus, Isolation of transmissible gastroenteritis virus
    from lungs of market-weight swine, Am. J. Vet. Res., 35:1209-1216
    (1974).

19. D. J. Garwes, F. Stewart, S. F. Cartwright and I. Brown, Differentiation
    of porcine coronavirus from transmissible gastroenteritis virus,
    Vet. Rec., 122:86-87 (1988).

20. P. Callebaut, I. Correa, M. Pensaert, G. Jimenez and L. Enjuanes,
    Antigenic differentiation between transmissible gastroenteritis
    virus of swine and a related porcine respiratory coronavirus, J. Gen.
    Virol., 69:1725-1730 (1988).

21. M. B. Pensaert, Transmissible gastroenteritis virus (Respiratory
    variant), In: "Virus Infections of Vertebrates, Vol. 2. Virus
    Infections of Porcines," M. B. Pensaert, ed., Elsevier, Amsterdam,
    Oxford, New York and Tokyo (1989).

446

Chapter 10

Turkey and Bovine Coronaviruses

CHARACTERIZATION AND LOCATION OF THE STRUCTURAL POLYPEPTIDES OF TURKEY ENTERIC CORONAVIRUS USING MONOCLONAL ANTIBODIES AND ENZYMATIC TREATMENTS

Serge Dea, Simon Garzon and Peter Tijssen

CRMC, Institute Armand-Frappier, University of Quebec

Laval-des-Rapides, Quebec, Canada, H7N 4Z3

INTRODUCTION

Turkey enteric coronavirus (TCV) is one of the major causes of epidemic diarrhoea in turkey poults (1, 2). The morphological and physicochemical characteristics of TCV resemble those of other members of the family Coronaviridae (3, 4). However, little is known with respect to the molecular and antigenic structure of the TCV virion, due to difficulties in propagating TCV strains in tissue cultures and lack of highly specific immunological probes (1, 4). Field isolates can be propagated by oral inoculation and intestinal infections of young turkey poults, or by inoculation into embryonating turkey eggs (4, 5). TCV possesses a hemagglutinating (HA) activity which may be associated to short granular projections located near the base of the characteristic larger bulbous peplomers (6). Recently, we adapted TCV isolates in HRT-18 cells, an established cell line derived from human rectum adenocarcinoma (7). In these cells, TCV induces cytopathic changes, including polykaryocytosis, which depended on trypsin in the culture medium (8).

We describe here the polypeptide structure of tissue culture-adapted TCV. We also begun to explore the antigenic features of the virus by producing monoclonal antibodies (MAbs) to its structural proteins.

RESULTS

Viral purification

The prototype egg-adapted Minnesota strain (4) of TCV was obtained from Dr B.S. Pomeroy, College of Veterinary Medicine, St-Paul, Minn., USA. The virus was serially propagated on HRT-18 cells in the presence of 10 U/ml bovine trypsin (Grade X, Sigma). The extracellular virus was purified by isopyknic ultracentifugation on sucrose gradients (6).

High yields of viral infectivity, ranging from 10^8 to 10^{10} TCID50/mL were recovered after less than 3 to 4 successive passages in HRT-18 cells. Maximal infectivity and HA activity, with rat erythrocytes, were recovered in sucrose-gradient fractions corresponding to a buoyant density of 1.18-1.20 g/ml. These fractions contained viral particles with a morphology consistent with that of coronaviruses, and possessed surface projections of two distinct sizes (Fig. 1).

Coronaviruses and Their Diseases
Edited by D. Cavanagh and T.D.K. Brown
Plenum Press, New York, 1990

449

An anti-TCV hyperimmune serum was obtained after immunization of rabbits with density gradient-purified egg-adapted Minnesota strain. The presence of anti-TCV antibodies was confirmed by IEM and HAI tests (6), and by the use of an indirect protein A-colloidal gold immunolabelling technique (PAG-IEM) (9). After incubation with antiserum, gold granules were usually located near to, or on, the tip of both types of surface projections (Fig. 1b). Control experiments, where pre-immune serum was used or where the anti-TCV serum was omitted, showed that the viral particles in the test were specifically labelled.

Structural polypeptides of TCV

Analysis by SDS-PAGE under non-reducing conditions of purified [³⁵S]methionine-labelled TCV revealed consistently four major and two minor polypeptide species (Fig. 2). The major components were estimated to possess Mr of 140K, 100K, 52K, and 24K, while two minor components had Mr of 200K and 120K. Polypeptide 24K was resolved as a group of 2 to 3 closely migrating bands. Labelling with [³H]glucosamine revealed that the 200K, 140K, 100K, and 24K species were glycosylated. Under reducing conditions, the gp140 species decreased in intensity concomitant with the appearance of a new gp66 species in the gel. The gp140 was thus suggested to be a disulphide-linked dimer of two gp65-70 molecules.

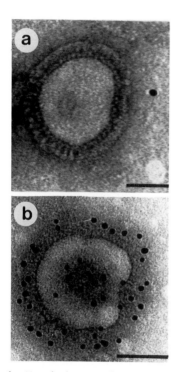
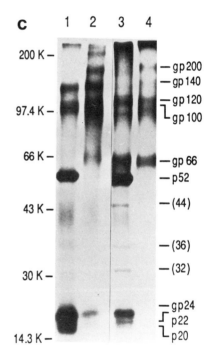

Fig. 1. Morphology and polypeptide structure of TCV. (a) Negatively stained TCV particles with a double fringe of surface peplomers; (b) Protein A-gold immunolabelling of TCV after incubation with rabbit anti-TCV hyperimmune serum. Bars= 50 nm.
(c) Sucrose-gradient purified TCV labelled with either [³⁵S]methionine (lanes 1 and 3) or [³H]glucosamine (lanes 2 and 4) was electrophoresed after solubilization with sample buffer in the absence (lanes 1 and 2) or the presence (lanes 3 and 4) of 5% 2-mercaptoethanol. Positions of molecular weight standards are shown on the left.

Table 1. Characterization of monoclonal antibodies to TCV.

No.of MAbs directed against				Biological properties		
gp200/100	gp140	p52	gp24	SN	HAI	IFA
–	3	–	–	+	+	Cyto + Mb
–	1	–	–	–	+	Cyto + Mb
5	–	–	–	+	–	Cyto + Mb
11	–	–	–	–	–	Cyto + Mb
–	–	8	–	–	–	Cyto
–	–	–	1	–	–	Perinuclear

Characterization of TCV-specific MAbs

For the production of anti-TCV MAbs, BALB/c mice were immunized either with purified whole virus or SDS-denaturated virus. Splenocytes from these mice were fused with SP2/0-Ag14, as described (9). Hybridoma supernates were screened against TCV virions in a solid phase ELISA (10) and subcloned twice by a limiting dilution method. Working preparations of antibodies were obtained by production of ascitic fluids in BALB/c mice primed with pristane. The polypeptide specificities of anti-TCV MAbs were determined by Western immunoblotting with purified virus or by immunoprecipitations with radiolabelled TCV-infected cell lysates, according to Laude et al. (11) and Deregt and Babiuk (12). SN, HAI, and IFA tests were done as previously described (8, 9).

Twenty-nine hybridoma cell lines, producing MAbs directed to TCV were obtained (Table 1). Sixteen hybridomas produced MAbs that recognized either gp200 or gp100, or both protein species. MAbs of 4 other hybridomas reacted only with gp140. In addition, 8 MAbs were specific to the major unglycosylated p52 protein, and only one hybridoma produced antibodies that reacted with gp24. MAbs directed against gp200/100 immunoprecipitated TCV-induced intracellular proteins 200K, 170 to 180K, and polypeptide species between 90 and 120K, whereas, anti-gp140 MAbs immunoprecipitated a 130K polypeptide species, only (data not shown).

Neutralization studies showed that eight anti-TCV MAbs had SN titres between 80 and 10,240; three were specific to gp140, while the five others were specific to gp200/100 (Table 1). Only MAbs to gp140 inhibited HA activity of TCV. MAbs of a given specificity also induced characteristic patterns of fluorescence. Anti-p52 Mabs gave a weak fluorescence that was evenly distributed in the cytoplasm of TCV-infected cells. With anti-gp24 MAb, the fluorescence appeared as fine granulation, essentially limited to the perinuclear area. With MAbs directed to gp200/100 and gp140, the fluorescence was diffuse throughout the cytoplasm, but appeared more intense around the nucleus. Both anti-gp200/100 and anti-gp140 MAbs induced a cell surface fluorescence.

Location and biological properties of TCV structural proteins

To determine the location on the TCV virion of the various proteins identified by SDS-PAGE, aliquots of purified virus were mock-digested or digested with 1 mg/ml of pronase, trypsin, α-chymotrypsin or bromelain, repurified by isopycnic sedimentation, and analysed by EM and SDS-PAGE. Protease-treated TCV was tested also for residual HA activity (Table 2).

Virions treated with pronase lost their HA activity after 45 min, coincidentally with the disappearance of the high mol. wt. glycoproteins from the gel and loss of both types of surface projections. Incubation for 1 hour with eithe trypsin or α-chymotrypsin did not alter the HA activity of TCV. However, complete or nearly complete dissappearance of the gp200 species from the gel was observed and the viral particles apparently lost the bulbous part of their large peplomers. Digestion of TCV with bromelain for two hours did not alter the HA activity of the virus, but caused the loss of the high mol.wt. glycoproteins, except gp140 or gp66, when virus was electrophoresed under reducing conditions. This treatment also left the internal p52 protein intact, but reduced the amounts of gp24. Bromelain-treated viral particles progressively lost their large bulbous peplomers, but their small granular projections persisted even after a 3 hour-exposure period.

Effects of glycosylation inhibitors on the synthesis of TCV glycoproteins

Extracellular virions purified from the supernatant fluids of TCV-infected cells, cultivated in the presence of 0.5 to 1.0 μg/ml of tunicamycin, lacked both infectivity and HA activity (Table 2). The extracellular viral particles were devoid of both types of surface projections. By SDS-PAGE, high mol.wt. structural glycoproteins (gp200/100 and gp140) could no longer be detected with TM-treated virion. Furthermore, the gp2⁄ species was reduced to its unglycosylated form p20, and it was no longer detectable by Western immunoblotting or immunoprecipitation with polyclonal antiserum. Similar results were obtained by immunoprecipitation with TM-treated TCV-infected cells (13).

Cultivation in the presence of sodium monensin (SM) at concentrations up to 2.5 μM neither affected the virulence (cytopathogenicity) of the virus, nor changed the morphology of the extracellular progeny viral particles (data not shown). The virus enveloppe-glycoproteins, including gp24, could be immunoprecipitated from extracts of SM-treated TCV-infected cells and strongly incorporated [³H]glucosamine (13).

Table 2. Hemagglutinating activity and TCV polypeptides detected by Western immunoblotting after treatment with proteases and tunicamycin (TM).

TCV polypeptides	Treatments				
	Trypsin 1000μg/ml	Chymotrypsin 1000μg/ml	Pronase 1mg/ml	Bromelain 1.3mg/ml	TMᵃ 1μg/ml
gp180-200	−	−	−	−	−
gp140	++	++	−	++	−
gp120	+	+	−	−	−
gp100	++	++	−	−	−
gp66	++	++	−	++	−
p52	++	++	++	++	++
gp24-26	++	++	+/−	+/−	−
p20	++	++	++	+	+
HA	++	++	−	++	−

ᵃ TM was added to the culture medium of TCV-infected cells after the adsorption period and extracellular virus was harvested at 24 h p.i.

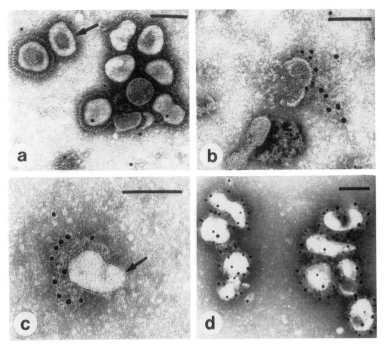

Fig. 2   Protein A-gold immunolabelling of TCV by anti-TCV monoclonal
antibodies (see legend in the text).

Location of the antigenic determinants on the virion

Distinct immunogold-labelling patterns of TCV particles were obtained by MAbs (Fig. 2). With anti-p52 MAbs, no labelling of intact virions
was observed. However, gold granules were found near filamentous-like
structures (helicoidal nucleocapsid) which appeared to exit the damaged
viral particles (Fig. 2b). With anti-gp200/100 MAbs, the gold granules
were located near the tips of the large bulbous projections (Fig. 2d).
Bromelain-treated viral particles were found to be labelled by anti-
gp200/100 MAbs only on a few large projections still remaining on their
enveloppe (Fig. 2c). With anti-gp140 MAbs, a specific labelling pattern
could not be defined with certainty (data not shown). No labelling was
obtained using pre-immune mouse serum (Fig. 2a).

DISCUSSION

The structural nature of the proteins resolved by SDS-PAGE of purified virus was confirmed by Western immunoblotting and immunoprecipitation, using antiserum to the original egg-adapted virus. Furthermore, 29
anti-TCV MAbs were characterized with respect to polypeptide specificity,
capacity to neutralize virus, and ability to inhibit its HA activity.

Four major viral protein species were identified and their location
on the TCV virion was deduced from digestion studies with proteolytic enzymes and by immunogold-labelling with MAbs. The TCV structural proteins
consist of three glycoproteins of 180-200,000, 140,000 and 24,000 which
were shown to correspond to the peplomer (E2 or S), hemagglutinin (E3)
and matrix (E1 or M) proteins, and a predominant unglycosylated 52,000
species that apparently represents the nucleocapsid (N) protein. A similar polypeptide pattern has been described previously with virus purified
from the intestinal contents of turkey embryos (7).

The largest virion glycoproteins of TCV thus appear to differ fundamentally from the largest glycoproteins of the avian infectious bronchitis virus (IBV) (14, 15). The presence of additionnal short granular projections on the surface of the TCV virion, and a hemagglutinin glycoprotein that appeared as a dimer of two smaller 65-70,000 molecules, are features that have been described so far only for viruses belonging to the group of mammalian hemagglutinating coronaviruses (16, 17, 18). The observation that bromelain treatment removed all glycoproteins from the virion except gp140, and that only small granular projections were retained on the particles, further suggested gp140 and small granular projections to correspond to the virion hemagglutinin.

In the presence of TM, non-infectious TCV virions lacking both types of surface peplomers were produced and released by infected cells. Biochemical data confirmed the absence of the high mol. wt. glycoproteins (gp200/100, gp140/66) consistent with a glycosylation process that involves attachement of oligosaccharide side chains via N-glycosidic bonds to asparagine residues, as demonstrated for other coronaviruses (19, 20). The matrix protein of TCV is apparently glycosylated by a similar process. In this respect, TCV resembles the avian infectious bronchitis virus (14, 21), but differs from the mammalian coronaviruses MHV-A59 and BCV. The matrix glycoprotein of these mammalian coronaviruses undergoes O-linked glycosylation by a process which is resistant to TM, but sensitive to SM, and involves attachment of oligosaccharides to serine residues (18, 22, 23). The enveloppe glycoproteins of TCV, including the matrix protein, were normally synthesized in the presence of SM. As previously reported for IBV and MHV (14, 22, 23), E1 appeared to be the only glycoprotein required for the formation of TCV virions, and its glycosylation is apparently not essential.

Antigenic determinants located on both E2 and E3 reacted with MAbs involved in TCV neutralization, as previously described for bovine enteric coronavirus (12). Both hemagglutinin and peplomer glycoproteins also were expressed at the cell surface and may thus represent potential targets for specific antibody-dependent or cell-mediated cytotoxicity.

ACKNOWLEDGEMENTS

This research was supported in part by grants from the Conseil des Recherches et Services Agricoles du Quebec and the Quebec Federation of Poultry Producers (VOLBEC). S.Dea has received a Fellowship from the Medical Research Council of Canada. These results were taken from a PhD thesis submitted by the senior author to the Department of Virology, Institute Armand-Frappier, University of Quebec, Canada.

REFERENCES

1. B. S. Pomeroy. Coronaviral enteritis of turkeys, in: Disease of poultry, 8th ed. M. S. Holstad, H. J. Barnes, B. W. Calnek, W. M. Reid, and H. W. Yoder, ed., Iowa State Univ. Press, Ames (1984).
2. S. Dea and P. Tijssen. Viral agents associated with outbreaks of diarrhea in turkey flocks in Quebec. Can. J. Vet.Res. 52:53 (1988)
3. D. R. Deshmukh and B. S. Pomeroy. Physicochemical characterization of a bluecomb coronavirus of turkeys. Am. J. Vet. Res. 35:1549 (1977).
4. A. E. Ritchie, D. R. Deshmukh, C. T. Larsen, and B. S. Pomeroy. Electron microscopy of coronavirus-like particles characteristic of turkey bluecomb disease. Avian Dis. 17:546 (1973).
5. D. R. Deshmukh, C. T. Larsen, and B. S. Pomeroy. Survival of Bluecomb agent in embryonating turkey eggs and cell cultures. Am. J. Vet. Res. 34:673 (1973).

6. S. Dea and P. Tijssen. Identification of the structural proteins of turkey enteric coronavirus. Arch. Virol. 99:173 (1988).
7. W. A. F. Tompkins, A. W. Watrach, J.D. Schmale, R.M. Schultz, and J.A. Harris. Cultural and antigenic properties of newly established cell strains derived from adenocarcinomas of the human colon and rectum. J. Natl. Cancer Inst. 52:101 (1974).
8. S. Dea, S. Garzon, and P. Tijssen. Isolation and trypsin-enhanced propagation of turkey enteric (Bluecomb) coronaviruses in a continuous human rectal tumor (HRT-18) cell line. Am. J. Vet. Res. (In press).
9. S. Dea and P. Tijssen. Antigenic and polypeptide structure of turkey enteric coronaviruses as defined by monoclonal antibodies. J. Gen. Virol. (In press).
10. S. Dea and P. Tijssen. Detection of turkey enteric coronavirus by enzyme-linked immunosorbent assay and differenhtiation from other coronaviruses. Am. J. Vet. Res. 50:226 (1989).
11. H. Laude, J.M. Chapsal, J. Gelfi, S. Labiau, and J. GrosClaude. Antigenic structure of transmissible gastroenteritis virus. I. Properties of monoclonal antibodies directed against virion proteins. J. Gen. Virol. 67:119 (1986).
12. D. Deregt and L. A. Babiuk. Monoclonal antibodies to bovine coronavirus: characteristics and topographical mapping of neutralizing epitopes on the E2 and E3 glycoproteins. Virology 161:410 (1987).
13. S. Dea, S. Garzon, and P. Tijssen. Intracellular synthesis and processing of the structural glycoproteins of turkey enteric coronavirus. Arch. Virol. (In press).
14. D. F. Stern and B.M. Sefton. Coronavirus proteins: structure and functions of the oligosaccharides of the avian infectious bronchitis virus glycoproteins. J. Virol. 44:804 (1982).
15. D. Cavanagh, P. J. Davis, D. J. C. Pappin, M. M. Binns, M. E. G. Boursnell, and T. D. K. Brown. Coronavirus IBV: partial amino terminal sequencing of spike polypeptide S2 identifies the sequence Arg-Arg-Phe-Arg-Arg at the cleavage site of the spike precursor polypeptide of IBV strains Beaudette and M41. Virus Res. 4:133 (1986).
16. B. G. Hogue, B. King, and D. A. Brian. Antigenic relationships among proteins of bovine coronavirus, human respiratory coronavirus OC 43, and mouse hepatitis coronavirus A59. J. Virol. 51:384 (1984).
17. B. King, B. J. Potts, and D.A . Brian. Bovine coronavirus hemagglu-tinin protein. Virus Res. 2:53 (1985).
18. W. Lapps, B. G. Hogue, and D. A. Brian. Sequence analysis of the bovine coronavirus nucleocapsid and matrix protein genes. Virology 157:47 (1987).
19. W. Luytjes, L. S. Sturman, P. J. Bredenbeek, J. Charite, B. A. M. Van der Zeijst, M. C. Horzinek, and W. J. M. Spaan. Primary structure of the glycoprotein E2 of coronavirus MHV-A59 and identification of the trypsin cleavage site. Virology 161:479 (1987).
20. L. S. Sturman and K. V. Holmes. The molecular biology of coronaviruses. Adv. Virus Res. 56:904 (1983).
21. M. E. G. Boursnell, T. D. K. Brown, and M. M. Binns. Sequence of the membrane protein gene from avian coronavirus IBV. Virus Res. 1:303 (1984).
22. P. J. M. Rottier, M. C. Horzinek, and B. A. M. Van Der Zeijst. Viral protein synthesis in mouse hepatitis virus strain A59-infected cells: effect of tunicamycin. J. Virol. 40:350 (1981).
23. H. Nieman and H. D. Klenk. Coronavirus glycoprotein E1, a new type of viral glycoprotein. J. Mol. Biol. 153:993 (1981).

EVIDENCE OF CLOSE RELATEDNESS BETWEEN TURKEY AND BOVINE CORONAVIRUSES

Peter Tijssen, Arnold J. Verbeek and Serge Dea

CRMC - Institute Armand-Frappier, University of Quebec

Laval-des-Rapides, Quebec, Canada, H7N 4Z3

INTRODUCTION

Immunoelectron microscopy and indirect immunofluorescence studies in 1973 showed that turkey enteric coronavirus (TCV or "Bluecomb agent") is unrelated to another avian coronavirus IBV, and to mammalian coronaviruses (1, 2). Coronaviruses have thus been classified, according to antigenic cross-reactivity, into four distinct subgroups within the family, two subgroups of avian viruses and two subgroups of non-avian viruses (3, 4, 5).

TCV is one of the major causative agents of epidemic diarrhea in turkey poults (6, 7). Studies on TCV have long been hampered by the failure to obtain sufficient virus and by the lack of a suitable tissue culture system (6, 8). Recently, however, we have been able to adapt this virus to HRT-18 cells, an established human rectal tumor cell line (9, 10). Studies on tissue culture- and egg-adapted TCV demonstrated that this virus shares many morphological, biological and molecular properties with bovine coronavirus (BCV; 11, 12), such as (i) the presence of additional short granular surface projections (hemagglutinating glycoprotein), (13, 14); (ii) antigenic relatedness as demonstrated by ELISA, (15); and (iii) intestinal tropism (in respective animals and replication "in vitro" in HRT-18 cells) (9, 16).

Here, we report studies undertaken to establish the extent of relatedness between BCV and TCV. These studies led us to conclude that these viruses are very closely related and that they should be reclassified.

RESULTS

TCV and BCV readily adapted to HRT-18 cells. Although the yield of infective viral particles were comparable for the two viruses, the cytopathic effect of TCV was considerably more pronounced (polykaryocytosis).

Monoclonal antibodies were raised against both TCV (12) and BCV (manuscript in preparation). About 30 MAbs were obtained against the five major structural proteins of each virus. These MAbs were used in Western immuno-blotting, neutralisation, and hemagglutination inhibition studies.

The structural polypeptide profiles after electrophoresis under denaturing conditions were comparable for the two viruses. In the presence of 2-mercapto-ethanol, the 140K polypeptide of TCV was split into two monomers (65K), as

Coronaviruses and Their Diseases
Edited by D. Cavanagh and T.D.K. Brown
Plenum Press, New York, 1990

457

Table 1.   Characteristics of MAbs distinguishing BCV and TCV

MAb	Immunizing Virus	Polypeptide Specificity	Reactivity by					
			ELISA		SN		HAI	
			TCV	BCV	TCV	BCV	TCV	BCV
M23	TCV	gp200/100	5.6[a]	3.8	-	-	-	-
43C3	TCV	p52	4.0	-	-	-	1280[c]	-
M31	TCV	gp140	5.0	5.0	5120[b]	-	-	-
M33	TCV	gp200/100	6.2	6.2	10230	-	-	-
VIF4E6	BCV	gp200/100	3.8	4.7	-	320	-	-
VIF4E5	BCV	gp200/100	3.8	4.7	40	640	-	-
VIA5	BCV	gp200/100	3.8	6.2	40	160	-	-
VIF3A	BCV	gp140	3.8	4.7	-	-	-	-
VIF3B	BCV	gp140	2.6	4.7	-	-	-	80
314C	BCV	p52	2.6	5.3	-	-	-	-
V27	BCV	p52	2.6	5.9	-	-	-	-

[a] Log 10 of the highest dilution of ascitic fluid giving an A492 value   2.5 X A492 value of a buffer control.

[b] Seroneutralization titers were expressed as the reciprocal of the highest dilution of ascitic fluid neutralizing CPE produced by 100 TCID50 of virus.

[c] Hemagglutination-inhibition titers were expressed as the reciprocal of the highest dilution ascitic fluid neutralizing 8 HA units of virus.

previously described for BCV (13, 17). Western immunoblotting of these proteins was used to establish the protein specificity of 29 anti-TCV MAbs and 20 anti-BCV MAbs. Neutralising antibodies were directed to gp 200, gp 120 and gp 100 or gp 140. MAbs inhibiting hemagglutinating activity were all directed to gp 140. The gp 200, gp 120 and gp 100 were shown by MAbs to be interrelated. Polyclonal antisera to TCV and BCV cross-reacted strongly with the proteins of the hetero-logous virus. Anti-BCV and anti-TCV MAbs revealed also an extensive hetero-logous activity. Most MAbs reacted similarly against both viruses by ELISA, SN, and HAI tests. At least four anti-TCV and at least seven anti-BCV MAbs could distinguish the two viruses (Table 1). On the other hand, we have shown recently that even among TCV strains, the variation in reactivity exists among the anti-TCV MAbs towards their homologous virus (12).

Different radio-isotopically labelled recombinant plasmids, containing both the matrix and the nucleocapsid gene, and other sequences obtained by cloning random-primed cDNA, were independently able to detect TCV under rather stringent hybridization conditions, optimized for BCV detection (17). TCV could also be detected in clinical specimens, using BCV-specific cDNA probes either labeled by nicktranslation or by amplification of BCV specific fragments using the polymerase chain reaction. These data and sequencing studies in progress demonstrated the presence of strong homologies between both viral genomes.

Experimental inoculation studies of turkey poults with TCV revealed that egg-adapted and tissue culture-adapted TCV isolates still caused the typical symptoms of enteritis (9, 19). Infection of poults with BCV (either from diarrheic fecal samples or from tissue culture strains) did not cause diarrhea, and poults killed after one week p.i. did not show any histologic lesions. However, coronavirus particles were detected by EM and by hybridization with cDNA probes in the clarified intestinal contents from poults from two different groups of seronegative poults.

It can be concluded from these studies that TCV and BCV are, on a molecular basis, almost indistinguishable, although they infect different animal species. Therefore, these viruses should be reclassified into a single subgroup.

ACKNOWLEDGMENTS

We would like to thank Drs P. Talbot and J.P. Descoteaux (Institut Armand-Frappier), and Dr. A., Bouffard (Animal Disease Research Center, Agriculture Canada, Nepean, Ontario, Canada) for providing rabbit anti-HCV 229E and anti-RECV (rabbit coronavirus) hyperimmune sera, and pig anti-HEV sera.

This report was taken in part from a dissertation submitted by S. Dea to the Department of Virology, Institute Armand-Frappier, University of Quebec, in partial fulfillment of the requirements for the Ph.D. degree.

This research was supported in part by grants from the Quebec Federation of Poultry Producers (VOLBEC) and the Conseil des Recherches et Services Agricoles du Quebec. S. Dea has received a Fellowship from the Medical Research Council of Canada.

REFERENCES

1. K.A. Pomeroy, B.L. Patel, C.T. Larsen, and B. S. Pomeroy. Combined immunofluorescence and transmission electron microscopic studies of se-quential intestinal samples from turkey embryos and poults infected with turkey enteritis coronavirus. Am. J. Vet. Res. 39:1348 (1978).

2. A.E. Ritchie, D.R. Deshmukh, C.T. Larsen, and B.S. Pomeroy. Electron microscopy of coronavirus-like particles characteristic of turkey bluecomb disease. Avian Dis. 17:546 (1973).

3. N.C. Pedersen, I. Wark and W.L. Mengeling. Antigenic relationships of the feline infectious peritonitis virus to coronaviruses of other species. Arch. Virol. 58:45 (1978).

4. M.C. Horzinek, H. Lutz, and N.C. Pedersen. Antigenic relationships among homologous structural polypeptides of porcine, feline and canine coronaviruses. Infect. Immun. 37:1148 (1982).

5. S. Siddell, H. Wege and V. Ter Meulen. The biology of coronaviruses. J. Gen. Virol. 64:761 (1983).

6. B.S. Pomeroy. Coronaviral enteritis of turkeys, In M.S. Holstad, H.J. Barnes, B.W. Calnek, W.M. Reid, and H.W. Yoder (eds), "Diseases of poultry", 8th ed. Iowa's State Univ. Press, Ames (1984).

7. S. Dea and P. Tijssen. Viral agents associated with outbreaks of diarrhea in turkey flocks in Quebec. Can. J. Vet. Res. 52:53 (1988).

8. D.R. Deshmukh, C.T. Larsen, and B.S. Pomeroy. Survival of bluecomb agent in embryonating turkey eggs and cell cultures. Am. J. Vet. Res. 34:673 (1973).

9. S. Dea and P. Tijssen. Isolation and trypsin-enhanced propagation of turkey enteric (bluecomb) coronaviruses in a continuous human rectal tumor (HRT-18) cell line. Am. J. Vet. Rec. (in press)

10. W.A.F. Tompkins, A.W. Watrach, J.D. Schmale, R.M. Schultz, and J.A. Harris. Cultural and antigenic properties of newly established cell strains derived from adenocarcinomas of the human colon and rectum. J. Natl. Cancer Inst. 52:101 (1974).

11. S. Dea and P. Tijssen. Identification of the structural proteins of turkey enteric coronavirus. Arch. Virol. 99:173 (1988).

12. S. Dea and P. Tijssen. Antigenic and polypeptide structure of turkey enteric coronaviruses as defined by monoclonal antibodies. J. Gen. Virol. (in press).

13. B. King, B.J. Potts, and D.A. Brian. Bovine coronavirus hemagglutinin protein. Virus Res. 2:53: (1985).

14. B.G. Hogue, B. King, and D.A. Brian. Antigenic relationships among proteins of bovine coronavirus, human respiratory coronavirus OC43, and mouse hepatitis coronavirus A59. J. Virol. 51:384 (1984).

15. J. Laporte and P. Bobulesco. Polypeptide structure of bovine enteric coronavirus: comparison between a wild strain purified from feces and a HRT-18 cell-adapted strain. Adv. Exp. Med. Biol. 142:171 (1981).

16. W. Lapps, B.G. Hogue, and D.A. Brian. Sequence analysis of the bovine coronavirus nucleocapsid and matrix protein genes. Virology 157:47 (1987).

17. A. Verbeek, and P. Tijssen. Biotinylated and radioactive cDNA probes in the detection by hybridization of bovine enteric coronavirus. Molecular Probes 2:209 (1988).

18. N.R. Adams, R.A. Ball, and M.S. Hofstad. Intestinal lesions in transmissible enteritis of turkeys. Avian Dis. 14:392 (1970).

A COMPARISON OF BOVINE CORONAVIRUS STRAINS USING MONOCLONAL ANTIBODIES

M.A. Clark, I. Campbell, A.A. El-Ghorr, D.R. Snodgrass
F.M.M. Scott

Moredun Research Institute
408 Gilmerton Road, Edinburgh

ABSTRACT

Eight monoclonal antibodies (MAbs) were raised against a bovine coronavirus (B.C.V.) which had been isolated in Scotland and was designated S2. The MAbs were divided into two groups on the basis of their reactions with S2 virus in indirect immunofluorescence (I.F.), neutralisation and haemagglutination inhibition (H.A.I.) tests. Five of the MAbs were positive by all three tests but failed to bind to proteins in Western immunoblotting experiments. The remaining three MAbs were positive in I.F. tests only, two of which were shown to bind to the 52K nucleocapsid protein by Western immunoblotting. Different patterns of antigen distribution within infected cells were demonstrated when the MAbs were used in the I.F. test. However only minor strain variations were detected by I.F. and H.A.I. tests when the MAbs were tested against each of five cell culture adapted strains of B.C.V. Twenty-nine isolates of B.C.V. have been grown in neonatal calf tracheal organ cultures: attempts are being made to further characterise these isolates.

INTRODUCTION

The structural proteins of B.C.V. have been well defined.[1, 2] Four proteins are described: the internal nucleocapsid protein N, the matrix glycoproteins E1, the peplomer glycoproteins E2 and the haemagglutinin glycoprotein E3. Monoclonal antibodies to both E2 and E3 have been found to neutralise the virus in vitro[3] and in vivo[4]. The E3 protein is responsible for the ability of B.C.V. to haemagglutinate red blood cells (R.B.C.'s).[5, 6]

Only minor strain variations have been found between different isolates of B.C.V. using both polyclonal antisera and MAbs.[7, 8, 9] The number of isolates available for such studies is limited because of the difficulties involved in the adaptation of B.C.V. to growth in cell culture systems. However organ cultures of foetal and neonatal calf tracheas have been used successfully as an alternative method for the primary isolation and growth of B.C.V.[10, 11, 12]

This report describes the characterisation of eight MAbs raised to the Scottish S2 isolate of B.C.V. and the use of these MAbs in the

Coronaviruses and Their Diseases
Edited by D. Cavanagh and T.D.K. Brown
Plenum Press, New York, 1990

identification of variations between five cell culture adapted isolates of B.C.V. A further four MAbs raised against a different isolate of B.C.V. were kindly supplied by the Central Veterinary Laboratory (C.V.L.) at Weybridge.

Twenty-nine isolates of B.C.V. from faecal samples were grown in neonatal calf tracheal organ cultures.

MATERIALS and METHODS

Viruses

Human rectal tumour cells, HRT-18, were used to culture B.C.V. The Scottish isolates of B.C.V., S1 and S2, had been isolated in tracheal organ culture and adapted to grow in HRT-18 cells.[13] Three reference strains i.e. M,[14] PQ[15] and CK[16] were also used.

Production of the monoclonal antibodies

MAbs to B.C.V. S2 isolate were produced from Balb-C mice essentially following a procedure described by Deregt et al.[2] Hybridoma cells were screened for antibody production by indirect I.F., neutralisation and H.A.I. tests. Antibody producing cells were terminally diluted three times before inoculation into the peritoneal cavity of pristane (2, 6, 10, 14-tetramethylpentadecane) primed mice. Ascitic fluid was collected, pooled, aliquoted and stored at -70°C.

Western immunoblotting

S2 viral proteins were separated by P.A.G.E. employing a vertical discontinuous gel system with a 3% stacking and a 10% resolving gel. The proteins were electroblotted overnight on to nitrocellulose membranes. The membranes were cut into strips and incubated for one hour at room temperature with a blocking solution of PBS/0.5% Tween 20. Bound viral proteins were detected by incubation with ascitic fluid diluted at 1:40 in PBS/T followed by Protein A labelled with I^{125}. The strips were then processed for autoradiography and incubated for 9 days at -70°C before developing.

Tracheal organ culture/Faecal Samples

Tracheal organ cultures were derived from neonatal Jersey bull calves.[17] The organ cultures were set up as described by Thomas and Howard,[17] except that each tracheal ring was placed in an individual petri dish.

Faecal samples from diarrhoeic calves were prepared as 10% suspensions in PBS and tested for B.C.V. in an indirect ELISA. BCV positive samples were inoculated on to tracheal organ cultures using a method similar to that described by Stott et al.[10]. Media was harvested twice a week and monitored for H.A. activity.

RESULTS

Production of hybridomas

Eight hybridoma cell lines secreting antibodies to B.C.V. detectable by at least one of the 3 screening tests were successfully cloned from two fusions.

The MAbs could be divided into two groups based on the results of these tests. In one group the MAbs (S2/1, S2/2, S2/3, S2/4 and S2/7) were positive by all 3 tests. In the other group the remaining 3 MAbs (S2/5, S2/6 and S2/8) were positive by I.F. only (Table 1).

Table 1. Characterisation of the MAbs

MAb	Indirect I.F.*[1]	Neutralisation*[1]	H.A.I.*[1]	Protein specificity*[2]
S2/1	+	+	+	N.R.
S2/2	+	+	+	N.R.
S2/3	+	+	+	N.R.
S2/4	+	+	+	N.R.
S2/5	+	−	−	52K protein
S2/6	+	−	−	N.R.
S2/7	+	+	+	N.R.
S2/8	+	−	−	52K protein

*[1] as determined with S2 virus
*[2] protein specificity determined by Western immunoblotting
N.R. signifies there was no reaction of the MAb with nitrocellulose bound viral proteins

Patterns of immunofluorescence

Different patterns of fluorescence were observed when the MAbs were reacted with S2 virus infected HRT-18 cells at 20 hrs post infection. The MAbs positive by all 3 of the screening tests gave a mainly perinuclear pattern of I.F. The MAbs positive by I.F. only gave a more even distribution of fluorescence throughout the cell cytoplasm. Distinctive large granules were seen with MAb S2/4. On membrane fluorescence tests, a clear bright membrane fluorescence was observed when the MAbs positive by all 3 of the screening tests were used. The MAbs positive by I.F. only were negative.

Isotype/Western immunoblotting

The immunoglobulins secreted by the hybridoma cell lines all belonged to the IgG class of antibody. Only 2 of the MAbs bound to blotted proteins (Table 1). These were MAbs S2/5 and S2/8 which both bound to a protein with a molecular weight of about 52 K (Fig. 1). This value agrees closely with that reported by other workers for the nucleocapsid N protein.[1,2]

Comparison of different strains of B.C.V.

Using the 8 MAbs directed against S2 virus, differences were shown by I.F. using S2/5 MAb only and in H.A.I. by S2/2 MAb (Table 2). No differences were demonstrated with the 4 MAbs supplied by C.V.L.

Isolation of B.C.V. from faecal samples in tracheal organ culture

H.A. titres obtained from consecutive harvests from a series of tracheal organ cultures are shown in Table 3.

Table 2. Differences detected by indirect I.F. and H.A.I.

Virus	TEST	
	Indirect I.F.*[1] S2/5 MAb	H.A.I.*[2] S2/2 MAb
S1	<100	1280
S2	9051	320
CK	<100	<20
M	<100	<20
PQ	<100	<20

*[1] Titres given are the reciprocal of the highest dilution of
MAb ascitic fluid giving clear fluorescence with virus
infected cells

*[2] Titres given are the reciprocal of the highest dilution of
ascitic fluid causing complete inhibition of haemagglutination
by 8 H.A. units of virus.

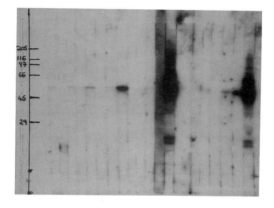

Fig. 1.   Autoradiograph of Western immunoblot.

The   reaction   of MAbs S2/5 and S2/8 with a 52K   molecular   weight
protein may be seen in lanes 5, 19 and 8, 20 respectively.

Table 3. H.A. titres of B.C.V. in tracheal organ culture

Faeces	Harvest No				
	1	2	3	4	5
L3317	-	-	-	-	-
L3032	16	≥128	≥128	≥128	8
L2759	-	-	-	-	-
N339	≥128	≥128	32	32	16
K2472	-	-	-	-	-
N164	-	-	-	-	-
L1096	-	64	≥128	≥128	32
L1121	16	≥128	64	64	16
Negative control	-	-	-	-	-

H.A. titres are the reciprocal dilutions

Out of a total of 60 faecal samples inoculated onto tracheal organ cultures, 29 have grown to give H.A. titres of at least 32. All isolates reacted positively when tested in an indirect ELISA for the detection of B.C.V. antigen.

DISCUSSION

Eight MAbs were raised against the S2 isolate of B.C.V. These were divided into two groups on the basis of their reactions with S2 virus in I.F., neutralisation and H.A.I. tests. Five of the MAbs gave positive reactions in all 3 of these tests whilst the remaining 3 were positive on I.F. tests only. Since the E3 protein has been confirmed as the viral haemagglutinin[5,6] it is reasonable to suggest that the MAbs positive in H.A.I. tests are directed against this protein. Confirmation of this has yet to be obtained.

It was demonstrated in Western immunoblotting that 2 of the MAbs which were I.F. positive only were directed against the nucleocapsid N protein. This is consistent with the negative results obtained in neutralisation and H.A.I. tests with these MAbs.

Using MAbs in immunofluorescence tests distinct patterns of B.C.V. antigen distribution within infected HRT-18 cells were defined. The putative anti E3 MAbs gave a mainly perinuclear pattern of fluorescence and showed positive membrane fluorescence. The anti-N MAbs gave a more even distribution of cytoplasmic fluorescence and were membrane fluorescence negative. Similar patterns have been described for murine hepatitis virus (M.H.V.)[18], transmissible gastroenteritis virus of swine (T.G.E.V.)[19] and turkey enteric coronavirus (T.C.V.).[20]

Only minor variations between the 5 cell culture adapted isolates of B.C.V. were demonstrated using MAbs. In order to gain a more complete understanding of the possible antigenic variations between B.C.V. strains it is desirable to test a larger number of isolates. The use of neonatal calf tracheal organ cultures has proved a useful method for the primary isolation of virus from faecal samples and should provide a sufficient number of isolates to allow a more thorough investigation of antigenic variation to be made.

REFERENCES

1. B. King and D.A. Brian. Bovine coronavirus structural proteins. J. Virol. 42:700 (1982).
2. D. Deregt, M. Sabara, and L.A. Babiuk. Structural proteins of bovine coronavirus and their intracellular processing. J. gen. Virol. 68: 2863 (1987).
3. D. Deregt and L.A. Babiuk. Monoclonal antibodies to bovine coronavirus: Characteristics and topographical mapping of neutralising epitopes on the E2 and E3 glycoproteins. Virology, 161: 410 (1987).
4. D. Deregt, G.A. Gifford, M.K. Ijaz, T.C. Watts, J.E. Gilchrist, D.M. Haines, and L.A. Babiuk. Monoclonal antibodies to bovine coronavirus glycoproteins E2 and E3: Demonstration of in vivo virus - neutralizing activity. J. gen. Virol. 70: 993 (1989).
5. B. King, B.J. Potts, and D.A. Brian. Bovine coronavirus haemagglutinin protein. Virus Res. 2: 53 (1985).

6. M.D. Parker, G.J. Cox, D. Deregt, D.R. Fitzpatrick, and L.A. Babiuk. Cloning and in vitro expression of the gene for the E3 haemagglutinin glycoprotein of bovine coronavirus. J. gen. Virol. 70: 155 (1989).

7. A.A. El-Ghorr, D.R. Snodgrass, F.M.M. Scott, and I. Campbell. A serological comparison of bovine coronavirus strains. Arch. Virol. 104: 241 (1989).

8. J.F. Vautherot, J. Laporte, M.F. Madelaine, P.Bobulesco, and A. Roseto. Antigenic and polypeptide structure of bovine enteric coronavirus as defined by monoclonal antibodies. Adv. Exp. Med. Biol. 173: 117 (1984).

9. S. Dea, R.S. Roy, and M.A.S.Y. Elazhary. Antigenic variations among calf diarrhoea coronaviruses by immunodiffusion and counterimmunoelectrophoresis. Ann. Rech. Vet. 13(4): 351 (1982).

10. E.J. Stott, L.H. Thomas, J.C.Bridger, and N.J. Jebbett. Replication of a bovine coronavirus in organ cultures of foetal trachea. Vet. Microbiol. 1: 65 (1976).

11. J.C. Bridger, G.N. Woode, and A. Meyling. Isolation of coronaviruses from neonatal calf diarrhoea in Great Britain and Denmark. Vet. Microbiol. 3:101 (1978).

12. M.S. McNulty, D.G. Bryson, G.M. Allan, and E.F. Logan. Coronavirus infection of the bovine respiratory tract. Vet. Microbiol. 9:425 (1984).

13. A.A. El-Ghorr, D.R. Snodgrass, and F.M.M. Scott. Evaluation of an immunogold electron microscopy technique for detecting bovine coronavirus. J. Virol. Methods. 19:215 (1988).

14. C.A. Mebus, E.L. Stair, M.B. Rhodes, and M.J. Twiehaus. Neonatal calf diarrhoea: Propagation, attenuation, and characteristics of a coronavirus-like agent. Am. J. Vet. Res. 34:145 (1973).

15. S. Dea, R.S. Roy, and M.E. Begin. Physicochemical and biological properties of neonatal calf diarrhoea coronaviruses isolated in Quebec and comparison with the Nebraska calf coronavirus. Am. J. Vet. Res. 41:23 (1980).

16. D.J. Reynolds, T.G. Debney, G.A. Hall, L.H. Thomas, and K.R. Parsons. Studies on the relationship between coronaviruses from the intestinal and respiratory tracts of calves. Arch. Virol. 85: 71 (1985).

17. L.H. Thomas and C.J. Howard. Effect of mycoplasma dispar, mycoplasma bovirhinis, acholeplasma laidlawii and T-mycoplasmas on explant cultures of bovine trachea. J. Comp. Path. 84: 193 (1974).

18. A.R. Collins, R.L. Knobler, H. Powell, and M.J. Buchmeier. Monoclonal antibodies to murine hepatitis virus-4 (strain JHM) define the viral glycoprotein responsible for attachment and cell-cell fusion. Virology, 119:358 (1982).

19. H. Laude, J-M. Chapsal, J. Gelfi, S. Labiau, and J. Grosclaude. Antigenic structure of transmissible gastroenteritis virus. I. Properties of monoclonal antibodies directed against virion proteins. J. gen. Virol. 67: 119 (1986).

20. S. Dea and P. Tijssen. Antigenic and polypeptide structure of turkey enteric coronaviruses as defined by monoclonal antibodies. J. gen. Virol. 70: 1725 (1989).

ANALYSIS OF DIFFERENT PROBE-LABELING SYSTEMS FOR DETECTION BY HYBRIDIZATION OF BOVINE CORONAVIRUS

J.A. Verbeek, S. Dea, and P. Tijssen

CRMC - Institute Armand-Frappier - University of Quebec

Laval-des-Rapides, Quebec, Canada, H7N 4Z3

INTRODUCTION

Several methods for the detection of bovine coronavirus (BCV) in clinical specimens have been developed (1-5). The notoriously difficult diagnosis by EM has recently been improved by the use of immunogold (3), whereas other methods have been described, based on serological detection (2,5) or on the hemagglutinating capacity of the virus (6,7). Even though increased specificity in immunological detection assays can be obtained using monoclonal antibodies, sensitivity and detectability still remain to be improved.

It has been shown that cDNA probes can be applied to detect viral RNA, isolated from tissue culture-propagated virus (8), whereas in a subsequent study (9), conditions were optimized for BCV detection without previous RNA isolation. Purified virus was directly applied in low-salt concentrations to the nitrocellulose membrane and denaturation and RNA fixation was conveniently achieved by baking the blots under vacuum.

In this report, we discuss different probe-labeling systems for BCV detection by hybridization. Furthermore, data are provided on the adaptation of this test system for clinical sample processing and virus detection, and for virus-specific sequence amplification by the polymerase-chain-reaction (PCR).

MATERIALS AND METHODS

Virus and cells

The NCDC strain (Mebus) of BCV was obtained from the American Type Culture Collection and propagated in human rectal tumor (HRT-18) cells (10). Virus purification was as in previously described methods (11).

Probes

Recombinant plasmids (vectors) used in probing assays, were selected from genomic-cDNA libraries, obtained by cloning oligo-dT or random primed-cDNA (9) or by cloning of polymerase-chain-reaction (PCR) amplified BCV-specific fragments.

Probe selection was based on the capacity of clones to hybridize strongly in colony-filter hybridization assays (12). Two other vectors, containing inserts, representing the translational reading frames for the nucleocapsid (N) and the matrix (E1) protein, as shown by sequence analysis, were also chosen as they have already been characterized (13).

Coronaviruses and Their Diseases
Edited by D. Cavanagh and T.D.K. Brown
Plenum Press, New York, 1990

Vectors were purified on CsCl gradients and their corresponding cDNA inserts were obtained by electro-elution, after separation of the restriction-enzyme digested DNA on an agarose gel.

Probe-labeling

Vectors or purified cDNA inserts were labeled by nick-translation (14) or random priming (15) in the presence of radioactive precursors α^{32}P dCTP, 3000 Ci/mmol). Biotinylated probes were obtained as described by Leary et al (16).

PCR-synthesized probes were principally labeled as described by Schowalter et al. (17), using as template, a vector that contained the 3' end of the genome until position 817 (13). Primers used in the amplification system were 5' GGC TCT ACT GGA TGC GCG TGA AGT AGA TCT GG and 5' ATG TCT TTT ACT CCT GGT AAG CAA, respectively, to amplify a 624 bp fragment. The synthesis of radio-isotopically labeled single-stranded (ss) probes by PCR, was done by incubation of the same, but linearized vectors with an RNA complementary primer, resulting in a linear rather than exponential amplification without any plasmid sequences. All labeled probes were separated from non-incorporated radionucleotides by spun-column chromatography, using Sephadex-G50.

Hybridization

Hybridization was done under optimized conditions (9) for 2 days at 42°C. Washing of the blots was done according to standard procedures (12) and auto-radiograms were exposed at -70°C overnight, using intensifying screens.

Sample application and processing

Serially-diluted purified virus was spotted on nitrocellulose membranes in final concentrations of 1xSSC (9), by means of a slot-blot apparatus (Schleicher and Schuell Inc.). Ten times diluted clinical specimens were directly applied to the membrane or after extraction with either of the following organical solvents; (phenol/chloroform (1:1), Freon (1,1,2 trichloro-1,2,2,-trifluorethane), carbon tetrachloride or chloroform).

Viral RNA, used for cDNA synthesis and PCR amplification (18), was isolated from clinical specimens by means of acid guanidium thiocyanate-phenol-chloroform (19).

Selective virus capture methods for detection by hybridization are discussed in the Results and Discussion section.

RESULTS AND DISCUSSION

BCV detection by nick-translated probes

Several cDNA inserts, varying in size fom 0.6 to 2.0 kb, and their corresponding vectors were labeled with radio-isotopes by nick-translation and independently used to detect serial dilutions of purified virus (one example is given in Fig. 1). Although probe inserts yielded specificities, sensitivities and detectabilities were reduced 5 to 8 times, respectively (Fig. 1). Two hours exposure of the autoradiograms to the blots showed detection signals obtained by vector probing that equalled those obtained by insert probing after a 24 h exposure time. Larger size insert-probes gave slightly better results than smaller ones. When using a pool of three non-overlapping insert-probes in the same hybridization assay, sensitivity and detectability levels still did not reach those obtained by probing with one single, radiolabeled vector. However, detectability and sensitivity was increased 14 and 6 times respectively, when using a probe-pool of 6 vectors containing non-overlapping cDNA sequences, thus hybridizing to different locations on the genome. These data demonstrate the significance for detection by hybridization of labeled plasmid fragments, attached to the cDNA-probe sequences involved in target hybridization. The formation of hyperpolymers

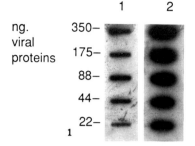

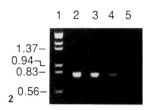

Fig. 1   Detection by hybridization of BCV with a nick-translated cDNA insert (600 bp; lane 1) or its corresponding vector (lane 2). An amount of 100 pg viral protein correspond to about 1.1×10^5 virus particles and about 1.1 pg genomic RNA.

Fig. 2   Agarose-gel electrophoresis of BCV-specific fragments, amplified by PCR, using isolated genomic RNA as template. Amounts of RNA-molecules used in the amplification systems were 10^3 (lane 2), 10^2 (lane 3), 10 (lane 4) and 1 molecule, respectively. One tenth of the PCR reaction volume was analyzed. Lane 1, DNA markers.

by vector sequences on the target sites likely plays a role in detection signal amplification. It was already established in previous studies (9) that pUC-9 sequences did not cause background signals, thus ensuring the specificity of the signals obtained.

Random-primed probes

Probes, labeled by random priming showed superior sensitivities and at least 7 times increased detectabilities than corresponding nick-translated probes, but at the same time, background signals were similarly increased, resulting in a more difficult determination of the detection-limit.

Background signals, likely due to non-specific probe trapping, and strongly amplified detection signals of spotted plasmid DNA, might lead to misinterpretation and an increased score of false-positive identifications, when probing clinical specimens, although this was not further investigated.

Biotinylated probes

Biotinylated probes (16) were shown to be superior for detection of BCV-RNA, isolated from purified virions (9). About 3×10^3 particles could be detected using amplification systems (9). However, probing of clinical specimens with these probes resulted in strong background hybridization signals, thus increasing the score of false-positive identifications significantly.

Incubation of blots, on which fecal specimens were spotted, with biotin-analogs alone, was already sufficient to reveal strong detection-signals, indicating the uselessness of these probes, when samples were spotted directly onto nitrocellulose membranes without previous RNA extractions.

Probes synthesized by PCR

Double-stranded probes, synthesized in an exponential amplification system

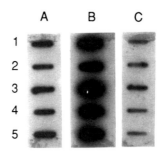

Fig. 3. Detection of BCV in 5 clinical specimens (nrs 1-5) with a probe-pool, consisting of 6 radiolabeled vectors (lane A) or with a PCR-synthesized single-stranded probe (lane B).
Detection signals of the PCR amplified products synthesized on viral RNA, isolated from the clinical specimens, are shown in lane C.

$((1+a)^n$; a=efficiency of PCR, n=number of cycles), gave 2 to 3 times increased sensitivities and at least 15 times higher detectabilities. However, background signals were very high, even after only 8 h exposure time. An exposure time of two hours did not result in background development and in this case detectabilities equalled those obtained by nick-translated probes, after a 24 h exposure period.

PCR, performed on the same, but linearized vector template, and in the presence of only the RNA complementary primer, resulting in a linear amplification $(n(1+a))$ of radio-isotopically-labeled single stranded probes, resulted in strongly improved sensitivities and detectabilities. These probes were directly added to the prehybridization solution, without any previous denaturation. No background signals were seen even after overnight exposure of the autoradiograms.

Determination of the detection limit after amplification by PCR

Isolated viral RNA was serially diluted in DCEP treated water.
Four dilutions, approximately containing 1 to 10^3 genomic-RNA molecules respectively, were processed for cDNA synthesis and PCR amplification of an 810 bp fragment, representing the translational reading frame of E1 and a part of the N-gene. cDNA synthesis was done by use of the RNA-complement primer (5' GAA CAT TTC TAG ATT GGT CGG ACT G) annealing at position 925 to 901 (13), followed by PCR after the addition of the upstream RNA-sense primer (5' ATG AGT AGT GTA ACT ACA CCA GCA) from position 115 to 138.

About 10 RNA genomes could be detected after agarose-gel electrophoresis of the amplified products (Fig. 2). The PCR products, except the one obtained from the highest dilution, could also be detected by hybridization with a nick-translated probe. Isolated RNA, resuspended in DCEP treated water and stored for several month at -20°C, was still usable for amplification purposes.

Application of molecular probes for BCV-detection in clinical specimens

Detection by hybridization of BCV in clinical specimens required several adaptations. Addition of purified virus to different BCV-negative clinical specimens, diluted 1:10 in TBS, resulted in strong variation of detection signals due to competition for binding sites on the membrane between the virus and other extraneous molecules. Several approaches were envisaged to either selectively capture the virus from specimens, or to eliminate macromolecules by extraction with organic solvents. Virus capture, by incubation of samples with rat red blood cells (7) or by protein-A immunobeads, coated with polyclonal or monoclonal antibodies, was feasible but the amounts of virus captured or released were relatively poor for detection by hybridization. Similarly, captures were assayed by incubation of samples on immunoblots (i.e. blots coated with different dilutions of polyclonal or monoclonal antisera or with $(NH_4)_2SO_4$ concentrated immuno-globulins).

Although immunoblot-captures were better than the other methods described above, simpler extractions of the samples with organic solvents were superior with respect to the detection signals obtained. Among the organic solvents tested, Freon appeared to be the most adequate concerning macro-molecule elimination and nucleocapsid preservation. BCV detection in Freon extracted samples with a probe-pool of 6 vectors, containing non-overlapping sequences, resulted in an increased sensitivity and test accuracy of 17% and 15 % respectively, compared to data obtained by indirect ELISA. The use of PCR synthesized probes, either single or double stranded, for detection of the virus in clinical specimens also significantly improved the sensitivity and detectability, when compared to corresponding nick-translated probes. The detection signals obtained by probing 5 BCV-positive clinical specimens with the pool of vector probes (Fig. 3, lane A) and the hybridization signals, revealed after probing with a single-stranded probe, synthesized by PCR (Fig. 3, lane B) are shown in Fig. 3. Incubation of blots, on which clinical samples were spotted, with nick-translated radiolabeled pUC-19 sequences did not cause background hybridization.

Detection by hybridization of PCR-amplified products, synthesized on genomic-RNA templates,isolated from clinical specimens

Viral-RNA was isolated from five clinical specimens that were identified previously as positive. PCR was performed during 30 cycles using primers, described as above. Analysis by agarose-gel electrophoresis was not sufficient to visualize the amplified products. Detection by hybridization with a nick-translated probe, however, showed that amplification had occured in all the samples analysed (Fig. 3, lane C). RNA, isolated from the specimens and which was 50 times more concentrated than the fraction used in the PCR amplification, was not detected. Although the probe used for detection was viral specific, radiolabeling of the amplified fragment(s) followed by size analysis would reveal the specificity of amplification. Studies are currently underway for application of PCR as a sensitive tool for clinical diagnosis of BCV.

Acknowledgements

P. Tijssen acknowledges the financial support for this project from CORPAQ. A. Verbeek acknowledges support from WUSC.

These studies will be submitted as a part of a PhD thesis.

References

1. Barnett, B.B., R.S. Splendlove, M.W. Peterson, L. Y. Hsu, V.A. La Salle, and L.N. Egbert. 1975. Immunofluorescent cell assay of neonatal calf diarrhea virus. Can. J. Comp. Med. 39:462-465.

2. Crouch, C.F., T.J.G. Raybould, and S.D. Acres. 1984. Monoclonal antibody capture enzyme-linked immunosorbent assay for detection of bovine enteric coronavirus. J. Clin. Microbiol. 19:388-393.

3. El-Ghorr, A.A., D.R. Snodgrass, and F.M.M. Scott. 1988. Evaluation of an immunogold electron microscopy technique for detecting bovine coronavirus. J. Virol. Meth. 19:215-224.

4. Flewett, T.H. 1978. Electron microscopy in the diagnosis of infectious diarrhea. J. Am. Vet. Med. Ass. 173:538-543.

5. Reynolds, D.J., D. Chasey, A.C. Scott, and J.C. Bridger. 1984. Evaluation of ELISA and electron microscopy for the detection of coronavirus and rotavirus in bovine faeces. Vet. Rec. 114:397-401.

6. Sato, K., Y. Inaba, S. Tokuhisa, Y. Miura, N. Kanedo, M. Asagy, and M. Matumoto. 1984. Detection of bovine coronavirus in feces by reversed passive hemagglutination. Arch. Virol. 80:23-31.

7. Van Balken, J.A.M., P.W. de Leeuw, D.J. Ellens, and P.J. Straver, 1978/79. Detection of coronavirus in calf faeces with haemadsorption-elution-haemagglutinating assay (HEHA). Vet. Microbiol. 3:205-211.

8. Shockley, L.J., P.A. Kapke, W. Lapps., D.A. Brian, L.N.D. Potgieter, and R. Woods. 1987. Diagnosis of porcine and bovine enteric coronavirus infections using cloned cDNA probes. J. Clin. Microbiol. 25:1591-1596.

9. Verbeek, A., and P. Tijssen. 1988. Biotinylated and radioactive cDNA probes in the detection by hybridization of bovine enteric coronavirus. Mol. and Cell. Probes 2:209-223.

10. Laporte, J.P., P. Bobulesco, and F. Rossi. 1980. Une lignée cellulaire particulièrement sensible à la réplication du coronavirus entérique bovin: Les cellules HRT 18. Comptes Rendus Acad. Sc. (Paris). 290:623-626.

11. Dea, S., R. Roy, and M.E. Begin. 1980. Physicochemical and biological properties of neonatal calf diarrhea coronaviruses isolated in Quebec and comparison with the Nebraska calf corona virus. Am. J. Vet. Res. 41:23-29.

12. Maniatis, T., E.F. Fritsch, and J. Sambrook. 1982. Molecular cloning: a Laboratory Manual: Cold Spring Harbor, New York: Cold Spring Harbor Laboratory.

13. Lapps W., B.G. Hogue, and D.A. Brian. 1987. Sequence analysis of bovine coronavirus nucleocapsid and matrix protein. Virol. 157:47-57.

14. Rigby, P.W.J., M. Dieckmann, C. Rhodes, and P. Berg. 1977. Labeling deoxyribonucleic acid to high specific activity in vitro by nick translation with DNA polymerase I. J. Mol. Biol. 113:237-251.

15. Feinberg, A.P., and B. Vogelstein. 1983. A technique for radiolabeling DNA restriction endonuclease fragments to high specific activity. Anal. Biochem. 132:6-13.

16. Leary, J.J., D.J. Brigati, and D.C. Ward. 1983. Rapid and sensitive colorometric method for visualizing biotin-labeled DNA probes hybridized to DNA or RNA immobilized on nitrocellulose: bioblots. Proc. Natl. Acad. Sci., USA 80:4045-4049.

17. Schowalter, D.B., and S.S. Sommer. 1989. The generation of DNA and RNA probes with polymerase chain reaction. Anal. Biochem. 177:90-94.

18. Saiki, R.U., D.N. Gelfand, S. Stoffel, S.J. Scharf, R. Higuchi, G.T. Horn, M.B. Mullis, and H.A. Erlich. 1988. Primer-directed enzymatic amplification of DNA with a thermostable DNA polymerase Science 239:487-491

19. Chomczynski, P., and N. Sacchi. 1987. Single step method of RNA isolation by acid guanidium thiocyanate-phenol-chloroform extraction. Anal. Biochem. 162:156-159.

Chapter 11

Non-Neurological Diseases

CANINE CORONAVIRUS INFECTION IN CATS; A POSSIBLE ROLE IN FELINE

INFECTIOUS PERITONITIS

F. McArdle*, M. Bennett*†, R.M. Gaskell*, B. Tennant*,
D.F. Kelly* and C.J.Gaskell†

Departments of Veterinary Pathology* and Veterinary
Clinical Science†, University of Liverpool
'Leahurst', Neston, Wirral, L64 7TE, U.K.

INTRODUCTION

Feline infectious peritonitis virus (FIPV) and canine
coronavirus (CCV) are serologically closely related viruses with
at least some genome sequence homology (Pedersen et al, 1978;
Horzinek et al, 1982; Shockley et al, 1987). They are
distinguished mainly by their host species of origin, and there
are also some accounts of minor or one-way serological
differences between the two groups (e.g. Pedersen et al, 1978).
However some strains, at least, of CCV can infect cats
(Barlough et al, 1984; Stoddart et al, 1988) and it is not known
how consistent the serological differences are when applied to a
large number of canine and feline isolates.

Antibody to FIPV, whether actively or passively acquired,
is known to enhance the development of disease in most cats upon
subsequent FIPV infection (Pedersen and Boyle, 1980; Weiss and
Scott, 1981). However, enhancement of FIP by previous infection
with CCV has not been found (Barlough et al, 1984; Stoddart et
al, 1988). In this paper we describe some preliminary
experiments in which previous exposure to two strains of CCV
appeared to cause enhancement of FIP, and, furthermore,
sequential systemic inoculation of two cats with a further
strain of CCV caused FIP without exposure to FIPV.

MATERIALS AND METHODS

The CCV isolates used in this study were CCV-171, the
original American strain (Binn et al, 1974) with unknown passage
history, CCV-C54 and CCV-INSAVC-1, geographically distinct UK
strains at sixth and fifth passage respectively, and CCV-INSAVC-

1/c, a ninth passage clone of CCV-INSAVC-1. The feline isolate used was FIPV-CVR1036, originally isolated from the faeces of an adult British cat with acute diarrhoea and kindly supplied by Dr DA Harbour, University of Bristol. Except where stated, CCV isolates were grown in A-72 (canine) cells (Binn et al, 1980) and FIPV isolates in FEA (feline) cells (Jarrett et al, 1973). Virus neutralisation (VN) tests were as described by Stoddart et al (1988b).

The overall design of the experiments is shown in Table 1. Briefly, eight six-months-old, specific pathogen free cats, with no detectable antibody to CCV and FIPV, were divided into four groups of two (A, B, C and D) and housed in separate, barrier maintained rooms within an isolation unit. Groups A to C were inoculated orally with $10^{6.8}$ TCID$_{50}$ CCV-171, CCV-C54 or $10^{7.3}$ CCV-INSAVC-1/c respectively, and group D inoculated orally with uninfected A-72 cells and media as controls. After 26 days, cats in groups A-C were again inoculated orally with homologous virus in an attempt to increase serum VN antibody.

On day 57, cats in groups A, B and D were inoculated orally with 10^6 TCID$_{50}$ FIPV-CVR1036. As the cats in group C still had not developed antibody to CCV, they were inoculated with 10^7 TCID$_{50}$ CCV-INSAVC-1/c, this time intramuscularly and intraperitoneally, and intramuscularly again on day 78. All the cats were examined for clinical signs, and samples were taken regularly for attempted virus isolation and VN antibody assays.

Table 1

Summary of experimental design; Cats were inoculated orally with CCV or FIPV on the days indicated, except * indicates intramuscular and † indicates intraperitoneal inoculation.

Group of cats	Days into experiment			
	0	26	57	78
A	CCV-171	CCV-171	FIPV-CVR1036	–
B	CCV-C54	CCV-C54	FIPV-CVR1036	–
C	CCV-INSAVC -1/c	CCV-INSAVC -1/c	CCV-INSAVC -1/c*†	CCV-INSAVC -1/c*
D	cells/media	–	FIPV-CVR1036	–

RESULTS

Following the first inoculation with CCV, no clinical signs were observed in any cats apart from mild diarrhoea in cats in group B (C54 virus) at 4-12 days post-inoculation (dpi). Virus was isolated sporadically between 4-20 dpi from oropharyngeal

476

and rectal swabs of all cats, except one cat in group A and the uninfected cats in group D. Homologous VN antibody titres at 21 dpi were 64 in groups A and B, and <2 in groups C and D. Further oral inoculation with CCV on day 21 was not associated with any clinical signs. On day 57, cats in groups A and B had VN titres to homologous viruses of 128, but cats in groups C and D did not have antibody to any CCV strain.

After oral inoculation with FIPV on day 57, cats in groups A and B rapidly developed severe disease, and by 5-7 days after challenge serum VN titres had reached a mean of 1024. Virus was isolated four days after challenge from oropharyngeal swabs from cats in group B only. Clinical signs such as inappetence, neurological signs and jaundice became apparent on days 6-12, and cats were killed as soon as they became ill. Cats in groups A and B had minimal gross lesions at necropsy, but histological lesions consistent with FIP. In contrast, cats in group D, which had not been previously exposed to CCV, remained healthy for much longer. One cat in group D developed 'wet' FIP at 30 days post-challenge; 100mls of abdominal fluid were collected at necropsy and microscopic examination revealed typical granulomatous lesions in the serosa. The other cat in group D did not become ill, apart from mild pyrexia at 12-18 days post-challenge, but microscopic focal lymphocytic accumulations were found in the mesentery and peritoneum at necropsy 94 days post-challenge. Virus was isolated post-mortem from one cat in each of groups A, B and D. Virus was isolated on FEA cells mostly from the gut, but also occasionally from other tissues including lung, spleen and peritoneum.

No clinical signs were observed in the cats in group C but by 35 days after the first intramuscular and intraperitoneal inoculations the cats had mean serum VN antibody titres to CCV-INSAVC-1/c of 768. Both cats were killed, and gross lesions of 'wet' FIP were found in both at necropsy. Twenty and 75 mls abdominal fluid were collected from each cat, and both cats had a fibrinous serositis. Microscopic examination confirmed an exudative serositis typical of 'wet' FIP. Virus was isolated from both cats mainly from the gut and tonsils. Virus was isolated on A-72 cells, but not high passage FEA cells.

Aliquots of the viruses used to inoculate cats and samples of viruses isolated from the cats post-mortem were compared in VN assays using cat antisera to FIPV-CVR1036 and CCV-171 and dog antisera to CCV-INSAVC-1. The two CCV antisera did not distinguish between any of the viruses. However, the FIPV antiserum had a significantly higher titre against FIPV and viruses isolated from cats in groups A, B and D than against CCV-INSAVC-1/c and virus isolated from cats in group C.

DISCUSSION

Infection of cats with CCV isolates has been demonstrated previously (Barlough et al 1984, Stoddart et al 1988), although we do not know of any previous report of diarrhoea in cats associated with CCV infection. There is some evidence of natural dog-to-cat transmission of CCV via contaminated faeces (Dr W Baxendale, personal communication). Thus it is possible that dogs may be a source of coronavirus infection to cats in the field, and some cases of symptomatic feline enteric coronavirus (FECV) infection may, in reality, be due to CCV infection.

Furthermore, although only preliminary in nature, these studies show that infection with at least some strains of CCV can predispose cats to enhanced development of FIP upon subsequent exposure to FIPV. These findings contrast with those of Barlough et al (1984) and Stoddart et al (1988), who found that previous infection with one strain of CCV did not predispose cats to enhanced FIP. This may be because of differences in the strains of CCV and FIPV used in the various studies, or due to differences in route of virus inoculation.

It is interesting that the FIPV strain used in these experiments was originally isolated from a cat with enteritis, and might therefore have been described as a feline enteric coronavirus (FECV). That one cat without CCV antibody developed clinical 'wet' FIP after inoculation with FIPV-CVR1036 and the other had only mild FIP-like lesions post-mortem, might suggest that FIPV-CVR1036 is of relatively low pathogenicity. However, it is well-known that some cats can be resistant to some FIPV strains (Pedersen and Floyd, 1985), and age may also play a role in susceptibility to disease.

CCV-INSAVC-1/c did not appear to be infectious to kittens by oral inoculation, but two intraperitoneal and intramuscular inoculations did produce 'wet' FIP in both cats. That the lesions in these cats were due to infection with CCV-INSAVC-1/c and not contamination with FIPV is borne out by the ability of the virus isolated from the cats in group C to grow on A-72 cells only, and by VN assays using FIPV-CVR1036 antisera.

To ascertain whether some CCV strains can cause FIP in cats following oral inoculation will require further research. However, we believe that these studies, albeit involving only small numbers of animals, suggest a closer relationship between FIPV and CCV than is generally assumed and have considerable epidemiological implications. Further studies, probably involving sequencing of several canine and feline coronavirus isolates, are required in order to to better understand the taxonomic relationship of FIPV and CCV. Further work is required to discover how frequently coronaviruses are transmitted from dogs to cats in the field. The ability of CCV to infect cats obviously may have a bearing on the use of serology to diagnose FIPV infection, on measures for controlling FIP in cat colonies and may also affect the use of live CCV vaccines in dogs.

REFERENCES

Barlough, JE., Stoddart, CA., Sorresso, GP., Jacobson, RH & Scott, FW. (1984) Experimental inoculation of cats with canine coronavirus and subsequent challenge with feline infectious peritonitis virus. Laboratory Animal Science 34: 592-597.

Binn, LN., Lazar, EC., Keenan, KP., Huxsoll, DL., Marchwicki, RH. and Strano, AJ. (1974) Recovery and characterisation of a coronavirus from military dogs with diarrhoea. Proceedings of the Annual Meeting of the U.S. Animal Health Association, 78: 359-366.

Binn, LN., Marchwicki, RH. and Stephenson EH (1980) Establishment of a canine cell line: Derivation, characterisation and viral spectrum. American Journal of Veterinary Research 41: 855-860.

Horzinek, MC., Lutz, H. and Pedersen, N. (1982) Antigenic relationships among homologous structural polypeptides of porcine, feline and canine coronaviruses. Infection and Immunity 37: 1148-1155.

Jarrett, O., Laird, HM. and Hay, D. (1973) Determinants of the host range of feline leukaemia viruses. Journal of General Virology 20: 169-175.

Pedersen, NC. and Floyd, K. (1985) Experimental studies with three new strains of feline infectious peritonitis virus: FIPV-UCD2, FIPV-UCD3 and FIPV-UCD4. Compendium on Continuing Education 7: 1001-1011.

Pedersen, NC., Ward, J. and Mengeling, WL. (1978) Antigenic relationship of feline infectious peritonitis virus to coronaviruses of other species. Archives of Virology 58: 45-53.

Shockley, LJ., Kapke, PA., Lapps, W., Brian, DA., Potgeiter, LND. and Wodds, R. (1987) Diagnosis of porcine and bovine enteric coronavirus infections using cloned cDNA probes. Journal of Clinical Microbiology 25: 1591-1596.

Stoddart, CA,. Barlough, JE., Baldwin, CA. and Scott, FW. (1988) Attempted immunisation of cats against feline infectious peritonitis using canine coronavirus. Research in Veterinary Science 45: 383-388.

Stoddart, ME., Gaskell, RM., Harbour, DA. and Gaskell, CJ. (1988b) Virus shedding and immune responses in cats inoculated with cell-culture-adapted feline infectious peritonitis virus. Veterinary Microbiology 16: 145-158.

CHARACTERIZATION OF AN ATTENUATED TEMPERATURE SENSITIVE FELINE INFECTIOUS

PERITONITIS VACCINE VIRUS

J.D. Gerber, N.E. Pfeiffer, J.D. Ingersoll, K.K. Christianson,
R.M. Landon, N.L. Selzer, and W.H. Beckenhauer

Biological Research and Development
Norden Laboratories, Inc.
Lincoln, NE USA 68501-0809

INTRODUCTION

Feline infectious peritonitis (FIP) is a complex and fatal disease of cats caused by infection with feline infectious peritonitis virus (FIPV). The FIPV is a coronavirus related to transmissible gastroenteritis virus of pigs, enteric coronavirus of dogs, and respiratory coronavirus of man. There is also a feline enteric coronavirus (FECV) that replicates mainly in the intestine and causes only a mild diarrheal disease.[1]

Primary FIP may be mild consisting of a febrile response and a slight nasal and ocular discharge. Secondary FIP may develop following the primary infection and appears in two forms. The exudative or wet form is characterized by peritonitis and pleuritis with ascites and pleural effusion. The dry form is characterized by granulomatous inflammation of different organs and no or little exudate. Both forms may appear together. The pathogenesis of FIP is complicated and not fully understood. Evidence suggests that FIP is an immune-mediated disease.[1] The virus replicates initially in the upper respiratory tract and small intestine.[2] The primary target of FIPV is the macrophage which may cross the mucosal barrier and spread the virus systemically.[3,4,5] A correlation has been observed between FIPV virulence in vivo and the ability to infect macrophages in vitro.[6] It has been suggested that a strong cell-mediated immune (CMI) response to FIPV is important to protect cats against this disease.[7,8] However, the local immune responses in the upper respiratory tract and intestinal tract have not been carefully evaluated and may represent an important immune defense system against FIPV.

An effective FIP vaccine should stimulate a strong mucosal immune response to stop systemic spread of the virus and a CMI response that would immediately halt the systemic spread of FIPV if the virus did cross the mucosa. To stimulate a mucosal immune response a temperature sensitive (ts) FIPV vaccine to be administered intranasally (IN) was developed. The ts-FIP vaccine virus was developed by first serial passaging the wild type (wt) DF2 strain of FIPV to give a high passage attenuated (hpa) FIPV. The hpa-FIPV was made temperature sensitive by ultraviolet irradiation. The virus will propagate at 31°C, its permissive temperature, but not at 39°C, its non-permissive temperature. Attenuation and temperature sensitivity were accompanied by the appearance of characteristics that

Coronaviruses and Their Diseases
Edited by D. Cavanagh and T.D.K. Brown
Plenum Press, New York, 1990

distinguish ts-FIPV from its virulent parent strain. The purpose of this report is to present these distinguishing characteristics and show how intranasal (IN) administration of this vaccine virus protects cats against FIPV infection and subsequent FIPV mediated immune pathology.

RESULTS AND DISCUSSION

Plaque Characterization

Morphological as well as temperature sensitive differences were found between wt-FIPV, hpa-FIPV, and ts-FIPV. Wild type-FIPV had large distinct plaques at 39°C ranging in size from 1.0 to 2.2 mm but no plaques at 31°C. Temperature sensitive-FIPV had smaller plaques at 31°C ranging in size from 0.5 to 1.0 mm but no plaquing was observed at 39°C. High passage attenuated-FIPV showed plaques at both temperatures ranging in size from 0.2 to 0.8 mm at 31°C and from 0.3 to 1.2 mm at 39°C.

Larger plaques may be associated with virulence. Tupper et al.[9] reported that two virulent FIPV strains (79-1146 and NOR 15, a plaque purified DF2 wt-FIPV) produced larger plaques than the nonvirulent FECV strain 79-1683. McKeirnan and co-workers[10] also documented this difference in plaquing profiles between these same feline coronavirus strains.

Thermolability of wt-FIPV and ts-FIPV

Thermolability studies were done to determine if differences existed in the thermolability of ts-FIPV and wt-FIPV. The ts-FIPV was more sensitive to high temperature. ts-FIPV was rapidly inactivated at 54°C.[11] ts-FIPV titers decreased by five logs in 15 minutes whereas the titer of the more stable wt-FIPV decreased by only two logs.

Virus Growth and RNA Synthesis

Virus growth and synthesis of RNA, as measured by 3H-uridine incorporation, was compared at permissive and nonpermissive temperatures. ts-FIP viral RNA synthesis at 31°C and 39°C was similar 12 hours after infection indicating viral entry and viral RNA synthesis had started at the nonpermissive temperature. However, there was a difference in virus titer by 12 hours. Temperature sensitive-FIPV grown at the permissive temperature had a virus titer of $10^{5.00}$ $TCID_{50}$/ml and 3H-uridine incorporation of 98,920 cpm. When ts-FIPV was grown at the non-permissive temperature, and subsequently titered at 31°C, the virus titer was only $10^{3.33}$ $TCID_{50}$/ml while the 3H-uridine incorporation was still 95,913 cpm. At the nonpermissive temperature, it appears that early viral RNA synthesis occurred without a concomitant virus maturation process. The absence of intact virion production in the presence of RNA synthesis at 39°C suggests a defect in the maturation and assembly of the virion which has been shown in other temperature sensitive viruses.[12,13,14]

Western Blot Analysis of ts-FIPV, hpa-FIPV, and wt-FIPV Structural Proteins

The structural proteins of ts-FIPV, hpa-FIPV, and wt-FIPV were compared by Western blot using coronavirus specific monoclonal antibodies. The structural protein profiles were characteristic of that reported for other coronaviruses.[15] All viruses showed similarities in peplomer (200 kd) and nucleocapsid (63 kd) proteins but there were differences in the envelope protein (Fig. 1). The wt-FIPV envelope protein consisted of a 30 kd and a 28 kd component. High passage attenuated FIPV and ts-FIPV had the 28 kD and 30 kd components and additional higher molecular weight components (46 kd, 42 kd, 38 kd, 34 kd) that were not identified in wt-FIPV. The 28 kd component in wt-FIPV appeared more intense than in either the ts-FIPV or the hpa-FIPV. Differences in the molecular weights of envelope polypeptides were also observed between two virulent strains of FIPV; UCD1 did not have the low molecular weight component that was present in the Dahlberg strain of FIPV.[16] These observed differences in the envelope protein may be due to differences in glycosylation. Further investigation by two-dimensional gels is needed to clearly differentiate the envelope proteins of ts-FIPV and wt-FIPV.

The culture supernatant from ts-FIPV infected cells was examined for the appearance of structural proteins at both the permissive and nonpermissive temperatures. All three structural proteins were detected in the culture supernatant of ts-FIPV grown at 31°C for 24, 48, 72, or 96 hours.[11] Only nucleocapsid was found when ts-FIPV was grown at 39°C for the same period of time. Nucleocapsid may be the only protein released at 39°C or the peplomer and envelope proteins were not present at detectable levels. The nucleocapsid protein released at 39°C is associated with infectious RNA or a few viral particles were released a 39°C because these culture supernatants were infective at 31°C. However, at 24 hours the infectivity of the supernatant fluids from 39°C was almost three logs less than the supernatant fluids from 31°C. No detectable virus titer was found when assayed at 39°C.

Immunofluorescent Antibody (IFA) Analysis of Intracellular and Surface Structural Proteins

Intracellular synthesis of ts-FIPV, hpa-FIPV, and wt-FIPV was examined by IFA using coronavirus specific monoclonal antibodies on acetone-fixed, infected cells. All three structural proteins of the ts-FIPV were detected in the cells at both the permissive and non-permissive temperatures (Table 1). The ts-FIPV proteins appeared at both temperatures within 6 hours postinfection. Similar results were obtained at 39°C with the wt-FIPV. However, at 31°C, wt-FIPV structural proteins appeared somewhat later. Nucleocapsid was detected at 8 hours while peplomer and

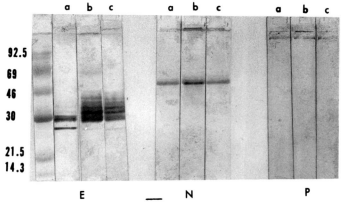

Figure 1. Western blot comparison of envelope (E), nucleocapsid (N), and peplomer (P) of wt-FIPV (a), hpa-FIPV (b), and ts-FIPV (c). Molecular weight markers are at the left.

Table 1. Immunofluorescent Antibody Analysis of Intracellular and
Surface Structural Proteins

Location	Structural Protein	ts-FIPV		hpa-FIPV		wt-FIPV	
		31°C	39°C	31°C	39°C	31°C	39°C
Intracellular	Peplomer	++[1]	++	++	++	+	++
	Nucleocapsid	++	++	++	++	+	++
	Envelope	++	++	++	++	+	++
Surface	Peplomer	++	−	++	++	+	+++
	Nucleocapsid	−	−	−	−	−	−
	Envelope	+	−	+	++	+	++

[1]Intensity of immunofluorescence.

envelope proteins were apparent at 9 hours. All three structural proteins
of hpa-FIPV were present at both temperatures.

Surface immunofluorescence of infected cells was examined using non-
fixed cells. Peplomer and envelope proteins were observed on the cell
surface of ts-FIPV infected cells at 31°C, but not at 39°C. Peplomer was
present by 12 hours post-infection and small areas of envelope surface
fluorescence were observed by 18 hours. Nucleocapsid was not detected at
either temperature. Wild type-FIPV peplomer and envelope surface immunofluorescence was observed after 12 hours at 39°C. At 31°C only weak peplomer surface fluorescence was detected after 15 hours. Again, nucleocapsid was not detected at either temperature. High passage attenuated-
FIPV peplomer and envelope, but not nucleocapsid surface immunofluorescence, was observed at both temperatures. Surface expression of ts-FIPV
and wt-FIPV peplomer and envelope proteins but not nucleocapsid at the
permissive temperature for each virus resembles that observed in FIPV
infected macrophage-like cells.[3] Thus initial synthesis of ts-FIPV
viral proteins appeared normal at the non-permissive temperature, as detected by IFA of acetone-fixed cells. However, the lack of surface immunofluorescence at 39°C indicates a breakdown in the normal maturation
process. In vivo, the expression of viral antigen on the cell surface
may be necessary for the pathogenesis of FIPV. The absence of ts-FIPV
structural proteins at 39°C may account for the lack of hypersensitivity
to FIPV infection in ts-FIPV vaccinated cats.

In-Vivo Fate of the Virus

To determine if the temperature sensitive characteristics of the ts-
FIPV observed in vitro were the same as growth of the virus in vivo, cats
were inoculated with either ts-FIPV or wt-FIPV. At predetermined times
postinoculation, cats were sacrificed and tissues were examined for the
presence of virus. Evidence to suggest that ts-FIPV replication was
limited to the upper respiratory tract was found by virus isolation and
immunofluorescence (Table 2). Temperature sensitive-FIPV was isolated
from the cervical lymph node, tonsil, trachea, and turbinate at 1, 2, or
4 days postvaccination. Temperature sensitive-FIPV antigen was also
identified by direct IFA in the mandibular lymph node and the tonsil. In
contrast, wt-FIPV had disseminated throughout the cat 4 days after oral
infection. Wild type-FIPV was isolated from four different lymph nodes
(cervical, mandibular, mediastinal, and mesenteric), the oral/nasal/
pharyngeal area, as well as from the thymus and spleen. All of these
tissues except the thymus were positive for viral antigen by direct IFA.

Table 2. Virus Isolation (VI) from Tissue Homogenates of Cats Vaccinated IN with ts-FIPV or Inoculated Orally with wt-FIPV. Also Shown is the Detection of FIPV Antigen in Tissues by Direct IFA.

Tissue	ts-FIPV VI	ts-FIPV IFA	wt-FIPV VI	wt-FIPV IFA
Kidney	−	−	−	−
Liver	−	−	−	−
Mediastinal Lymph Node	−	−	+	ND
Mesenteric Lymph Node	−	−	+	+
Pharynx	−	−	+	ND
Salivary Gland	−	−	−	+
Spleen	−	−	+	+
Cervical Lymph Node	+	−	+	+
Mandibular Lymph Node	−	+	+	+
Thymus	−	−	+	−
Tonsil	+	+	+	+
Trachea	+	−	+	+
Turbinate	+	−	+	+

ND = Not Done.

The ability of the ts-FIPV to replicate at its permissive temperature (31°C) allows it to grow in the cooler upper respiratory tract of cats. Replication of ts-FIPV in the upper respiratory tract may stimulate mucosal and cell mediated immune (CMI) responses that may be required to protect cats against FIPV challenge. Mucosal immunity, stimulated by intranasal administration of ts-FIPV may be important in stopping the primary infection of FIPV since Stoddart et al.[2] has shown that FIPV administered orally replicated initially in the tonsil and small intestine. The temperature preference of ts-FIPV may prevent vaccine-induced hypersensitization of the cat. Pedersen and Black (17) reported that vaccination with a modified-live FIPV not only failed to protect cats against disease, but made the cats more susceptible to FIPV challenge. Since ts-FIPV structural proteins are not present on the surface of infected cells at 39°C, the body temperature of the cat, and ts-FIP vaccine virus is not detected in tissues outside of the oral/pharyngeal area, ts-FIPV vaccine induced hypersensitivity would most likely not occur.

Immune Response and Results of Challenge of Vaccinated and Nonvaccinated Cats

Specific pathogen free cats, negative for anti-coronavirus antibodies, were used in vaccination and challenge studies. A scoring system that included symptoms associated with FIP was devised to judge the extent of disease (Table 3). This scoring system included the following symptoms: 1) eosinopenia; 2) lymphopenia; 3) leukopenia; 4) Doehle bodies; 5) icterus; 6) vacuolated neutrophils; 7) decreased packed cell volume; 8) febrile response; and 9) death. The total clinical score of each cat was an accumulation of scores of 4 to 6 observations of blood clinical symptoms, febrile responses monitored for 11 to 19 days and of deaths through 8 weeks postchallenge.

Cats that were vaccinated twice intranasally, three weeks apart, with the ts-FIPV vaccine developed antibody and CMI responses to wt-FIPV.[18] Serum IgG and IgA and local IgA responses were shown by an ELISA. Virus

485

neutralizing antibody was also detected. A CMI response was demonstrated by a lymphocyte blastogenesis response to wt-FIPV following vaccination and challenge. The vaccinated cats were protected against two oral challenges of virulent wt-FIPV. Seventeen of 20 vaccinated cats (85%) survived a rigorous wt-FIPV challenge that caused FIP in 12 of 12 control cats (100%), 10 of which died within 8 weeks of challenge (Figure 2). Vaccinated cats were challenged a second time to determine if the first exposure to wt-FIPV would make the cats more susceptible to subsequent FIPV exposure. This was clearly not the case. Sixteen of the 17 vaccinated cats (94%) that survived the first challenge survived the second challenge. In contrast, 4 of 6 naive control cats (67%) developed FIP and died. Cats vaccinated IN with the hpa-FIPV also acquired protection against virulent FIPV challenge. However, reduction of clinical symptoms was not as great as obtained with the ts-FIPV vaccine (results not shown).

Interestingly, the VN titers of vaccinated cats were much lower than the titers of nonvaccinated cats following challenge (Figure 3). High concentrations of virus neutralizing antibody, presumably to peplomer epitopes, may play a significant role in the pathogenesis of FIP. Indeed, Vennema et al.[19] reported that cats vaccinated with a recombinant peplomer vaccine developed FIP and died sooner than nonvaccinated control cats.

Table 3. Scoring of Clinical Symptoms of FIPV.

Symptom	Point Value[1]
Eosinopenia	2
Lymphopenia – <1200 (absolute count)	2
– <10% Lymphocytes (relative count)	1
Leukopenia – Decrease of $\geq$50%	1
– $\leq$6000	3
Doehle Bodies – 5-9/100 WBC's	1
– 10-24/100 WBC's	3
– $\geq$25/100 WBC's	4
Icterus – +	1
– ++	2
– +++ or ++++	4
Vacuolated Neutrophils $\geq$5	3
Decreased PCV – $\leq$25% of whole blood	3
Febrile Response – 103.1 – 103.9	1
– 104.0 – 104.9	2
$\geq$105.0	4
Death	25

[a]The higher the number the more severe the symptom.

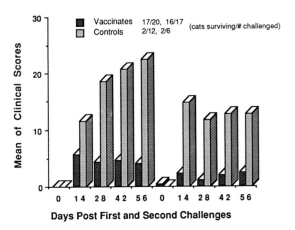

Figure 2. Mean clinical scores following wt-FIPV challenge of ts-FIPV
vaccinated and nonvaccinated cats.

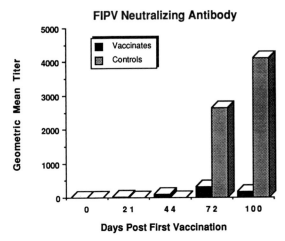

Figure 3. Geometric mean of serum VN titers of nonvaccinated cats and
cats vaccinated on day 0 and day 21. Cats were challenged with
wt-FIPV on day 44.

SUMMARY AND CONCLUSIONS

Intranasal administration of a ts-FIPV vaccine protected cats against two rigorous challenges of immunity. Investigations showed that ts-FIP viral RNA synthesis was normal at 39°C and structural proteins were synthesized, but not expressed at the cell surface. Lack of surface expression combined with decreased virus titer indicate that, although structural viral proteins were initially synthesized, they were not packaged into intact virions at the nonpermissive temperature. The ts-FIP vaccine virus was shown to replicate exclusively in the upper respiratory tract, where lower temperatures allow maturation of the virus. Viral proteins expressed on cells in the upper respiratory tract probably stimulate the development of local IgA and CMI responses and a systemic CMI response which in turn may stop the dissemination of virulent FIPV if it crosses the mucosal barrier. Investigations are ongoing to study the protective mechanism of ts-FIPV induced immunity.

ACKNOWLEDGEMENT

The authors thank Cindy Rollins for her help in preparing this manuscript.

REFERENCES

1. H. Lutz, B. Hauser, and M. C. Horzinek, Feline infectious peritonitis (FIP)--The present state of knowledge, J. Small Animal Pract. 27:108 (1986).
2. M. E. Stoddart, R. M. Gaskell, D. A. Harbour, and G. R. Pearson, The sites of early viral replication if feline infectious peritonitis, Vet. Microbiol. 18:259 (1988).
3. H. L. Jacobse-Geels and M. C. Horzinek, Expression of feline infectious peritonitis coronavirus antigens on the surface of feline macrophage-like cells, J. Gen. Virol. 64:1859 (1983).
4. R. C. Weiss and F. W. Scott, Pathogenesis of feline infectious peritonitis: nature and development of viremia, Am. J. Vet. Res. 42:382 (1981).
5. R. C. Weiss and F. W. Scott, Pathogenesis of feline infectious peritonitis: pathogenic changes and immunofluorescence, Am. J. Vet. Res. 42:2036 (1981).
6. C. A. Stoddart and F. W. Scott, Intrinsic resistance of feline peritoneal macrophages to coronavirus infection correlates with in vivo virulence, J. Virol. 63:436 (1989).
7. N. C. Pedersen and K. Floyd, Experimental studies with three new strains of feline infectious peritonitis virus: FIPV-UCD2, FIPV-UCD3, and FIPV-UCD4, Comp. Cont. Educ. Prac. Vet. 7:1001 (1985).
8. M. E. Stoddart, R. M. Gaskell, D. A. Harbour, and C. J. Gaskell, Virus shedding and immune responses in cats inoculated with cell culture-adapted feline infectious peritonitis virus, Vet. Microbiol. 16:145 (1988).
9. G. T. Tupper, J. F. Evermann, R. G. Russell, and M. E. Thouless, Antigenic and biological diversity of feline coronaviruses: feline infectious peritonitis and feline enteritis virus, Arch. Virol. 96:29 (1987).
10. A. J. McKeirnan, J. F. Evermann, E. V. Davis, and R. L. Ott, Comparative properties of feline coronaviruses in vitro, Can. J. Vet. Res. 51:212 (1987).
11. K. K. Christianson, J. D. Ingersoll, R. M. Landon, N. E. Pfeiffer, and J. D. Gerber, Characterization of a temperature sensitive feline infectious peritonitis coronavirus, submitted for publication.

12. B. W. Burge and E. R. Pfefferkorn, Isolation and characterization of conditional-lethal mutants of sindbis virus, _Virol._ 30:204 (1966).
13. P. D. Cooper, R. T. Johnson, and D. J. Garwes, Physiological characterization of heat-defective (temperature-sensitive) poliovirus mutants: preliminary classification, _Virol._ 30:638 (1966).
14. K. B. Tan, J. F. Sambrook, and A. J. D. Bellet, Semlike forest temperature-sensitive mutants: isolation and characterization, _Virol._ 38:427 (1969).
15. S. G. Siddell, H. Wege, V. ter Meulen, The biology of coronaviruses, _J. Gen. Virol._ 64:761 (1983).
16. M. C. Horzinek, J. Ederveen, H. Egberink, H. E. L. Jacobse-Geels, T. Niewold, and J. Prins, Virion polypeptide specificity of immune complexes and antibodies in cats inoculated with feline infectious peritonitis virus, _Am. J. Vet. Res._ 47:754 (1986).
17. N. C. Pedersen and J. W. Black, Attempted immunization of cats against feline infectious peritonitis, using avirulent live virus or sublethal amounts of virulent virus, _Am. J. Vet. Res._ 44:229 (1983).
18. J. D. Gerber, J. D. Ingersoll, K. K. Christianson, N. L. Selzer, R. M. Landon, N. E. Pfeiffer, and W. H. Beckenhauer, Protection against feline infectious peritonitis (FIP) by a temperature sensitive FIP-virus vaccine inoculated intranasally, Submitted for publication.
19. H. Vennema, R. deGroot, P. Harbour, M. Dahlberg, M. C. Horzinek, and W. Spaan, Early death after challenge with feline infectious peritonitis virus (FIPV) of kittens immunized with a recombinant vaccine virus expressing the FIPV spike protein. (Abstract) Modern Approaches to New Vaccines. Cold Spring Harbor Laboratory, 155 (1988).

INVESTIGATIONS INTO RESISTANCE OF CHICKEN LINES TO INFECTION WITH

INFECTIOUS BRONCHITIS VIRUS

Jane Cook, Koichi Otsuki, Michael Huggins, Nat Bumstead

IAH Institute for Animal Health, Houghton Laboratory
Houghton, Huntingdon
Cambridgeshire, PE17 2DA, United Kingdom

ABSTRACT

Although nine inbred and partially inbred lines of chickens were equally susceptible initially to infection with infectious bronchitis virus (IBV), the outcome of that infection varied considerably between the lines. A more detailed study of a line which was resistant (line C) and one which was highly susceptible (line 15I) confirmed that both lines could be infected initially with IBV but showed that the respiratory tract epithelium of line C chicks recovered more rapidly than that of line 15I chicks. Whereas more virus could be recovered from tissues of line 15I chicks following IBV inoculation, explants of tissues from each line inoculated in vitro appeared equally susceptible. The possibility of a different immunological response to IBV infection in the two lines is discussed and it is clear that further work is required to elucidate the mechanism involved in the differing susceptibility of the inbred chicken lines to inoculation with IBV.

INTRODUCTION

Infectious bronchitis (IB) has been an important disease of poultry of all ages and types worldwide since it was first described in the USA in the early 1930s[1]. It is a major pathogen of the respiratory and reproductive tracts and some strains can cause nephritis[2]. Because of its major importance, the pathogenesis and epizootiology have been widely studied yet there are few reports on the susceptibility of different breeds or lines of chicken to IBV infection and the genetics of resistance has not been studied in detail. One reason for this may have been the lack of a reliable assay to quantify the disease caused by IBV. The development of a model IBV and E.coli infection[3] facilitated such studies and has recently enabled us to investigate the inheritance of resistance[4]. One surprising outcome of this work was the observation that in certain lines of chicken, high mortality occurred following inoculation with IBV alone. This finding has enabled a study of the nature of resistance to IBV infection to be initiated.

MATERIALS AND METHODS

Chickens

Six inbred lines of White Leghorn (lines 6_1,7_2,15I,N,W1,C) and three partially inbred Houghton laboratory flocks (Brown Leghorn, Rhode Island Red, Light Sussex) were used. Their properties have been described

Coronaviruses and Their Diseases
Edited by D. Cavanagh and T.D.K. Brown
Plenum Press, New York, 1990

previously[4]. They were maintained under conditions of strict isolation and shown to be free from evidence of IB infection. They were used at between 4 and 11 days of age.

IB Viruses

Either the IBV Pool[3] or the M41 strain[5], both grown and assayed in chick embryo tracheal organ cultures (OC)[5], were used. Virus was administered intranasally (i.n.), each bird receiving $\log_{10}$ 4.0-5.0 median ciliostatic doses (CD_{50}).

Assessment of ciliary activity

Tracheas were removed carefully from groups of line C and line 15I chicks killed by intravenous injection of sodium barbitone at intervals after inoculation with IBV (M41). Ten 1-2mm thin rings were prepared from each trachea (3 from the upper and lower parts and 4 from the middle portion). They were examined by low power microscopy and ciliary activity scored on a scale from 0 (100% ciliary activity) to 4 (total ciliostasis).

Virus recovery from tissues of IBV inoculated lines C and 15I chicks

At intervals after inoculation with IBV (M41) three chicks from each line were killed as described above and trachea, lung, airsac, liver, spleen and kidney removed asceptically for attempted virus recovery[3].

In vitro susceptibility of tissues from lines C and 15I chicks to IB infection

Trachea, lung, liver and kidney were removed asceptically from three 4-day-old chicks of each line. Explants of each tissue were prepared[6] and inoculated with $\log_{10}$ 2.6 CD_{50} of IBV (M41). To minimise individual variation, 3 explants of each organ was selected from each of the 3 chicks to provide 9 replicates of each organ. The medium was harvested daily for 7 days and replaced. Fluids from like explants were pooled and assayed in OC.

Serum neutralisation tests

Blood samples were collected at intervals after inoculation of groups of 8 lines C and 15I chicks with IBV (M41) and pooled sera examined for IBV neutralising antibodies in OC[7].

RESULTS

Respiratory infection of inbred and partially inbred lines of chicken inoculated with IBV alone

Table 1. Effect of inoculating inbred and partially inbred lines of chicken intranasally with the IB Pool

Line of chicken	% of chickens with airsac lesions	% Mortality
LS	43	0
N	33	0
C	13	0
BrL	43	3
Wl	57	3
RIR	23	10
6_1	77	10
$15\dot{1}$	73	47
7_2	100	83

When groups of 30 eleven-day-old chicks from nine inbred and partially inbred lines were inoculated with the IBV Pool alone all lines initially appeared equally susceptible to infection, in that respiratory signs i.e. tracheal rales, coughing and nasal discharge were observed in all chicks for a similar time. The results presented in Table 1 show that although the incidence varied, airsac lesions were recorded in all lines. However, appreciable mortality occurred only in lines 15I and 7, indicating a considerable variation between lines in the likely outcome of an IBV infection.

This finding prompted a study of the mechanisms of resistance to IBV infection. For this study lines which were highly resistant to infection, (line C), or highly susceptible (line 15I), were selected and different parameters investigated.

Table 2. Duration of clinical signs and airsac lesions in lines C and 15I chicks following intranasal inoculation with IBV (M41)

	Duration (days) of persistence of		
	respiratory signs	Nasal exudate	Airsacculitis
Line C	2 – 7	2 – 11	7 – 14
Line 15I	2 – 14	2 – 14	7 – >21

Following inoculation with IBV (M41 strain), respiratory infection was first observed at the same time in both lines (Table 2). However, line C chicks recovered more rapidly than did line 15I chicks and, in general, the severity of clinical signs and of airsac lesions was greater in the line 15I chicks.

The degree of damage which IBV caused to the tracheal epithelium of the two lines was examined in more detail by quantifying the ciliary activity at intervals after inoculation. The results (Table 3) show that complete ciliostasis had occurred by two days post inoculation (p.i.) in line 15I chicks and by 4 days p.i. in line C. Ciliary activity was restored in line C chicks by 11 days p.i. In line 15I, only partial recovery was observed by 14 days p.i. and considerable variation was observed in the time required for regeneration of the ciliated epithelium in that line, in that at 22 days, recovery was complete in only 3 of 7 chicks examined.

Table 3. Duration of tracheal ciliostasis in lines C and 15I chicks following intranasal inoculation with IBV (M41)

	Mean ciliary activity score per chick	
Days post inoculation	Line C	Line 15I
1	0	0
2	0.4	4.0
3	3.2	4.0
4–9	4.0	4.0
11	0	4.0
14	0	3.0
17	0	2.8
22	0	0.4

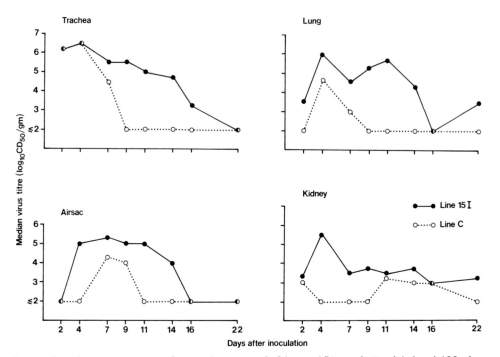

Figure 1. Virus recovery from tissues of lines 15I and C chicks killed at intervals after intranasal inoculation with IBV (M41). Median values of 3 chicks sampled at each time ●——● line 15I, o------o line C.

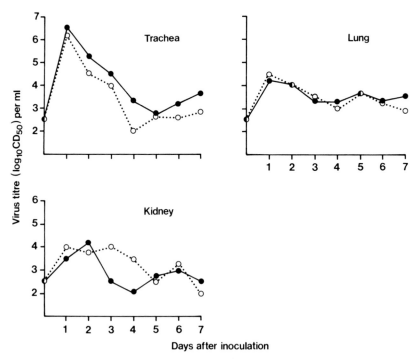

Figure 2. Daily release of IBV (M41) into the supernatant of explants of tissues derived from lines 15I and C chicks. Each explant was inoculated with $\log_{10}$ 2.5 CD_{50} of virus ●——● line 15I o-----o line C.

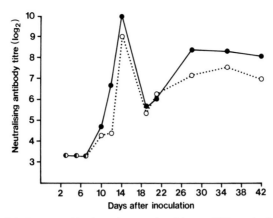

Figure 3. Neutralising antibody titres in lines 15I and C chicks inoculated intranasally with IBV (M41). Values are for pools of 8 sera tested at each time. ●_____● line 15I   o-----o line C.

Virus recovery from tissues of line C and 15I chicks following IBV inoculation

Groups of three chicks from each line were killed at intervals after inoculation with IBV (M41) and virus recovery attempted from selected tissues. In the case of trachea, similar amounts of virus were recovered initially from chicks of both lines (Figure 1), but by 9 days p.i., IBV could no longer be recovered from the trachea of line C chicks whereas it was detected in line 15I chicks until at least 16 days p.i. Throughout the study, considerably more virus was recovered from the lungs, airsacs and kidneys of line 15I chicks. Little virus was recovered from the spleen or liver of either line. The experiment was repeated with similar results.

In vitro susceptibility of tissues from lines C and 15I chicks to IBV infection

The results (Figure 2) show that, in vitro, IBV grew to a similar titre in explants of trachea, lung and kidney from each line. No IBV replication was demonstrated in explants of liver.

Serum neutralising antibody response of lines C and 15I chicks to IBV inoculation

The results (Figure 3) show that following inoculation of IBV (M41) similar levels of neutralising antibodies were produced by each line of chicken throughout the 42 days period studied.

DISCUSSION

It has previously been found possible, using a model IBV and E.coli infection, to identify lines of chicken which are highly resistant or highly susceptible to that infection[4]. Examination of crosses and back crosses between pairs of resistant and susceptible lines suggested the involvement of a single autosomal dominant resistance gene. However, the behaviour of two highly resistant lines suggested a more complex situation in that in one of them (line C) little invasion of the pathogenic E.coli occurred whilst in the other (BrL), the E.coli invaded and proliferated in the visceral organs but without causing mortality.

This study also indicated that in some lines, IBV on its own could cause a lethal infection, thereby providing the opportunity to study the mechanism of resistance to the virus in more detail. In that work, the IBV Pool, a pool of eight strains of the Massachusetts serotype, was used.

However, in studies to examine various parameters of an IBV infection in resistant and susceptible chickens, high mortality or a high incidence of moribund chicks would adversely affect our ability to quantify these parameters. Therefore, for most of the current experiments, the M41 strain was used as it has previously been shown[3] to be less virulent than the IBV Pool. In both cases it was possible to show that whilst all lines of chicken appeared susceptible to IBV infection initially, the outcome of that infection varied between lines and ones which were highly susceptible or highly resistant to infection could be identified.

The more detailed studies carried out on lines C and 15I chicks confirmed these findings and showed that, whilst equally susceptible initially, line C chicks recovered more rapidly. This was shown by the ability of line C chicks to recover clinically more quickly, by the more rapid regeneration of the ciliated tracheal epithelium in that line and by the reduced rate of virus recovery from their tissues. It has also been shown[8] that, although body weight gain was depressed initially in both lines, line C chicks subsequently grew more rapidly than did line 15I chicks.

Despite the difference found in vivo between the two lines in the amount and duration of virus recovery, explants of tissues of each line, when inoculated in vitro, yielded similar amounts of virus. This suggests that the different response of the two lines to IBV infection is not a result of differing susceptibilities of tissues to IBV infection, for example the lack of specific viral receptors by target cells of resistant lines, as has been suggested with murine hepatitis coronavirus[9]. It is possible that differing immunological responses to IBV infection by the two lines is an important factor. Since both lines are initially susceptible, it may be that the rate of response varies between the two lines. The role of cell mediated and local antibody remains to be investigated as does the possibility of different antibody class responses in the resistant and susceptible lines.

REFERENCES

1. A.F. Schalk and M.C.Hawn. An apparently new respiratory disease of baby chicks. J. Amer. vet. med. Ass., 78:413 (1931).
2. M.S. Hofstad. Avian infectious bronchitis, in: "Diseases of Poultry" M.S. Hofstad, ed., Publisher, Iowa State University Press, Ames, Iowa, USA. (1984).
3. H.W. Smith, J.K.A. Cook and Z.E. Parsell. The experimental infection of chickens with mixtures of infectious bronchitis virus and Escherichia coli. J. gen. Virol. 66:777. (1985).
4. N. Bumstead, M.B. Huggins and J.K.A. Cook. Genetic differences in susceptibility to a mixture of avian infectious bronchitis virus and Escherichia coli. Br. Poult. Sci. 30:39 (1989).
5. J.K.A. Cook, J.H. Darbyshire and R.W. Peters. The use of chicken tracheal organ cultures for the isolation and assay of avian infectious bronchitis virus. Arch. Virol. 50:109 (1976).
6. J.H. Darbyshire, J.K.A. Cook and R.W. Peters. Organ culture studies on the efficiency of infection of chicken tissues with avian infectious bronchitis virus. Br. J. exp. Path. 57:443 (1976).
7. J.H. Darbyshire, J.G. Rowell, J.K.A. Cook and R.W. Peters. Taxonomic studies on strains of avian infectious bronchitis virus using neutralisation tests in tracheal organ cultures. Arch. Virol. 61:227 (1979).
8. K. Otsuki, M.B. Huggins and J.K.A. Cook. Comparison of the susceptibility to avian infectious bronchitis virus infection of two inbred lines of White Leghorn chickens. Avian Path.
9. J.F. Boyle, D.G. Weismiller and K.V. Holmes. Genetic resistance to mouse hepatitis virus correlates with absence of virus-binding activity on target tissues. J. Virol. 61:185 (1987).

COMPARISON OF THE REPLICATION OF DISTINCT STRAINS OF HUMAN CORONAVIRUS OC43

IN ORGANOTYPIC HUMAN COLON CELLS (Caco-2) AND MOUSE INTESTINE

A. R. Collins

Dept. of Microbiology
State University of New York at Buffalo
Buffalo, NY 14214

Abstract

Three strains of human coronavirus (HCV) OC43 were compared for their ability to cause enteric infections and to induce interferon alpha (IFNα) using the Caco-2 human colon carcinoma cell line which exhibits spontaneous epithelial differentiation in vitro. MRC-5 cell culture grown stocks were prepared from: 1. CV Paris, a strain of OC43 recovered from an outbreak of necrotizing enterocolitis in newborns. 2. CV Mb, a neurotropic strain of OC43 which exhibits strict neuronal specificity in murine neuronal cell cultures. 3. CV Rd, a strain of OC43 which grows to a high titer in human rhabdomyosarcoma (RD) cells. Immunofluorescent staining for nucleocapsid antigen and plaque assay in MRC-5 cells was used to detect viral replication. BG-9 (human foreskin) cells challenged with vesicular stomatitis virus were used to detect IFNα production by human peripheral blood monocytes (PBMC) stimulated by virus infected Caco-2 cells.

Caco-2 cells infected with virus at a multiplicity of infection of 0.5 yielded $10^{4.6}$ and $10^{4.4}$ plaque forming units/ml (pfu/ml) with CV Rd and CV Paris respectively, while CV Mb yielded only 10^3 pfu/ml. Caco-2 cells infected with CV Rd induced 64 IU/ml of IFNα in PBMC while these cells infected with CV Paris induced <2 IU/ml IFNα. In cells infected with CV Mb 4 IU/ml IFNα was detected. The results suggest that a lack of IFNα induction by CV Paris may be an indicator of its enteropathogenic potential.

When newborn Balb/c mice were given 10 μl of CV Paris orally, viral antigens could be demonstrated in intestinal homogenates inoculated onto RC cells and an antibody titer of 40 at three weeks post infection was shown by immunodot blot. Some virus was recovered from mice given mouse neurotropic CV Mb strain orally but the serum antibody titer was <20. Therefore CV Paris but not CV Mb is enterotropic and induces immunity in mice given the virus orally.

Introduction

Infection with human coronaviruses 229E and OC43 generally produces only mild upper respiratory tract infections which are not life threatening and therefore no special management is required. A few reports have suggested lower respiratory involvement in some cases, especially young children. Routine diagnosis is non-existent in most laboratories (1). Treatment of common colds due to coronaviruses has met with some success. Recombinant IFNα reduced the number of colds in volunteers given IFNα over three to four weeks (2).

Coronaviruses and Their Diseases
Edited by D. Cavanagh and T.D.K. Brown
Plenum Press, New York, 1990

Table 1

Human Coronaviruses

Strain	Illness	Serologic Specificity
229E	respiratory	distinct
OC43	respiratory	cross reactive
CV Paris	necrotizing enterocolitis	cross reacts with OC43
HEC A4 HEC C14	necrotizing enterocolitis	distinct
HECV-24 HECV-35	acute gastroenteritis	cross reacts with OC43

Human enteric coronaviruses (HEC) were found in stools from infants with necrotizing enterocolitis (3,4). HEC were also shed in stools from patients with non-bacterial gastroenteritis (5) and an increased incidence of shedding of virus was found to occur from homosexual men with diarrhea who were symptomatic and seropositive for human immunodeficiency virus (6). Two studies of necrotizing enterocolitis yielded cultivable virus. In one study (3), the HEC A14 and HEC C14 virus isolates recovered from the stool were serologically unrelated to OC43 and 229E coronaviruses by immunoblotting. The HEC A14 and HEC C14 isolates produced destructive effects in culture on the brush border of the intestinal epithelium and caused degeneration of the villi. In another case (4), the CV Paris isolate was serologically related to OC43 and bovine coronavirus. In a study of non-cultivable coronaviruses, two isolates HECV-24 and HECV-35 from children with acute gastroenteritis, reacted with antiserum to OC43 by immune electron microscopy. Convalescent sera in the study showed reactivity with a 62kd and a 56kd protein. No antigenic relatedness to OC43 virus was detected by immunoblotting (7,8). Molecular and pathogenic comparison of the human coronaviruses is not available due largely to the difficulty of obtaining isolates of the enteric viruses. A summary of the current strains is shown in Table 1. We have begun to examine what we propose to be several distinct strains of OC43 which could be cultured in MRC-5, human diploid lung fibroblasts. We sought to identify differences in the biological behavior of these strains. Interaction of the viruses with immune system cells was of interest, specifically the stimulation of interferon. Interferon induction by viruses is strictly a property of type 1 (α and β) interferons. However, both interferon gamma (IFNγ) and IFNα are induced in sensitized lymphocytes exposed to viral antigens. In the present study, enteropathology and interferon induction was examined with the possibility in mind that IFNα may be used to ameliorate the symptoms of chronic diarrhea in individuals with immune system disorders (9,10).

Materials and Methods

Cells: Caco-2 cells, a line of human colonic carcinoma cells, were obtained from the ATCC and maintained in Eagle's MEM with 10% fetal bovine serum (fbs). MRC-5 cells were maintained in Eagle's MEM with 5% fbs.
Virus: CV Paris, a strain of OC43 of probably human origin isolated from the feces of an infant with necrotizing enterocolitis, was obtained from D.A.J. Tyrell, Clinical Disease Center, Harrow, Middlesex, England (4). CV Mb, a

strain of OC43 passaged in suckling mouse brain, was obtained from Cedric Mims, St. Guys Hospital, London, England (11). CV Rd, a strain of OC43 propagated in human rhabdomyosarcoma cells, was obtained from G. Gerna, Pavia, Italy (7). For plaque assay, MRC-5 cell monolayers grown in 24-well tissue culture trays (Costar, Cambridge, MA) were inoculated with 0.2 ml of virus inoculum. After adsorption for 1 h at 37°C, an overlay of 0.5 ml of EMEM with 0.2% fbs and 0.5% agarose was added and the cultures incubated at 33°C. Plaques were visualized on day 4 after addition of a second overlay containing 0.2 mg/ml neutral red. In the 50% plaque reduction assay, 100 plaque forming units (pfu) of virus in 0.2 ml were added to 0.2 ml serial dilutions of heat inactivated antiserum and the mixtures incubated at room temperature for 1 h. Two culture wells were then inoculated with 0.2 ml of each mixture. Plaques were allowed to develop and counted after staining. The titer was defined as the reciprocal of the highest dilution of serum which reduced the number of plaques by 50% of the virus control.

Immunofluorescent staining was performed on acetone fixed cells using a monoclonal antibody (mab) to nucleocapsid (4B-6) obtained from Dr. Michael Buchmeier, Scripps Research Institute, San Diego, CA as previously described (12).

For dot immunoblot assay, microsol protein (10 μg/3.5 μl) extracted from virus-infected cells was spotted onto a nitrocellulose membrane (0.45 μm pore size prewet with 0.1 M phosphate buffered saline (PBS) pH 7.2 and allowed to adsorb for 90 min at room temperature in a Biodot Microfiltration apparatus (BioRad Laboratories, Richmond, CA). Following the BioRad procedure, briefly the wells were blocked with 1% BSA, washed, then 100 μl of antibody dilution (1:16,000 for mab 4B-6) was allowed to flow through by gravity for 30-40 min. After three washes, 100 μl of goat anti-mouse IgG, horseradish peroxidase conjugated, at 1:3000 was filtered through the membrane. The washed membrane was placed in substrate solution containing 4-chloro-1-naphtol (Kirkegaard and Perry Laboratories, Gaithersburg, MD) to develop for 10-20 min.

Peripheral blood mononuclear cells were obtained from heparinized human type O donor blood by Ficol density centrifugation on Lymphoprep (Nyegaarde, Oslo, Norway).

Interferon assays were performed on BG-9 (human foreskin) cells grown in 24-well tissue culture trays by treatment of lightly confluent monolayers overnight with supernatant medium which had been clarified by centrifugation at 1000 xg for 10 min and left at pH 2 for 48 h and returned to neutral pH. The medium was removed and the cultures were challenged with 100 pfu of vesicular stomatitis virus. The cultures were graded for cytopathic effect after 48 h incubation at 37°C and the interferon units (IU) were determined by comparison with an IFNα reference standard (12).

Mice: Pregnant Balb/c mice were obtained from West Seneca Laboratories, West Seneca, NY. All mice tested serologically negative for antibody to OC43 by the plaque reduction assay and the dot immunoblot assay.

Results

Caco-2 cells are highly polarized cells which form microville, resembling colonic crypt cells and form domes which are typical transporting epithelial monolayers (13,14,15). These properties favor expression of antigens and infectious virus as it occurs in vivo although the virus inoculum is from cultured cells. Monolayers of Caco-2 cells showing typical dome formation were infected with each strain of OC43 at a multiplicity of infection (m.o.i.) of 0.5. After adsorption of virus for 1 h at 37°C, monolayers were washed twice and maintenance medium with 0.2% fetal bovine serum was added. After 48 h the cells were fixed in acetone and stained by immunofluorescence using monoclonal antibody to nucleocapsid. Figure 1 shows virus antigen in CAco-2 cells infected with CV Paris. Cells containing virus antigen were observed to occur in foci and appeared as aggregates of fused cells which pulled away from the monolayer. Antigen containing cells but no focal destruction were observed in cells infected with CV Rd and scant antigen was evident in Caco-2 cells infected with CV Mb.

To determine if virus-infected Caco-2 cells will induce interferon in peripheral blood monocytes, cells were infected with each strain at an m.o.i. of 0.5. After 18 h the supernatant medium was removed for virus assay and replaced with medium containing human peripheral blood mononuclear cells (PBMC) at a concentration of 1×10^8 per culture of infected and uninfected cells. After 24 h at 37°C, the supernatants were collected, the PBMC were removed by centrifugation and the supernatant medium was tested for interferon activity. As shown in Table 2, Caco-2 cells infected with CV Paris produced 2.5×10^4 pfu/ml of virus but induced no detectable interferon in PBMC whereas Caco-2 cells infected with CV Rd strain produced 4.5×10^4 pfu/ml and induced 64 IU/ml of interferon in PBMC. The interferon titer was not reduced by pH 2 treatment for 48 h, and was not present in infected Caco-2 cells suggesting that it was IFNα. Only 10^3 pfu/ml of virus was present in the supernatant medium from CV Mb-infected Caco-2 cells and 4 IU/ml of IFNα were induced. No interferon was induced by uninfected Caco-2 cells.

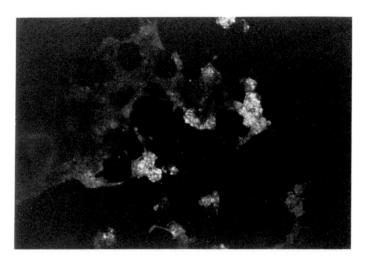

Figure 1.   Immunofluorescent staining of Caco-2 cells 48 h after infection with CV Paris at an moi of 0.5. Cells were fixed in acetone, reacted with mab 4B-6 to nucleocapsid, then with biotinyllated goat antiserum to mouse IgG and avidin FITC. (magnification: 160x)

Table 2

Interferon α induction by human colon cells
infected with coronaviruses

Virus Strain	Virus Yield (pfu/ml)	IFNα titer (U/ml)
CV Paris	2.5×10^4 [a]	<2[b]
CV Rd	4.5×10^4	64
CV Mb	3.0×10^3	4

[a] At 18 h after infection
[b] After 24 h incubation with PBMC (25×10^6/ml)

In order to compare CV Paris and CV Mb strains for their enteropathogenicity in newborn mice, Balb/c strain mice two to four days old were given 10 μl orally of a suspension containing 3 to 10 x 10^3 pfu/ml of virus. Intestinal homogenates were prepared from animals taken on day 2, 4 and 7 and virus recovery was sought by plaque assay on MRC-5 cells and by inoculation of RD cell cultures. As shown in Table 3, virus was recovered on day 2 and day 4 from intestinal homogenates of newborn mice given CV Paris and on day 4 from mice given CV Mb. Recovery of CV Paris was confirmed by examination of immunofluorescent-stained RD cells inoculated with the intestinal homogenates. Serum taken three weeks after inoculation was tested for antiviral activity by the plaque reduction assay. Neutralizing antibody to OC43 virus was present at a titer of 80 PRD 50/ml in the serum of mice given CV Paris while no significant neutralization was found in serum from mice given CV Mb. CV Paris antiserum also gave a reaction titer of 40 with the microsol fraction of OC43 virus-infected RD cells in a dot immunoblot assay (Figure 2).

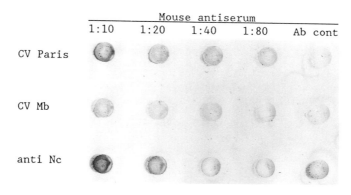

Figure 2

Discussion

We have observed that CV Rd-infected Caco-2 cells induce IFNα in PBMC. The process of induction may be due to viral proteins as has been shown for transmissible gastroenteritis coronavirus (TGEV) (18) or due to the RNA of

Table 3

Enteropathogenicity of human coronaviruses in newborn mice

Virus inoculum[a]	Virus recovery[b]			Antibody titer (PRD$_{50/ml}$)
	d2	d4	d7	
CV Paris	++++	++	--	80
CV Mb	--	+	--	<20
Uninfected	--	--	--	<20

[a] 10 μl (10^3 PFU) orally
[b] Plaque assay of 10% intestinal homogenate

the infectious virus. The fact that the interferon induction was not a potent response suggests that a mechanism dependent on virus penetration into producer cells is involved. The interferon induced by infected Caco-2 cells was acid stabile and therefore considered to be alpha type.

The lack of antibody production and the low level of virus recovered show that CV Mb is not significantly infectious for newborn mice by the oral route. This observation supports the work of Pearson and Mims (15) which showed that this strain of OC43 was neurotropic in newborn mice. The presence of neutralizing antibody and the recovery of virus indicate that CV Paris is infectious for newborn mice by the oral route. To account for the selective tropism of this strain for mouse intestine, a difference in tissue specificity may be postulated. It would be of value to correlate the IFN-inducing capacity of OC43 strains with the development of enteropathogenicity. A protective role of interferon in mice infected with mouse hepatitis type 3 was demonstrated by the use of anti-interferon serum (16). Furthermore, a regulatory role for interferon in coronavirus infections of mice may be inferred from the experience of Weiser and Bang (17) which showed that the supernatant from a mixed lymphocyte reaction (presumably containing interferon and other lymphokines) rendered macrophages from C3H mice susceptible to mouse hepatitis virus. The experiments presented here suggest that CV Paris lacks the ability to induce interferon. Whether the induction depends on viral dose or prior exposure to certain OC43 strains and what is the role of specific lymphocyte subpopulations in induction requires determination. We hypothesize that absence of a vigorous immune response as in individuals with immune disorders, strains of coronaviruses which do not stimulate interferon may have the ability to cause persistent enterocolitis.

References

1. McNaughton, M.R. Coronaviruses in Principles and Practice of Clinical Virology. A.J. Zuckerman, J.E. Banatvala and J.R. Pattison eds John Wiley and Sons Ltd. 1987.

2. Tyrell, D.A.J. Interferons and their clinical value. Rev. Inf. Dis. 9:243 (1987).

3. Resta, S., Luby, J.P., Rosenfeld, C.R. and D.J. Siegal. Isolation and propagation of a human enteric coronavirus. Science 229:978 (1985).

4. Sureau, C., Amiel-Tison, C., Moscovici, O., Lebon, P., Laporte, J. and C. Chany. Une epidemie d'enterocolitis ulceronecrosantes en maternite. Arguments en facor de son origine virale. Bull Acad. Nat. Med. 163:286.

5. Caul, F.O. and S.K.R. Clark. Coronaviruses propagated from a patient with non bacterial gastroenteritis. Lancet 1975-II, 953.

6. Cunningham, A.L., Grohman, G.S., Harkness, J., Law, C., Marriott, D., Tindall, B. and D.A. Cooper. Gastrointestinal viral infections in homosexual men who were symptomatic and sero-positive for human immunodeficiency virus. J. Infect. Dis. 158:386 (1988).

7. Gerna, G., Passarini, N., Cerida, P.M., and M. Battaglia. Antigenic relatedness of human enteric coronavirus strains to human coronavirus OC43: a preliminary report. J. Infect. Dis. 150:618 (1984).

8. Battaglia, M., Passarini, N., DiMatteo, A. and G. Gerna. Human enteric coronaviruses: Further characterization and immunoblotting of viral proteins. J. Infect. Dis. 155:140 (1987).

9. Carlin, J.M. and E.C. Borden. Interferons and their induction in Interferon and Nonviral Pathogens. G.I. Byrne and J. Turco eds Marcel Dekker, Inc., New York (1987).

10. Rossol, S., Voth, R., Laubenstein, P., Muller, W.E.G., Schroder, H.C., Meyer zum Buschenfelde, K.H. and G. Hess. Interferon production in patients infected with HIV-1. J. Infect. Dis. 59:815 (1989).

11. Rousset, M. The human colon carcinoma cell lines HT 29 and Caco-2: two in vitro models for the study of intestinal differentiation. Biochemie 68:1035 (1986).

12. Collins, A.R. and O. Sorenson. Regulation of viral persistence in human glioblastoma and rhabdomyosarcoma cells infected with coronavirus OC43. Microbial Pathogenesis 1:573 (1986).

13. Pinto, M., Robine-Leon, S., Appay, M.-D., Kedinger, M., Triadou, N., Dussaulx, E., Lacroix, B., Simon-Assmann, P., Haffen, K., Gogh, J. and A. Zweibaum. Enterocyte-like differentiation and polarization of the human colon carcinoma cell line Caco-2 in culture. Biol. Cell 47:323 (1983).

14. Dharmsathaphorn, K., McRoberts, J.A., Mandel, K.G., Tisdale, L.D. and H. Maui. A human colonic tumor cell line that maintains vectorial electrolyte transport. Am. J. Physiol. 246:G204 (1984).

15. Pearson, J. and C.A. Mims. Selective vulnerability of neural cells and age-related susceptibility to OC43 virus in mice. Arch. Virol. 77"109 (1983).

16. Virelizier, J.L. and I. Gresser. Role of interferon in the pathogenesis of viral diseases of mice as demonstrated by the use of anti interferon serum. V. Protective role in mouse hepatitis type 3 infection of susceptible and resistant strains of mice. J. Immunol. 120:1616 (1989.

17. Weiser, W.Y. and F.B. Bang. Macrophages genetically resistant to mouse hepatitis converted in vitro to susceptible macrophages. J. Exp. Med. 145:690 (1976).

18. Charley, B. and H. Laude. Induction of alpha interferon by transmissible gastroenteritis coronavirus: role of transmembrane glycoprotein El. J. Virol. 52:8 (1988).

DETECTION OF CORONAVIRUS RNA IN CNS TISSUE OF

MULTIPLE SCLEROSIS AND CONTROL PATIENTS

Ronald S. Murray[+], Bonnie MacMillan[+],
Gary Cabirac[+*], and Jack S. Burks[+]

Rocky Mountain Multiple Sclerosis Center[+],
Colorado Neurological Institute, AND Swedish
Medical Center, Englewood, Colorado, and
Dept. of Biochemistry[*], Univ. of Colorado
Health Sciences Center, Denver, Colorado

The cause of multiple sclerosis (MS) remains unknown. One of the leading hypothesis states that MS may result from the direct or indirect effects of a CNS viral infection. The hallmark of MS is the demyelinating lesion which may represent the final immunopathological reaction to many viral or non-viral precipitants. We are investigating coronaviruses in MS. Previously, two CV's were isolated from the brains of two patients with MS after passage through murine systems (1). CV are widely distributed in nature and are common human and animal pathogens. In addition, CNS demyelination results from CV infection of rodents (2,3) and in one report primates (4). The putative MS isolates (CV-SD and CV-SK) are antigenically related to the human CV OC43 and the murine CV A59 (5). To date no species specific marker has been identified and serologic data have not definitively resolved the species origin of CV-SD or CV-SK (5-7). Direct virus isolation from tissue is difficult, therefor to evaluate whether CV are present in human CNS tissue, the method of _in situ_ hybridization (ISH) was performed using cDNA probes to detect CV-RNA. We report here the presence of CV-RNA sequences in human CNS tissue. In addition, CV-RNA is much more frequent in MS than non-MS tissue. These findings raise the question of a potential role for CV in MS.

We previously reported the following ISH results utilizing a cDNA probe prepared from purified CV-SD RNA by the randon primer method (8-11). Tissue from 21 MS patients, 16 non-neurological disease (NND) and 5 other neurological disease (OND) control patients were examined. The OND cases included one of each of the following: amyotrophic lateral sclerosis (ALS), post-infectious encephalomyelitis, bacterial meningitis, subacute sclerosing panencephalitis (SSPE) and radiation-induced cerebral vasculitis.

All tissues were rapidly frozen and stored at -80°C. Average duration from patient death to tissue acquisition and freezing (autolysis time) for MS and control patients was 5.0 hours and 6.1 hours, respectively. The total number of MS and control tissue sections tested was 442 and 404 respectively.

Results for each experimental group are shown in Table I. CV RNA was detected in the CNS from 11 of 21 MS patients (52%) and 2 of 21 non MS patients (9.5%). Significance was determined by chi square $(X^2)= 9.02$, 1 degree of freedom with $p < 0.005$. Specifically, CV RNA was detected in CNS tissue from 1 of 16 (6%) NND patients and in 1 of 5 (20%) OND patients. The OND patient positive for CV RNA genome had radiation induced cerebral vasculitis. Both multiple sclerosis patients' CNS tissue from which CV-SD and CV-SK were originally isolated were found positive for CV RNA.

Table 1. PATIENTS POSITIVE FOR CV RNA

Patients	N	# positive(%)
MS	21	11[*](52)
Non-MS	21	2 (9.5)
-NND	16	1 (6)
-OND	5	1 (20)

* p< 0.005

Tables 2 and 3 summarize the total number of brain sections sampled from MS and control patients. The positive NND and OND patients were both found to have CV RNA in frontal cortex. CV RNA was not easily detected in the CNS of MS patients as only 49 (11.1%) of 442 sections tested contained viral genome. Genome was identified in both plaque and non-plaque areas of cortex, brainstem and spinal cord. CV RNA was found in only 3 (0.8%) frontal white matter sections of 376 sections examined from the 21 control patients.

We then repeated the above experiment utilizing cloned MHV-A59 cDNA (12) (kindly provided by S. Weiss and J. Leibowitz) as a probe. MHV-A59 has extensive homology with CV-SD (6). The 1800 base pair fragment was excised from pstl site of clone g344, agarose purified, and end labelled (13) with ^{32}P-ATP to high specific activity (1×10^9 cpm/ng). The probe was shown to be specific for CV-SD and MHV-A59 (Fig. 1). There was no cross reactivity to human or murine nucleic acids.

MS and control brains were cut into four micron frozen sections, placed onto pretreated slides, fixed with 3:1 v/v ethanol/acetic acid solution, dehydrated through graded alcohols and pretreated to improve probe diffusion (10). The hybridization mixture contained 0.6M NaCl, 50% foramamide, 10% dextran sulphate, 1x Denhardt's, and 100ug/ml of denatured human nucleic acids to decrease any nonspecific tissue background (9). ISH was carried out at 42°c for 24 hours with 1×10^6 cpm's of probe per tissue section. Coverslips were removed and all sections washed

Table 2. MS TISSUES POSITIVE FOR CV RNA

CNS REGIONS	positive/total (%)
CORTEX PLAQUE	17/230 (7.4)
CORTEX NON-PLAQUE	16/142 (11.3)
BRAIN STEM PLAQUE	2/16 (12.5)
BRAIN STEM NON-PLAQUE	6/20 (30.0)
SPINAL CORD PLAQUE	8/32 (25.0)
SPINAL CORD NON-PLAQUE	NOT DONE
TOTAL	49/440 (11.1)

Table 3. NON MS TISSUE POSITIVE FOR CV RNA

CNS REGION	positive/total (%)
CORTEX	3/376 (0.8)
BRAINSTEM	0/58 (0.0)
TOTAL	3/404 (0.7)

for 8 hours in 50% formamide; .01M Tris and 0.6M NaCl. Sections were then dehydrated in graded alcohols containing 0.3M ammonium acetate, air dried, coated with NTB-2 photographic emulsion (Eastman Kodak Co., Rochester, N.Y.), air dried, and placed in a desiccated container at 4°C. Slides were developed 3 to 5 days later and counter stained with hematoxylin and eosin. Positivity was determined by finding a significant number of silver grains developed over cells compared with background. Pretreatment of all tissues with ribonuclease significantly decreased or abolished the amount of positive hybridization.

Results with the MHV-A59 probe were similar to those obtained with the CV RNA probe. Fig.1 shows areas of positive hybridization in the white matter cells from MS patients brains. These patients were the donors from which CV RNA and CV-SK were isolated.

These results indicate that CV RNA is present in human CNS tissue and in a significantly higher proportion of MS patients than controls. There was no predilection for plaque or non-plaque areas. Even in sections that contained viral genome, there was a paucity of positive cells. This may explain previously negative results by less sensitive technology (14) and the difficulty of consistent successful CV isolations from human CNS tissue.

Although human CV's are generally associated with upper respiratory infections, more recent reports indicate that these viruses may cause gastroenteritis (15) and childhood meningitis (16). In humans, CV are ubiquitous with 100% of some populations seropositive for CV-OC43 by the age of 6 years (17). Human CV's are difficult to grow, presumably due to restrictive species and/or tissue tropisms. However, human CV OC43 productively infects suckling mice and _in vitro_ infects and persists both in mouse astrocytes and human embryonic astrocytes (18,19). Murine coronaviruses are known to cause demyelination in rodents (2,3)

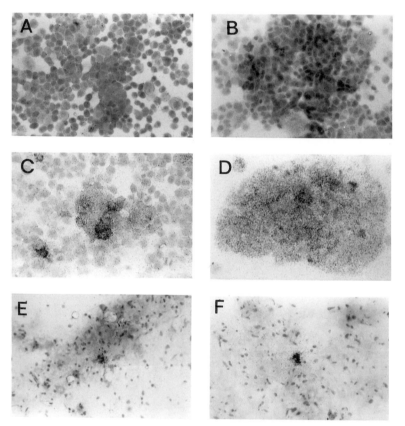

Fig. 1.   Results of ISH with 32-P labelled A59 cDNA probe. All photos are 400x magnification before reduction. All sections were developed after 3 days of exposure.   A) Uninfected DBT cells.   B) A59 infected DBT cells treated with RNAse resulting in no detectable signal. C) A59 infected DBT cells showing positive cytoplasmic signal. D) CV-SD infected DBT cells showing a multinucleated giant cell with diffuse positive cytoplasmic signal. E and F) MS patients SD and SK showing positive signal within the cerebral white matter.

and in one reported study primates (4). CV-SD also causes demyelination in mice (3). Murine coronaviruses are also capable of inducing class II antigen expression on cultured rat astrocytes rendering them capable of participating in the immune response (20). Demyelination can also be adoptively transferred to naive rodents from CV infected rodents suggesting a role for cross reactive epitopes between CV antigens and myelin proteins (21). The above suggest that the full spectrum of CV induced human disease may not be fully appreciated and that CV may play a role in MS.

Acknowledgement

This work was supported by the Fausel Foundation, Swedish Medical Foundation, and the National MS Society Tissue Bank Grant #RG1627-B-4.

References

1. Burks, J.S., DeVald, B.L., Jankovsky, L.D. and Gerdes, J.C., Two coronaviruses isolated from central nervous system tissue of two multiple sclerosis patients. (1980) Science 209:933-934.
2. Weiner, L.P., Pathogenesis of demyelination induced by a mouse hepatitis virus (JHM virus). (1973) Arch. Neurol. 28:298-303.
3. Mendelman, P.M., Jankovsky, L.D., Murray, R.S., Licari, P., Devald, B., Gerdes, J.C., Burks, J.S., Pathogenesis of Coronavirus SD in Mice I. Prominent Demyelination in the Abscence of Infectious Virus Production. (1983) Arch Neurol 40:493-498.
4. Kersting, G. and Pette, E. Deutsche Zeitschrift f. Nervenheilkunde., Zur Pathohistologie und Pathogenese der experimentellen JHM-Virusencephalomyelitis des Affen. (1956) Eingegangen 174:283-304.
5. Gerdes, J.C., Klein, I., DeVald, B.L. and Burks, J.S., Coronavirus isolates SK and SD from multiple sclerosis patients are serologically related to murine coronaviruses A59 and JHM and human coronavirus OC43; but not to human coronavirus 229E. (1981) J. Virology 38:231-238.
6. Weiss, S.R. Coronaviruses SD and SK share extensive nucleotide homology with murine coronavirus MHV-A59, more than that shared between human and murine coronavirus. (1983) Virology 126:669-677.
7. Burks, J.S., DeVald, B.L., Gerdes, J.C., McNally, I.T. and Kemp, M.C., (1984) In: Advances in Experimental Medicine and Biology. Rottier, P. et al. eds. 173:393-394.
8. Haase, A.T., Ventura, P., Gibbs, C.J. and Tourtellotte, W.W., Measles virus nucleotide sequences: detection by hybridization in situ. (1981) Science 212:672-675.
9. Stroop, W.G., Brahic, M., Baringer, J.R., Detection of tissue culture-adapted Theiler's virus RNA in spinal cord white matters cells throughout infection. (1982) Infect Immunity 37:763-770.

10. Haase, A.T., Stowring, L., Ventura, P., Burks, J., Ebers, G.,Tourtellotte, W., and Warren, K.: Detection by hybridization of viral infection of the human central nervous system. Ann. N.Y.Acad. Sci. 436:103-108, 1984.

11. Murray, R.S., MacMillan, B., Burks, J.S., Detection of Coronavirus Genome in the CNS of MS Patients and Control Patients (1987) Neurology 37:109.

12. Budzilowicz, C.J., Wilczynski, S.P., Weiss, S.R., Three Intergenic Regions of Coronavirus Mouse Hepatitis Virus Strain A59 Genome RNA Contain a Common Nucleotide Sequence That is Homologous to the 3' End of the Viral mRNA Leader Sequence. (1985) Virology 53:834-840.

13. Feinberg, A.P., Vogelstein, B., A Technique for Radiolabeling DNA Restriction Endonuclease Fragments to High Specific Activity. (1983) Analytical Biochemistry 132:6-13.

14. Sorenson, O., Collins, A., Flintoff, W., Ebers, G., Dales, S. Probing for the human coronavirus OC43 in multiple sclerosis. (1986) Neurology 36:1604-1606.

15. Resta, S., Luby, J.P., Rosenfeld, C.R., Siegel, J.D., Isolation and Propagation of a Human Enteric Coronavirus. (1985) 229:978-981

16. Malkova, D., Holubova, J., et al. Isolation of tettnang coronavirus from man? (1980) Acta Virol (Prague) (Engl Ed) 24 (5):363-366.

17. Hovi, T., Kainulainen, H., Ziola, B., Salmi, A., OC43 Strain-Related Coronavirus Antibodies in Different Age Groups (1979) J. Med. Virol 3:313-320.

18. Pearson, J., Mims, C.A., Selective vulnerability of neural cells and age-related susceptibility to OC43 virus in mice. (1985) Arch. Virol 77:109-118.

19. Pearson, J., C. A. Mims. Differential susceptibility of cultured neural cells to the human coronavirus. (1985) J. Virol. 53:1016-1019.

20. Massa, P.T., Dorries, R. and ter Meulen, V. Viral particles induce Ia antigen expression on astrocytes. (1986) Nature 320:543-546.

21. Watanabe, R., Wege, H. and ter Meulen, V. Adoptive transfer of EAE-like lesions from rats with corona virus-induced demyelinating encephalomyelitis.(1983) Nature 305:150-153.

RABBIT DILATED CARDIOMYOPATHY

Ralph S. Baric[*1], Suzanne Edwards[1] and J. David Small[2]

University of North Carolina at Chapel Hill
Department of Parasitology and Laboratory Practice[1]
Glaxo Corporations, Research Triangle Park North Carolina[2]

INTRODUCTION

Viruses have long been recognized as important etiologic agents of heart disease in man and experimental animals[1]. Epidemiologic evidence suggests that between 2-5% of a virus-infected population experiences some degree of cardiac involvement[2]. Virus infection may result in degeneration and necrosis of myocytes by direct cytotoxicity and cause myocarditis, or inflammation of the heart muscle[3]. Myocarditis may progress to arrhythmias, conduction disturbances, circulatory collapse and/or acute congestive (dilated) cardiomyopathy[4]. Clinically, dilated cardiomyopathy is diagnosed by an increase in the heart weight, heart weigh/body weight weight ratios, enlargement of the left and/or right ventricular cavities, thinning/hypertrophy of the ventricular walls, and low ejection fractions. In humans particularly ominous signs of dilated cardiomyopathy include the presence of pulmonary edema, pleural effusion, and congestion of the lungs and liver [4,5]. The incidence of idiopathic dilated cardiomyopathy is estimated between 3-5 cases/100,000 population/year and accounts for about 30% of all heart disease related deaths in some areas of the world[6]. The mechanism(s) by which virus infection progresses to myocarditis and dilated cardiomyopathy is unclear.

Animal model systems provide considerable insight into the mechanisms of virus-induced heart disease. Coxsackie B virus(CBV) and encephalomyocarditis virus(EMC) infection in mice results in and/or dilated cardiomyopathy[7,8,9]. CBV and EMC-induced myocarditis is primarily immune-mediated rather than caused by direct virus cytotoxicity to myocytes. The mechanism(s) by which other viruses cause myocarditis and dilated cardiomyopathy is unknown.

Recently, a new model system for virus-induced heart disease was described in rabbits. Rabbit cardiomyopathy is characterized by: (1) multifocal to diffuse myocardial degeneration and necrosis, (2) myocarditis, (3) and death in 60-70% of the infected animals[11]. In this article, we demonstrate that RbCV infection is associated with increases in heart weight, heart weight/body weight ratios, dilation of the right and left ventricles, and alternations in a variety of parameters consistent with the development of dilated cardiomyopathy.

Coronaviruses and Their Diseases
Edited by D. Cavanagh and T.D.K. Brown
Plenum Press, New York, 1990

MATERIALS AND METHODS
Animals and Virus

Rabbit coronavirus (RbCV) was originally obtained from Dr. James D. Small (Glaxo Inc., Research Triangle Park, NC). Virus stocks were diluted to 10^4-10^5 rabbit infectious dose (RID) and stored at $-145^{\circ}C$. Male New Zealand white rabbits (2.5-3.0Kg) were inoculated intravenously via the marginal ear vein with 0.2ml of virus. Daily records were kept on body weight, temperature, and the animals observed for clinical signs of infection. Clinical signs of infection included severe congestion of the conjunctivae, temperatures in excess of $40^{\circ}C$, and weight loss.

Pathology and Measurement Studies

Moribund animals were euthanized by intravenous injection with 60mg/Kg sodium pentobarbital (nembutal) and weighed. Necropsies were performed as previously described[11],[12], and the heart excised, trimmed of fat and excess connective tissue, and weighted. The heart was immersed in 10% buffered formalin and sectioned transversely at the midpoint of the ventricles. Sections were stained with hemotoxylin-eosin or Masson's Trichrome and mounted for measurement studies and histology. Heart tissue was also stained for the presence of calcification with the von Kossa stain, or the presence of monocytes with DE histochemical staining techniques[13],[14],[15]. A computerized Zeiss Videoplan was used to calculate the dimensions of the cardiac walls and cavities as well as determining the area within each ventricular section. Mean values were averaged between animals which had died during the acute and subacute phases of infection and reported as means$\pm$SD. Student's test for unpaired observations were used to evaluate differences in the cardiac dimensions.

RESULTS
Clinical Course of RbCV Infection

New Zealand white rabbits were inoculated with approximately 10^3 RID and examined daily for clinical signs of infection. Mortality rates peaked at 4 days post-infection, decreased, and then increased again by day 7 or 8. No animals died after 12 days post-infection, and the overall mortality rate was about 60% (Figure 1). Heart from animals dying between days 3-5 were enlarged and characterized by the presence of right ventricular dilation. Rabbits dying between days 9-12 contained pleural effusion, pulmonary edema, ascites, enlarged hearts and congestion of the lungs and liver. The cause of death appeared to be congestive heart failure. From these data, we have divided RbCV infection into an acute(2-5) and subacute(6-12) phases based upon day of death and pathologic findings in infected animals. These findings are similar to previous studies of RbCV and PEDV infection in rabbits and EMC-induced myocarditis in mice[15],[7],[8],[11].

Heart Weight, Heart Weight/Body Weight Ratio's during RbCV Infection

During EMC-induced dilated cardiomyopathy, heart weight, heart weight/body weight ratio's increase following infection[78]. Since RbCV infection results in a similar clinical course of infection and pathology in the heart muscle, we examined body weight, heart weight, and heart weight/body weight ratios during the acute and subacute stages of infection. Body weights slowly decreased during the course of infection and were notable decreased (~0.5kg) during the subacute phase of the disease (data not shown).

Uninfected controls sacrificed between days 3-5 or 6-12 had heart weights of 6.1$\pm$0.3g and 6.1$\pm$0.5g between days 3-5 and 6-12, respectively.

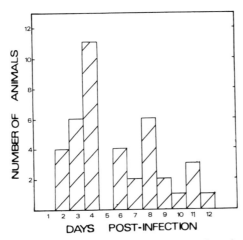

FIGURE 1. Clinical Course of RbCV Infection in Rabbits.

Following RbCV infection, heart weights were significantly increased during the acute (8.4±1.4g; p <0.001) and the subacute phase of infection (8.7±1.6g; p<0.001)(Table 1). Heart weight/body weight ratios were also increased during the acute and subacute phases of the infection, and were 3.07+0.33 x 10^{-3} (p<0.001) and 3.46+0.61 x 10^{-3} (p<0.001), respectively. Conversely, the heart weight/body weight ratios of uninfected controls were 2.19±0.23 x 10^{-3} (3-5 days) and 2.16+0.20 x 10^{-3} (6-12 days), respectively (Figure 2b). Chronological changes in the size of the heart and dimensions of the ventricles were evident through day 36 and are illustrated in Figure 2. These data suggest that right ventricular dilation is prominent during the acute and subacute phase of infection and that dilation of the left ventricle increases progressively throughout the subacute phase of infection.

Dimensions of the Cardiac Walls and Cavities during RbCV Infection

The dimensions of the ventricular walls were measured through the coronal axis at the midpoint of the ventricules. During the acute phase of infection, the dimensions of the right ventricular wall were significantly decreased from 2.037±0.292 x 10^3 um(uninfected) to 1.545±0.248 x 10^3 um; p<0.001 (infected). Thinning of the right ventricular wall continued through the subacute stage of infection and was decreased from 2.065±0.300 x 10^3 um(uninfected) to 1.295±0.319 x 10^3 um; p<0.001 (infected) (Table 1). The dimensions of the intraventricular septum were not significantly altered during the acute stage of infection between the uninfected (4.470±0.676 x 10^3 um) and infected animals (4.419±0.740 x 10^3 um; p<0.87). However, some thinning of the intraventricular septum was noted during the subacute phase of the disease (uninfected-4.471±0.503 x 10^3 um; infected-3.579±0.604 x 10^3 um; p<0.002) (Table 1). The dimensions of the left ventricular wall were also similar during the acute phase of the disease (uninfected-4.188±0.547 x 10^3um; infected-4.369±0.512 x 10^3um; p<0.442), and were reduced slightly during the subacute phase of infection (uninfected-4.410±0.617 x 10^3 um; infected-3.776±0.718 x 10^3 um; p<0.044) (Table 1). Dilated cardiomyopathy is also characterized by increases in the dimensions of the left and/or right ventricular cavity. Consequently, we measured the widest portion of the right and left ventricular cavity in animals dying during the acute or subacute stage of infection (Table 1). During the acute phase, the dimensions of the right ventricular cavity were significantly increased as compared to the uninfected controls (uninfected-3.571±1.07 x 10^3 um; infected-7.334±1.707 x 10^3 um; p<0.001), and markedly increased during the subacute stage of infection

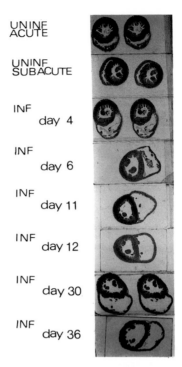

UNINF ACUTE

UNINF SUBACUTE

INF day 4

INF day 6

INF day 11

INF day 12

INF day 30

INF day 36

FIGURE 2. Progression of Dilated Cardiomyopathy during RbCV Infection.
Transverse sections through the midpoint of the ventricles were
prepared and stained with hemotoxylin-Eosin or Massons Trichrome.
Representative sections are shown from days 4-36 post-infection.

(uninfected-3.127$\pm$1.167 x 10^{3}um; infected-8.669+2.084 x 10^{3}um; p<0.001).
Dimensions of the left ventricular cavity were not significantly altered
during the acute stage (uninfected-8.537$\pm$0.996 x 10^{3}um; infected-
9.361$\pm$1.427 x 10^{3}um; p<0.115), and significantly dilated during the
subacute stage (uninfected-8.488$\pm$1.143 x 10^{3}um; infected-10.027$\pm$0.986 x
10^{3}um; p<0.004)(Table 1).

Table 1. Alternations in cardiac sturcutres during RbCV infection.

	Acute		Subacute	
	Uninfected	Infected	Uninfected	Infected
Body Weight (kg)				
Heart Weight (g)	6.1$\pm$0.3g	8.4$\pm$1.4	6.1$\pm$0.5g	8.7$\pm$1.6
Heart Wt/Body Wt. (x10^{-3})	2.19$\pm$0.23	3.07$\pm$0.33	2.16$\pm$0.20	3.46$\pm$0.61
Right Vent. Wall (umx10^3)	2.04$\pm$0.30	1.55$\pm$0.25	2.06$\pm$0.30	1.30$\pm$0.32
Intravent. Septum (umx10^3)	4.47$\pm$0.70	4.42$\pm$0.74	4.47$\pm$0.50	3.58$\pm$0.60
Left Vent. Wall (umx10^3)	4.20$\pm$0.55	4.37$\pm$0.50	4.41$\pm$0.62	3.77$\pm$0.70
Right Vent. Cavity (umx10^3)	3.57$\pm$1.07	7.33$\pm$1.70	3.13$\pm$1.17	8.67$\pm$2.08
Left Vent. Cavity (umx10^3)	8.54$\pm$1.0	9.36$\pm$1.43	8.48$\pm$1.14	10,027$\pm$1.0
Right Vent. Area (um^{2}x10^6)	38.82$\pm$11.8	100$\pm$39.74	41.23$\pm$13.1	146.2$\pm$51.8
Left Ventr. Area (um^{2}x10^6)	57.56$\pm$6.1	66.18$\pm$25.0	59.95$\pm$11.0	77.56$\pm$20.3

   To obtain a more accurate estimate of the dilation of the right and
left ventricular cavities during infection, we also examined the effects
of virus infection on right and left ventricular area. In the uninfected
controls, the area within the right ventricular cavity was 38.82$\pm$11.76 x
10^{6}um^2 and 41.23$\pm$13.11 x 10^{6}um^2 between days 3-5 and 6-12, respectively.
Following RbCV infection, area in the right ventricular cavity increased

dramatically during the acute (100 ± 39.74 x 10^6um^2; p<0.001), and during the subacute phases of infection (146.20 ± 51.79 x 10^6um^2; p<0.001) (Table 1). Area within the left ventricular cavity was similar between the uninfected control animals sacrificed between days 3-5 or 6-12 (uninfected acute-57.56 ± 6.09 x 10^6um^2; uninfected subacute-59.95 ± 11.03 x 10^6um^2). Viral infection did not result in significant increases in the area within the left ventricular cavity during the acute phase (66.18 ± 25.04 x 10^6um^2; p<0.29), but significant increase were evident during the subacute phase of infection (77.56 ± 20.29 x 10^6um^2; p<0.025) (Table 1).

Pathologic Findings during RbCV Infection

Yellowish-white patches were seen on the surface of the ventricles of infected rabbits after 3-4 days post-infection. Histological changes in the heart consisted of degeneration and necrosis of myocytes and interstitial edema through day 12 post-infection. Little if any myocarditis was detected through day 8 or 9 post-infection consistent with previous findings by our group[11]. However, animals examined after day 9 had increasing amounts of myocarditis in the heart muscle (Figure 3a). Calcification was rarely present, but occasionally detected in animals dying late in the subacute phase of the disease (Data not shown). Congestion of the lungs and liver was common in about 12% of the animals dying during infection especially in the latter phase of the subacute stage of infection (Figure 3b). Myocarditis was present in 100% of the survivors through 65 days post-infection and a significant percentage (~30%) had evidence of right and/or left-sided dilated cardiomyopathy.

A   **B**

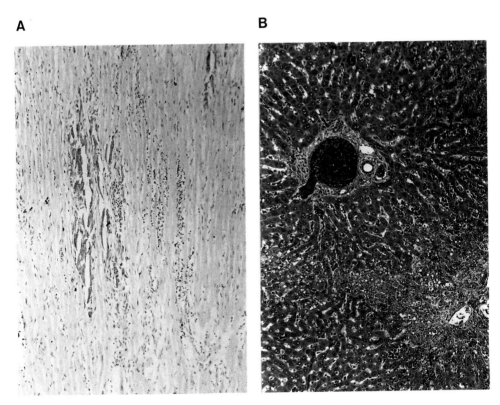

FIGURE 3. Pathologic Examination of RbCV-Infected Animals
Panel A: Myocardititis 12 days post-ingection; Panel B: congestion of the liver.

DISCUSSION

Heart disease is associated with a variety of viral infections in man and experimental animals. Viral infections may cause degeneration and necrosis of myocytes, myocarditis, and/or progress to dilated cardiomyopathy[1,2,3]. Dilated cardiomyopathy is probably a common end product of a variety of cardiac disorders including viral infections, alcohol and other conditions[1,4]. Few model systems for virus-induced myocarditis and dilated cardiomyopathy are amenable to experimental analysis and have been limited to picornavirus infection in mice[7,8,9]. In this article, we describe a new model system for virus-induced myocarditis and dilated cardiomyopathy in rabbits. The etiologic agent is probably a enveloped RNA virus antigenically related to the group II human and porcine coronaviruses[11]. RbCV is also antigenically related to the etiologic agent responsible for pleural effusion disease in rabbits (PEDV) and both viruses produce similar diseases in vivo[12].

Rabbit coronavirus infection produces a similar disease as EMC infection in mice. EMC infection in BALB-C mice results in myocarditis, extensive calcification, dilation of the heart and ventricles and about 15% of the animals die from congestive heart failure. EMC-infected DBA-2 mice develop dilation and hypertrophy of the heart muscle, myocarditis, extensive calcification and fibrosis by 3 months post-infection. This model represents the best studied system for virus-induced dilated cardiomyopathy. In the rabbit model, animals dying during the acute stage of infection are characterized by right-sided degeneration and necrosis of myocytes and dilation of the right ventricle. The left ventricle is also infected but to a lesser extent. The most logical explanation for the increase in heart weight, heart weight/body weight ratios during the acute stage of infection is due to interstitial edema. Little or no myocarditis was evident through day 8 post-infection. During the subacute stage of the disease, a more global involvement of the heart muscle is noted, and interstitial edema is probably responsible for the increases in heart weight, heart weight/body weight ratios. Myocarditis peaks by 12-13 days post-infection after exposure to the virus. Calcification is rarely detected during infection and is only present in a small percentage of animals dying late in the subacute phase of the disease. Dilation of the ventricles, pleural effusion, ascites, pulmonary edema, and congestion of the lungs, liver, heart, and spleen are common findings in animals that die late in the subacute stage of infection (9 days). Death is probably due to congestive heart failure. Myocarditis (2 to ~15 foci) and fibrosis are detected in all survivors examined through 64 days post-infection. Roughly 30% of these animals have evidence of dilated right and/or left hearts. In contrast to findings in EMC infected animals, no calcification is detected in survivors. In this regard, pathologic findings in the rabbit are more typical of findings in humans suffering from dilated cardiomyopathy and consist of few inflammatory foci, dilated hearts, and little, if any, calcification. It is unclear whether dilation and hypertrophy of the heart muscle persists beyond 64 days post-infection.

Virus-induced congestive heart failure has been reported accompanying chicken pox, mumps, CBV, poliomyelitis, dengue and chikungunya fever viruses and influenza virus infection[1,2,3,4]. A mouse model system for CBV-induced dilated cardiomyopathy has been described in which infected mice are forced to swim during infection. Cardiac damage is concentrated in the left ventricle and intraventricular septum, particularly at the atrioventricular junction[10]. The mechanism by which EMC-induces myocarditis and dilated cardiomyopathy in mice is probably immune-mediated rather than due to direct virus cytotoxicity in myocytes[4]. In the rabbit model, significant cardiac damage is occurring prior to immune induction suggesting that direct virus cytotoxicity to myocytes is primarily responsible for the disease. This is supported by recent findings in our laboratory that cortisome-immunosuppressed animals are not protected from infection and are characterized by necrosis and degeneration of myocytes and right ventricular dilation (Edwards, et al, manuscript in preparation).

Dilated cardiomyopathy is normally recognized by ventricular dilation, hypertrophy of the heart muscle, and low ejection fractions[1,2,3,4]. In most patients, the left ventricle is more severely effected. However, a variety of right-sided disorders have been reported in man and experimental animals. Right-sided perimyocarditis has been described previously during CBV3 infection of BALB-C mice[20], and idiopathic right ventricular myocardial hypoplasia in association with right ventricular dilation (Uhl's anomaly) is well documented in children[21]. Right ventricular dilated cardiomyopathy occurs in humans and is characterized by a male preponderance, syncope, ventricular tachycardia and right heart failure. Clinically, right-sided heart failure has a poor prognosis in humans[22]. The mechanism by which RbCV produces a predominantly right-sided disease is unclear. This model will provide new insight into the mechanism by which viruses cause heart disease and right-sided dilated cardiomyopathy in rabbits. This model is particularly important since rabbits are amenable to a variety of experimental techniques not available in mice and will allow us to measure hemodyamic alterations and muscle contractibility at different times post-infection.

ACKNOWLEDGEMENTS

This work was supported by grants from the National Institute of Health (AI 23946) and the American Heart Association (AHA 871135). This work was done during the tenure of an Established Investigator from the American Heart Association (AHA 890193)(RSB).

REFERENCES

1. Woodruff, J.F.(1980). Am. J. Path. 101:427-478.
2. Abelmann, W.H.(1973). Ann. Rev. Med. 24:145-152.
3. Bolte, H.-D. eds.(1984). In: Viral Heart Disease, Springer-Verlag, New York, New York, pgs. 1-247.
4. Kishimoto, C. et al.(186) Cardiovascular Res. 20:665-671.
5. Hudson, E.B.(1972). In: Cardiomyopathy, G.E. Burch eds, Philadelphia Davis Co., p4.
6. Burch, G.E. and DePasquale, N.P.(1970). Circulation 42:A-47-53.
7. Woodruff, J.F. and Woodruff, J.J.(1974). J.Imm. 113:1726-1734.
8. Matsumori, A., and Kawai, C.(182). Circulation 66:355-360.
9. Matsumori,A., and Kawai, C.(1982). Circulation 64:1230-1235.
10. Reyes, M.P. et al.(1981). J. Inf. Dis. 144:232-236.
11. Small, J.D. et al.(1979). Am. J. Path. 95:707.
12. Fennestad, R.L. Et al.(1986). J. Gen. Virol. 67:993-1000.
13. Matsumori, A. and Kawai, C.(1984). In: Viral Heart Disease, Bolte, H.-D ed, New York, NY pgs 35-56.
14. Kishimoto, M.D. et al.(1985). Circul. 71:1247.
15. Matsumori, A. and Kawai, C.(1982). Circulation 66: 1349-1350.
16. Wolf, D.K.(1981). In: Int. of Electropheretic pattern of proteins and isoenzymes. Masson Pub., New York, NY, pp56-60.
17. Lukehart, S.A. et al(1981). J. Imm. 127:1361.
18. Fennestad, R.L.(1983). Arch. of Virol. 76:179-187.
19. Mackarthur, C.G.C. et al(1984). J. 5:1023-1035.
20. Matsumori, A. and Kawai, C.)1980) J. Path. 131:97-106.
21. Uhl, H.S.M.(1952) Bull. John Hopkins Hosp. 91:197-209.
22. Fitchett, D.H. et al(1984).

RETINOPATHY FOLLOWING INTRAVITREAL INJECTION OF MICE WITH MHV STRAIN JHM

Susan G. Robbins, Barbara Detrick and John J. Hooks

National Eye Institute, National Institutes of Health

Bethesda, Maryland

INTRODUCTION

The causes of many human degenerative and inflammatory diseases of the retina are unknown. Some are genetic in origin; others are preceded by viral infections (Ryan and Maumenee, 1972; Annesley et al., 1973; Fitzpatrick and Robertson, 1973; Bos and Deutman, 1975; Wright et al., 1978). These diseases are difficult to study since eye tissue from patients is rarely available. Thus, animal models are considered useful for understanding their pathogenesis.

The neurotropic coronavirus mouse hepatitis virus (MHV) strain JHM causes both acute and chronic CNS disease in rodents (Cheever et al., 1949; Bailey et al., 1949; Weiner, 1973; Herndon et al., 1975; Goto et al., 1977; Nagashima et al., 1978; Stohlman and Weiner, 1981). Prior to our studies, it had also been shown to cause abnormalities in the posterior pole of the eye. In the earliest studies of JHM-induced disease in mice, Bailey and colleagues detected small retinal lesions confined to the nerve fiber layer (Bailey et al., 1949); this was also mentioned by Barthold and Smith (1987). Furthermore, it was shown that the virus caused demyelination of the optic nerve in rats after intracranial inoculation (Sorensen et al., 1980, 1981). That JHM was associated with retinal necrosis and optic neuritis suggested it could be a good candidate for studying virus-induced retinal degeneration. To study its effects on the retina, we chose to inoculate the virus directly onto the retina, i.e., intravitreally.

MATERIALS AND METHODS

The complete materials and methods have been described (Robbins et al., submitted). To summarize, twelve-week-old BALB/c mice were inoculated with MHV strain JHM (ATCC) grown in 17 Clone 1 cells (Sturman et al., 1980). Mice were anesthetized and sedated, then injected behind the lens. Extremely thin 33-gauge needles were used, and the eye punctured just behind the ciliary body. Left eyes were inoculated with 1.5×10^4 PFU of JHM in 5 ul, whereas right eyes were inoculated with mock-infected cell supernatant. Eyes were removed on specific days p.i. and either embedded for freezing or fixed with glutaraldehyde for methacrylate embedding and hematoxylin and eosin staining. Frozen sections were stained by an immunoperoxidase technique (Hsu et al., 1981), using a polyclonal rabbit serum (a gift from Dr. Kathryn V. Holmes) raised against NP40-disrupted MHV strain A59 virions.

Coronaviruses and Their Diseases
Edited by D. Cavanagh and T.D.K. Brown
Plenum Press, New York, 1990

MHV-specific serum IgG titers were determined by indirect ELISA.

RESULTS

Before describing the pathologic effects of the virus on the retina, we will describe the microanatomy of this organ, moving from its outer to inner layers (Fig. 1A). Exterior to the neural retina and adjacent to the choroid, lies the retinal pigment epithelium (RPE), which nourishes the photoreceptors, engulfs used outer segments and absorbs excess light. Interior to this layer lie the photoreceptor outer (OS), then inner (IS), segments. Next to these structures in the outer nuclear layer (ONL), lie the photoreceptor cell bodies. The cell bodies of the secondary neurons (bipolar, horizontal and amacrine) and supporting Müller (glial) cells are located in the inner nuclear layer (INL). Visual information is transmitted from them to the ganglion cells (GCL) and passed along the nerve fibers to the optic nerve.

Following intravitreal injection of JHM, histopathologic changes were evident by day 3, consisting of a few focal retinal lesions (Fig. 1B). Lesions were characterized by disorganization of the retinal layers, nuclear pyknosis, loss of inner and outer segments, abnormal RPE cells, and infiltration of macrophages to the subretinal space. From days 3-15, cells derived from the RPE were found accumulated at the periphery of the retina (Fig. 1C). The disease progressed to five or more lesions (containing macrophages) by day 6 (Fig. 1D). Enlarged RPE cell nuclei were apparent on day 10 (Fig. 1E). Long-term effects at one month included breaks in the RPE, reduction in the thickness of the photoreceptor layer, and abnormal ganglion cells (Fig. 1F). Because of the degenerative effects of the virus on the retina, we have termed this disorder "JHM retinopathy."

JHM antigens were detected in frozen sections of eyes by immunoperoxidase staining using both polyclonal and monoclonal antibodies, with similar results. The results from staining with polyclonal antiserum specific for viral structural proteins are shown in Figure 2. Sections of mock-injected eyes showed no reactivity (Fig. 2A). In virus-injected eyes on day 1, the iris and ciliary body contained viral antigen; by day 2, infection had spread to include the RPE and optic nerve. The RPE was stained very strongly on days 3 and 4 (Fig. 2B). In the neural retina, small areas of the ganglion cell and nerve fiber layers were antigen-positive and the other layers were beginning to express antigen. On day 6, radial staining patterns strongly resembling Müller cells lay across the neural retina (Fig. 2C). The photoreceptor inner and outer segments and optic nerve (Fig. 2E) also reacted with the virus-specific antiserum. On day 7, little antigen was detected in the inner and outer nuclear layers, and none was detectable by immunoperoxidase staining on subsequent days. Virus-specific serum IgG was first detected on day 5 and reached the maximum which could be measured, on day 8.

DISCUSSION

We have shown that mice inoculated intravitreally with MHV-JHM develop an acute infection of the retina (as well as anterior structures) which peaks at about 6 days. Infection of the retina appears to begin in both the RPE and ganglion cells, from which it spreads to the photoreceptors, Müller cells, inner layers of the retina and optic nerve. Thus, the retinal aspect of this disease is probably a primary pigmentary retinopathy, such as congenital rubella retinopathy (Zimmerman, 1968) and measles retinitis (Nelson et al., 1970). Our model of virus-induced retinopathy is interesting and distinct from other viral diseases of the retina in that it is more degenerative than inflammatory, it occurs in adult animals, and the retinal disease is prolonged after the apparent disappearance of viral

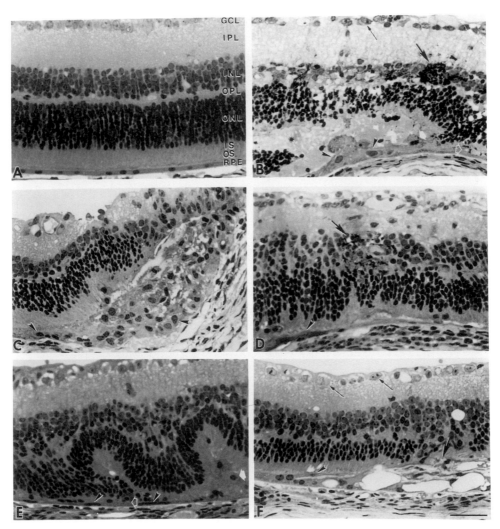

Fig. 1. Retinal changes after intravitreal inoculation with JHM. (A) Retina of mock-injected eye, day 3, showing normal architecture (RPE,
retinal pigment epithelium; OS, photoreceptor outer segments; IS,
photoreceptor inner segments; ONL, outer nuclear layer; OPL, outer
plexiform layer; INL, inner nuclear layer; IPL, inner plexiform
layer; GCL, ganglion cell layer). (B-F) Retinas of virus-injected
eyes. (B) Day 3. There are abnormalities in RPE cells (arrowheads),
loss of outer segments (open arrow), red blood cells (*), an occasional macrophage in the subretinal space (white arrow), nuclear
pyknosis (large arrow), and abnormal ganglion cells (small arrow).
(C) Periphery of the retina, day 3. Cells derived from the RPE had
accumulated (arrowheads). (D) Day 6. A lesion is shown (arrow).
RPE abnormalities continued to be present (arrowhead). (E) Day 10.
Pathologic changes, by then diffuse, included enlarged RPE nuclei
(arrowheads), loss of many outer segments (open arrow) and subretinal macrophages (white arrow). (F) Day 30. The photoreceptor
layer had narrowed significantly. In a few places the RPE had
thinned (arrowhead) and breaks in the RPE and Bruch's membrane
had occurred (arrow). Abnormal ganglion cells were still present
(small arrows). Hematoxylin and eosin stains. Bar = 5 microns.

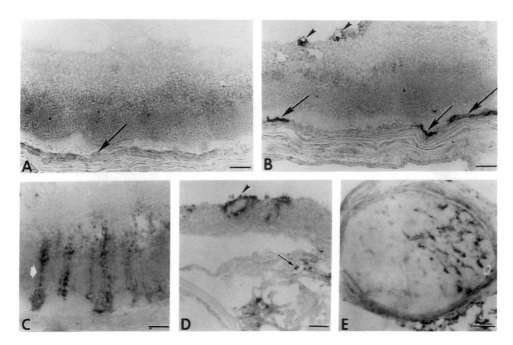

Fig. 2. Localization of viral antigens in JHM-infected eyes by immunoperoxidase staining. (A) Retina of mock-injected eye, day 4, revealing no reactivity with virus-specific antiserum. (B) Retina of
virus-injected eye, day 4. The RPE and two areas in the ganglion
cell layer stained with anti-viral antibody. (C) Retina of virus-
injected eye, day 5. The fibers spanning the layers of the neural
retina, which are most likely Müller cells, were stained with
virus-specific antiserum. (D) Iris and ciliary body of virus-injected eye, day 4. The iris endothelium (arrowhead) and stroma, as
well as the ciliary body (arrow) contained viral antigen.
(E) Optic nerve in cross section, extending from virus-injected
eye, day 6. Antibody staining occurred in septal (glial) cells of
nerve bundles (open arrow). Bars = 5 microns.

antigen. We plan to investigate the possibility of viral RNA persistence
using in situ hybridization.

Coronaviruses clearly cause very different ocular diseases in different
species. JHM retinopathy in mice involves a mild uveitis (ocular inflammation) which resembles slightly the "non-effusive" uveitis seen in some
feline infectious peritonitis virus (FIPV) infections (Doherty, 1971). The
two diseases have very different causes, however; the former primarily results from the direct effects of the virus, whereas the latter is immune-
mediated (August, 1984). FIPV causes a variety of symptoms in the central
nervous system, of which the eye is a direct extension developmentally
(Slauson and Finn, 1972). The major ocular symptom is a necrotizing and
pyogranulomatous uveitis involving blood vessels, brought on by an Arthus-
type reaction (Krebiel et al., 1974). Ocular symptoms sometimes occur in
the absence of systemic disease symptoms (Kern, 1984).

Superficially, JHM retinopathy and sialodacryoadenitis virus (SDAV) infection share the characteristic of retinal atrophy, but they probably occur
by different means. SDAV classically causes inflammation of the salivary
and harderian glands in rats. Also, keratoconjunctivitis has been observed,
lasting 3-5 weeks (Lai et al., 1976; Weisbroth and Peress, 1977). Retinal
atrophy may occur in rats with enlarged eyes; the retinal lesions are either
focal or diffuse. Paradoxically, no viral antigen was detected in retinas
by immunofluorescence staining, although it was found in harderian glands.

Therefore, the retinal changes may be only secondary to the glaucoma-like disease (Lai et al., 1976).

Infectious bronchitis virus may be transmitted to birds by aerosol/droplet inoculation of the eye (Cowen et al., 1971), from which the virus drains into the respiratory tract. However, replication of the virus in the eye or its supporting tissues has not been reported.

There is one study of eye infection in piglets infected with hemagglutinating encephalomyelitis virus (HEV) (Andries and Pensaert, 1980). Eye tissue from one of two piglets infected with HEV strain VW572 was positive for viral antigen in immunofluorescence tests. This was attributed to centrifugal spread of the virus from the CNS. HEV causes early gastrointestinal effects, followed by encephalitis. One of its numerous CNS effects is blindness (Andries and Pensaert, 1981). The existing data suggest that blindness could be due to lesions in the CNS and/or eye.

Unfortunately, there are no data as yet indicating whether coronaviruses infect human eyes. Because they are neurotropic for human cells in tissue culture (Pearson and Mims, 1985), one can speculate that, given the right circumstances (e.g., damage to the choroid coupled with viremia), introduction of a coronavirus into the retina could lead to retinal disease and optic neuritis.

ACKNOWLEDGMENTS

We thank Dr. W. Richard Green, Wilmer Eye Institute, Johns Hopkins University, for consultation on the ocular pathologic effects of the virus. The technical assistance of Mary Alice Crawford and Nicole Newman is also appreciated.

REFERENCES

Andries, K., and Pensaert, M.B., 1980, Immunofluorescence studies on the pathogenesis of hemagglutinating encephalomyelitis virus infection in pigs after oronasal inoculation, Am. J. Vet. Res., 41:1372.

Andries, K., and Pensaert, M., Vomiting and wasting disease, in: "Biochemistry and Biology of Coronaviruses," V. ter Meulen, S. Siddell, and H. Wege, ed., Plenum Press, New York (1981).

Annesley, W.H., Tomer, T.L., and Shields, J.A., 1973, Multifocal placoid pigment epitheliopathy, Am. J. Ophthalmol., 76:511.

August, J.R., 1984, Feline infectious peritonitis. An immune-mediated coronaviral vasculitis, Vet. Clin. N. Amer: Sm. Anim. Prac., 14:971.

Bailey, O.T., Pappenheimer, A.M., Cheever, F.S., and Daniels, J.B., 1949, A murine virus (JHM) causing disseminated encephalomyelitis with extensive destruction of myelin. II. Pathology, J. Exp. Med., 90:195.

Barthold, S.W., and Smith, A.L., 1987, Response of genetically susceptible and resistant mice to intranasal inoculation with mouse hepatitis virus JHM, Virus Res., 7:225.

Bos, P.J.M., and Deutman, A.F., 1975, Acute macular neuroretinopathy, Am. J. Ophthalmol., 80:573.

Cheever, F.S., Daniels, J.B., Pappenheimer, A.M., and Bailey, O.T., 1949, A murine virus (JHM) causing disseminated encephalomyelitis with extensive destruction of myelin. I. Isolation and biologic properties of the virus. J. Exp. Med. 90:181.

Cowen, B.S., Hitchner, S.B., and Lucio, B., 1971, Characterization of a new infectious bronchitis virus isolate. I. Serological and pathogenicity studies of Clark 333, Avian Dis., 15:518.

Deutman, A.F., 1974, Acute retinal pigment epitheliitis, Am. J. Ophthalmol., 78:571.

Doherty, M.J., 1971, Ocular manifestations of feline infectious peritonitis, J. Am. Vet. Med. Assn., 159:417.

Fitzpatrick, P.J., and Robertson, D.M., 1973, Acute posterior multifocal placoid pigment epitheliopathy, Arch. Ophthalmol., 89:373.

Gass, J.D.M., 1968, Acute posterior multifocal placoid pigment epitheliopathy, Arch. Ophthalmol., 80:177.

Goto, N., Hirano, N., Aiuchi, M., Hayashi, T., and Fugiwara, K., 1977, Nasoencephalopathy of mice infected intranasally with a mouse hepatitis virus, JHM strain, Jpn. J. Exp. Med., 47:59.

Herndon, R.M., Griffin, D.E., McCormick, U., and Weiner, L.P., 1975, Mouse hepatitis virus-induced recurrent demyelination: A preliminary report, Arch. Neurol., 32:32.

Hsu, S., Raine, L., and Fanger, H., 1981, Use of avidin-biotin-peroxidase complex (ABC) in immunoperoxidase techniques: a comparison between ABC and unlabeled antibody (PAP) procedures, J. Histochem. Cytochem., 29:577.

Kern, T.J., 1984, Intraocular inflammation in cats as a manifestation of systemic diseases, Cornell Feline Hlth. Ctr. News, Winter, p.4.

Krebiel, J.D., Sanger, V.L., and Ravi, A., 1974, Ophthalmic lesions in feline infectious peritonitis: gross, microscopic and ultrastructural changes, Vet. Path., 11:442.

Lai, Y.L., Jacoby, R.O., Bhatt, P.N., and Jonas, A.M., 1976, Keratoconjunctivitis associated with sialodacryoadenitis in rats, Invest. Ophthalmol., 15:538.

Nagashima, K., Wege, H., Meyermann, R., and ter Meulen, V., 1978, Coronavirus induced subacute demyelinating encephalomyelitis in rats: A morphological analysis, Acta Neuropathol. (Berl.)., 44:63.

Nelson, D.A., Weiner, A., Yanoff, M., and de Peralta, J., 1970, Retinal lesions in subacute sclerosing panencephalitis, Arch. Ophthalmol., 84:613.

Pearson, J., and Mims, C.A., 1985, Differential susceptibility of cultured neural cells to the human coronavirus OC43, J. Virol., 53:1016

Robbins, S.G., Hamel, C.P., Detrick, B., and Hooks, J.J., submitted, Murine coronavirus induces an acute and long-lasting disease of the retina, Lab. Invest.

Ryan, S.J., and Maumenee, A.E., 1972, Acute posterior multifocal placoid pigment epitheliopathy, Am. J. Ophthalmol., 74:1066.

Slauson, D.O., and Finn, J.P., 1972, Meningoencephalitis and panophthalmitis in feline infectious peritonitis, J. Am. Vet. Med. Assn., 160:729.

Sorensen, O., Perry, D., and Dales, S., 1980, In vivo and in vitro models of demyelinating diseases. III. JHM virus infection of rats, Arch. Neurol., 37:478.

Sorensen, O., Coulter-Mackie, M., Percy, D., and Dales, S., 1982, In vivo and in vitro models of demyelinating diseases, in: "Biochemistry and Biology of Coronaviruses," V. ter Meulen, S. Siddell, and H. Wege, eds, Plenum Press, New York (1981).

Stohlman, S.A., and Weiner, L.P., 1981, Chronic central nervous system demyelination in mice after JHMV virus infection, Neurology, 31:38.

Sturman, L.S., Holmes, K.V., and Behnke, J.N., 1980, Isolation of coronavirus envelope glycoproteins and interaction with the viral nucleocapsid, J. Virol., 33:449.

Weiner, L.P., 1973, Pathogenesis of demyelination induced by a mouse hepatitis virus (JHM virus), Arch. Neurol., 28:298.

Weisbroth, S.H., and Peress, N., 1977, Ophthalmic lesions and dacryoadenitis: a naturally occurring aspect of sialodacryoadenitis virus infection of the laboratory rat, Lab. Animal. Sci., 27:466.

Wright, B.E., Bird, A.C., and Hamilton, A.M., 1978, Placoid pigment epitheliopathy and Harada's disease, Br. J. Ophthalmol., 62:609.

Zimmerman, L.E., 1968, Histopathologic basis for ocular manifestations of congenital rubella syndrome, Am. J. Ophthalmol., 65:837.

REPRODUCTIVE DISORDERS IN FEMALE SHR RATS INFECTED WITH

SIALODACRYOADENITIS VIRUS

Kenjiro Utsumi, Yutaka Yokota, Takashi Ishikawa,
Kunio Ohnishi and Kosaku Fujiwara*

Research Laboratories
Dainippon Pharmaceutical Ltd.
Suita 564 and
*Nihon University School of Veterinary Medicine
Fujisawa 252
Japan

ABSTRACT

Effects of sialodacryoadenitis virus infection on the
reproduction of female SHR rats were studied. The oestrous cycle
was considerably perturbed in most infected rats, the per-
turbation was observed initially between Days 0 to 10 post
infection and the effect persisted for 6 to 18 days. About half
of the foetuses of dams infected on Day 0 of gestation were
found dead while only 4% of the foetuses from non-infected dams
were found dead. Five or six days after infection on Day 0 of
gestation, some infected dams were shown to have metritis, and
virus antigen was detectable within the endometrium as well as
exudate cells. In dams infected on Day 5 or later of gestation
and severely diseased, the offspring showed a low survival rate
possibly because of inadequate nursing.

INTRODUCTION

In pregnant mice infected with mouse hepatitis virus (MHV)
foetal death due to vertical transmission of the virus was observed (1,2,3). We previously reported that breeder rats
naturally infected with sialodacryoadenitis virus (SDAV),
another member of coronaviridae, showed apparent disorders in
the oestrous cycle and lowered reproduction rate (4). The
experiments described below were designed to effects of experimental SDAV infection on the oestrous cycle as well as gestation
of female SHR rats; this strain of rat is known to be highly
susceptible to the infection (4).

MATERIALS AND METHODS
Animals. Male and female SHR rats, F14 of brother-sister mating,
were supplied in 1968 by the Department of Pathology, Kyoto
University Medical School. They were randomly bred at this
laboratory, and a Caesarean-derived colony was established in
1972 (5). The colony had been serologically monitored for

freedom from SDAV infection (6). Animals were kept on a commercial bedding (White Flake, Charles River Japan, Atsugi) in metal cages (200x305x130mm) and given pellets(CA-1, Japan CLEA, Tokyo) and tap water. The animal room was kept at $24\pm2°C$, $55\pm5\%$ relative humidity and lighting for 12 hours per day. The air was exchanged ten times/hour. Animals were used for experiments at 13 to 19 weeks of age. Each morning Giemsa-stained vaginal smear preparations were examined microscopically and females found to be at the pro-oestrus were mated.

SDAV. Strain TG of SDAV (7) from a naturally infected rat was subjected to seven passages in rats by intranasal (i.n.) inoculation of infected sub-maxillary gland tissue. The affected gland tissue was homogenized in phosphate buffered saline, pH 7.2, and i.n. inoculation into dams was made with $2.5\text{x}10^2$ LD_{50} in 0.05 ml between Days 6 and 15 of gestation. LD_{50} was determined for suckling ICR mice inoculated intracerebrally (i.c.). For detecting infectious virus in tissue samples from dams, 2-day-old suckling ICR mice from an MHV-free breeder (Japan CLEA, Tokyo) were used.

Complement fixation(CF) test. The TG strain of SDAV, which was grown on LBC cells (8), was treated with diethylether and used in the CF test (6).

Histopathology: Tissues of the salivary gland, pregnant uterus, brain and other major organs were sampled from infected dams and foetuses as well as suckling mice, and they were fixed in phosphate-buffered formalin, pH 7.2. Paraffin sections were made and stained with hematoxylin and eosin (HE).For detecting SDAV antigen on tissue sections the avidin-biotin-complex(ABC) method (9) was applied using rabbit or mouse antiserum to MHV-2 sharing common antigens with SDAV (6,10,11) and a commercial kit (Stravingen, Bio-Genex, California). Anti-MHV rabbit serum was kindly supplied by Prof. N. Goto, Department of Veterinary Pathology, University of Tokyo. The results of the immuno-histochemistry were confirmed by immunofluorescence (12) using fluorescein-conjugated goat antiserum to rabbit or mouse IgG (Serotec, Oxford).

RESULTS

After i.n. inoculation of SDAV into twenty 13-week-old female SHR rats, all the animals showed apparent clinical signs of sialoadenitis on Days 4 to 7 post-inoculation (p.i.)(Fig. 1). Through the course of observation one of them had a regular oestrous cycle of 4 days, but 19 of 20 (95%) were found to have signifcant disorder in the cycle starting on Days 0 to 10 p.i. and persisting for 6 to 18 days.

The next experiment was carried out to study effect of SDAV infection on pregnancy. Three groups of 7 female rats of age 14 weeks received i.n. inoculation of the virus 2, 3 or 4 days before gestation, while two groups of 7 rats received i.n. inoculation on Day 0 or 2 of gestation. Another group of 10 rats remained uninfected. On Day 14 of pregnancy all animals were sacrificed and examined for foetuses. As presented in Table 1 and Fig.2, 16 of 83 (19%), 33 of 68 (49%) and 10 of 44 (23%) foetuses were found aborted or dead in dams infected on Days -2, 0 and 2 of gestation, respectively. Only 7 of 108 (6%) foetuses were dead in non-infected dams. Similar results were obtained in another experiment using 19-week-old females (Table 1). In dams infected on Day 0 of gestation, 43 of 94 (46%) foetuses were aborted or dead on Day 14 p.i.

```
              SDAV   Clinical
Case  Day p.i.  ↓     SDA
No.    -5        0   ←—5—→    10        15
 1   - E - - - E - - - E - - - E - - - E - - - E - - - E
 2   - - - E - - - E M D D P E M M D P E - - - E - - - E
 3   - - - E - - - E E D D P E M D P E E D D P E E M P P
 4   - E - - - E - - - E M D P M M P P E - - - E - - - E
 5   - E - - - E - - - E M D D D D D P E - - - E - - - E
 6   - E - - - E - - - E M D P M M E E D D P E E - - - E
 7   - - E - - - E - - - E M M D D P E - - - E - - - E -
 8   - - E - - - E - - - E E M D D D P E - - E - - - E -
 9   - - E - - - E - - - E M M P E E M D P E E - - - E -
10   - - E - - - E - - - E E D D D D P E D D P E - - - E
11   - - - E - - - E - - - E M M D P E - - - E - - - E -
12   - - - E - - - E - - - E M M M D D P P E - - - E - -
13   - - - E - - - E - - - E M D D D P E E D D P E - - -
14   E - - - E - - - E - - - E M D D P E - - - E - - - E
15   E - - - E - - - E - - - E M D D P E E - - - E - - -
16   E - - - E - - - E - - - E M D D P E D D P E - - - E
17   E - - - E - - - E - - - E M D D P E E M D P E - - -
18   E - - - E - - - E - - - E M M D D M E E M D P E - -
19   - E - - - E - - - E - - - E D D P E E - - - E - -
20   - E - - - E - - - E - - - E - - - E E M D P E E D D
```

Fig. 1. Irregular estrous cycles in 13-week-old SHR rats infected with SDAV. P:Proestrus, E:Estrus, M:Metestrus, D:Diestrus, determined by vaginal smear examination.

Table 1. Mortality of embryos in SDAV-infected SHR dams

Age of dams	SDAV[a] (i.n.)	Number of dams		Number of implanted embryos[c]		
		Mated[b]	Gestated	Mean±S.D.	Total	Dead(%)
14W	Day -4 of gestation	7	7	7.7±4.1	54	8(15%)
	-3	7	7	10.9±1.4	76	4(5%)
	-2	7	7	11.9±1.5	83	16(19%)
	0	7	6	11.3±3.5	68	33(49%)
	2	7	5	8.8±5.2	44	10(23%)
	Not inoculated	10	10	10.8±1.6	108	7(6%)
19W	Day -5 of gestation	7	7	12.3±2.2	86	9(10%)
	-4	6	5	11.2±2.1	56	12(21%)
	-3	6	6	12.8±1.9	77	11(14%)
	-2	5	5	12.2±4.3	61	6(10%)
	0	8	8	11.8±2.0	94	43(46%)
	2	6	6	12.3±2.0	74	5(7%)
	Not inoculated	10	10	11.4±2.2	114	2(2%)

a) 2.5×10^2 LD_{50} for suckling mice(i.c.).
b) Positive for sperms on vaginal smear.
c) On Day 14 of gestation.

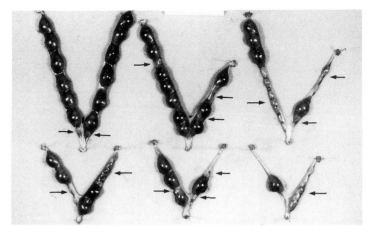

Fig. 2. Pregnant uteruses from dams inoculated i.n. on Day 0 of gestation, showing implanted, but dead or aborted embryos (arrows) present at Day 14.

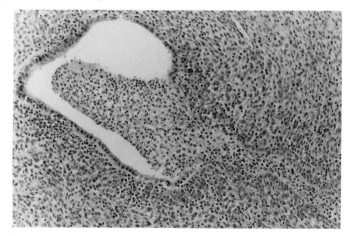

Fig.3. Exudative and desquamative endometritis in a dam infected on Day 0 of gestation.Day 6 p.i. HE stain.

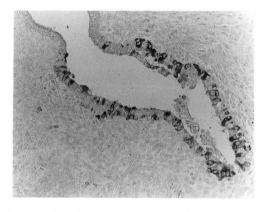

Fig.4. SDAV antigen within the endometrium of a dam infected on Day 0 of gestation. Day 6 p.i. Anti-MHV rabbit serum-ABC and methyl green stain.

Table 2. Effect of diet restriction on the mortality of
embryos

SDAV[a] (i.n.)	Diet	Number of dams	Number of implanted embryos[b]		
			Mean±S.D.	Total	Dead(%)
−	Restricted[c]	6	11.5±2.1	69	0
−	ad libitum	6	9.8±2.6	59	1(2%)
+	ad libitum	7	12.1±2.9	85	22(26%)

a) 2.5×10^2 LD_{50} for suckling mice(i.c.).
b) On Day 14 of gestation.
c) 4 g pellets per day for 4 days(Days 3 to 6 of gestation).

Table 3. Mortality of youngs from SDAV-infected SHR dams

Age of dams	SDAV[a] (i.n.)	Gestation period in days	Number of dams		Number of youngs		
			Delivered	Nursing	Litter size[b]	Total	Dead(%)[c]
13W	Day 2 of gestation	21,22	6	5	11.5	69	17(25%)
	5	22	6	5	11.7	70	14(20%)
	10	21,22	6	5	11.2	67	36(54%)
	15	23,24	4	0	8.8	35	35(100%)
	Not inoculated	22	5	4	11.0	55	19(35%)
16W	Day 2 of gestation	21–23	5	5	6.8	34	3(9%)
	5	22,23	6	5	8.7	52	5(10%)
	10	22,23	5	5	12.0	60	3(5%)
	15	22–25	5	2	9.0	27	13(48%)
	Not inoculated	22,23	6	5	11.2	67	15(22%)

a) 2.5×10^2 LD_{50} for suckling mice(i.c.).
b) Mean.
c) At 2 weeks of age.

To see whether the death of embryos described above
resulted from SDAV infection *in utero*, 10 dams were inoculated
i.n. with the virus on Day 0 of gestation, and they were sacrificed 5 or 6 days later and examined for pathology of the
pregnant uterus. The uteruses from 3 dams were shown to have
severe endometritis with desquamated endometrium and accumulation of neutrophils and mononuclear cells in the lumen
(Fig.3). By immunohistochemistry SDAV antigen was detectable
within the endometrium as well as exudate cells (Fig.4). By i.c.
inoculation of affected uterine tissue into suckling mice,
infectious virus was recovered which produced fatal encephalitis
with viral antigen within neurons. Such viral metritis could not
be produced in non-pregnant females, which had received the same
virus inoculation and showed apparent sialoadenitis. Since food
consumption was noticed to decrease during clinical mani-

festation of sialoadenitis, the effect of dietary restriction on
the viability of embryos was studied. Nineteen females aged 13
weeks were mated with males, and 6 of them were given 4g of
pelleted diet per day for 4 days between Days 3 and 6 of gestation. The remaining 13 rats were fed *ad libitum* and 7 of them
received i.n. inoculation of SDAV on Day 0 of gestation. All the
animals were sacrificed and examined for the number of dead
embryos on Day 14 of gestation. As shown in Table 2, 22 of 85
(26%) embryos were found dead in SDAV-infected dams given full
diet. However, there was no fetal death in dams with dietary
restriction.

In the foregoing experiments, dams infected on Day 2 of
gestation showed a lower rate of fetal death than those infected
on Day 0 (Table 1). The next experiment was done to see the
survival rate of sucklings from dams infected on Day 2 or later
of gestation. Thirty females were divided into 5 groups of 6
animals after mating, and 4 groups were exposed to i.n. inoculation of SDAV while the remaing one remained uninoculated.

Clinical signs of sialoadenitis were apparent in all dams 4
to 9 days after virus inoculation, that is, on Days 6 to 11,
Days 9 to 14, Days 14 to 19 or Days 19 to 24 of gestation in
each infected group. As shown in Table 3, dams infected on Day
15 of gestation had a considerably decreased number of newborns
and none of the pups survived for 2 weeks. In other groups which
were infected at an earlier stage of gestation, the mortality of
newborns was rather lower than in non-infected controls which
showed unexpectedly high mortality in this experiment. No
specific lesions were observed in any organs of sucklings from
infected and non-infected dams. Dams in all the groups were
shown to have CF antibody to SDAV at a titer of 1:160 or 1:320.

Similar results were obtained in another experiment using
16 week-old females, and 13 of 27(48%) sucklings from dams
infected on Day 15 of gestation were found dead before 2 weeks
of age.

DISCUSSION

The SHR rat is known to be difficult to breed and rear
because of high susceptibility to infectious agents (13, 14).
Natural SDAV infection in laboratory rats has been revealed to
cause disorders in the oestrous cycle and to lower the gestation
rate to 50% resulting in poor reproductive performance (4,11).
In this study with SHR rats the disorder was shown to appear
already at the first estrus after inoculation of SDAV, persisting for more than 6 days. The oestrous cycle was disturbed
in 40% of Wistar and Sprague-Dawley rats after infection with
SDAV (unpublished observation). In SHR rats, however, almost all
infected females showed remarkably irregular cycles, persisting
as long as 19 days.

When the virus was inoculated on the Day 1 of gestation,
almost a half of embryos were found dead, possibly as a result
of viremia and infectious metritis occurring at the early stage
of embryonic development. Most embryonic deaths seemed to occur
on Day 6 or 7 of gestation when the virus titer in the maternal
blood circulation was reported to be declining (15). At this
stage of infection, affected dams were shown still to have
severe inflammation in the submaxillary glands with the presence

of a great deal of virus, which might be the source of viremia. Moreover, the feto-maternal communication in the uterus should be close enough to cause the involvement of embryos in the local inflammation. In the uteruses of infected dams, which had dead or aborted embryos, viral antigen was detectable within *in situ* and desquamated endometrial cells as well as in exudate cells in the lumen. Infectious virus was successfully recovered from the affected uterine tissue by inoculation into the brains of suckling mice. These findings suggested that the death or abortion of embryos in SDAV-infected dams might be due to viral metritis involving the embryos implanted shortly before the onset of maternal illness.

No correlation was found between embryonic death and decreased diet consumption of the dams having severe signs of sialoadenitis.

The embryonic death rate was lower when dams were infected before or shortly after the start of gestation than when infected at the start of gestation. The number of dead embryos was not so great in dams inoculated at a later stage in gestation. However the delivery of young was retarded and most newborns died within 2 weeks of birth. Such retarded delivery and delayed death of young might result from inadequate nursing by seriously diseased dams infected shortly before parturition. Some dams who delivered normally were shown to have high serum antibody titres and to protect their young by transfer of maternal antibody via milk as described previously (15,16).

Reproductive performance has been reported to be adversely affected in mice infected with MHV (1) as well as in the fowl infected with avian infectious bronchitis virus (17). In the case of SDAV infection in rats, early abortion due to viral endometritis is a feature of the virus pathogenicity which manifests itself as sialodacryoadenitis in adult animals.

REFERENCES

1. K. Fujiwara, S. Tanaka and S. Shumiya, Carrier state of anti-bodies and viruses in a mouse breeding colony persistently infected with Sendai and mouse hepatitis virus, Lab. Anim. Sci., 26: 153 (1976).
2. H. Iwai, T. Ito, J. Yamanaka, Y. Ishihara, and S. Shumiya, Sero-epidemiological observation on mouse hepatitis virus in a mouse breeder colony, Exp. Anim., 22:259 (1973).
3. K. Katami, F. Taguchi, M. Nakayama, N. Goto, and K. Fujiwara, Vertical transmission of mouse hepatitis virus infection in mice, Jpn. J. Exp. Med., 48:481 (1978).
4. K. Utsumi, T. Ishikawa, T. Maeda, S. Shimizu, H. Tatsumi, and K. Fujiwara, Infectious sialodacryoadenitis and rat breeding, Lab. Anim. 14:303 (1980).
5. A. Nagaoka, K. Kikuchi, and Y. Arakawa, Production of specific pathogen free spontaneously hypertensive rats, Jpn. J. Const. Med., 30:135 (1967).
6. K. Fujiwara, Y. Tanishima, and M. Tanaka, Seromonitoring of laboratory mouse and rat colonies for common murine pathogens, Exp. Anim., 28:297 (1979).
7. R. Yamaguchi, F. Taguchi, A. Yamada, K. Utsumi, and K. Fujiwara, Pathogenicity of sialodacryoadenitis virus for rats after brain passages in suckling mice, Jpn. J. Exp. Med., 52:45 (1982).

8. N. Hirano, Y. Suzuki, K. Ono, T. Murakami, and K. Fujiwara, Growth of rat sialodacryoadenitis virus in LBC cell culture, Jpn. J. Vet. Sci., 48:93 (1986).

9. S. M. Hsu, and L. Raine, The use of avidin-biotin-peroxydase complex (ABC) in diagnostic and research pathology, in: "Advances in Immunohistochemistry", R. A. Delellis, ed., Masson Publ. USA, New York (1984).

10. M. Nakagawa, M. Saito, E. Suzuki, K. Nakayama, J. Matsubara, and T. Muto, Ten-years-long survey on pathogen status of mouse and rat breeding colonies, Exp. Anim., 33:115 (1984).

11. K. Utsumi, T. Maeda, H. Tatsumi, and K. Fujiwara, Some clinical and epizootiological observation of infectious sialoadenitis in rats, Exp. Anim., 27:283 (1978).

12. D. G. Brownstein, and S. W. Barthold, Mouse hepatitis virus immunofluorescence in formalin- or Bouin's-fixed tissues using trypsin digestion, Lab. Anim. Sci., 32:37 (1982).

13. N. Takeichi, Development of auto-antibodies in spontaneously hypertensive rats (SHR), Metabol. Dis., 20:997 (1983).

14. K. Tuch, T. Matthiesen, and F. Helm, Sialoadenitis in spontaneously hypertensive rats, Z. Versuchstierk., 19:40 (1977).

15. R. O. Jacoby, P. N. Bhatt, and A. M. Jonas, Pathogenesis of sialodacryoadenitis in gnotobiotic rats, Vet. Pathol., 12:196 (1975).

16. M. Maru, and K. Sato, Characterization of a coronavirus isolated from rats with sialoadenitis, Arch. Virol., 73:33 (1982).

17. M. S. Hofstad, Avian infectious bronchitis, in: "Diseases of Poultry, 6th ed.", M. S. Hofstad, ed., Iowa State Univ. Press, Ames (1972).

MECHANISM OF PROTECTIVE EFFECT OF PROSTAGLANDIN E IN MURINE HEPATITIS VIRUS STRAIN 3 INFECTION: EFFECTS ON MACROPHAGE PRODUCTION OF TUMOUR NECROSIS FACTOR, PROCOAGULANT ACTIVITY AND LEUKOTRIENE B4

S. Sinclair[1], M. Abecassis[1], P.Y. Wong[2], A. Romaschin[2], L.S. Fung[1] and G. Levy[1]

Departments of Medicine[1] and Biochemistry[2] University of Toronto, Toronto, Canada

INTRODUCTION

Murine hepatitis virus strain 3 (MHV-3) produces a strain dependent spectrum of liver disease. Mice of the A strain are fully resistant whereas Balb/cJ mice die of fulminant hepatic failure (1). The susceptibility of inbred mice to MHV-3, is dependent on host factors which are under strict genetic control. Differences in viral replication both in-vivo and in-vitro do not appear to account for strain-dependent differences in resistance to MHV-3 and it has been suggested that variation in susceptibility/resistance of inbred mice reflects defects in the host's immune response (2). Experimental ablation of the immune cell populations by X irradiation (3), antilymphocyte serum (4), or infection with frog virus-3 (5) renders resistant A/J mice susceptible. Furthermore, reconstitution of susceptible neonatal A/J mice with adult immune cells requires both T lymphocytes and an adherent cell population (6). More recently, it has been demonstrated that clearance of virus from the central nervous system is dependent upon the presence of both CD4+ and CD8+ cells that recognize viral antigens in the context of H-2D gene products (7).

Previously we have shown that susceptibility to MHV-3 in Balb/cJ mice is associated with an impaired early activation of the immune system as demonstrated by the failure of lymphocyte proliferation during in-vitro culture (8). At the same time however, macrophages from susceptible animals were able to produce a significant interleukin 1 response suggesting that macrophage activation may play a role in the pathogenesis of the disease (8). We have demonstrated that macrophages from susceptible animals upon stimulation with MHV-3 with T cell cooperation produce a protease which activates the coagulation system resulting in microcirculatory disturbances (9). The production of this protease is genetically linked to the resistance/ susceptibility genes and is not H-2 linked (10). We have shown that infusion of prostaglandin E_2 prevents fulminant viral hepatitis without altering viral replication (11).

Coronaviruses and Their Diseases
Edited by D. Cavanagh and T.D.K. Brown
Plenum Press, New York, 1990

Thus, it appears that following MHV-3 infection, activation of macrophages occurs with resultant production of monokines leading to immune activation of the coagulation system which appears to be important in the pathogenesis of MHV-3 infection. Macrophage activation results in production of specific inflammatory mediators including tumour necrosis factor (TNF) and leukotrienes (LTB_4). Early expression of these monokines has been implicated in a number of specific inflammatory processes. TNF can induce endothelial cell expression of procoagulant activity, down regulation of expression of thrombomodulin, adhesion of neutrophils, suppression of tissue plasminogen activator(s) and phospholipase A2 activity (12). The present studies were designed to determine whether differences occur in production of these monokines in peritoneal macrophages from susceptible (Balb/cJ) and resistant (A/J) mice following MHV-3 infection and to study the effects of exogenous $dmPGE_2$ on their production.

MATERIALS AND METHODS

Cells

The origin and growth of L2, DBT and 17CL1 cells has been described previously.

Peritoneal macrophages were obtained from A/J and Balb/cJ mice three days after intraperitoneal innoculation with 2 ml thioglycollate. Cells were adjusted to 1 x 10^6/ml of RPMI on 24 well plates (Costar, Cambridge, MA) for studies of TNF and eicosanoid (PGE_2, LTB_4) production.

Virus

MHV-3 was purified on monolayers of DBT cells as previously described. Stock virus was propagated to a titer of 1.2 x 10^7 plaque-forming units (PFU) per ml in 17CL1 cells. The virus was then assayed on monolayers of L2 cells in a standard plaque assay. Monolayers of macrophages were infected with 10^4 and 10^5 PFU of plaque purified MHV-3.

Prostaglandins

Dimethyl prostaglandin E_2 ($dmPGE_2$) was kindly provided by the Upjohn Co., Kalamazoo, MI and was reconstituted in absolute ethanol to a stock concentration of 10 mg/ml. Dilutions were then made using a 0.1 M phosphate buffer (pH 7.4). Vehicle controls were prepared using an identical amount of absolute ethanol diluted in 0.1 M phosphate buffer (pH 7.4) and this resulted in an equivalent final concentration of ethanol.

Procoagulant Activity (PCA)

Samples of macrophages, after three cycles of freeze thawing and sonication, were assayed for the capacity to shorten the spontaneous clotting time of normal citrated human plasma in a 1-stage clotting assay. The time for appearance of a fibrin gel was recorded. Clotting times were converted to units of PCA by comparison to a rabbit brain thromboplastin standard (Dade Div., American Hospital Supply, Miami, FL).

Tumour Necrosis Factor

The activity of TNF was monitored using a semi-automated L929 fibroblast modified lytic assay according to the method of Kunkel et al. (13). The amount of cell lysis was determined using a micro ELISA autoreader. Units of TNF activity were defined as the reciprocal of the dilution necessary to lyse 50% of the L929 target cells. An internal standard of recombinant mouse TNF (Genzyme, Boston, MA) was included in each assay.

Assay for Eicosanoids

Prostaglandin E_2 (PGE_2)

Supernatants from control and MHV infected macrophages in culture were collected and frozen at $-70^{\circ}C$ until assayed. PGE_2 was determined by a standard RIA (New England Nuclear, Boston, MA) (14). Tubes were then counted in a gamma counter with an efficiency of 44% for 1 minute.

Leukotriene B_4 (LTB_4)

LTB_4 was determined in a competitive inhibition RIA (New England Nuclear, Boston, MA) (14).

RESULTS AND DISCUSSION

In these experiments, we have demonstrated that macrophages from fully susceptible Balb/cJ mice produced procoagulant activity (PCA), tumour necrosis factor (TNF) and leukotriene B_4 (LTB_4) in a dose dependent fashion to MHV-3 whereas no such increment was seen in macrophages from the fully resistant A/J mice. The fact that dimethyl prostaglandin E_2 ($dmPGE_2$), which we have previously shown to be capable of preventing fulminant murine hepatitis, blocks induction of these inflammatory monokines supports their importance to the disease process.

When peritoneal macrophages from Balb/cJ mice were infected in culture with 1×10^5 PFU of MHV-3, infectious virus could be recovered within 12 hours which continued to increase in titre at 24 hours. A similar pattern of viral replication was observed in macrophages from resistant A/J mice; although the titre of virus recovered was significantly less at all time points studied (24 hours). This is in keeping with previous data (15). However, at later time points (48-72 hours) the viral titres in A/J macrophages reached equivalent titres seen in Balb/cJ macrophages. This would suggest that differences in viral replication solely do not account for susceptibility/resistance to MHV-3 infection (Figure 1).

PGE_2 treatment both in vitro and in vivo failed to reduce the infectious titre of MHV-3, despite the fact that PGE_2 prevented the cytopathic effect both in liver in-vivo and in hepatocytes in-vitro. This provides further evidence that replication does not in itself account for disease activity.

Macrophages from Balb/cJ mice which were infected with MHV-3 showed a dose dependent increase in expression of

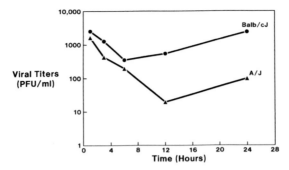

Figure 1. Growth of MHV-3 in peritoneal macrophages from
(▲————▲) A/J and (●————●) Balb/cJ mice.   1 x 10^6
thioglycollate elicited macrophages were infected with 10^5
PFU of MHV-3 and supernatants recovered and assayed for MHV-
3.

procoagulant activity (PCA).   In contrast, no such increase
was seen in MHV-3 infected macrophages from the resistant A/J
mice (Figure 2).   The induction of PCA has previously been
shown to be a lymphocyte dependent event (16), although MHV-3
can induce 20-30% of maximum PCA in macrophages isolated and
infected in the absence of lymphocytes (data not shown).

DmPGE$_2$ was able to inhibit the induction of PCA in a dose
dependent fashion (Figure 3).   Ninety four (94) percent
inhibition was observed at 10^{-3}M dmPGE$_2$ however, significant
inhibition was seen even at 10^{-11}M (Figure 3).

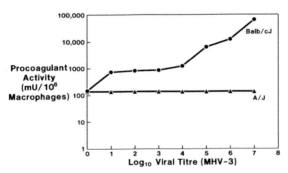

Figure 2.   Induction of macrophage procoagulant activity.   1
x 10^6 thioglycollate elicited (●———●) Balb/cJ and (▲—▲) A/J
macrophages were incubated with 1 x 10^3 PFU of MHV-3 and
assayed for PCA.

Previously, we suggested that induction of PCA, a potent coagulant, may account for disturbances in microcirculation seen early in the course of MHV-3 infection (15). The observation that dmPGE$_2$ prevents induction of PCA underscores the importance of this monokine in the pathogenesis of MHV-3 induced liver disease since no such disturbances in microcirculation were seen in animals treated with dmPGE$_2$.

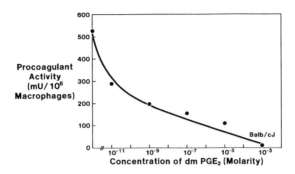

Figure 3. Inhibition of MHV-3 induced macrophage PCA by dmPGE$_2$.

Macrophages from both A/J and Balb/cJ mice in response to endotoxin (LPS) produced a marked augmentation in tumour necrosis factor (TNF) within four hours increasing to maximal levels by 24 hours (Figure 4A). In contrast, only macrophages from Balb/cJ mice produced TNF to MHV-3 (Figure 4B).

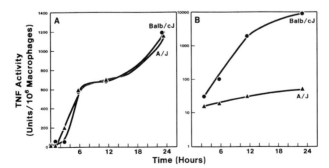

Figure 4. Induction of tumour necrosis factor (TNF) in peritoneal macrophages from (▲——▲) A/J and (●——●) Balb/cJ mice by (A) LPS and (B) MHV-3.

TNF (cachectin) has been implicated as an important inflammatory mediator in a number of diseases (17). The shock-promoting effects of cachectin and its ability to produce hemorrhagic necrosis appear to depend largely upon its vascular effects. TNF down regulates endothelial cell expression of thrombomodulin and causes the elaboration of procoagulant activity as well as the release of interleukin 1 (IL-1) from endothelial cells in-vitro and prompts the adhesion of neutrophils to vascular endothelium (12), a

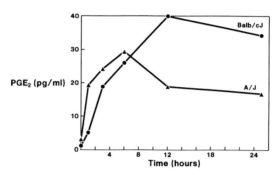

Figure 5. Induction of PGE$_2$ in peritoneal macrophages from (▲———▲) A/J and (●———●) Balb/cJ mice by MHV-3.

prominent feature of murine hepatitis virus infection. Thus, the margination and transudation of neutrophils that occurs only in livers of susceptible mice during MHV-3 infection appears to be secondary to production of cachectin/TNF. Furthermore, it has been reported that cachectin stimulates the release of IL-1 and PGE$_2$ from resting macrophages (18). Following MHV-3 infection marked increases in PGE$_2$ were seen in macrophages from both resistant and susceptible strains of mice (Figure 5).

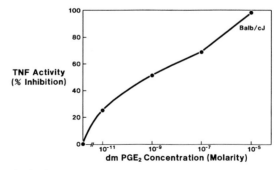

Figure 6. Inhibition of MHV-3 induced tumour necrosis factor by dmPGE$_2$ in peritoneal macrophages from Balb/cJ mice.

The production of PGE_2 in the Balb/cJ, may not be related directly to MHV-3 infection, but rather may occur as a consequence of viral induced production of TNF. In contrast, A/J mice, production of PGE_2 probably is a direct result of infection by MHV-3 as no induction of TNF occurred. $DmPGE_2$ abrogated MHV-3 induced TNF in a dose dependent fashion with 50% reduction at 10^{-9}M $dmPGE_2$ and 100% at 10^{-5}M (Figure 6).

The fact that prostaglandins have previously been shown capable of blocking TNF production to endotoxin (LPS) stimulation suggests that PG may be regulating TNF production in the A/J mice. However, the mechanism by which PG blocks TNF production is not well understood.

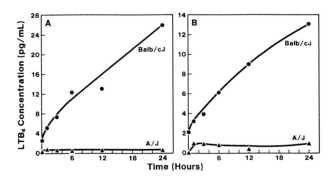

Figure 7. Induction of leukotriene B_4 (LTB_4) in peritoneal macrophages from (●——●) Balb/cJ and (▲——▲) A/J mice by (A) LPS and (B) MHV-3.

Leukotriene B_4 is a potent chemotactin, especially for polymorphonuclear leukocytes the production of which results in cell adhesion and aggregation. Furthermore, LTB_4 induces an increase in vascular permeability. The immunoregulatory activities of LTB_4 include activation of cytotoxic/suppressor T cells and inhibition of the proliferation of helper/inducer T cells. LTB_4 furthermore augments human monocyte-mediated cytoxicity and enhances production of TNF by human monocytes (19). Following addition of LPS or MHV-3, macrophages from Balb/cJ mice produced increasing concentrations of LTB_4 whereas no response was seen in A/J mice to either stimulus (Figure 7). $DmPGE_2$ markedly reduced production of LTB_4 from macrophages infected with both 10^4 and 10^5 PFU of MHV-3 (Figure 8).

Prostaglandins E_1 and E_2 have been previously shown to inhibit LTB_4 release from polymorphonuclear cells in a dose related manner with a 50% inhibition at a concentration of 10^{-8}M (20). These results are somewhat in conflict with the present studies as higher concentrations of PGE_2 were required in order to observe this 50% inhibition. This may reflect either variation in stimuli (MHV-3 vs. fMET-LEU-PHE) or a relative refractoriness of macrophages to inhibition of

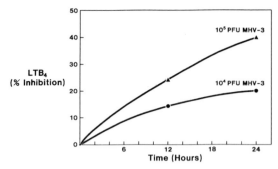

Figure 8. Inhibition of LTB_4 by $dmPGE_2$ in peritoneal macrophages from Balb/cJ infected with (●——●) 10^4 PFU or (▲——▲) 10^5 PFU MHV-3.

production of LTB_4 by PG compared to polymorphonuclear cells.

The results of these experiments show that early in the course of infection with MHV-3, macrophages from susceptible Balb/cJ mice express high concentrations of potent inflammatory mediators. Subsequently, a marked increase in both class I and II MHC antigens is observed in livers of infected mice. The fact that $dmPGE_2$ blocks the induction of inflammatory mediators and class II antigens at a time when in vivo $dmPGE_2$ prevents tissue necrosis supports a role for these mediators in the initiation of the inflammatory process. As TNF and IL-2 can both induce procoagulants in endothelial cells and adhesion of neutrophils, the production of these monokines may account for the histologic abnormalities observed in livers of susceptible mice and are probably important in the pathogenesis.

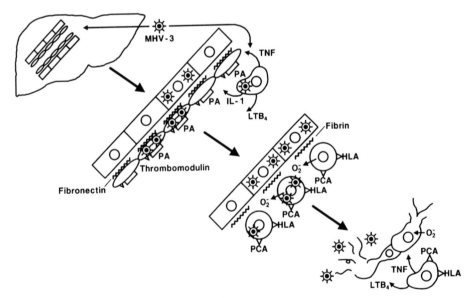

Figure 9. A proposed mechanism for the pathogenesis of MHV-3 induced fulminant hepatitis.

REFERENCES

1. Levy, G.A., Leibowitz, J.L., Edgington, T.S. 1982. Lymphocyte-instructed monocyte induction of the coagulation pathways parallels the induction of hepatitis by the murine hepatitis virus. Prog. Liver Dis. 7:393-409.

2. MacNaughton, M.R. and S. Patterson. 1980. Mouse hepatitis virus strain 3 infection of C57, A/Sn and A/J strain mice and their macrophages. Arch. Virol. 66:71.

3. Dindzans, V.J., MacPhee, P., Fung, L.S., Leibowitz, J.L. and Levy, G.A. 1985. The immune response to mouse hepatitis virus: Expression of monocyte procoagulant activity and plasminogen activator during infection in vivo. J. Immunol. 135:4189.

4. Dupuy, J.M., Levy-Leblond, E., Le Provest, C. 1975. Immunopathology of mouse hepatitis virus type 3 infection. II. Effect of immunosuppression in resistant mice. J. Immunol. 114:226.

5. Pereira, C.A, Steffan, A.M. and Kirn, A. 1984. Kupffer and endothelial liver cell damage renders A/J mice susceptible to mouse hepatitis virus type 3. Virus Res. 1:557.

6. Levy-Leblond, E. and Dupuy, J.M. 1977. Neonatal susceptibility to MHV-3 infection in mice. I. Transfer of resistance. J. Immunol. 118:1219.

7. Sussman, M.A., Shubin, R.A., Kyuwa, S. and Stohlman, S.A. 1989. T-cell mediated clearance of mouse hepatitis virus strain JHM from the central nervous system. J. Virol. 63:3051-3056.

8. Dindzans, V.J., Zimmerman, B., Sherker, A. and Levy, G.A. 1987. Susceptibility to mouse hepatitis virus strain 3 in Balb/cJ mice: Failure of immune cell proliferation and interleukin 2 production, in: Coronaviruses, Michael M.C. Lai and Stephen A. Stohlman, ed., Plenum Publishing Corp, New York.

9. Levy, G.A. and Abecassis, M. 1989. Activation of the immune coagulation system by murine hepatitis virus strain 3. The Reviews of Infectious Diseases. 11:S712-S721.

10. Dindzans, V.J., Skamene, E. and Levy, G.A. 1986. Susceptibility/resistance to mouse hepatitis virus strain 3 and macrophage procoagulant activity are genetically linked and controlled by two non-H-2-linked genes. J. Immunol. 137:2355-60.

11. Abecassis, M., Falk, J.A., Makowka, L., Dindzans, V.J., Falk, R.E. and Levy, G.A. 1987. 16, 16 dimethyl prostaglandin E_2 prevents the development of fulminant hepatitis and blocks the induction of monocyte/macrophage procoagulant activity after murine hepatitis virus strain 3 infection. J. Clin. Invest. 80:881-889.

12. Stern, D.M. and Nawroth, P.P. 1986. Modulation of endothelial hemostatic properties by tumor necrosis factor. J. Exp. Med. 163:740-45.

13. Kunkel, S.L., Wiggins, R.C., Chensue, S.W. and Larrick, J. 1986. Regulation of macrophage tumor necrosis factor production by prostaglandin E_2. Biochem. and Biophys. Res. Comm. 137:404-410.

14. Hagmann, W., Steffan, A., Kirn and Keppler, D. 1987. Leukotrienes as mediators in frog virus 3-induced hepatitis in rats. Hepatology. 7:732-736.

15. MacPhee, P.J., Dindzans, V.J., Fung, L.S. and Levy, G.A. 1985. Acute and chronic changes in the microcirculation of the liver in inbred strains of mice following infection with mouse hepatitis virus type 3. Hepatology. 5:649-60.

16. Levy, G.A., Leibowitz, J.L., Edgington, T.S. 1981. Induction of monocyte procoagulant activity by murine hepatitis virus type 3 parallels disease susceptibility in mice. J. Exp. Med. 154:1150-63.

17. Beutler, B. and Cerami, A. 1989. The biology of cachectin/TNF- A primary mediator of the host response. Ann. Rev. Immunol. 7:625-55.

18. Bachwich, P.R., Chensue, S.W., Larrick, J.W., Kunkel, S.L. 1986. Tumor necrosis factor stimulates interleukin-1 and prostaglandin E_2 production in resting macrophages. Biochem. Biophys. Res. Commun. 136:94-101.

19. Keppler, D., Huber, M. and Baumert T. 1988. Leukotrienes as mediators in diseases of the liver. Seminars in Liver Disease. 8:357-366.

20. Ham, E.A., Soderman, D.D., Zanetti, M.E., Dougherty, H.W., McCauley E, Kuehl Jr., F.A. 1983. Inhibition by prostaglandins of leukotriene B_4 release from activated neutrophils. Proc. Natl. Acad. Sci. USA. 80:4349-4353.

MOUSE HEPATITIS VIRUS 3 PATHOGENICITY AND B AND T

LYMPHOTROPISMS

Pierre Jolicoeur and Lucie Lamontagne

Département des Sciences Biologiques
Université du Québec à Montréal
C.P.8888 Succ A, Montréal, Qué. Canada H3C 3P8

INTRODUCTION

Viral pathogenicity may be regulated by a host defense mechanism during virus-cell interaction at the immune system level. When the virus is lymphotropic, understanding the pathogenic process of the viral disease is complicated by the virus-lymphocyte interaction which may alter the integrity of the cell and induce a subsequent immunodeficiency.

Mouse hepatitis virus type 3 (MHV3), a hepatolytic virus, is a member of the coronavirus group. Its inoculation in mice induces an acute infection characterized by an hepatic necrosis, killing the animal within a couple of days (1). The outcome of the MHV3 infection varies according to the mouse strain: resistant A/J mice support a subclinical infection, while the other strains, including C57BL/6 mice, are fully susceptible to acute disease. The immune system plays an important role in the outcome of acute disease induced by MHV3. Resistant A/J mice become fully susceptible to accute hepatitis after immunosuppressive treatments (2,3). The genetically-determined resistance of A/J mice develop as the cell populations mature, as non-adherent spleen cells, T lymphocytes, and a third population present in bone marrow (4,5). Efficient cellular and humoral immune responses to viral infection depend on normal B or T lymphopoiesis which take place in bone marrow or thymus (6,7). The specific anti-viral humoral and cellular immune responses act as mechanisms in viral elimination, promoting cellular and antibody-mediated dependent cell cytotoxicity or neutralization of infectious viral particles (8-10).

Lymphoid cells are believed to be the target host for MHV3 replication (11) and at the same time, the effectors of the elimination of the virus. Humoral and cellular immunodeficiencies previously observed in MHV3 chronically-infected (12) related to the loss of non-adherent cells in spleen and thymus despite the stimulation of bone marrow precursor cells (13). No information is available on the mechanism which causes cell depletions in lymphoid organs and subsequently develops into humoral and cellular immunodeficiency, and the role of MHV3 lymphotropism in the pathogenic process of acute disease.

To evaluate the role of B and T lymphotropisms in the MHV3 pathogenicity, B and T lymphoid subpopulations have been studied in vivo in pathogenic MHV3 (L2-MHV3) and its non-pathogenic variant, derived from a chronically

Coronaviruses and Their Diseases
Edited by D. Cavanagh and T.D.K. Brown
Plenum Press, New York, 1990

infected YAC cell line (YAC-MHV3), acutely-infected susceptible C57BL/6 or resistant A/J mice or _in vitro_ in purified T and B cell subpopulations.

METHODS

Mice: A/J and C57BL/6 mouse strains were purchased from the Jackson Laboratories (Bar Harbor, ME). Before being used, the animals were tested for the presence of anti-MHV antibodies, by ELISA by using MHV3 preparation as Ag. During experiments the animals were housed in a sterile atmosphere (Forma Scientific, Marietta, OH).

Viruses: Pathogenic MHV3 was a cloned substrain in L2 cells (L2-MHV3) as previously described (14). YAC-MHV3 variant was a cloned virus derived from persistently infected lymphoid YAC cells (15). Viruses were passaged in L2 cells before use and their pathogenic properties were verified regularly.

Cells: L2 cells, a continous mouse fibroblast cell line, were grown in Eagle's MEM with glutamine (2mM), 5% FCS (GIBCO Laboratories, Grand Island, NY), and antibiotics. L2 cells were used for propagation, cloning and titration of viruses. The thymic cells were obtained by teasing of the thymuses apart in HBSS with 10% FCS at room temperature by using needles. The bone marrow cells were collected from femurs. Femoral shafts were flushed four times with 1 ml. cold Eagle's MEM supplemented with 10% FCS. Large particles were removed by sedimentation on a cushion of 1 ml. of FCS for 5 minutes. The cell suspension was then centrifugized and resuspended in 1 ml. of Eagle's MEM with 10% FCS. Cell preparations were electronically counted (Coulter Counter, Coulter Electronics, Hialeah, FL) and cell viability was assayed by the trypan blue exclusion test. B Cell purification was done by panning according to the Wysocki and Sato's method (16) with some modifications. Before purification, adherent monocytes were removed by incubating the cell suspension (supplemented with 20% FCS) in a petri dish for 1 h at 37°C with 5% CO_2. After incubation, the dish was washed thoroughly with HBSS. The non-adherent cell suspension (10^7/ml) was pipetted into an anti-IgM coated plastic dish and incubated twice at room temperature for 30 min. Non-adherent cells were sucked off from the dish and the remaining adherent cell layer was washed four times with Ca-Mg-free PBS and then removed with a policeman. Immunofluorescence study revealed that the final cell population contained around 94% of sIg+cells.

Histopathological examination: Groups of mice from strains, inoculated i.p. of 10^4TCID$_{50}$ with L2-MHV3 or YAC-MHV3 were necropsied at 72 h p.i. The spleen were collected, fixed in Perfix (Fisher Scientific, Montréal, Qué, Can.) and processed for routine light microscopic examination (hematoxylin-eosine stain).

Virus titration and virus-producing cell assay. Viral suspensions were serially diluted in 10-fold steps and tested in L2 cells cultured in 96-well microtiter plates. CPE characterized by syncytia formation and cell lysis were recorded at 72 h.p.i. and virus titers expressed as TCID$_{50}$. The titrations were made in triplicate. Single cell suspensions of B lymphocytes or thymic cells, prepared as above, were deposited on a gradient of Lymphoprep (Cedarlane, Hornby, Ont. Canada). The suspensions were collected in RPMI 1640 medium supplemented with 10% heat-inactivated FCS, antibiotics and glutamine. Cell preparations consisted of extensive washings (at least three times) to remove free virus and count the cells electronically. The cells were diluted at a concentration of 10^4 cells/ml and measured for virus-producing cell assay by 10-fold step dilutions until 100 cells/ml; thus by 2-fold step in RPMI 1640 medium. Virus production by each cell dilution was tested in L2 cells as described for viral titration. The percentage of virus-producing cells were calculated by the ratio between the number of cells in the last dilution causing 50% of CPE and the initial concentration.

Immunofluorescence analysis. Double labeling of u chains (pre-B and B cells) was done as per Park and Osmond (17). Briefly described, bone marrow samples (100ul of 4×10^7 nucleated cells/ml suspension) were incubated for 30 min on ice an optimal dilution of FITC anti-u chains (Cappel Biomedical, Malvern, PA) for surface (su) labeling. The cells were washed twice by centrifugation through FCS at 200g at 4^0C for 7 min. Cells were resuspended in PBS with EDTA (2.7mM) supplemented with 5% BSA. Bone marrow cells were cytocentri-fugized at 1000 rpm for 5 min. (Cytospin; Shandon Southern Instrument Inc. Sewickly, PA) and fixed in precooled acetic acid-methanol (5% v/v) for 12 min on ice and then washed 4-5 times in cooled PBS. Cytoplasmic u (cu) chains were labelled with an optimal dilution of TRITC anti-u directly on the cell spots, then incubated 30 min at room temperature in a humidified chamber, then washed 4 times and mounted on a medium containing 90% glycerol in PBS and 0.1% p-phenylenediamine.

Double labeling of CD4 and CD8 thymic cells (4×10^7 cells/mL) were incubated for 30 min on ice with rat-FITC anti-CD4 (Dimension Laboratories, Missisauga Ont. Canada). The cells were washed twice by centrifugation through FCS at 200 g at 4^0C for 7 min. Cells were then resuspended in RPMI 1640 medium and, incubated with anti-CD8 (Dimension Laboratories, Missisauga, Ont. Canada) for 30 min on ice. Cells were washed and re-incubated with mouse TRITC anti-IgG (Cappel Biomedical, Malvern, PA, USA) for an additional 30 min on ice. Cells were resuspended in PBS with EDTA supplemented with 5% BSA.

Percentage of labelled cells was determined by counting a total of 1000 cells. The absolute numbers were calculated by the percentage of posi-tive labeled cells and the total bone marrow count. A diameter of at least 100 cells at each subpopulation was measured using a calibrated micrometer scale.

RESULTS

Microscopic evaluation of spleen in resistant A/J or susceptible C57BL/6 mice

To determine the role of the immune system in genetic resistance or in viral nonpathogenicity, microscopic evaluation of spleen of pathogenic L2-MHV3 or nonpathogenic YAC-MHV3 infected resistant A/J or susceptible C57BL/6 mice have been studied. A splenic atrophy characterized by disappea-rance of lymphoid follicles has been noted in L2-MHV3 infected A/J and C57BL/6 mice. The lesions observed were more severe in C57BL/6 mice than in A/J mice. The YAC-MHV3 variant also produced lesions in spleen of C57BL/6 mice, but were less severe.

Pre-B and B cell subpopulations in bone marrow from L2-MHV3 or YAC-MHV3 infected C57BL/6 or A/J mice

We have recently observed a decrease in the number of splenic B lym-phocytes in susceptible C57BL/6 mice infected with the pathogenic L2-MHV3 virus (19). This decrease may reflect the virus-induced cell lysis or the inability of animal to compensate the loss of splenic lymphoid cells. Lym-phopoiesis disorders during the maturation process of B cell subpopulations in the bone marrow may explain the absence of splenic B cells. To verify this hypothesis, we have evaluated the absolute number of the B (cu+su+) and pre-B (cu+su-) cell subpopulations in the bone marrow. Groups of three susceptible C57BL/6 or resistant A/J mice have been infected intraperito-neally (i.p.) with 10^4 TCID$_{50}$ of pathogenic L2-MHV3 or nonpathogenic YAC-MHV3 viruses. Groups of uninfected mice received i.p. with similar

Table 1. Absolute number of mature B cells in bone marrow
from pathogenic L2-MHV3 or non-pathogenic YAC-MHV3
infected resistant A/J or susceptible C57BL/6 mice.

Mice	Virus	Time postinfection (days)			
		0	1	3	7
A/J	L2-MHV3	2.2 ± 0.2^a	2.7 ± 0.3	3.0 ± 0.2	2.3 ± 0.3
	YAC-MHV3	2.2 ± 0.2	2.3 ± 0.3	2.2 ± 0.2	2.1 ± 0.2
C57BL/6	L2-MHV3	2.1 ± 0.2	3.0 ± 0.3	0.3 ± 0.5	n.a.^{b}
	YAC-MHV3	2.1 ± 0.2	2.4 ± 0.3	2.3 ± 0.2	2.2 ± 0.2

a: x 10^6 cells
b: n.a. not applicable

volume of PBS. Absolute number of B cells rapidly decreased in the bone
marrow of C57BL/6 mice infected with L2-MHV3 until the death of mice
(Table 1). Slight increases have been noted at days 1 and 3 in L2-MHV3
resistant A/J mice but returned to normal values at day 7. No significant
changes has been detected in both strain mice infected with YAC-MHV3 virus.

Similarly, absolute number of pre-B cells decreased in the bone marrow
of C57BL/6 mice infected with L2-MHV3 only (Table 2). These results indicate
that depletion of bone marrow pre-B and B cells is responsible for the
maintenance of low number of splenic B cells. In addition, the B lineage
cell disorder in bone marrow correlates with viral pathogenicity or genetically-determined sensitivity to MHV3 viral infection.

Diminished number of B cell subpopulations in the bone marrow during the
viral infection is perhaps caused by a blockade of cell mitosis or a viral-
induced cell lysis. To verify this hypothesis, size distribution of the

Table 2. Absolute number of pre-B (cu+ su-) cells in bone marrow
from pathogenic L2-MHV3 or nonpathogenic YAC-MHV3
infected resistant A/J or susceptible C57BL/6 mice.

Mice	Virus	Time postinfection (days)			
		0	1	3	7
A/J	L2-MHV3	0.8 ± 0.2^a	0.9 ± 0.1	0.8 ± 0.1	0.8 ± 0.1
	YAC-MHV3	0.8 ± 0.1	0.8 ± 0.1	0.8 ± 0.2	0.8 ± 0.2
C57BL/6	L2-MHV3	0.8 ± 0.1	0.9 ± 0.1	0.5 ± 0.2	n.a.^{b}
	YAC-MHV3	0.8 ± 0.2	0.8 ± 0.2	0.8 ± 0.1	0.8 ± 0.1

a: x 10^6 cells
b: n.a. not applicable

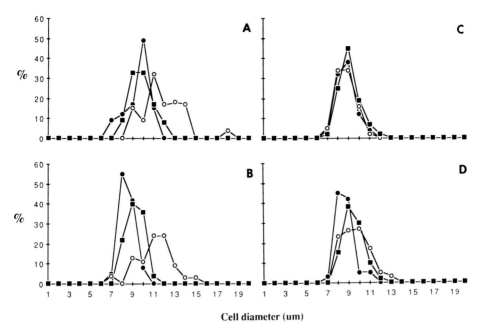

Fig. 1. Size distribution of bone marrow pre-B (cu+su-) (A,C) and B (cu+su+) (B,D) cell subpopulations from uninfected (●), pathogenic L2-MHV3 (O) or non-pathogenic YAC-MHV3 (■) infected susceptible C57BL/6 (A,B) or resistant A/J (C,D) mice. Groups of three susceptible C57BL/6 or resistant A/J mice have been infected with 10^4 TCID$_{50}$ of pathogenic L2-MHV3 or non-pathogenic YAC-MHV3. Groups of uninfected mice received i.p. a similar volume of PBS. Bone marrow cells were stained with a FITC anti -u chain for su labeling, cytocentrifugized, fixed in acetic acid/methanol solution, and labeled with a TRITC anti-u (cu). Diameter of at least 100 cells of each subpopulation was measured using a calibrated micrometer scale (standard deviation < 3%).

different B cell subpopulations were analyzed at 48 h.p.i. in bone marrow of L2-MHV3 or YAC-MHV3 infected C57BL/6 or A/J mice (Fig. 1). Size distribution of B cell subpopulations in the bone marrow from uninfected mice varied from 7 to 12 um. Normal-sized pre-B and B cells decreased in L2-MHV3 infected C57BL/6 mice, contrary to the A/J mice or YAC-MHV3 infected mice. In addition, an abnormally larger-sized cell subpopulation, with a cell diameter varying from 12 to 17 um, occurred in L2-MHV3 infected C57BL/6 mice.

In vitro infection of purified bone marrow mature B cells

To determine the permissivity role of B cells to MHV3 viral replication, upon cell depletion accompanied by cell enlargement, we performed in vitro L2-MHV3 or YAC-MHV3 viral infection (1 m.o.i.) in mature B cells (cu+su+) collected from uninfected C57BL/6 and A/J mice and purified by a panning method using anti-u chains antibodies. Cellularity, percentage of virus-producing cells and viral titer were recorded at 48 h.p.i. (Table 3).

The number of L2-MHV3 infected B cells from C57BL/6 mice greatly decreased whereas B cells from A/J mice were slightly affected. Majority of L2-MHV3 infected B cells from C57BL/6 mice were productively infected (>80%) and virus titer in the supernatant reached 4.1+0.3 TCID$_{50}$/ml. Few B cells from A/J mice were also successfully L2-MHV3 infected and lower

Table 3. Cellularity, percentage of virus producing cells, and viral titers in in vitro pathogenic L2-MHV3 or nonpathogenic YAC-MHV3 infected purified bone marrow mature B (cu+su+) cells from resistant A/J or susceptible C57BL/6 mice.

Mouse strain	Virus	Cellularity (10^5)	Virus producing cells (%)	Viral titers ($TCID_{50}/ml$)
A/J	Uninfected	3.0+0.2	n.a.[a]	n.a.
	L2-MHV3	2.4+0.1	0.02+0.02	2.8+0.3
	YAC-MHV3	2.6+0.3	<0.005	>1.6
C57BL/6	Uninfected	4.0+0.2	n.a.	n.a.
	L2-MHV3	1.4+0.1	>80	4.1+0.3
	YAC-MHV3	3.8+0.2	<0.005	<1.6

a: n.a. not applicable

virus titers in supernatants detected. No cell depletion or viral replication were found in YAC-MHV3 infected cells. Similar results were obtained with pre-B cells (results not shown). These results demonstrate that lytic viral infection occurs in B lineage cell subpopulations and is responsible for cell depletions as observed in vivo in L2-MHV3 infected C57BL/6.

To determine if the viral replication generates the abnormal-sized cells, size distribution of in vitro infected mature B cells was analyzed. Majority (>95%) of L2-MHV3 infected B cells from C57BL/6 mice expressed abnormal increase in cell diameters (11 to 19 um) with a simultaneous decrease in the percentage of normal sized cells. Normal-sized distribution of B cells was observed in L2-MHV3 infected A/J or in YAC-MHV3 infected cells. These results demonstrate that L2-MHV3 viral replication induces in vitro the formation of abnormally large lymphocytes as detected in the bone marrow of in vivo infected C57BL/6 mice.

T cell subpopulations in thymus from pathogenic L2-MHV3 or non-pathogenic YAC-MHV3 infected susceptible C57BL/6 or resistant A/J mice

We have recently demonstrated that viral pathogenicity or susceptibility to MHV3 infection correlated with viral replication in vivo in thymus and in vitro in isolated thymocytes (20). To evaluate the immune disorders induced in thymus by the viral infection, the thymic T cell subpopulations have been analyzed in L2-MHV3 or YAC-MHV3 infected ($10^4 TCID_{50}$i.p.) C57BL/6 or A/J mice at 48 hrs p.i.. As shown in Table 4, CD4+CD8+, CD4+CD8- and CD4-CD8+ thymic cell subpopulations decreased in pathogenic L2-MHV3 infected susceptible C57BL/6 mice whereas no significant depletions of these subpopulations were detected in resistant A/J mice or in both strain mice infected with YAC-MHV3. In addition, the ratio CD4/CD8, representing the functional level of the immune system, also decreased in L2-MHV3 infected C57BL/6 mice, indicating that the diseased mice not only express an immunodeficient state, they are also immunosuppressed (Table 5).

Table 4. Percentage of CD4+CD8+, CD4+CD8-, and CD4-CD8+ cells
from the thymus of pathogenic L2-MHV3 or nonpathogenic
YAC-MHV3 infected resistant A/J or susceptible C57BL/6
mice.

Mouse strain	Virus	Thymic cell subpopulations (x 10^6)		
		CD4+CD8+	CD4+CD8-	CD4-CD8+
A/J	Uninfected	57+5	12+1	6.2+0.5
	L2-MHV3	62+5	12+2	7.0+0.5
	YAC-MHV3	60+3	12+1	7.0+0.6
C57BL/6	Uninfected	60+3	11+1	6.0+0.3
	L2-MHV3	45+4	6.0+0.3	4.1+0.2
	YAC-MHV3	66+5	11+0.4	6.1+0.3

These results indicate that T immunodeficiency occurs in acutely-infected
mice and relates to depletion of all thymic lymphoid cell subpopulations.
In addition, the T lineage cell disorder in thymus correlates with viral
pathogenicity or genetically-determined sensitivity to MHV3 viral infection.

In vivo viral replication in thymocytes from L2-MHV3 or YAC-MHV3 infected
resistant A/J or susceptible C57BL/6 mice

The loss of thymic T cell subpopulations in diseased mice may be
related to a cytolytic MHV3 infection. To verify this hypothesis, viral
replication was evaluated by the percentage of thymocytes expressing intracellular viral proteins, detectable by an indirect immunofluorescent assay,
or of thymocytes producing infectious virions, in L2-MHV3 or YAC-MHV3 infected A/J or C57BL/6 mice at 48h. p.i.(Tableau 6). Interestingly, the
majority of thymic cells from L2-MHV3 infected C57BL/6 mice expressed
intracellular viral proteins, however, a nominal amount of cells produced
infectious viruses. This interaction suggests that an abortive viral replication, blocked at the level of virion assembly, occured in T cells.

Table 5. CD4/CD8 ratio of thymic cells in pathogenic L2-MHV3
or nonpathogenic YAC-MHV3 infected resistant A/J or
susceptible C57BL/6 mice.

Mouse strain	Virus	CD4/CD8 ratio
A/J	Uninfected	1.72+0.10
	L2-MHV3	1.60+0.09
	YAC-MHV3	1.63+0.17
C57BL/6	Uninfected	1.83+0.15
	L2-MHV3	1.08+0.12
	YAC-MHV3	1.63+0.20

Tableau 6. L2-MHV3 or YAC-MHV3 viral replication in thymocytes
from in vivo infected A/J or C57BL/6 mice.

Mouse strain	Virus	Intracellular viral proteins expressing cells (%)	Virus producing cells (%)
A/J	L2-MHV3	< 1	< 0.002
	YAC-MHV3	< 1	< 0.002
C57BL/6	L2-MHV3	81+4	0.08+0.04
	YAC-MHV3	< 1	< 0.002

No viral replication was detected in thymic T cells from L2-MHV3 infected
A/J mice or YAC-MHV3 infected mice.

DISCUSSION

We have demonstrated, in this work, that the B and T lymphocytes are
the target cells in vivo and in vitro for the pathogenic L2-MHV3 viral
replication. The specific virus-lymphocyte interactions correlate with
viral pathogenicity. In vivo results reveal that bone marrow and thymus
to be the other target organs for MHV3 virus infection. These results on
bone marrow B lymphocytes extend the previous works of Piazza et al. (1)
which demonstrated that MHV3 replication accompanied by decrease in number
of lymphocytes, monocytes and polymorphonuclear cells occurred in acutely-
infected mice. In addition, thymic atrophy, previously observed in MHV3
infected C57BL/6 mice (2,3), results in loss of the thymic cells in the
first days of viral infection. On the other hand, the absence of detectable
hematopoietic disorders in the bone marrow and cell depletions in the
thymus of L2-MHV3 infected resistant A/J mice or in nonpathogenic YAC-MHV3
infected mice confirm the integral role played by the primary lymphoid
organs in inducing a resistance to acute disease (2,18). Analysis of B
lymphocyte subpopulations in the bone marrow revealed depletions of pre-B
and B lymphocytes in L2-MHV3 infected susceptible C57BL/6 mice only. Abnormal forms of B lineage cells were also observed in the bone marrow of
diseased mice. These large mononucleated cells may have resulted from an
impairment of cell metabolism following viral infection and leading to
cell lysis. In determining the number of splenic B lymphocytes in L2-MHV3
susceptible C57BL/6 mice, we found that the cell depletion (18) reconciles
our previous findings on the correlation between impairment of B cells (12)
and the loss of cellularity in the lymphoid organs (13). The mechanism
against MHV3 viral infection is controlled under H-2 or non-H-2 related
genes (20) and expressed as hemopoietic cells, mature splenic cell or
thymic cells and macrophages (5,19).

The in vitro results of B lymphocytes thus correlate and explain the
in vivo observations. L2-MHV3 infection of bone marrow purified B cells
from C57BL/6 revealed that these cells are productively infected, expressed
abnormal morphology and lead to subsequent cell lysis. The permissivity
of T lymphocytes to MHV3 replication, however, remains unclear. No viral
replication can be detected in vitro in purified T cells from thymocytes
preparation, despite the high percentage of viral protein expressing cells
in thymus from diseased mice. Preliminary result on in vitro viral replication in enriched thymic epithelial cell preparation indicates that viral
infection primarly occurs in thymic epithelial cells, also present in the
thymocyte preparation. The infection is then transmitted to T lymphocytes

by a yet unknown mechanism. Thus the lack of lymphoid repopulation in the spleen following an MHV3 infection explains the depletion of mature B and T cells into bone marrow and thymus.

As the result of a viral permissivity of B and T lymphocytes, two immunological consequences occur. First, B and T lymphocytes partially act as a natural barriers to MHV3 replication in producing no or low level of infectious virions in extracellular media, and second, in inducing B and T lymphocyte cell lysis and subsequent cellular and humoral immunodeficiencies. As previously demonstrated, MHV3 viral replication is restricted in splenic or thymic lymphoid cells in resistant A/J mice and delayed in susceptible C57BL/6 mice (19). Such immunodeficiencies is perhaps responsible for the inefficient viral elimination process. Virus titers continue to increase until death in C57BL/6 mice whereas they decrease in A/J mice despite similar virus titers observed in various organs in susceptible C57BL/6 or resistant A/J mice infected with L2-MHV3 or YAC-MHV3 for the first 72 h.p.i. (18). In addition, virus-induced cell lysis of lymphocytes was ineffective in the viral elimination process. This situation has been previously observed in (C57BL/6 x A/J)F1 mice surviving an acute disease (21).

Further work will be performed to determine the mechanism involved in T cell depletion during the acute disease and the occurrence of immunodeficiency in chronically-infected mice.

ACKNOWLEDGEMENTS

The authors thank D. Décarie for excellent technical assistance. This work was supported in part by grant from the NSERC (Canada), and grant from FCAR (Québec).

REFERENCES

1. Piazza, M., F. Piccinino, and F. Matano. 1965. Haematologic changes in viral (MHV3) murine hepatitis. Nature 205: 1034.
2. LePrevost, C., E. Levy-Leblond, J.L. Virelizier, and J.M. Dupuy. 1975. Immunopathology of mouse hepatitis virus type 3 infection. I. Role of humoral and cell-mediated immunity in resistance mechanisms. J. Immunol. 114: 221.
3. Dupuy, J.M., E. Levy-Leblond, and C. LePrevost. 1975. Immunopathology of mouse hepatitis virus type 3 infection. II. Effect of immunosuppression in resistant mice. J. Immunol. 114: 226.
4. Tardieu, M., C. Hery, and J.M. Dupuy. 1980. Neonatal susceptibility to MHV3 infection in mice. II. Role of natural effector marrow cells in transfer of resistance. J. Immunol. 124: 418.
5. Dupuy, J.M., C. Dupuy, and D. Décarie. 1984. Genetically-determined resistance to mouse hepatitis virus 3 expressed in hematopoietic donor cells in radiation chimeras. J. Immunol. 133: 1609.
6. Osmond, D.G., and G.V.J. Nossal. 1974. Differenciation of lymphocytes in mouse bone marrow. II. Kinetics of maturation and renewal of antiglobulin binding cells studied by double labeling. Cell. Immunol. 13: 137.
7. Raff, M.C., and Owen, J.J.T. 1971. Thymus derived lymphocytes: their distribution and role in the development of peripheral lymphoid tissues of the mouse. Eur. J. Immunol. 1: 27.
8. Collins, S.W., and J.S. Portefield. 1986. A new mechanism for the neutralization of enveloped viruses by antiviral antibody. Nature 321: 244.

9. Borysiewicz, L.K., and J.G.P. Sissons. 1986. Immune response to virus infected cells. Clin. Immunol. Allergy 6: 159.

10. Sissons, J.P.G., R.D. Schreiber, N.R. Couper, and M.B.A. Oldstone. 1982. The role of antibody and complement in lysing virus-infected cells. Med. Microbiol. Immunol. 170: 221.

11. Krystyniak, K., and J.M. Dupuy. 1981. Early interaction between mouse hepatitis virus 3 and cells. J. Gen. Virol. 57: 53.

12. Leray, D., C. Dupuy, and J.M. Dupuy. 1982. Immunopathology of mouse hepatitis virus type 3 infection. IV. MHV3- induced immunodepression. Clin. Immunol. Immunopathol. 23: 223.

13. Lamontagne, L., C. Dupuy, D. Leray, J.P. Chausseau, and J.M. Dupuy. 1985. Coronavirus-induced immunosuppression: Role of mouse hepatitis virus 3-lymphocyte interaction. Prog. Leuk. Biol. 1: 29.

14. Dupuy, J.M., and D. Rodrigue. 1981. Heterogeneity in evolutive pattern of inbred mice infected with a cloned substrain of mouse hepatitis virus type 3. Intervirology 16: 116.

15. Lamontagne, L., and J.M. Dupuy. 1984. Persistent in vitro infection with mouse hepatitis virus type 3 in mouse lymphoid cell lines. Infect. & Immun. 44: 716.

16. Wysocki, L.J., and V.L. Sato. 1978. Panning for lymphocytes: a method for cell selection. Proc. Natl. Acad. Sci. USA 75: 2844.

17. Park, Y.H., and D.G. Osmond. 1987. Phenotype and proliferation of early B lymphocyte precursor cells in mouse bone marrow. J. Exp. Med. 165: 444.

18. Lamontagne, L., J.P. Descoteaux, and P. Jolicoeur. 1989. Mouse hepatitis virus 3 replication in T and B lymphocytes correlate with viral pathogenicity. J. Immunol. 142: 4458.

19. Lamontagne, L., D. Décarie, and J.M. Dupuy. 1989. Host cell resistance to mouse hepatitis virus type 3 is expressed in vitro in macrophages and lymphocytes. Viral Immunol. 2: 37.

20. Levy-Leblond, E., D. Oth, and J.M. Dupuy. 1979. Genetic study of mouse sensitivity to MHV3 infection: influence of the H-2 complex. J. Immunol. 112: 1359.

21. LePrevost, C., J.L. Virelizier, and J.M. Dupuy. 1975. Immunopathology of mouse hepatitis virus type 3. III. Clinical and virologic observations of a persistent viral infection. J. Immunol. 115: 640.

Chapter 12

Neurological Consequences of Murine Hepatitis Virus Infection of Mice

BACKGROUND PAPER

ADVANCES IN THE STUDY OF MHV INFECTION OF MICE

Shigeru Kyuwa and Stephen Stohlman

Departments of Neurology and Microbiology
University of Southern California School of Medicine
Los Angeles
CA 90033
USA

Since the last International Coronavirus Meeting a number of very intriguing papers have appeared. These papers have provided insight into what continues to be a very exciting and complex interaction between MHV strains and their natural hosts and include studies of viral tropism, pathogenesis, the role of immune system and genetic factors. MHV infections in mice have been studied mainly as models of viral hepatitis (4,7,9,11,13) and both acute and chronic viral infection of the central nervous system (CNS) (2,5,6,8,15-17,19,20).

MHV strains with selective tropism for cells within the CNS continue to provide information of the interactions of the immune system and the CNS as a target of infectious processes. Studies with the JHM strain (2,5) suggest that the E2 is a major, if not the major, determinant of cellular tropism. The definition of the target cell in the CNS has also been brought into question. Previous data were consistent with the oligodendroglial cell as the major target; however, it has been recently suggested that the astrocyte may be a more important target during the acute infection as well as the cell in which MHV infections persist within the CNS (16). The immune response to CNS infection with MHV has also taken some interesting turns. It is now clear that antibodies specific to all three structural proteins can prevent death following a lethal infection with MHV (6,13). Similarly, some T cell subsets can also prevent death (19). However, neither the antibodies, even if they are able to neutralize the virus *in vitro*, nor the CD4+ DTH effector T cells can reduce virus replication in the CNS. Prolongation of life in the face of unrestricted virus replication results in increased evidence of disease. Finally, a recent paper has ascribed the reduction of virus in the CNS to the CD8+ T cell subset (20).

Because CD8+ and CD4+ T cells recognize antigen in the context of the major histocompatibility (MHC) class I and class II antigens, respectively, the expression of MHC antigens on the cells within the CNS during MHV infection is another intriguing issue. Although their expression in the CNS of normal mice is relatively low, some cytokines have been reported to up-regulate expression of class I antigens on glial cells (21). However, MHV infection shuts off cellular protein synthesis of established cell lines. This complex interaction between the immune enhancement of MHC gene expression and the virus ability to suppress the expression may be important, not only in virus clearance from the brain, but also in establishment of acute and chronic demyelinating disease (12).

Genetic factors, which may control the virus replication strategy involving virus receptor and the immune response, are one of restricting elements of MHV pathogenicity (1). One well-known phenomenon is the resistance to A59 and JHM virus of SJL mice, perhaps due to a deficiency of a proteolytic activity necessary for dissemination(22). On the other hand, A/J and C57BL/6 mice are respectively resistant and susceptible to the acute hepatitis induced by MHV-3. Using recombinant strains, the susceptibility to MHV-3 induced hepatitis has been shown to correlate with the expression of lymphocyte-controlled prothrombin cleaving activity which facilitates necrosis (4).

Finally, it is important to remember that MHV infection of mouse colonies is still a prevalent and intractable problem (7). Recent papers have demonstrated that the infection of mice by MHV leads to a number of immune dysregulations. These include the loss of ability of spleen cells to secrete some lymphokines early in acute infection (18) as well as the hypersecretion following infection (10). Moreover, additional papers (3,14) appear frequently demonstrating the adverse effect of MHV infection on the analysis of a variety immune effector mechanism, including tumor clearance and macrophage activation.

REFERENCES

1. Barthold, S.W. 1987. Lab. Anim. Sci. 37:36-40.
2. Buchmeier, M.J., R.G. Dalziel, and M.J.M. Koolen. 1988. J. Neuroimmunol. 20: 111-116.
3. Casebolt, D.B., D.M. Spalding, T.R. Schoeb, and J.R. Lindsey. 1987. Cell.Immunol. 109: 97-103.
4. Dindzans, V.J., E. Skamene, and G.A. Levy. 1986. J. Immunol. 137: 2355-2360.
5. Fleming, J.O., M.D. Trousdale, J.Bradbury, S.A. Stohlman, and L.P. Weiner. 1987. Microb. Pathog. 3: 9-20.
6. Fleming, J.O., R.A. Shubin, M.A. Sussman, N. Casteel, and S.A. Stohlman. 1989. Virology 168: 162-167.
7. Fujiwara, K. 1988. Jpn. J. Exp. Med. 58: 115-121.
8. Goto, N., Y. Tsutsumi, A. Sato, and K. Fujiwara. 1987. Jpn. J. Vet. Sci. 49: 779-786.
9. Goto, N., K. Doi, T. Inoue, Y. Murai, and K. Fujiwara. 1988. Jpn. J. Vet. Sci. 50: 879-885.
10. Kyuwa, S., K. Yamaguchi, M. Hayami, J. Hilgers, and K. Fujiwara. 1988. J. Virol. 62: 2505-2507.
11. Kyuwa, S., K. Yamaguchi, Y. Toyoda, and K. Fujiwara. 1989. Jpn. J. Vet. Sci. 51: 219-221.
12. Lavi, E., A. Suzumura, E.M. Murray, D.H. Silberberg, and S.R. Weiss. 1989. J. Neuroimmunol. 22: 107-111.
13. Lecomte, J., V. Cainelli-Gebara, G. Mercier, S. Mansour, P.J. Talbot, G. Lussier, and D. Oth. 1987. Arch. Virol. 97: 123-130.
14. Li, L.H., T.F. DeKoning, J.A. Nicholas, G.D. Kramer, D.Wilson, T.L. Wallace, and M.J. Collins. 1987. Lab. Anim. Sci. 37: 41-44.
15. Perlman, S., R. Schelper, E. Bolger, and D. Ries. 1987. Microb. Pathog. 2: 185-194.
16. Perlman, S., and D. Ries. 1987. Microb. Pathog. 3: 309-314.
17. Perlman, S., G. Jacobsen, and S. Moore. Virology 166: 328-338.
18. Smith, A.L., K. Bottomly, and D.F. Winograd. 1987. J. Immunol. 138: 3426-3430.
19. Stohlman, S.A., M.A. Sussman, G.K. Matsushima, R.A. Shubin, and S.S. Erlich. 1988. J. Neuroimmunol. 19: 255-268.
20. Sussman, M.A., R.A. Shubin, S. Kyuwa, and S.A. Stohlman. 1989. J. Virol. 63: 3051-3056.
21. Suzumura, A., E. Lavi, S. Bhat, D. Murasko, S.R. Weiss, and D.H. Silberberg. 1988. J. Immunol. 140: 2068-2072.
22. Wilson, G.A.R., and S. Dales. 1988. J. Virol. 62: 3371-3377.

T CELL-MEDIATED CLEARANCE OF JHMV FROM THE CENTRAL NERVOUS SYSTEM

J. Williamson, S. Kyuwa, F.-I. Wang and S. Stohlman

Departments of Neurology and Microbiology
University of Southern California School of Medicine
Los Angeles, CA 90033

INTRODUCTION

Infection with the JHM strain of mouse hepatitis virus (JHMV) results in acute encephalomyelitis accompanied by primary demyelination in the central nervous system (CNS; 1). Animals that survive show evidence of persistent viral infection in the CNS that is associated with ongoing demyelination (2). Infection of immunocompromised animals suggests that the immune response is important not only in survival, but also as a determinant of whether the infection is cleared or progresses to become persistent. We initially demonstrated that the addition of anti-viral antibody to in vitro cultures of cells persistently infected with JHMV stopped the release of infectious virus (3,4). These in vitro data suggested that anti-viral antibody might play an important role in the ability of JHMV to establish a persistent infection in the CNS. Subsequent work has demonstrated that the passive transfer of monoclonal antibodies specific for all three structural proteins prevents death due to acute infection (5,6,7,8). Two very surprising findings were made. First, none of the transferred antibodies inhibited the replication of the virus in the CNS. Second, these antibodies altered the cellular tropism of the virus by preventing infection of neurons, which is associated with the death of the animals. The outcome of this altered tropism is an increase in the demyelination and the establishment of persistent infection.

Our laboratory initially used T cell clones to examine the role of cell-mediated immunity in the pathogenesis of JHMV infection. The adoptive transfer of CD4$^+$ delayed-type hypersensitivity (DTH) inducer T cell clones specific for JHMV is, like the passive transfer of antiviral antibody, able to prevent death due to a lethal infection (9). These clonal T cells prevented death without limiting the replication of the virus and resulted in more severe

demyelinating disease than untreated animals.   Virus
replication was not due to infection of the infiltrating
mononuclear cells (10). Hence, neither the anti-viral
antibody response nor the anti-viral DTH response, while able
to protect from death, inhibited JHMV replication.

In contrast, adoptive transfer of spleen cells from
immunized mice effectively reduced the replication of JHMV
in the CNS of infected mice (11).   Separation of spleen
cells into T cell and monocyte/B cell enriched populations
by nylon wool showed that the anti-viral activity partitioned
to the nylon wool adherent (NWA) population.   Analysis of
this population by negative selection demonstrated that a
subset of NWA T cells were mediating the reduction of virus
titer in the CNS. These T cells express the CD4 cell surface
marker, similar to the DTH-inducer T cells clones previously
described (9,10); however, this CD4+ T cell population does
not mediate a DTH response (11).   In addition, while the
expression of the CD4 cell surface marker suggested a major
histocompatibility (MHC) class II restricted cell, protection
was found to be MHC class I restricted. We suggested that
this apparent anomaly was because this cell functioned as a
helper-inducer of CD8$^+$ T cells, rather than as an effector
of anti-viral function (11).

RESULTS AND DISCUSSION

EFFECT OF CD8 AND CD4 T CELL DEPLETION ON JHMV INFECTION.
Abrogation of the immune response by irradiation results in
uncontrolled virus replication in the CNS (12). To examine
the role of the CD4$^+$ and CD8$^+$ subsets of T cells on JHMV
infection, mice were passively transferred with approximately
250 ug of anti-L3T4 and anti-Lyt-2 monoclonal antibodies
(Mab) on days -2, 0 and +2. Mice were infected with JHMV at
5 x 10^3 pfu i.c. on day 0. Recipients were sacrificed at the
days indicated in Figure 1. On days 9 and 11 p.i. both Mab

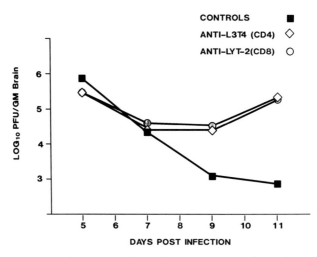

Figure 1. Impaired reduction in JHMV replication in the CNS
following in vivo treatment with anti-CD4 and anti-CD8 Mab.
Virus titer was determined as previously described (9)

treatments inhibited the reduction of JHMV titer in infected mice compared to untreated controls. This finding is consistent with our previous data suggesting that the adoptive transfer of NWA CD4[+] spleen cells mediate the reduction of virus by activating a CD8[+] T cell population. The finding that neither Mab altered the initial drop in virus replication, suggests the possibilities that another cell in the CD4[-], CD8[-] population maybe responsible for the early reduction in titer or that the Mab treatments were not effective.

To determine if the anti-L3T4 Mab was effective in blocking the immunological effector mechanisms attributed to CD4[+] T cells we examined the synthesis of anti-viral IgG by ELISA as previously described (13). Figure 2 shows that no anti-JHMV IgG was detectable in the serum of mice treated with anti-L3T4 Mab. The untreated and anti-Lyt-2 treated mice produced equivalent amounts of anti-JHMV IgG. These data suggest that the anti-L3T4 Mab was effective in inhibiting CD4[+] T cells. We have shown that similar treatment with anti-Lyt-2 Mab is effective in eliminating the anti-lymphocytic choriomengitis virus (LCMV) cytotoxic T cell response(11). These data suggest that the Mab treatments were indeed effective. The demonstration of effective depletion of CD4[+] and CD8[+] T cells reinforces the possibility that another irradiation sensitive effector mechanism may be reducing JHMV replication in the CNS early in infection.

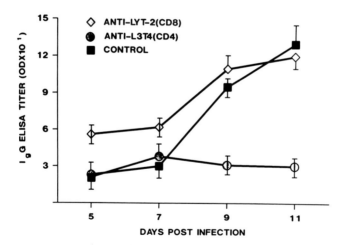

Figure 2. Abrogation of virus-specific IgG in mice following in vivo treatment with anti-CD4 Mab. Results show the mean OD obtained from 3 mice per group at each time point.

Histological examination of the CNS showed that there was a reduction in viral antigen in the untreated mice, comparable to the reduction in recoverable virus (see Figure 1). In contrast, mice treated with either Mab had significantly more viral antigen in the white matter tracks of the brain and spinal cord. Figure 3 shows representative

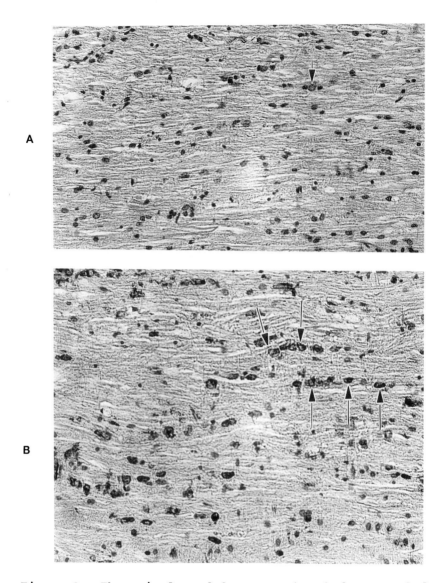

Figure 3. The spinal cord from an untreated mouse at day 11 post infection (Panel A: immunoperoxidase, X250). Panel B shows the spinal cord from a mouse treated with anti-Lyt-2 Mab demonstrating the abundant viral antigen within the cytoplasm of oligodendrocytes (immunoperoxidase, X250). Arrows indicate antigen positive cells.

photomicrographs of the spinal cords of untreated mice and mice treated with the anti-Lyt-2 Mab. Surprisingly, the amount of inflammation in the brains and spinal cords in all groups was not apparently different. These data suggest the possibility that gamma interferon, which is secreted by both CD4[+] and CD8[+] T cells, may play a role in the induction of inflammation in the CNS of mice infected with JHMV. Taken together these data suggest that the CD8[+] population is a critical component in the reduction of virus in the CNS.

EXPRESSION OF CLASS I ON INFECTED CELLS. While our data
suggests that CD8[+] T cells play a crucial role in reducing
JHMV replication in the CNS, it is presently unclear how this
is achieved. Cells in the CNS express little if any MHC
encoded molecules. Neurons, a primary target of JHMV
infection in dying mice (5), not only fail to express MHC
class I molecules, the restricting element for CD8[+] T cells,
but in contrast to cells of glial origin, these molecules
cannot be induced by gamma interferon (13,14). The clearance
of LCMV from the periphery and CNS is mediated by CD8[+] T
cells (15,16). However, because of the lengthy time required
for clearance from the CNS compared to the periphery and the
absence of cellular infiltration it has been suggested that
clearance from the CNS might be effected by lymphokines
rather than by direct cytolysis of infected cells. To
determine if JHMV can alter the expression of class I
molecules on the surface of potential targets of CD8 T cell
mediated cytotoxicity, the expression of class I MHC
molecules on the surface of J774.1 cells was examined using
Mab and ^{125}I-protein A. Cells were infected with JHMV at an
MOI of 4 and the expression of class I molecules was
determined. The data in Figure 4 show that there is a

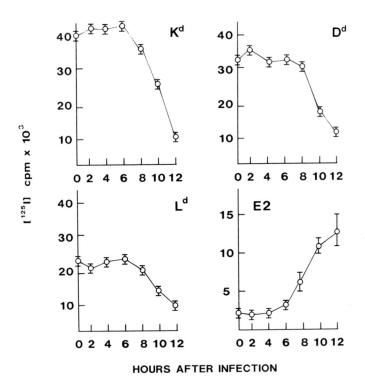

HOURS AFTER INFECTION

Figure 4. The time course of the loss of MHC class I
antigen expression from the surface of cells infected with
JHMV.

dramatic drop between 8 and 12 hours post infection in class I antigen on the surface of infected J774.1 cells compared to uninfected cells. At the same time there is an increase in JHMV E2 expression. We have also detected the loss of Fc receptor from the surface of these cells at 12 hours post infection (data not shown). These data indicate that JHMV infection may indeed inhibit the expression of MHC class I molecules on the surface of infected cells. This suggest the possibility that JHMV may escape the direct CD8$^+$ mediated cytolysis of cells in the CNS by suppressing the induction of MHC class I molecules on cells which constitutively express little or no class I.

CONCLUSION

The current and previously published data demonstrate a number of very unique aspects of the interaction between the replication of JHMV in the CNS of infected mice and the immune system. First, in contrast to other well characterized viruses which replicate predominantly outside the CNS, JHMV requires CD4$^+$ helper T cells that function as helper/inducers to activate a population of CD8$^+$ class I restricted T cells. Second, the down regulation of MHC class I molecules on the surface of infected cells suggests that the mechanism of protection afforded by these cells may not be through the direct cytolysis of infected CNS cells. Finally, another radiation sensitive cell, possibly an NK cell, may initially mediate the reduction of JHMV in the CNS. This final point will require the direct demonstration of NK cells in the CNS of infected mice. The observation of inflammation in the CNS of mice treated with anti-Lyt-2 or anti-L3T4 Mab suggests that gamma interferon may be present locally and either suppress virus itself or activate NK cells. Although the mechanism of JHMV-induced demyelination associated with persistent infection is not clear, the role(s) of the immune response in modulating this infection are beginning to be understood. Clearly, further work in this exciting area will be required to complete our understanding of how this virus is able to establish a chronic infection in its natural host.

REFERENCES

1. Weiner, L.P. 1973. Pathogenesis of demyelination produced by mouse hepatitis virus (JHM virus). Arch. Neurol. 28: 298-303.
2. Stohlman, S. A. and L. P. Weiner. 1981. Chronic central nervous system demyelination in mice after JHM virus infection. Neurology 31: 38-44.
3. Stohlman, S. A. and L. P. Weiner. 1978. Stability of mouse hepatitis virus (JHM strain) during chronic infection of neuroblastoma cells. Arch. Virol. 57:53-61.
4. Stohlman, S. A., Sakaguchi, A. Y. and L. P. Weiner. 1979. Rescue of a positive stranded RNA virus from antigen negative neuroblastoma cells. Life Sci. 24:1029-1036.

5. Buchmeier, M. J., Lewicki, H. A., Talbot, P. J., and R. L. Knobler. 1984. Mouse hepatitis virus-4 (strain JHM)-induced neurologic disease is modulated in vivo by monoclonal antibody. Virology 132:261-270.

6. Fleming, J. O., Shubin, R. A., Sussman, M. A., Casteel, N. and S. A. Stohlman. 1989. Monoclonal antibodies to the matrix (E1) glycoprotein of mouse hepatitis virus protect mice from encephalitis. Virology 168:162-167.

7. Nakanaga, K., Yamanouchi, K. and K. Fujiwara. 1986. Protective effect of monoclonal antibodies on lethal mouse hepatitis infection in mice. J. Virol. 59:168-171.

8. Wege, H., Dorries, R. and H. Wege. 1984. Hybridoma antibodies to the murine coronavirus JHM: characterization of the epitopes on the peplomer glycoprotein (E2). J. Gen. Virol. 65:1931-1942.

9. Stohlman, S., Matsushima, G., Casteel, N. and L. Weiner. 1986. In vivo effects of coronavirus-specific T cell clones: DTH-inducer cells prevent a lethal infection but do not inhibit virus replication. J. Immunol. 136:3052-3056.

10. Erlich, S., Matsushima, G. and S. Stohlman. 1989. Studies on the mechanism of protection from acute viral encephalomyelitis by delayed-type hypersensitivity inducer T cell clones. J. Neurol. Sci. 90:203-216.

11. Sussman, M., Shubin, R., Kyuwa, S. and S. Stohlman. 1989. T-cell-mediated clearance of mouse hepatitis virus strain JHM from the central nervous system. J. Virol. 63:3051-3056.

12. Sussman, M., Kachuck, N., Allen, H. and S. Stohlman. Immune mediated clearance of JHM from the CNS. Adv. Exp. Biol. Med. 218: 399-410.

13. Wong, G., Barteltt, P., Clark-Lewis, I., Battye, F. and J.W. Schrader. 1984. Inducible expression of H-2 and La antigens on brain cells. Nature 310: 668-670.

14. Main, E., Monos, D., and L. Lampson. 1988. IFN-treated neuroblastoma cells remain resistant to T cell-mediated allo-killing, and susceptible to non-MHC restricted cytotoxicity. J. Immunol. 141:2943-2950.

15. Oldstone, M., Blount, A., Southern, P. and P. Lampert. 1986. Cytoimmunotherapy for persistent virus infection: unique clearance pattern from the central nervous system. Nature 321:239-243.

16. Ahmed, R., Jamieson, E. and D. Porter. 1987. Immune therapy of a persistent and disseminated viral infection. J. Virol. 61:3920-3929.

IMMUNOPATHOGENESIS OF DEMYELINATION INDUCED BY MHV-4

J.O. Fleming[1,2], F.I. Wang[1,2], M.D. Trousdale[2,4],
D.R. Hinton[3], and S.A. Stohlman[1,2]

Departments of Neurology[1], Microbiology[2], Pathology[3]
and the Estelle Doheny Eye Institute[4]
University of Southern California Medical School
Los Angeles, CA 90033

INTRODUCTION

Mouse hepatitis virus-4 (MHV-4 or JHM) is a murine coronavirus which causes central nervous system (CNS) demyelination in rodents (1). Experimental MHV-4 infection has been used as a model of human demyelinating diseases, such as multiple sclerosis. One of the major questions relating to MHV-4 pathogenesis is the degree to which demyelination caused by this virus is due either to 1) direct viral cytopathology, especially for oligodendrocytes, the cells which produce and maintain myelin, or 2) immunological responses elicited by viral infection.

We have examined this issue by using a neutralization-resistant variant of MHV-4, designated 2.2-V-1 (2). This variant, immunoselected by a monoclonal antibody to the major glycoprotein (E2), has little neurovirulence but causes marked paralytic-demyelinating disease in at least 70% of mice inoculated intracerebrally (3). The role of immunity in experimental demyelination of mice during MHV-4 infection was explored in two ways. First, immunity was abrogated by X-irradiation of MHV-4-infected mice. Second, immunity was reconstituted by adoptive transfer of spleen cells into irradiated, infected recipient mice. Both approaches indicated that immune responses play a critical, essential role during demyelination induced by this virus.

RESULTS

Six-week old C57BL/6J male mice (Jackson Laboratories) seronegative (4) for MHV, were inoculated intracerebrally (i.c.) with 10^3 plaque forming units (pfu) of MHV-4, variant 2.2-V-1, as previously described (2). These mice developed marked paralytic-demyelinating disease, and at day 12 post-inoculation (p.i.) viral antigen and infectious virus were not detectible in the CNS (Fig. 1; Group 1, Table). In a second experiment, infected mice were immunosuppressed with 850 rads of X-irradiation on day 3 p.i. and observed daily until sacrifice at day 12 p.i. Despite the presence of abundant CNS virus, most prominently in oligodendrocytes, these mice did not develop paralytic-demyelinating disease (Fig. 2; Group 2, Table). Irradiation of mice infected with another variant of MHV-4, JHMV-DS (5) also blocked demyelination (data not shown). Similarly, paralytic-demyelinating disease was abrogated after immunosuppression of 2.2-V-1-infected mice with cyclophosphamide (200 mg/kg intraperitoneally (i.p.) on day 3 p.i.) (data not shown). Thus, unrestrained viral replication in oligodendrocytes during immunosuppression is insufficient to cause demyelination.

To explore the role of immune cells, mice were inoculated with MHV-4 i.c. and irradiated at day 3 p.i. as before; subsequently, these mice were reconstituted by the adoptive transfer of approximately 5×10^7 donor spleen cells intravenously. In the first adoptive transfer, recipient mice were given splenocytes from 6-week old C57BL/6 mice which had been immunized with 3×10^6 pfu of MHV-4 i.p. six days previously, that is, MHV-4-immune donors. Disease was fully reconstituted by this transfer (Fig. 3; Group 3, Table). However, when the adoptive transfer was repeated with MHV-4-immune donor cells which had been depleted of T lymphocytes by prior treatment with complement and anti-Thy-1.2 monoclonal antibody (5a-8, Cedarlane), disease was not restored (Group 4, Table), indicating that MHV-4-immune T cells are necessary for demyelination. Preliminary studies indicate that the cell predominantly responsible for adoptive transfer of disease may have the CD8[+] phenotype (Fig. 4).

In following experiments, spleen cells from naive, unimmunized donor mice were transferred to MHV-4-infected, irradiated mice (Group 5, Table). The majority (75%) of these mice were normal clinically and histologically at d. 12 p.i.; the remaining mice showed signs of disease which developed less rapidly and with less intensity than in virally-infected (Group 1) or immune-reconstituted (Group 3) mice. Similar results were obtained with transfers in which keyhole limpet hemocyanin (KLH) (Sigma) was used to immunize donor mice (Group 6), indicating that robust, efficient transfer of disease requires cells which have been specifically sensitized to MHV-4. Transfer of MHV-4-immune cells into uninfected, irradiated recipients (Group 7) did not result in disease, indicating that immunopathological responses are primarily directed against virus or virus-altered determinants, not self. In other experiments, the transfer of allogenic immune spleen cells from BALB/c ($H-2^d$) mice into infected, irradiated C57BL/6J $H-2^b$) mice did not result in paralysis or demyelination, suggesting that adoptive transfer of disease is restricted by the major histocompatibility complex.

Low levels (approximately 1:100 end point titers) of anti-MHV-4 IgM antibody were detected in all groups of mice, except number 2 (infected, irradiated mice that were not reconstituted by splenocytes). The finding that group 4 mice, lacking T cells but positive for antibody, do not develop paralytic-demyelinating disease indicated that antibody alone is insufficient to cause disease.

Table 1. Outcome at 12 days post-inoculation, after Irradiation and Adoptive Transfers

Group	[a]Experiment	[b]Paralysis	[b]Demyelination	[b]Virus	Antibody
1	virus only	+	+	-	+
2	virus, irradiation	-	-	++	-
3	virus-immune→ virus recipient	+	+	-	+
4	virus-immune (T cell depleted)→ virus recipient	-	-	+	+
5	non-immune→ virus recipient	+/-	+/-	+	+
6	KLH-immune→ virus recipient	+/-	+/-	+	+/-
7	virus-immune→ uninfected recipient	-	-	-	+

[a]Experimental groups, as explained in text; "virus" refers to MHV-4, variant 2⊙2-V-1, "irradiation" to 850 rads given on day 3 p.i., and arrows indicate the adoptive transfer of approximately 5×10^7 spleen cells intravenously into irradiated recipients on day 3 p.i. Donor mice were prepared by the intraperitoneal administration of 3×10^6 pfu of virus or 150 ug of KLH 6 days prior to adoptive transfer as indicated.

[b]Outcome of experiments, judged at 12 days p.i. Positive symbols indicate severe hindleg paralysis, marked demyelination on blinded histologic evaluations, infectious virus recovery from brain homogenates (2), and IgM antibody measured by enzyme-linked immunosorbent assay (4), respectively. Where positive results were obtained in occasional mice or were of low titer, a "+/-" symbol is used.

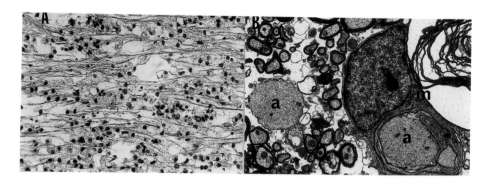

Figure 1. Mouse infected with virus and sacrificed at day 12 p.i. (Group 1, Table) A. Longitudinal section of spinal cord, stained immunohistochemically for MHV-4 antigen and counterstained with hematoxylin, as previously described (3), x 100. Note extensive white matter rarefaction, marked inflammatory infiltrate consisting primarily of lymphocytes and macrophages, and the absence of viral antigen. B. Epon-embedded transverse section of spinal cord, prepared as previously described (2). Note demyelinated axons (a) and macrophage stripping myelin (m). x 6,000.

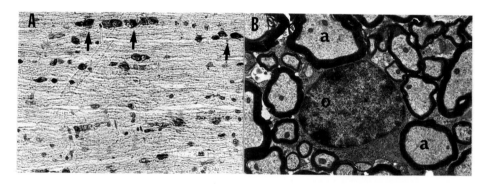

Figure 2. Mouse infected with virus, irradiated at day 3 pi., and sacrificed at day 12 p.i. (Group 2, Table). A. Spinal cord stained for viral antigen, as in Fig. 1A. Note abundant viral antigen in cells with the appearance of intrafascicular oligodendrocytes (arrows). x 200. B. epon-embedded spinal cord, prepared as in figure 1B. Note normal appearance of myelinated axons (a) and an oligodendrocyte (o) x 6,000.

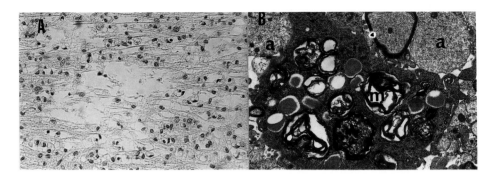

Figure 3. Adoptive transfer in which virus-immune donor splenocytes were given intravenously at day 3 p.i. to a virus-infected, irradiated recipient (Group 3, Table). A. spinal cord, prepared as in Fig. 1A. Note intense inflammation, similar to virus-only mouse shown in Fig. 1A x 200. B. Spinal cord, prepared as in 1B. Note demyelinated axons (a) and macrophage (m) with phagocytosed myelin debris. x 15,000.

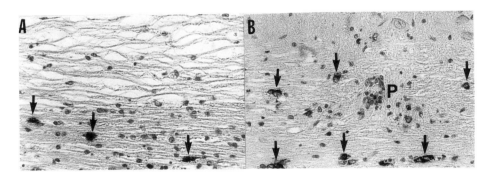

Figure 4. Longitudinal section of mouse spinal cords, stained immunohistochemically for viral antigen, as in Fig. 1A. Viral-immune donor splenocytes were depleted of different T cell subsets by incubation with complement and specific monoclonal antibodies prior to transfer into virus-infected, irradiated recipient mice. A. After depletion of donor CD4[+] cells (anti-L3T4 monoclonal antibody RL172.4 recognizing helper-inducer T cells (6)). Note demyelinated lesion at top of figure; although white matter rarefaction is severe, cellular·infiltration is less intense than virus-only control mice (Fig. 1A). Scanty viral antigen is seen outside of the borders of this lesion (arrows) x 200. B. After depletion of donor CD8[+] cells (anti-Lyt-2 monoclonal antibody recognizing cytotoxic-suppressor T cells (7)). Note perivascular infiltrate (P) and abundant antigen (arrows). White matter rarefaction and demyelination are not present. x 200 Treatment of donor splenocytes with complement only had no effect on the transfer of disease (data not shown).

DISCUSSION

MHV-4-induced demyelination has often been considered to be a direct consequence of viral infection of oligodendrocytes. This hypothesis is supported by three lines of evidence. First, many in vivo and in vitro studies have established the tropism of MHV-4 for oligodendrocytes and other CNS cells of rodents (1,8,9,10). Second, in an early study, mice infected with MHV-4 and treated with cyclophosphamide showed "small areas of demyelination" despite the apparent ablation of humoral and cellular immunity (11). Similarly, treatment of MHV-4-infected rats with cyclophosphamide (12) or with cyclosporin A (13) resulted in a panencephalitis in which foci of necrosis were noted in white matter, although the status of myelin was not specifically addressed in these reports. Third, immunodeficient, athymic mice (12) and rats (14) also develop small demyelinated foci after MHV-4 infection. It is important to note, however, that in the studies cited immunosuppression or immunodeficiency converted the normally non-fatal MHV-4 infection into an acute fatal panencephalitis. It is not clear that occasional demyelinating lesions in the setting of an overwhelming panencephalitis accurately reflect the natural disease as originally described by Bailey et al (15); in this case, MHV-4 produces a paralytic disease in which pathology is centered in the white matter and large demyelinating lesions are readily apparent.

We have studied MHV-4-induced demyelination under conditions in which acute encephalitis is minimized and does not confound the analysis of subacute white matter pathology. This was achieved by two means: 1) a relatively avirulent, less encephalitic, MHV-4 strain, MHV-4 2.2-V-1 (2), was used, and 2) immunosuppression was applied at day 3 p.i., that is, after the initial phase of viral replication, but before severe white matter pathology develops. Using this protocol, we were able to ablate demyelination by means of immunosuppression and reconstitute demyelination by the adoptive transfer of MHV-4-specific immune T cells. As noted, preliminary results indicate that T cells with the $CD8^+$, or cytotoxic-suppressor cell, phenotype may be the critical element which clears virus (J. Williamson et al, this volume) and contributes to the development of typical foci of primary demyelination (fig 4). Together with previous investigations, these results suggest two contrasting roles for the immune system during MHV-4 pathogenesis. First, as shown by studies of immunodeficient rodents (12,14) or animals immunosuppressed simultaneously with viral inoculation (11,12,13), immunocompetence is necessary early in MHV-4 infection in order to prevent an overwhelming, fulminant CNS infection. In other words, the primary role of the immune system is to protect mice from acute encephalitis and to clear virus from the CNS (16). Second, the results above indicate that participation of the immune system, especially T cells, is essential during subacute demyelination elicited by MHV-4. In this sense, the role of the immune system is a negative one, resulting in disease. Learning in detail how MHV-4 elicits this response may be an important step in understanding human diseases such as multiple sclerosis in which a viral etiology and an immunopathological basis for demyelination are suspected.

CONCLUSIONS

1. MHV-4-induced demyelination is not a direct, cytolytic consequence of virus infection of oligodendrocytes.

2. Immunosuppression abrogates MHV-4-induced demyelination.

3. MHV-4-specific T cells play a critical role in MHV-4-induced demyelination.

4. Preliminary evidence indicates that CD8[+] T cells may be the predominant cell in adoptive transfer of demyelination; transfer of disease also appears to be restricted by the major histocompatibility complex.

ACKNOWLEDGEMENTS

We thank Ligaya Pen, Cindy Fabricius-Segal, Wenqiang Wei, and Julie Adams for technical assistance and Carol Flores for preparation of the manuscript. This work was supported by grants from the NIH.

REFERENCES

1. H. Wege, S. Siddell, and V. ter Meulen: The biology and pathogenesis of coronaviruses. Curr. Top. Microbiol. Immunol. 99:265-200 (1982).

2. J.O. Fleming, M.D. Trousdale, F.A.K. El-Zaatari, S.A. Stohlman, and L.P. Weiner: Pathogenicity of antigenic variants of murine coronavirus JHM selected with monoclonal antibodies. J. Virol. 58:869-875 (1986).

3. J.O. Fleming, M.D. Trousdale, J. Bradbury, S.A. Stohlman, and L.P. Weiner: Experimental demyelination induced by coronavirus JHM (MHV-4): molecular identification of a viral determinant of paralytic disease. Microb. Pathogenesis. 3:9-20 (1987).

4. J.O. Fleming and L.B. Pen: Measurement of the concentration of murine IgG monoclonal antibody in hybridoma supernatants and ascites in absolute units by sensitive and reliable enzyme-linked immunosorbent assays (ELISA). J. Immunol. Methods 110:11-18 (1988).

5. S.A. Stohlman, P.R. Brayton, J.O. Fleming, L.P. Weiner, and M.M.C. Lai: Murine coronaviruses: isolation and characterization of two plaque morphology variants of the JHM neurotropic strain. J. Gen. Virol. 63:265-275 (1982.

6. R. Ceredig, J.W. Lowenthal, M. Nabholz, and H.R. MacDonald: Expression of interleukin-2 receptors as a differentiation marker in intrathymic stem cells. Nature 314:98-100 (1985).

7. M. Sarmiento, A.L. Glasebrook, and F.W. Tich: IgG or IgM monoclonal antibodies reactive with different determinants on the molecular complex bearing Lyt 2 antigen block T cell-mediated cytolysis in the absence of complement. J. Immunol. 125:2665-2672 (1980).

8. H.C. Powell, and P.W. Lampert: Oligodendrocytes and their myelin-plasma membrane connections in JHM mouse hepatitis virus encephalomyelitis. Lab. Invest. 33:440-445 (1975).

9. H.J.A. Fleury, R.D. Sheppard, M.B. Bornstein, and C.S. Raine: Further ultrastructural observations of virus morphogenesis and myelin pathology in JHM virus encephalomyelitis. Neuropath. Appl. Neurobiol. 6:165-179 (1980).

10. R.L. Knobler, M. Dubois-Dalcq, M.V. Haspel, A.P. Claysmith, P.W. Lampert, and M.B.A. Oldstone: Selective localization of wild type and mutant mouse hepatitis virus (JHM strain) antigens in CNS tissue by fluorescence, light and electron microscopy. J. Neuroimmunol. 1:81-92 (1981).

11. L.P. Weiner: Pathogenesis of demyelination induced by a mouse hepatitis virus (JHM virus). Arch. Neurol. 28:298-303 (1973).

12. O. Sorensen, R. Dugre, D. Percy, and S. Dales: In vivo and in vitro models of demyelinating disease: endogenous factors influencing demyelinating disease caused by mouse hepatitis virus in rats and mice. Infection Immunity 37:1248-1260 (1982).

13. M.J. Zimmer and S. Dales: In vivo and in vitro models of demyelinating diseases XXIV. The infectious process in cyclosporin A treated Wistar Lewis rats inoculated with JHM virus. Microb. Pathogenesis 6:7-16 (1989).

14. O. Sorensen, A. Saravani, and S. Dales: In vivo and in vitro models of demyelinating disease. XVII. The infectious process in athymic rats inoculated with JHM virus. Microb. Pathogenesis 2:79-90 (1987).

15. T.O. Bailey, A.M. Pappenheimer, F.S. Cheever, and J.B. Daniels: A murine virus (JHM) causing disseminated encephalomyelitis with extensive destruction of myelin II. Pathology. J. Exp. Med. 90:195-231 (1949).

16. M.A. Sussman, R.A. Shubin, S. Kyuwa, and S.A. Stohlman: T-cell-mediated clearance of mouse hepatitis virus strain JHM from the central nervous system. J. Virol. 63:3051-3056 (1989).

LOCALIZATION OF VIRUS AND ANTIBODY RESPONSE IN

MICE INFECTED PERSISTENTLY WITH MHV-JHM

Gary Jacobsen and Stanley Perlman

University of Iowa School of Medicine
Departments of Pediatrics and Microbiology
University of Iowa Hospitals and Clinics
Iowa City, Iowa 52242

ABSTRACT

Suckling mice infected intranasally with MHV-JHM and nursed by immunized dams develop a late onset demyelinating encephalomyelitis. Analysis by in situ hybridization revealed that MHV-JHM entered the central nervous system (CNS) via the olfactory and trigeminal nerves and spread over the next two weeks to the spinal cord, prior to amplification at this site. Serial measurements of neutralizing antibody titers showed that the late onset disease developed in some mice at levels of antibody which protected mice from the fatal, acute encephalitis, supporting the notion that cell-mediated and not humoral immunity is important in protecting mice from MHV-JHM persistence.

INTRODUCTION

Intranasal or intracerebral inoculation of weanling or suckling mice with the JHM strain of mouse hepatitis virus (MHV-JHM) causes an invariably fatal encephalitis. In previous reports, we have characterized a model in which suckling C57BL/6 mice are protected from the acute encephalitis if they are nursed by immunized dams (1-3). We have shown that:

1) After inoculation with MHV-JHM intranasally, all of the mice were protected from the fatal encephalomyelitis at 7 d p.i. However, histological evidence of encephalitis was present even though the mice remained asymptomatic. 40% of the maternal antibody-protected mice developed neurological disease expressed clinically by hindlimb paralysis and histologically by a demyelinating encephalomyelitis. Whereas viral antigen could be detected in all mice whether symptomatic or asymptomatic, virus could only be isolated from symptomatic mice. The serum antibody response in both asymptomatic and symptomatic mice was minimal.

2) The astrocyte was an important target cell in the CNS in both symptomatic and asymptomatic mice and accounted for 20-40% of the infected cells in nearly all mice.

3) Using in situ hybridization, we determined that MHV-JHM was present throughout the brain in mice dying from the acute encephalitis. On the other hand, virus could always be detected in the spinal cord and brainstem of mice with hindlimb paralysis. Additionally, it was also present in other

parts of the brain, including the hippocampus, the thalamus, the cerebral cortex and the optic chiasm, in some mice with the late onset disease.

In this report, we describe the localization of virus in asymptomatic mice at early and late times p.i. We also present experiments which show that high levels of anti-MHV-JHM antibody do not protect against the development of the late onset neurological disease.

MATERIALS AND METHODS

Animals, viruses, sera. MHV-JHM, MHV-A59 and C57BL/6 mice were obtained as previously described (1). In some experiments, mice were immunized with UV-inactivated MHV-JHM, prepared by treatment of MHV-JHM with 18,000 erg/mm^2. No residual virus could be detected by plaque assay. Sera were titered by either a neutralization assay (1) or by ELISA (manuscript in preparation).

In situ hybridization. This was performed as described previously (3).

RESULTS

Clinical studies: In our first study, we showed that suckling mice inoculated at ten days of age and suckled by unimmunized dams all died of an encephalitis, whereas mice suckled by immunized dams all survived. Forty percent of the latter developed hindlimb paralysis at 35 d p. i., with a range of 23 to 60 d (1).

In the present study, 103/114 (90%) of maternal antibody-protected offspring developed hindlimb paralysis. Of the 103 which developed hindlimb paralysis, 15 (15%) recovered with a mild residual paresis; some of these mice also had several additional relapses. Mean maternal antibody titers, as measured by plaque-reduction neutralization assay, were 1:550 in this study, as opposed to 1:2700 in the first one.

Hindlimb paralysis was noted at 25 d (S.D. 11 d) with a range of 9-83 d; only two mice were noted to develop hindlimb paralysis at an age greater than 60 d p.i. Most of the mice had only hindlimb paralysis, with no signs of encephalitis (hunching, ruffled fur, irritability and lethargy). However, some of the mice that developed clinical disease at earlier times after inoculation (less than 18 d p.i.) were observed to have mild encephalitic symptoms as well.

Since mice greater than 60 days of age generally did not develop clinical disease, this suggested that some type of maturation, whether in the immune system or otherwise, had occurred to prevent viral reactivation. To identify a possible active role of the immune system in this process, a group of older mice were immunosuppressed with cyclophosphamide. For this purpose, 12 mice greater than 100 days p.i. were divided into two groups. Six were treated with cyclophosphamide at a dosage shown previously to be immunosuppressive (200 mg/kg/d administered intraperitoneally every other day for three doses (4)). No neurological disease developed in any mouse from either group.

Regional localization of MHV-JHM in mice at early times p.i. In the first experiments, brains isolated from mice inoculated intranasally with MHV-JHM and nursed by unimmunized dams were analyzed by in situ hybridization with [35S] labelled antisense RNA probes (3). At 3 d p.i., viral RNA was readily detected in the olfactory lobes of all mice. By 4 d p.i., viral RNA could be detected in nearby areas of the olfactory system, and could also be detected in the brainstem at a site corresponding to the mesencephalic nucleus of the trigeminal nerve. By 5 d p.i., when the mice were nearly dead, viral RNA could be detected throughout the brain, with prominent labelling occurring in the hypothalamus, hippocampus, basal ganglia and thalamus. In the computerized version of these data shown in Figure 1, representative sagittal sections from each mouse were digitalized. Viral RNA was clearly present initially in the olfactory lobes and mesencephalic nucleus at 3 and 4 d p.i., with rapid spread to central portions of the brain at 5 d p.i.

Suckling mice nursed by immunized dams are completely protected from the acute encephalitis, but may develop hindlimb paralysis several weeks p.i.(1). When these mice were analyzed at early times p.i., MHV-JHM RNA could be detected in the olfactory lobes and mesencephalic nucleus of the trigeminal nerve, in the same distribution as observed in mice nursed by unimmunized dams. Similarly, the same distribution of viral RNA was observed at 3-4 d p.i. in mice infected with the attenuated A59 strain of MHV. These results suggested that MHV, whether the virulent JHM or avirulent A59 strain, entered the CNS via the olfactory and trigeminal nerves, both of which innervate the nose.

Regional localization in asymptomatic mice at 15 d p.i. Maternal antibody-protected mice remain asymptomatic at 15 d p.i., and MHV-JHM RNA could not be detected in the brains of these mice by in situ hybridization and film autoradiography. However, viral RNA could be detected in the cephalic part of the spinal cord in all mice that were examined. This result suggested that virus was transported from the olfactory/limbic or trigeminal systems to the spinal cord prior to the increase in viral replication which in turn led to clinical disease.

Relationship of serum antibody titer and the development of clinical disease. In the next set of experiments, we determined the level of neutralizing antibody protective against the acute disease, and also determined whether infected mice with low levels of antibody were capable of mounting any antibody response against MHV-JHM. To interpret experiments involving the decay of maternal anti MHV-JHM antibody, we first determined its rate of decay in uninfected suckling mice. Maternal anti-MHV-JHM

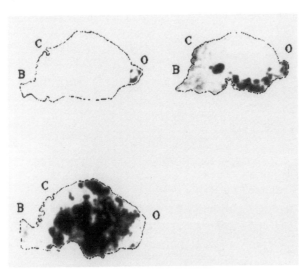

Figure 1-Computer digitalization of mice with acute encephalitis analyzed by in situ hybridization. Digitalization was performed using the LONISP program (Washington University, St. Louis). B-brainstem, O-olfactory lobe, C-cerebellum, arrow-mesencephalic nucleus of the trigeminal nerve. Upper left-3 dp.i.; upper right-4 d p.i.; lower left-5 d p.i.

antibody decayed with a half-life of 5.75 d (S.D. .88 d, range 4.76-6.88 d), in agreement with previous measurements of decay of total maternal antibody (5).

To determine the minimal level of neutralizing antibody protective against the acute encephalitis, antibody titers were measured at 3 and 7 d p.i. in 82 infected mice suckled by immunized dams. Fifty one (62%) had a titer >1:400, 22 (27%) had titers between 1:200 and 1:400 and 9 (11%) had titers between 1:100 and 1:200. These results suggested that titers greater than 1:100 were protective against the acute disease.

Serial titers were measured in 62 of these mice. Thirty six (69%) had neutralizing titers <1:100 when they developed hindlimb paralysis. The remainder had titers >1:100, with 4 mice (6%) developing hindlimb paralysis with serum titers >1:400 (Figure 2A). This result suggested that neutralizing titers effective against the acute disease did not protect against the development of hindlimb paralysis. For greater sensitivity, serial titers were also assayed by ELISA. Antibody titer decayed at the same approximate rate when measured by either neutralization assay or ELISA. However, measurement by ELISA showed that in most mice, the titer either remained constant or rose slightly at 20-30 days p.i. (Figure 2B). Thus, most mice were able to mount a minimal antibody response, which could only be detected by ELISA.

To determine whether the mice which exhibited a low antibody response were capable of mounting a greater response, a group of 18 mice greater than 40 d p.i. were immunized at weekly intervals with either live virus (two times) or UV-inactivated virus (three times) in Freund's adjuvant. 89% (16/18) of the mice so immunized developed an elevated antibody response with a titer (mean 1:692) similar to that observed in uninfected mice immunized as described previously (1).

Antibody response in young mice. The results presented thus far showed that maternal antibody-protected mice did not develop a significant antibody response to MHV-JHM, although they were capable of doing so if immunized in the presence of a strong adjuvant. To determine if younger mice were

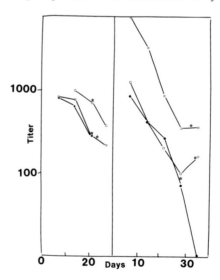

Figure 2-Serial neutralization and ELISA antibody titers in maternal antibody-protected mice. A) Neutralizing titers in 3 mice that developed hindlimb paralysis in the presence of elevated levels of serum antibody. B) Representative serial ELISA titers for three mice that developed hindlimb paralysis. *-time when hindlimb paresis was first noted.

capable of responding to MHV-JHM, uninfected suckling and young weanling mice, suckled by unimmunized dams, were immunized with live MHV-JHM in Freund's adjuvant. Five mice were immunized with MHV-JHM at weekly intervals for three weeks beginning at 14 d after birth. Four weeks later, neutralizing antibody titers ranged from 1:50 to 1:377, with a mean of 1:191. In comparison, mice immunized at 10-12 weeks of age developed mean titers of 1:692 (range 1:200 to 1:1500) as described in the previous section. Thus these mice were capable of mounting an antibody response, although the kinetics of response and maximal titer attained were less than that observed in older mice. Attempts made to immunize young infected mice with MHV-JHM were unsuccessful, probably because the presence of maternal antibody prevented any antibody response.

DISCUSSION

After intranasal inoculation, MHV enters the CNS via the olfactory and trigeminal nerves. If mice are susceptible to the acute encephalitis, virus spreads rapidly from these portals of entry to more central locations, causing death. On the other hand, if the fatal disease is prevented either by using an attenuated virus such as the A59 strain or by inoculating mice that are nursed by immunized dams, virus remains confined to the olfactory and trigeminal systems and their direct connections, such as the limbic system. Viral RNA disappears from the brain over the next few days, but can be detected in the spinal cord at 15 d p.i., although the mice remain asymptomatic.

In mice that develop hindlimb paralysis, viral RNA can always be detected in the spinal cord, suggesting that virus which has been previously transported to this structure is able to amplify and eventually cause clinical disease. At the same time, virus appears to amplify in some mice in other parts of the CNS which are either immediate or distant connections of the olfactory and trigeminal nerves and from there spread to other structures in the CNS.

The factors that are important for suppression of viral replication in asymptomatic mice, and those which facilitate viral amplification and resultant clinical disease have not been determined. One explanation would be that the virus has been modified during the period of clinical latency in mice, as has been shown to occur under certain conditions in rats infected with MHV-JHM (6-8). We have found that virus isolated from mice with hindlimb paralysis is identical to the initial stock of MHV-JHM by protein and RNA blot analysis, by radioimmunoprecipitation and polyacrylamide gel electrophoresis of infected cell proteins and by ELISA with a panel of monoclonal antibodies directed against 5 different epitopes of the E2 glycoprotein of MHV-JHM (antibodies provided by Dr. Michael Buchmeier).

A second explantion is that the immune system is not able to respond appropriately to MHV, thus allowing viral replication. Sufficient levels of maternal antibody protect mice from the acute encephalitis (1,9), but do not prevent viral persistence in the CNS. In this report, we show that after passively-acquired maternal antibody levels have decayed to low levels, antibody response in infected offspring is minimal, whether the mice have developed hindlimb paralysis or remain asymptomatic. Additionally, some of the mice become paralyzed at a time when their serum antibody titers are at a level which would protect against the acute encephalitis, suggesting that even if mice could mount a high antibody response, this would not protect against viral amplification and the development of clinical disease. One caveat is that these measurements were performed on serum, and may not reflect levels present in the CNS.

Neutralizing antibody may not be protective for one of several reasons.

Even though the envelope glycoprotein E2 is usually found on the surface of infected cells, less may be present in cells of the CNS (10). Another possibility is that MHV-JHM spreads primarily via cell to cell spread and is therefore not accessible to antibody.

Maternal antibody-protected C57BL/6 mice for the most part develop only a low level of neutralizing or total antibody, although they are capable of mounting a response if immunized with a strong adjuvant. This may reflect inadequate antigen presentation since the virus is present in the CNS, considered an immunologically protected site. The same difficulty may cause an inadequate cell-mediated immune response, which in turn might account for the inability of the host to eliminate MHV-JHM. An age-dependence exists as well, since antibody response is less in young mice and almost all mice which survive to ten weeks (60 d p.i.) do not develop hindlimb paralysis.

In previous studies, antibody response also has not correlated well with the development of clinical disease or demyelinating lesions in rodents infected with MHV-JHM (4,11). Our results suggest, as do other studies (12), that cellular immunity may be most important in protection of mice against MHV-JHM.

ACKNOWLEDGEMENTS: This research was supported by grant NIH NS24401 and by a Research Career Development Award to S.P.

REFERENCES

1. Perlman, S., Schelper, R., Bolger, E., Ries, D., 1987, Late onset, symptomatic, demyelinating encephalomyelitis in mice infected with MHV-JHM in the presence of maternal antibody. Microbial Pathog. 2:185.
2. Perlman, S., Ries, D., 1987, The astrocyte is a target cell in mice persistently infected with mouse hepatitis virus, strain JHM. Microbial Pathog. 3:309.
3. Perlman, S., Jacobsen, G., Moore, S., 1988, Regional localization of virus in the central nervous system of mice persistently infected with murine coronavirus JHM. Virology 166:328.
4. Stohlman, S., Weiner, L., 1981, Chronic central nervous system demyelination in mice after JHM virus infection. Neurology 31:38.
5. Pace, G., Dresser, D., 1961, The elimination of mouse and bovine globulins from the circulation of newborn and adult mice. Quart. J. Exp. Physiol. 46:369.
6. Taguchi, F. Siddell, S., Wege, H., ter Meulen, V.,1985, Characterization of a variant virus selected in rat brain after infection of mouse coronavirus JHM. J. Virol. 54:429.
7. Taguchi, F., Fleming, J., 1989, Comparison of six different murine coronavirus JHM variants by monoclonal antibodies against the E2 glycoprotein. Virology 169:233.
8. Morris, V., Tieszer, C., MacKinnon, J., Percy, D., 1989, Characterization of coronavirus JHM variants isolated from Wistar Furth rats with a viral-induced demyelinating disease. Virology 169:127.
9. Pickel, K., Muller, M., ter Meulen, V., 1985, Influence of maternal immunity on the outcome of murine coronavirus JHM infection in suckling mice. Med. Micro. Immunol. 174:15.
10. Parham, D., Tereba, A., Talbot, P., Jackson, D., Morris., V., 1986, Analysis of JHM central nervous system infections in rats. Arch. Neurol. 43:702
11. Watanabe, R., Wege, H., ter Meulen, V., 1987, Comparative analysis of coronavirus JHM-induced demyelinating encephalomyelitis in Lewis and Brown Norway rats. Lab. Invest. 57:375.
12. Sussman, M., Shubin, R., Kyuwa, S., Stohlman, S., 1989, T-Cell-Mediated clearance of mouse hepatitis virus strain JHM from the central nervous system. J. Virol. 63:3051

REGULATION OF MHC CLASS I AND II ANTIGENS ON CEREBRAL

ENDOTHELIAL CELLS AND ASTROCYTES FOLLOWING MHV-4 INFECTION

J. Joseph, R L. Knobler, F.D. Lublin and M.N. Hart [*]

Division of Neuroimmunology,
Department of Neurology, Jefferson Medical College
Philadelphia, PA, and *Department of Neuropathology
University of Iowa, Iowa City, IA, USA.

The direct induction of major histocompatibility complex coded molecules following virus infection of cerebral endothelial cells and astrocytes may play an important role in the pathogenesis of organ specific CNS disease. Mouse hepatitis virus type 4 (MHV-4)(JHM strain), a member of the coronavirus family, causes a spectrum of disease ranging from fatal acute encephalomyelitis to demyelination in susceptible murine hosts (Bailey et al., 1949). Massa et al., (1986, 1987a) demonstrated the ability of MHV-4 to directly induce Ia (class II) antigen expression on Lewis rat astrocytes in vitro. In contrast in the C57BL/6 mouse, Suzumura et al., (1986) showed that a related coronavirus, MHV-A59, induced class I but not class II antigens on mouse astrocytes and oligodendrocytes.

We were interested in studying the response of cerebral endothelial cells, a major structural component of the blood-brain barrier (BBB), to MHV-4 infection. These cells play an important role in regulating virus entry into the brain (Johnson 1974, 1982,; Wiley et al., 1986). Cerebral endothelial cells have also been shown to function in antigen presentation (McCarron et al., 1985, 1986) and therefore could potentially modulate immune mediated events occuring in the CNS following MHV-4 infection. We assessed the expression of class I and II MHC antigens following MHV-4 infection, in brain endothelial cells derived from strains of mice that differed in their susceptibility to MHV-4 induced disease. The response of astrocytes to MHV-4 infection was also studied in order to compare them with endothelial cells.

Our studies were performed using cultured brain endothelial cell lines derived from MHV-susceptible (Balb/c, B10.S and (Balb/c x SJL) F1) and MHV-resistant (SJL) strains of mice (Stohlman and Frelinger, 1978; Knobler et al., 1981). Astrocytes were isolated and cultured from Balb/c, CXJ-8, B10.S and SJL strains of mice. Cytopathic effects and the degree of expression of class I and II MHC antigens were examined after MHV-4 infection of cerebral endothelial cells and astrocytes. Our findings demonstrate that following MHV-4 infection, there was a differential modulation of the H-2K and

H-2D class I molecules on endothelial cells derived from Balb/c, but not SJL, B10.S and (Balb/c x SJL)F1 mice in which parallel modulation occurred. Parallel modulation of class I molecules was also seen in astrocytes derived from Balb/c, SJL, B10.S and CXJ-8 strains of mice. In contrast class II molecules did not fluctuate following MHV-4 infection of either endothelial cells or astrocytes. MHV-4 infection, however, selectively down regulated gamma interferon induced class II antigen expression in both endothelial cells and astrocytes. Gamma interferon induced class I antigen expression appears unaffected by MHV-4 infection.

MATERIALS AND METHODS

Endothelial cell culture

Cerebral endothelial cells were isolated from the brains of Balb/c, SJL, B10.S, (Balb/c x SJL)F1 strains of mice using a modification of the method described by DeBault et al., (1981). Endothelial cell lines obtained were maintained in Medium 199 with 20% fetal bovine serum and additional supplements that included (BME) Basal medium Eagle amino acids, BME vitamins, glutamine, Bacto-peptone and penicillin-streptomycin. Endothelial identity was established by studying the uptake of DiI-Ac-LDL (Biomedical Technologies, Stoughton, MA, USA) and specific binding of Bandeirea simplicifolia BSI-B_4 (Voyta et al., 1984; Schelper et al., 1985).

Astrocyte cultures Astrocyte cultures were established from Balb/c, SJL, B10.S and CXJ-8 strains of mice. Brain cortices derived from 14 day mouse embryos were mechanically dissociated through Nitex mesh bags (210 microns). Astrocytes were cultured in Hams F-10 medium containing 10% fetal bovine serum. Astrocytic identity of these cells was established by their positive reactivity to an antibody directed against glial fibrillary acidic protein.

Virus infection and interferon treatment of cultures

Endothelial cells or astrocytes grown in T25 flasks (1 x 10^6/flask) were infected for 1 hour at an MOI of 0.1 with MHV-4(JHM strain). After three washes the infected cultures were refed with either Med 199 (with added supplements) or 200U/ml recombinant rat gamma interferon (Amgen Biologicals, Thousand Oaks, CA). Control uninfected cultures treated with gamma interferon were also set up.

Monoclonal antibody labeling and flow cytometry

Four days after infection cells were removed from plates by trypsin-EDTA treatment. 5×10^5 cells were labeled with an antibody to H-2k^d, H-2D^d (Organon Teknika-Cappel, Malvern, PA), H-2K^s, H-2D^s (Dr. Chella David, Mayo Clinic, MN), I-A^d (Becton Dickinson, Mountain View, CA) or I-A^s (Dr. Larry Steinman, Stanford Univ.). Fluorescein conjugated F(ab)'$_2$ fragments of sheep anti-mouse or anti rat IgG were used as a secondary reagent at a 1:40 dilution. Percent positive cells were determined by analysis on the flow cytometer (EPICS C, Coulter diagnostics, Hialeah, FL) equipped with an argon laser tuned to 488nm. Only live cells were analyzed using ethidium bromide as an exclusion method for non viable cells. All values in the Result's section are presented by subtracting the reading measured on cells labeled with 2nd antibody alone.

RESULTS

MHV-4 infection of cerebral endothelial cells

The cell populations were identified as brain endothelial
cells by their uptake of DiI-Ac-LDL (Voyta et al., 1984), and
labeling of the lectin Bandeiraea simplicifolia BSI-B$_4$
(Schelper et al., 1985). Characteristic MHV-4 induced
cytopathic effects (multinucleate giant cells) were observed
2-4 days after infection of BALB/c (Fig.1), SJL, (BALB/c x
SJL)F1 and B10.S brain endothelial cells. Similar results were
observed with MHV-4 infected astrocytes

The MHV-susceptible BALB/c strain showed differential
modulation of class I antigen expression on both brain and fat
pad derived endothelial cells (Table 1). The down regulation
of the number of H-2K^d positive cells was not likely due to
shut down of host cell protein synthesis, since an increase in
the number of BALB/c derived brain and fat pad endothelial
cells expressing H-2D^d antigens was observed at the same time
(Table I). The observed differential response of class I
antigens on BALB/c derived brain endothelial cells in MHV-4
infection did not reflect defective regulation of the H-2K^d
antigen in these cells, since exposure to gamma interferon led
to a parallel increase in the number of cells expressing all
of the class I (H-2K^d and H-2D^d) and class II (I-A^d) antigens
measured (Table I).

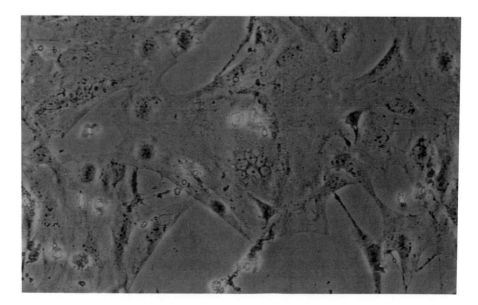

Figure 1.   Photomicrograph of Balb/c cerebral endothelial
             cells one day after infection with MHV-4 (JHM
             strain) at an MOI of 0.1. Multinucleate giant cell
             formation is evident.

TABLE I
Differential Modulation of Class I Antigens on BALB/c
Endothelial Cells Following MHV-4 Infection

	H-2K^d	H-2D^d	I-A^d
Cerebral Endothelial Cells			
Expt.1			
Untreated	54.26*	11.5	-0.13
MHV-4	25.72	20.77	-0.2
Expt.2			
Untreated	68.26	8.0	-0.94
MHV-4	45.75	14.3	-4.77
Expt.3			
Untreated	49.77	0.43	ND
MHV-4	17.54	11.03	ND
Expt.4			
Untreated	32.9	2.1	-2.3
Gamma IFN*	60.18	7.6	42.63
Expt.5			
Untreated	32.81	1.79	0.04
MHV-4	19.72	5.5	1.23
UV-Inact MHV-4	32.23	1.54	0.08
Expt.6 **Fat pad endothelial cells**			
Untreated	67.17	3.14	-1.23
MHV-4	61.91	27.47	1.01

All numbers represent percent positive cells and are averages of duplicate sample analysis on the flow cytometer.
* Cells were treated with 200U/ml of recombinant rat gamma interferon (Amgen,Thousand Oaks, CA) for 72 hrs.

In contrast to the findings for the BALB/c strain, brain endothelial cells derived from the SJL strain (MHV resistant) showed an increased number of cells expressing both H-2K^s and H-2D^s antigens following infection with MHV-4 (Table II). However this finding was not unique to the resistant phenotype, since B10.S derived brain endothelial cells (MHV susceptible, but with an H-2^s MHC haplotype) also had an increase in the number of cells expressing both the H-2K^s and H-2D^s antigens following infection with MHV-4 (Table III).

TABLE II

Parallel Modulation of Class I Antigens on SJL Cerebral Endothelial Cells

	H-2K^S	H-2D^S	I-A^S
Expt.1			
Untreated	4.64	0.56	0.72
MHV-4	18.14	3.75	0.73
Gamma IFN*	79.1	11.21	12.3
Expt.2			
Untreated	10.11	3.83	0.32
MHV-4	22.95	5.29	0.05
Expt.3			
Untreated	4.00	3.03	0.32
MHV-4	22.98	4.45	1.69

All numbers represent percent positive cells and are averages of duplicate sample analysis on the flow cytometer.

* Cells were treated with 200U/ml of recombinant rat gamma IFN (Amgen, Thousand Oaks, CA) for 72 hrs.

TABLE III

Parallel Modulation of Class I Antigens on B10.S Brain Endothelial Cells

	H-2K^S	H-2D^S	I-A^S
Expt.1			
Untreated	8.15	0.68	-0.8
MHV-4	11.41	4.31	-0.15
Gamma IFN*	40.27	1.04	13.83
Expt.2			
Untreated	3.4	0.41	0.54
MHV-4	10.52	2.46	-0.24

All numbers represent percent positive cells and are averages of duplicate sample analyses on the flow cytometer.

Additional studies were done with the MHV-4 susceptible (BALB/c x SJL)F1 cerebral endothelial cell line. In this particular cell line the H-2^d haplotype is preferentially expressed compared to the H-2^S haplotype (Table IV). However the pattern of modulation of the H-2K^d molecule following MHV-4 infection is different from that observed following infection of BALB/c derived brain endothelial cells with this virus. There is a parallel increase in the number of cells expressing H-2K^d and H-2D^d following infection with MHV-4.

MHV-4 infection of astrocytes

Unlike results obtained with endothelial cells, a parallel modulation of H-2K and H-2D antigens was observed following MHV-4 infection of astrocytes derived from susceptible (BALB/c, CXJ-8, B10.S) and resistant (SJL) strains of mice (Table V). The results obtained with BALB/c astrocytes are of particular interest since they contrasted with the differential modulation of class I antigens observed in brain and fat pad derived endothelial cells following infection with MHV-4.

TABLE IV

Parallel Modulation of Class I Antigens on
(BALB/c X SJL) F1 Cerebral Endothelial Cells.

	H-2K^d	H-2D^d	I-A^d	H-2K^s	H-2D^s	I-A^s
Expt.1						
Untreated	12.8	1.2	-0.28	-0.27	0.34	-0.44
MHV-4	17.96	7.7	-0.87	0.17	5.83	-12.2
Expt.2						
Untreated	19.3	6.53	ND	1.43	1.23	ND
MHV-4	31.23	10.00	ND	0.0	0.0	ND
Expt.3						
Untreated	8.93	0.47	-0.03	0.33	0.33	0.67
Gamma IFN*	73.94	0.21	5.08	0.16	0.18	0.75

All numbers represent percent positive cells and are averages of duplicate sample analyses on the flow cytometer.

* Cells were treated with 200U/ml of recombinant rat gamma interferon (Amgen,Thousand Oaks, CA) for 72hrs.

Effect of MHV-4 infection on gamma interferon induced class I and II antigens in endothelial cells and astrocytes

When endothelial cells were simultaneously treated with MHV-4 and gamma interferon, there is a reduced level of class II antigen expression compared to cells treated with gamma interferon alone (Table VI). These results were obtained with both I-A^s and I-A^d expressing cells. Similar observations were made with astrocytes that were simultaneously treated with MHV-4 and gamma interferon (Table VII). In contrast, the induction of class I antigens by interferon was not blocked by MHV-4 infection of either endothelial cells or astrocytes (Table VIII).

TABLE V

Parallel Modulation of Class I Antigens on Astrocytes
Following MHV-4 Infection

	$H-2K^d$	$H-2D^d$	$I-A^d$
BALB/C			
Untreated	24.82	7.07	2.65
MHV-4	54.69	8.15	0.87
CXJ-8			
Untreated	5.32	0.17	0.00
MHV-4	23.33	0.87	0.48
	$H-2K^s$	$H-2D^s$	$I-A^s$
SJL			
Untreated	10.6	-0.1	-2.44
MHV-4	33.36	6.35	-1.74
B10.S			
Untreated	34.93	3.62	1.53
MHV-4	55.92*	4.82	-3.61

* This number signifies the percent number of positive cells
as analyzed by the flow cytometer.

Table VI

Effect of MHV-4 Infection on Gamma Interferon Induced
Class II Expression on Cerebral Endothelial Cells

	BALB/c $I-A^d$	B10.S $I-A^s$	(BALB/c x SJL)F1 $I-A^d$
Untreated	0.78	0.56	0.33
Gamma IFN	*63.36	25.73	91.66
MHV-4	1.85	1.95	-1.0
MHV-4 + Gamma IFN	12.02	8.13	70.5

* This number signifies the percent number of positive cells
as analyzed by the flow cytometer.

Table VII

Effect of MHV-4 Infection on Gamma Interferon Induced
Class II Antigen Expression on Astrocytes

	BALB/c $I-A^d$	SJL $I-A^s$	B10.S $I-A^s$
Untreated	0.3	5.57	0.2
Gamma IFN	61.47	36.47	36.95
MHV-4	0.68	-1.57	-0.19
MHV-4 + Gamma IFN	23.73	14.47	14.43*

* This number signifies the percentage of positive cells as
analyzed by the flow cytometer.

Table VIII

Effect of MHV-4 Infection on Gamma Interferon Induced
Class I Antigen Expression on Endothelial Cells and
Astrocytes

	Balb/c astrocyte $H-2K^d$	B10.S astrocyte $H-2K^s$	(Balb/c x SJL)F1 endothelium $H-2K^d$
Untreated	12.89	14.3	5.27
Gamma IFN	60.73	52.66	52.3
MHV-4	34.53	28.87	16.9
MHV-4 + Gamma IFN	77.09	71.83	54.86*

* This number signifies the percent number of positive cells
as analyzed by the flow cytometer.

DISCUSSION

Cerebral endothelial cells are a major structural component
of the blood brain barrier (BBB). These cells can play an
important role in regulating virus entry into the brain
(Johnson, 1974,1982; Wiley et al., 1986) and in modulating
immune mediated events occurring within the CNS (McCarron et
al., 1985,1986). We have examined the effect of the
neurotropic coronavirus MHV-4 (JHM) infection on cerebral
endothelial cell class I and II expression because of the
potential role of these molecules in viral antigen
presentation and anti-viral cytotoxic T cell activity
(Zinkernagel and Doherty 1975, 1979; Paabo et al., 1986;
Burgert et al., 1987; Yamaguchi et al., 1988; McCarron et al.,
1985, 1986).

In the BALB/c derived brain and fat pad endothelial cells, we
observe differential modulation of MHC class I molecules
following infection with MHV-4. MHV-4 induced a decrease in
the percentage of $H-2K^d$ positive cells and an increase of H-
$2D^d$ expressing cells (Table I). This pattern of response to
MHV-4 infection does not appear to be a unique characteristic
of the BALB/c cerebral endothelial cell line since endothelial
cells derived from another organ source (fat pad) show
identical patterns of modulation. The BALB/c brain derived
endothelial cells also responds in a predicted manner to
treatment with gamma interferon. There is an increase in the
percentage of class I ($H-2K^d$, $H-2D^d$) and class II ($I-A^d$)
expressing cells as shown in Table II. This suggests that the
regulation of MHC gene expression in this cell line is not
defective. The differential modulation observed does not
appear to be a property of the $H-2^d$ haplotype since BALB/c
derived astrocytes respond with an increase in both $H-2K^d$ and
$H-2D^d$ expression following infection with MHV-4.

Infection of endothelial cells derived from MHV-4 resistant (SJL) or susceptible (B10.S) strains of mice leads to an increase in percent of H-2K^s and H-2D^s expressing cells. The (BALB/c x SJL) F1 derived brain endothelial cells show patterns of modulation similar to B10.S and SJL derived cells. There is an increase in the number of cells expressing H-2K^d and H-2D^d antigen. Unlike BALB/c derived endothelial cells, no differential modulation is observed.

Several conclusions can be drawn from this data. Differential modulation appears to be strain dependent, suggesting genetic regulation. Since both B10.S and Balb/c mice are susceptible to MHV-4 replication (Stohlman and Frelinger 1978; Knobler et al., 1981), this may suggest the involvement of a separate gene from the chromosome 7 locus (Knobler et al., 1984) determining susceptibility to MHV replication. A second gene regulating susceptibility to MHV-4 induced fatal encephalomyelitis had previously been proposed following studies comparing B10.S and SJL mice and their progeny (Stohlman and Frelinger., 1978; Stohlman et al., 1985). Recombinant-inbred mice between BALB/c and SJL strains, the CXJ series (Knobler et al., 1985), can be a useful tool to search for, sort and map the location of this gene through characterization of brain derived endothelial cell class I MHC responses to MHV infection.

Our preliminary studies on MHC modulation using (BALB/c x SJL) F1 endothelial cells indicate that although the H-2^d haplotype is preferentially expressed in this cell line, the pattern of modulation is not like that seen with BALB/c derived endothelial cells. An SJL background gene(s) appears to have an effect on class I antigen modulation since we observe an increase in the expression of both H-2K^d and H-2D^d following infection of the (BALB/c X SJL)F1 cerebral endothelial cell line. We are currently involved in generating endothelial cell cultures from a panel of MHV susceptible mice in order to better understand the genetic regulation of susceptibilty to MHV-4.

An important extension of our studies will also be to examine the role of endothelial class I modulation in regulating cytotoxic T cell (CTL) activity against MHV-4. Anti-viral CTL's have been demonstrated to be class I restricted (Zinkernagel and Doherty, 1975,1979). It has been difficult until recently to demonstrate cytotoxic T cells directed against MHV-4. However, Yamaguchi et al., (1988) have recently developed cytotoxic T cell clones that are MHV-4 (JHM) specific. We will examine if MHV infected endothelial cells can act as targets in an MHV specific cytotoxic T cell response. CTL activity against virus infected endothelial cells may have damaging effects on the host. For instance, if CTL's lyse virus infected blood brain barrier endothelial cells there might be damage to the barrier permitting the virus to more readily enter the brain. Alternatively, CTL's may aid in rapid clearing of the virus preventing further spread and infection.

Differential modulation of MHC class I antigens has been

reported previously. In the murine leukemia virus-induced AKR SL3 tumor cell line, a large increase in H-2D and no change or a slight decrease in H-2K^K is observed following exposure to gamma interferon (Green and Philips, 1986).

The mechanism of differential modulation of class I MHC expression as observed in the decline of H-2K^d expression on BALB/c derived brain endothelial cells is presently unknown. In other viral systems like adenoviruses, the mechanism of regulation of MHC antigens is better understood. The E3/19K protein of this virus binds directly to class I molecules preventing their terminal glycosylation and inhibiting cell surface expression. This reduced level of class I antigen has been correlated with reduced cellular immune response and target cell lysis (Paabo et al., 1986; Burgert et al., 1987).

Soluble factors released by infected cells may also have a role in MHC class I modulation. Such a factor has recently been characterized from infected mouse astrocytes (Suzumura et al., 1988). This factor was found to be, nondialyzable, heat and trypsin sensitive, but resistant to treatment at pH 2.0. The authors speculate based on molecular weight determination and antibody blocking experiments, that the factor is not interferon, but most likely tumor necrosis factor. The potential role of tumor necrosis factor in class I antigen modulation of virus infected endothelial cells is currently being investigated in our laboratory.

There is no change in the low level of class II expression on brain endothelial cells following infection with MHV-4 in all strains examined, regardless of their susceptibility or resistance to virus or immune mediated demyelinating disease. This is in contrast to the results reported for Lewis rat astrocytes which demonstrated an increase in class II expression following exposure to either live or UV-inactivated virus (Massa et al., 1986). It has been suggested that the late immune mediated demyelinating disease in the rat is correlated with the observed induction of class II antigens on astrocytes (Massa et al., 1986, 1987). Our results are identical to that observed with mouse astrocytes and oligodendrocytes by Suzumura et al. (1986), where no change in class II antigens were observed following MHV-A59 infection. Therefore, the absence of late immune mediated demyelinating disease in the mouse may in fact reflect the failure of induction of MHC class II antigens on brain endothelial cells and astrocytes.

The selective blocking of gamma interferon induced class II antigen by MHV-4 infection may also contribute to the absence of late immune mediated demyelinating disease in the mouse. It would of interest to study the interaction of lymphokines and MHV-4 infection in the rat system. The mechanism of blocking of gamma interferon induced class II antigen by MHV-4 infection is unclear. The effect may be mediated indirectly by induction of cytokines like interferon alpha/beta or tumor necrosis factor, both of which have been demonstrated to downregulate interferon gamma induced class II antigens (Joseph et al., 1988; Leeuwenberg et al., 1988).

In summary, we have demonstrated differential modulation of
MHC class I antigens on BALB/c derived endothelial cells _in
vitro._ In all other strains examined [SJL, B10.S, (BALB/c X
SJL) F1] we observed an increase in the percentage of H-2K and
H-2D antigen expressing cells. MHV-4 infection has no effect
on class II antigen expression in any of the strains examined.
However, gamma interferon induced class II, but not class I
antigen, is blocked by MHV-4 infection. The effects of
endothelial cell MHC modulation, by MHV-4, on the host immune
response to the virus is currently being investigated.

ACKNOWLEDGEMENTS

This work was supported by Research Grants RG-2072-A-1, RG
1772-B-4 and RG 1801-A-3 from the National Multiple Sclerosis
Society and NS 00961, NS 23081 and NS 22145 from the National
Institutes of Health.

REFERENCES

Bailey, O. T., Pappenheimer, A. M., and Cheever., F. S., 1949,
    J. Exp. Med., 90: 195.
Burgert, H. G., Marayanski, J. L., and Kvist, S., 1987, Proc.
    Natl. Acad. Sci. USA., 84:1356.
Crissman, H. A., and Steinkamp, J. A., 1982, Cytometry., 3:84.
Dasgupta, J. V., and Yunis, E. J., 1987, J. Immunol., 129:
    672.
DeBault, L. E., Henriquez, E., Hart, M. N., and Cancilla, P.
    A., 1981, In Vitro., 17:480.
Flyer, D. C., Burakoff, S. J., and Faller, D. V., 1982, J.
    Immunol., 135: 2287.
Fontana, A., Fierz, W., and Wekerle, H., 1984, Nature.,
    307:273.
Green, W. R., and Phillips, J. D., 1986, J. Immunol.,
    137:814.
Grundy, J. E., McKeating, J. A., and Griffiths, P. D., 1987,
    In: Abstracts VII International Congress of Virology,
    National Research Council Canada, Ottawa, Ont., 125.
Helenius, A., Morein, B., Fries, E., Simons, K., et al., 1978,
    Proc. Natl. Acad. Sci. USA., 75: 3846.
Johnson, R. T., 1974, Adv. Neurol., 6:27.
Johnson, R. T., 1982. Viral Infections of the Nervous System.
    Raven Press, New York, 49.
Joseph, J., Knobler, R. L., D'Imperio, C., Lublin, F.D.,
    1988, J. Neuroimmunol., 20:39.
Knobler, R. L., Haspel, M. V., and Oldstone, M. B. A. 1981,
    J.Exp. Med ., 153:832.
Knobler, R. L., Taylor, B. A., Wooddell, M.K., Beamer, W. G.,
    and Oldstone, M. B. A. 1984, Exp. Clin. Immunogenet .,
    1:217.
Knobler, R. L., Linthicum, D. S., and Cohn, M., 1985, J.
    Neuroimmunol., 8:15.
Knobler, R. L., Weismiller, D. G., Williams, R. K.,
    Cardellichio, C., and Holmes, K. V., 1987, In: Abstracts
    VII International Congress of Virology, National Research
    Council, Canada, Ottawa, Ont., 73.
Lavi, E., Suzumura, A., Murasko, D. M., Murray, E. M.,
Silberberg, D. H., and Weiss, S., 1988, J. Neuroimmunol.,
    18:245.
Leeuwenberg, J. F. M., Van Damme, J., Meager, T., Jeunhomme,
    T. M. A. A., and Buurman, W. A., 1988, Eur. J. Immunol.,
    18:1469.

Massa, P. T., Dorries, R., and ter Meulen, V, 1986, Nature.,
320:543.

Massa, P. T., Brinkmann, R., and ter Meulen, V., 1987a,
J.Exp.Med., 166:259.

Massa, P. T., Schimpl, A., Wecker, E., and ter Meulen, V.,
1987b, Proc. Natl. Acad. Sci. USA., 84:7242.

McCarron, R.M., Kempski, O., Spatz, M., and McFarlin, D. E.,
1985, J. Immunol., 134:3100.

McCarron, R. M., Spatz, M., Kempski, O., Hogan, R. N., Muehl,
L., and McFarlin, D. E., 1986, J. Immunol., 137: 3428.

Paabo, S., Nilsson, T., and Peterson, P. A., 1986, Proc. Natl.
Acad. Sci. USA., 83:9665.

Rodriguez, M., Pierce, M. L., and Howie, E. A., 1987,
J. Immunol., 138:3438.

Schelper, R. L., Whitters, E., and Hart, M. N., 1985, Fed.
Proc., 44:1261.

Stohlman, S. A., and Frelinger, J. A., 1978, Immunogenet.,
6:227.

Stohlman, S. A., Knobler, R. L., and Frelinger, J. A., 1985,
In: E. Skamene (Ed.), Genetic Control of Host Resistance to
Infection and Malignancy, Alan R. Liss, New York, 125.

Suzumura, A., Lavi, E., Weiss, S. R., and Silberberg, D. H.,
1986, Science., 232:991.

Suzumura, A., Lavi, E., Bhat, S., Murasko, D., Weiss, S. R.
and Silberberg, D. H, 1988, J. Immunol., 140:2068.

Tanaka, K., Isselbacher, K. J., Khoury, G., and Jay, G., 1985,
Science., 228:26.

Trauggot, U., Raine, C. S., and McFarlin, D. E., 1985, Cell.
Immunol., 91:240.

Voyta, J. C., Netland, P. A., Via, D. P., and Zetter, B. R.,
1984, J. Cell. Biol., 99:81A.

Wagner, R. C., and Mathews, M. A., 1975, Microvasc. Res.,
10:287.

Watanabe, R., Wege, H., and ter Meulen, V., 1983, Nature.,
305:150.

Wiley, C. A., Schrier, R. D., Nelson, J. A., Lampert, P. W.,
and Oldstone, M. B. A., 1986, Proc. Natl. Acad. Sci. USA.,
83:7089.

Yamaguchi, K., Kyuwa, S., Nakanaga, K., and Hayami, M, 1988,
J. Virol., 62:2505.

Zinkernagel, R. M., and Doherty, P. C., 1975, J. Exp.
Med.,141:1427.

MOUSE HEPATITIS VIRUS A59 INCREASES STEADY-STATE LEVELS

OF mRNAS ENCODING MAJOR HISTOCOMPATIBILITY COMPLEX ANTIGENS

James L. Gombold and Susan R. Weiss

Department of Microbiology

University of Pennsylvania School of Medicine, Philadelphia, PA 19104

INTRODUCTION

The murine hepatitis viruses (MHV) have been widely studied as models of human neurologic infections. MHV strains A59 and JHM cause an acute necrotizing encephalitis in mice when inoculated intracerebrally. Studies using low doses of virus, attenuated virus strains, or temperature-sensitive mutants have shown that animals surviving the acute infection develop a chronic disease characterized by inflammatory demyelination of neurons in the central nervous system (Haspel et al., 1978; Knobler et al., 1982; Lavi et al., 1986; Koolen et al., 1987).

Recovery from the acute encephalitis requires an active cell-mediated immune response. Stohlman et al. (1986, 1988) have shown that CD4[+], MHC class II-restricted T cell prevents death in JHM-infected mice. In addition, MHC class I-restricted T cells, possibly suppressor/cytotoxic T cells (CTL), have been isolated from mice infected with JHM (Kyuwa et al., 1987). However, the role of these CTLs in MHV pathogenesis is not clear.

The mechanism involved in MHV-induced demyelination is also not well understood. Some evidence suggests that MHV-induced demyelination may result from direct viral lysis of oligodendrocytes (Weiner, 1973; Beushausen and Dales, 1985). In contrast, Watanabe et al. (1983) have demonstrated adoptive transfer of subacute demyelination with T cells from JHM-infected rats. This strongly indicates that immune-mediated mechanisms may be active in demyelination.

The potential for MHC-restricted immune responses to modulate MHV infections is especially interesting given that both JHM and A59 induce the expression of MHC proteins. *In vitro* infection of glia with JHM induces the expression of class II (Ia) molecules (Massa et al., 1986,1987) while A59 induces class I molecules (Suzumura et al., 1986a,1986b). We show here that infection of glia by MHV-A59 increases the steady-state levels of H-2 mRNA both *in vivo* and *in vitro*. Furthermore, elevated expression occurs in cells that do not contain detectable amounts of viral RNA, consistent with previous data suggesting the role of a soluble factor in the induction.

Coronaviruses and Their Diseases
Edited by D. Cavanagh and T.D.K. Brown
Plenum Press, New York, 1990

MATERIALS AND METHODS

Virus and Cells

MHV strain A59 was propagated in a mouse fibroblast cell line (17 Cl1) and titered by plaque assay in mouse L cells. Virus for use in *in vivo* studies was also titered by end-point dilution in 4-6 week old male C57Bl/6 mice and contains approximately 5000 pfu per LD_{50}. Mixed glial cultures were made from dissociated brains of newborn mice and were used 10-15 days after plating. All cells were grown in Dulbecco's modified Eagles medium containing 10% fetal bovine serum.

Mice

MHV-free C57Bl/6 mice were purchased from Jackson Laboratories (Bar Harbor, ME). Mice were inoculated immediately upon arrival with 1 LD_{50} of A59 or mock- infected with a comparable dilution of 17 Cl1 cell lysate. All inoculations were intracerebral in a volume of 20 ul. Infected animals were house in a separate isolation room for the duration of the experiments.

RNA Isolation

RNA for northern blot analysis was isolated from primary glial cultures or from mouse brain using different but standard techniques.

Cytoplasmic RNA from cell cultures was obtained by lysing cells with 1% Nonidet P40. After removing nuclei by centrifugation, the lysate was digested with Proteinase K, extracted with phenol:chloroform and chloroform, and precipitated in ethanol.

Total brain RNA from virus- and mock-infected mice was obtained by homogenizing brains in 4M guanidinium isothiocyanate (BMB). RNA was collected by centrifugation through 5.7M CsCl. RNA pellets were then extracted and precipitated as described above.

Northern Blots

RNA (10ug) was fractionated by gel electrophoresis in 1% agarose containing 2.2M formaldehyde. RNAs were transferred to nylon membranes (Gene Screen Plus, New England Nuclear) and hybridized at 42C in 50% formamide. DNA probes for hybridization included an 800 bp H-2 class I cDNA (pH2II; Steinmetz et al., 1981), a 900 bp H-2 class II cDNA (obtained from S. Stohlman, UCLA), a 3kb viral cDNA from the 3' end of the A59 genome (cl320), and a 3kb actin specific cDNA (Khalili et al., 1983).

In Situ Hybridization

Hybridizations were done on frozen brain sections or on infected cells as described previously (Chesselet et al., 1987). Briefly, samples were fixed in 3% paraformaldehyde, incubated in 0.1M Tris/0.1 M glycine, acetylated, and dehydrated through graded ethanols. [^{35}S]-RNA probes were prepared by *in vitro* transcription of cDNAs subcloned into Gemini vectors (Promega). Hybridization was done at 50C in 50% formamide for 4 hours using $1x10^6$ cpm of probe per sample. Following hyridization, samples were washed in 2X SSC/50% formamide at 52C, digested with RNase A, rinsed in 2X SSC/50% formamide at 52C, and washed overnight in 2X SSC/0.05% Triton X-100. After dehydration through graded ethanols, the slides were coated with emulsion (NTB-2, Kodak) and exposed for 2-3 weeks at 4C.

RESULTS AND DISCUSSION

Mice were inoculated intracerebrally with 1 LD_{50} of A59 or mock-infected with uninfected cell lysate. At regular intervals after infection, one virus-infected and one mock-infected mouse was sacrificed and total brain RNA was isolated. Northern blots revealed that expression of both MHC class I and class II sequences increased in virus-infected mice but not in mock-infected controls (Fig. 1). The two groups of mice showed no difference in MHC expression when sacrificed immediately after infection.

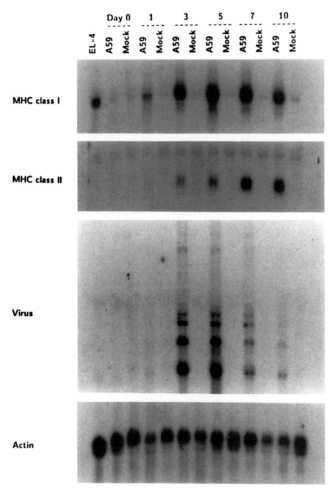

Figure 1. RNA from virus- and mock-infected mouse brain was extracted by homogenizing brains in guanidinium isothiocyanate and pelleted through CsCl. Total RNA (10 ug) was resolved by gel electrophoresis, blotted onto membranes, and hybridized for the indicated mRNA species. EL-4 is a control lane of RNA isolated from a murine lymphoma cell line known to express class I antigens. A59: virus-infected sample from the indicated day postinfection. Mock: mock-infected sample from the indicated day postinfection. MHC class I probe was an 800 bp cDNA from the 3 domain of class I antigens; MHC class II probe was a 970 bp fragment from the E chain of class II antigens; viral probe was a 3 kb cDNA derived from the 3' end of the viral genome and detects all virus-specific mRNAs; actin was a 3 kb cDNA from a domain conserved in alpha, beta, and gamma actin.

However, as early as 24 hr postinfection (pi), brains of infected animals contained increased levels of class I mRNA, which continued to increase until 5 days pi. Thereafter, the level of class I transcripts decreased to that observed in mock-infected mice (Fig. 1 and data not shown). Expression of class II genes was similar but lagged behind that of class I mRNA (Fig. 1). During this time, infected animals developed signs of disease characterized by paresis and ruffled fur. As expected, approximately 50% of the infected animals died. Remaining infected littermates recovered from disease. Expression of both class I and II genes again increased in animals examined at 8, 12, and 16 weeks pi (data not shown). This was accompanied by signs of disease similar to those observed during the acute infection. These changes in mRNA levels were not due to variations in the amount of RNA on the membranes as shown by the relatively constant signal obtained by probing for the cellular message for actin (Fig. 1).

Viral RNA was first detected at three days pi with peak levels occurring at 5 to 7 days pi (Fig. 1). After 2 weeks pi, viral RNA could not be detected, even in samples taken between 8 and 16 weeks after infection when animals experienced a recurrence of disease and when class I and class II transcripts were elevated.

Since lymphocytes and macrophages express class I and class II antigens, the observed increases in MHC expression could have been due to the influx of these cells during infection. If this were true, we expected that MHC expression would be restricted to inflammatory foci. To examine this possibility, *in situ* hybridization of brain sections was done. Negative-sense probes detected expression of class I mRNA in brains of both virus- and mock-infected animals that were sacrificed immediately following infection (Fig. 2). RNA levels appeared to be uniform throughout the brain, although epithelial cells usually hybridized more strongly than other cells. By 24 hr pi, virus-infected animals had slightly higher levels of class I mRNA compared to controls, and expression increased markedly by days 3 and 7 pi. Elevated expression occurred in most, if not all, cells but was highest in epithelial cells of the ependyma. In contrast, mock-infected animals displayed a relatively constant level of class I mRNA during this period. Hybridization using positive-strand probes was minimal regardless of the inoculum or the time after infection. In contrast to the rather unrestricted and elevated expression of class I genes, viral gene expression was focal and largely restricted to the limbic system. The number of foci containing viral RNA increased during the seven days over which animals were examined but remained mostly within the limbic system (data not shown).

Similar studies on primary glial cells in culture gave slightly different results. Dot blot hybridization of infected glial cell RNA with class I probes showed only minor elevation of these sequences during infection compared to uninfected cells (data not shown). Induction appeared to be maximum by 2 days pi and decreased thereafter. However, levels of class I mRNA was still higher than in uninfected cells at 2 weeks pi. Hybridization for viral RNA reveal similar kinetics in that expression increased to maximum at 2 to 3 days pi. Although the amount of viral RNA appeared to decrease slightly after this time, significant amounts of RNA were present 2 weeks pi. *In situ* hybridization revealed most cells in uninfected cultures expressed class I mRNA. When infected, a minor increase in expression was observed 3 to 7 days after infection, consistent with the increase detected by dot hybridization (data not shown).

These results demonstrate that MHV-A59 causes an increase in steady-state levels of mRNA encoding MHC antigens. This effect is most pronounced *in vivo* but occurs in cultured primary glial cells as well. Several conclusions can be drawn from these data: (1) The increased expression of MHC-specific RNAs in not the result of either the trauma of inoculation or an immune response to non-viral components in the inoculum since only virus-infected animals displayed elevated RNA levels; (2) the mechanism responsible for MHC induction, which is not yet identified, occurs in cells throughout the brain and is not restricted to infected cells. This observation suggests that the induction may be mediated by lymphokines or other related factors; (3) the increase in class I transcripts in primary glial cultures demonstrates that these cells are able to increase expression directly.

Previously, Suzumura et al. (1986a) observed by immunofluorescence that infection of astrocytes in culture or of glia *in vivo* prior to culturing resulted in expression of class I antigens over that seen in uninfected cells. This induction could be mediated by virus-free medium from infected astrocytes demonstrating the role of a diffusible factor. However, increased expression of MHC antigens was not observed when highly-enriched oligodendrocyte cultures were infected, but occurred only when cultures were treated with conditioned medium from infected astrocytes. This last observation strongly argues for the role of a soluble mediator in the induction of MHC antigens by virus, and is consistent with the data presented here: *In situ* hybridization showed that induction of H-2 expression occurred in regions of brain far removed from

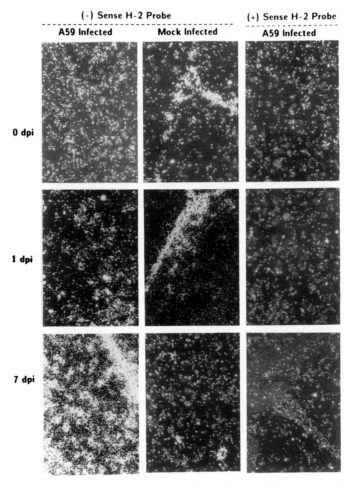

Figure 2. *In situ* hybridization of frozen sections with negative-sense or positive-sense H-2 class I RNA probes. Sections were cut from brains of virus- and mock-infected animals sacrificed immediately following inoculation (O dpi), 1 dpi, or 7 dpi, and all were hybridized in the same experiment and for the same amount of time. All panels were photographed at approximately 200X magnification.

the area of infection. Thus, even though glia are capable of responding to MHV infection with increases in expression of MHC class I genes, the widespread elevated levels of class I transcripts may be regulated by cytokines secreted by immune cells during infection.

It is not clear what role the heightened expression of MHC antigens may play in the pathogenesis of either acute or chronic MHV-induced disease. However, the identification of MHC-restricted T cell responses following infection (Kyuwa et al.,1988; Stohlman et al., 1988) suggests that expression of these antigens in the brain may be important. Demonstration that infected glia function as targets for such T cell populations may provide evidence that histocompatibilty antigens have a role in MHV pathogenesis.

ACKNOWLEDGEMENTS

We wish to thank Anita Jackson for cutting frozen sections, and Frank Baldino and Elane Robbins for help with the *in situ* hybridizations. We also wish to thank Crystal Thorpe for technical assistance. This work was supported by Public Health Service grants NS 21954 and NS 10037 from the National Institutes of Health. JLG was supported by National Research Service Award NS 07180.

REFERENCES

Bang, F.B. and A. Warwick. 1960. Mouse macrophages as host cells for the mouse hepatitis virus and genetic basis of their susceptibility. Proc. Natl. Acad. Sci. 46:1065-1075.

Beushausen, S. and S. Dales. 1985. *In vivo* and *in vitro* models of demyelinating disease. Virology 141:89-.

Chesselet, M-F.; L.T. Weiss; C. Wuenschell; A. Tobin; and H.U. Affolter. 1987. Comparative distrubution of mRNAs for glutamic acid decarboxylase, tyrosine hydroxylase, and tachykinins in the basal ganglia: An *in situ* hybridization study in the rodent brain. J. Comp. Neurol. 262:125-140.

Haspel, M.V.; P.W. Lampert; and M.B.A. Oldstone. 1978. Temperature-sensitive mutants of mouse hepatitis virus produce a high incidence of demyelination. Proc. Natl. Acad. Sci. 75:4033-4036.

Khalili, K.; C. Salas; and R. Weinmann. 1983. Isolation and characterization of human actin genes cloned in phage lambda vectors. Gene 21:9-17.

Knobler, R.L.; P.W. Lampert; and M.B.A. Oldstone. 1982. Virus persistence and recurring demyelination produced by a temperature-sensitive mutant and MHV-4. Nature 298:279-280.

Koolen, M.J.M.; S. Love; W. Wouda; J. Calafat; M.C. Horzinek; and B.A.M. van der Zeijst. 1987. Induction of demyelination by a temperature-sensitive mutant of the coronavirus MHV-A59 is associated with restriction of viral replication in the brain. J. Gen. Virol. 68:703-714.

Kyuwa, S.; K. Yamaaguchi; M. Hayami; and K. Fujiwara. 1987. Characterization of mouse hepatitis virus-reactive T cell clones. In: M.C. Lai and S.A., Stohlman (Eds.), Coronaviruses, Plenum Press, New York, pp. 391-398.

Lavi, E; D.H. Gilden; M.K. Highkin; and S.R. Weiss. 1986. The organ tropism of mouse hepatitis virus A59 is dependent on dose and route of inoculation. Lab. Animal Sci. 36:130-135.

Massa, P.T.; R. Brinkmann; and V. ter Meulen. 1987. Inducibility of Ia antigen on astrocytes by murine coronavirus JHM is rat strain dependent. J. Exp. Med. 166:259-264.

Massa, P.T.; R. Dorries; and V. ter Meulen. 1986. Viral particles induce Ia antigen expression on astrocytes. Nature 320:543-546.

Steinmetz, M.; D.W. Moore; J.G. Frelinger; B.T. Sher; F-W. Shen; E.A. Boyse; and L. Hood. 1981. A pseudogene homologous to mouse transplantation antigens: Transplantation antigens are encoded by eight exons that correlate with protein domains. Cell 25:683-692.

Stohlman, S.A.; G.K. Matsushima; N. Casteel; and L.P. Weiner. 1986. *In vivo* effects of coronavirus-specific T cell clones: DTH inducer cells prevent a lethal infection but do not inhibit virus replication. J. Immunol. 136:3051-3056.

Stohlman, S.A.; M.A. Sussman; G.K. Matsushima; R.A. Shubin; and S.S. Erlich. 1988. Delayed-type hypersensitivity response in the central nervous system during JHM virus infection requires viral specificity for protection. J. Neuroimmunol. 19:255-268.

Suzumura, A.; E. Lavi; S.R. Weiss; and D.H. Silberberg. 1986. Coronavirus infection induces H-2 antigen expression on oligodendrocytes and astrocytes. Science 232:991-993.

Suzumura, A.;D.H. Silberberg; and R.P. Lisak. 1986. The expression of MHC antigens on oligodendrocytes: Induction of polymorphic H-2 expression by lymphokines. J. Neuroimmunol. 11:179-190.

Watanabe, R.; H. Wege; and V. ter Meulen. 1983. Adoptive transfer of EAE-like lesions by BMP stimulated lymphocytes from rats with coronavirus-induced demyelinationg encephalomyelitis. Nature 305:150.

Weiner, L.P. 1973. Pathogenesis of demyelination induced by mouse hepatitis virus (JHM). Arch. Neurol. 28:298-303.

VACUOLAR DEGENERATION INDUCED BY JHM-CC VIRUS IN THE CNS OF CYCLO-

PHOSPHAMIDE-TREATED MICE

Yuzo Iwasaki, Norio Hirano*, Tetsuro Tsukamoto** and
Satoru Haga*

Department of Neurological Sciences, Tohoku University
School of Medicine, Sendai 980, Japan
*Department of Veterinary Microbiology, Iwate University
Morioka 020, Japan
**Department of Neurology, Fukushima Medical College
Fukushima 960, Japan

INTRODUCTION

The infection with JHM-CC virus (1), a small plaque mutant of neurovirulent JHM virus, is non-fatal in immunocompetent mice but constantly
induces vacuolar degeneration in the brain and spinal cord (2). To elucidate the role of host immune response in pathogenesis of JHM-CC induced
vacuolar degeneration in the central nervous system (CNS), the kinetics of
virus growth and the temporal sequence of viral antigen distribution were
correlated with histopathological changes in cyclophosphamide-treated
adult ICR mice.

MATERIALS AND METHODS

A total of 204 male ICR mice of 4 to 6 week-old of age were inoculated i.c. with 0.02 ml of undiluted JHM-CC virus preparation. The stock
virus of JHM-CC was prepared after 3 serial plaque-purifications in DBT
cell monolayer cultures. After centrifugation at 8,000 rpm for 10 min,
the supernatant of infected cultures was stored at $-80^{o}C$ until use. This
virus preparation had an infectivity of $5 \times 10^{8}PFU/ml$. Ninety-four out of
204 infected mice were given i.p. 100mg/kg of cyclophosphamide(Cy) 1, 3
and 5 days after virus inoculation. Both Cy-treated and untreated mice
were randomly sacrificed between day 1 and day 21 for virus titration,
immunohistochemistry and histological examinations.

For virus titration, the tissue homogenates were prepared from the
brain and spinal cord separately. The infectivity was assayed by plaqueing in the DBT culture as reported previously (1). For histological and
immunohistochemical examinations, mice were perfused with a 10% phosphate
buffered formalin solution. Multiple coronal sections of the brain and
longitudinal sections of the spinal cord were embedded in paraffin. Serial
paraffin sections were stained with H&E and by the Kluver-Barrera and
Bodian methods for myelin and axon. The viral antigen was detected in
paraffin sections with a hyperimmune rabbit serum raised against the DBT-
culture-grown JHM virus by the avidin-biotin peroxidase complex (ABC)
method. Some sections were also subjected to immunohistochemistry with
polyclonal antibodies against neurofilaments (150k) and GFAP.

Coronaviruses and Their Diseases
Edited by D. Cavanagh and T.D.K. Brown
Plenum Press, New York, 1990

RESULTS

Clinical symptoms and virus titer in the CNS

The JHM virus infection was usually dormant in immunocompetent mice, although approximately 20% of them developed mild hindlimb paralysis. On the contrary, the infection in Cy-treated mice was often fatal. Almost half of Cy-treated mice became very inactive between day 7 and day 12, and 40 out of 94 Cy-treated mice died with or without paraplegia.

The kinetics of virus titer in the CNS tissue is shown in Figure 1. Each point represents the average of 3 mice. In immunocompetent mice, the virus titer of the brain (closed circles with a dotted line) reached its peak on day 5 and then rapidly decreased. On the other had, the virus titer of the spinal cord (open circles with a dotted line) increased slowly and gradually decreased. In Cy-treated mice, the mean virus titer of the brain (closed circles with a solid line) rapidly rose with a peak on day 7. The high titer in the brain was sustained for another week, and then it appeared to decline gradually. The virus titer of the spinal cord in Cy-treated mice (open circles with a solid line) slowly increased reaching its peak on day 10 and then declined. In both groups, the highest titer in the spinal cord was always lower than that in the brain.

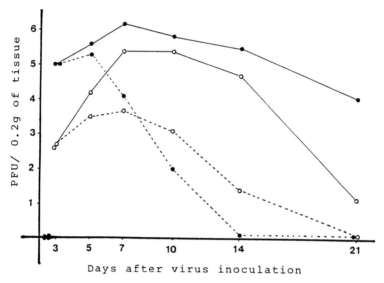

Fig.1. Virus titer in the brain and spinal cord.

Viral antigen distribution and histopathological changes in the CNS of Cy-treated mice

Since histopathology of this virus infection in immunocompetent mice is presented in another chapter of this book (T. Tsukamoto et al), only the findings in Cy-treated mice will be described in this chapter. In Cy-treated mice, inflammatory cell infiltration in the CNS was almost completely abrogated during an observation period of 3 weeks. Although a few mononuclear cells were seen in the subarachnoidal space of the mice sacrificed on days 3 and 5, and massive cell necrosis was often accompanied by a focal microglial reaction, heavy mononuclear cell infiltration into parenchymal tissues and in perivascular spaces was totally absent in Cy-treated mice.

The brain: In asymptomatic mice sacrificed on days 3 and 5, the viral antigen was readily detected in a large number of neurons in the brain. In addition to sporadic occurrence of viral antigen positive (Ag-positive) cells in the ependymal linings of the lateral, 3rd and 4th ventricles and of the choroid plexus, in the paraventricular tissue and the tissue adjacent to the needle tract, the viral antigen was detected in the majority of mitral cells of the bilateral olfactory bulb (Fig. 2). Some neurons in the anterior olfactory nuclei were also Ag-positive but the glomerular and internal granule layers of the olfactory bulb were virtually free of the viral antigen. Groups of Ag-positive cells were also found in the habenular nuclei, the perirhinal, pyriform and entorhinal and somatosensory cortices. Furthermore, a few Ag-positive neurons were always present in the mesencephalic reticular formation and the gigantocellular reticular nuclei of the pons. The number of Ag-positive cells apparently increased on day 5 but their distribution remained unchanged. In many neurons, not only their perikaryon but also the entire cellular processes were heavily labeled with anti-JHM antibody. No glial cells, however, were convincingly labeled with the antibody.

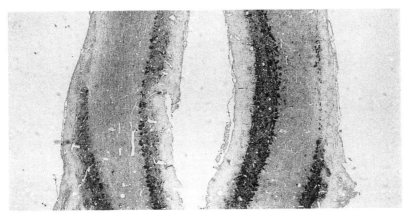

Fig. 2. JHM virus antigens are strongly expressed in the majority of mitral cells of the bilateral olfactory bulb while the glomerular and internal granule cell layers are free of the antigens. 5th post-inoculation day. ABC method.

At this stage of infection, the majority of Ag-positive cells showed no cytopathic changes. Necrotic cells were only rarely encountered among the largely normal ependymal lining cells, the medial habenular nucleus, the hypothalamic nuclei, the deep layer of the cerebral cortex and the roof of the 4th ventricle. Those cells had a deeply eosinophilic cytoplasm and their nuclei were often fragmented. In the 3rd and 4th ventricles, a few desquamated ependymal cells were found on the ventricular surface. Proliferation of microglial cells was evident at the sites of neuronal degeneration. In some mice, mild subarachnoidal mononuclear cell infiltration was seen.

On days 7 and 10, Ag-positive cells were more widely distributed in the brain. In the olfactory system, the viral antigen was not confined to the mitral cell layer. Many cells in the molecular and glomerular layers and in the anterior olfactory nuclei were also Ag-positive. The internal granule cell layer, however, was almost completely spared. In the midbrain and pons, Ag-positive large neurons were widely distributed (Fig. 3). The perikarya and neuritic processes of the Ag-positive neurons often appeared vesicular, and some had a ghost-like appearance (Fig. 3, arrows). On day 10, Ag-positive cells were more randomly distributed in the brain.

In some mice sacrificed on day 10, a large number of the Purkinje cell perikarya and their apical dendrites were heavily labeled. Furthermore, groups of Ag-positive neurons were randomly distributed in the neocortex, the hippocampus and entorhinal cortex. The thalamus and caudoputamen, however, were usually spared. Histological examinations disclosed that some neurons had already been lost and many of the remaining neurons were either chromatolytic or severely pyknotic in the mitral cell layer. In the mesencephalic and pontine reticular formation, swelling of large neurons was conspicuous. Both their perikarya and neuritic processes were markedly swollen and appeared watery, and the neuropil in these regions was grossly vesicular on day 10 (Fig. 4). Such vacuolar changes often involved the bilateral fasciculus retroflexus, the bilateral olfactory and mammillothalamic tracts. Although the majority of the Ag-positive cells randomly distributed in the brain showed little cytopathic change, massive neuronal degeneration was commonly seen in the bilateral entopeduncular and subthalamic nuclei. In addition, necrotic Purkinje and Golgi cells were sporadically found in the cerebellar cortex.

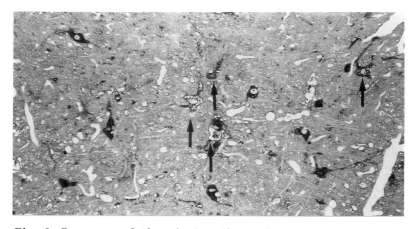

Fig. 3. Presence of the viral antigens in a large number of neurons in the gigantocellular reticular nuclei of the pons on day 7. Note the viral antigens in severely degenerated cells and their processes (arrows). ABC method.

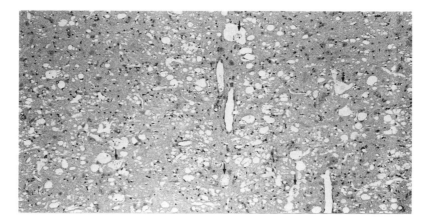

Fig. 4. Vacuolar degeneration of the pontine reticular formation on day 10. The presence of nuclear remnants in some vacuoles (arrows) could be suggestive of the neuronal cell origin of these vacuoles. H&E stain.

On day 14 and thereafter, the number of Ag-positive cells in the brain gradually decreased while vacuolar degeneration was steadily progressive. On day 21, the viral antigen was virtually absent in the olfactory bulb, and was sparsely distributed in the severely vacuolated midbrain and pons and rarely in the cerebral cortex. In some mice, however, a large number of Purkinje cells remained strongly Ag-positive while the antigen was hardly detectable in other parts of the brain. Histological examinations on day 21 disclosed foci of massive neuronal cell necrosis and loss, often accompanied by pseudocalcification. Such changes were commonly seen in the olfactory bulb and the subthalamic nucleus. Vacuolar change of the mesencephalic and pontine reticular formation was most extensive in the mice sacrificed on day 21.

The spinal cord: Development of the viral antigen was apparently retarded in the spinal cord. Although as early as 3 days after virus inoculation, the viral antigen was detected in a few neurons residing in the vicinity of the central canal and root entry zones, the majority of spinal neurons remained Ag-negative until day 7. The number of Ag-positive neurons reached its peak on day 10 and then decreased. Except for few swollen chromatolytic neurons in both the anterior and posterior horns, histopathological change of the spinal cord was inconspicuous.

Unlike the infection in the brain, however, groups of Ag-positive cells were found in the white matter on day 10 and thereafter. These Ag-positive cells were often clustered near the surface and mostly lined up along the myelinated fibers (Fig. 5a), but they were not necessarily accompanied by myelin degeneration. Most of them had a scanty cytoplasm and seemed to be GFAP negative (Fig. 5b). In all of 4 mice sacrificed on day 21, there were many foci of focal vacuolar degeneration in the white matter (Fig. 5c). These vacuoles were mostly associated with swollen axons and Ag-positive mass was occasionally localized to these vacuolar lesions (Fig. 5d).

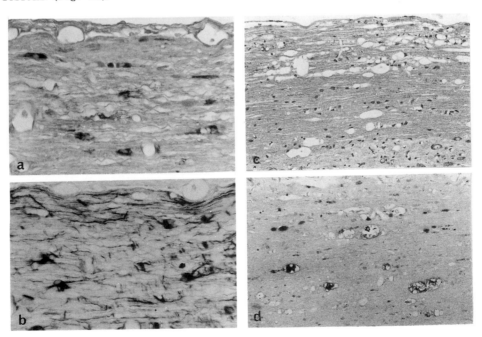

Fig. 5. Vacuolar change and viral antigens in the spinal white matter. Most of Ag-positive cells lining along myelinated fibers (a) appear to be GFAP-negative (b). Many vacuoles in the white matter (c) are apparently associated swollen axons and often contained Ag-positive mass(d).

DISCUSSION

Vacuolar change of the CNS tissue in mouse hepatitis virus (MHV) infection has long been recognized but the study on its mechanism was often hampered by a high mortality of the infection in mice. Unlike other strains of MHV, the JHM-CC virus infection in adult mice is not fatal and yet constantly induces vacuolar degeneration in the CNS tissue. In the present study, Cy-treatment effectively suppressed inflammatory reactions at least for 3 weeks at the expense of an increased mortality rate up to 40%. In the absence of inflammatory cell infiltration, Cy-treated mice developed vacuolar degeneration in the CNS. Although the absence of inflammatory cells gave superficially an impression of milder pathological changes in Cy-treated mice than those in immunocompetent mice, the severity and temporal and spatial sequences of vacuolar degeneration in Cy-treated mice was comparable to those in immunocompetent mice. Therefore, host immune response does not seem to be playing any major role in the pathogenesis of vacuolar degeneration induced by this JHM-CC virus.

Cy-treatment also resulted in the protraction of virus clearance from the CNS tissue, and this provided an opportunity to chase the spread of virus in the CNS for an extended period of time. After intracerebral virus inoculation, a portion of the inoculum apparently spread along the passage of the CSF resulting in the development of sporadic infections in the ventricular and paraventricular tissues. However, early and exclusive development of a large number of Ag-positive cells in the bilateral olfactory system and the brainstem reticular formation could be indicative of possible neural spread of the virus within the CNS as reported in an A59 virus infection in mice (3). Distribution of the viral antigen in the present study seemed to support the possibility of virus spread through the habenular nucleus, the fasciculus retroflexus and the interpeduncular nucleus to the brainstem reticular formation.

In the brain, the viral antigen was solely localized to neurons except for rare infection of ependymal cells at an early stage of the infection. Susceptibility of neuronal cells to this strain of virus is seemingly diverse. No viral antigens were detected in the internal granule cell layer of the olfactory bulb despite the severe infection and extensive necrosis in the neighboring mitral cell layer. Similarly, in the cerebellum, only Purkinje and Golgi cells were selectively infected leaving the granule cells totally uninvolved. The fate of infected cells was also variable. Comparing the number of Ag-positive cells with that of necrotic cells, many of the infected cells seemed to survive. Massive neural necrosis was found only in the mitral cell and molecular layers of the olfactory bulb, the subthalamic nucleus, the entopeduncular nucleus, and when they were involved, it occurred always bilaterally.

While pyknotic cells with karyorrhexis were occasionally found in the brain, the majority of the infected cells were rendered to marked swelling of both the perikarya and neuritic processes; a unique phenomenon in virus infection. The process was apparently slow but it was severe enough to make a substantial contribution to the development of vacuolar degeneration in the midbrain and pons. Similar vacuolar changes also involved small fiber tracts, anatomically related to the sites of severe infection, such as the fasciculus retroflexus and the olfactory tract. On the other hand, the callosal radiation and the pyramidal tract remained intact even on day 21. Therefore, the white matter does not seem to be the primary target of the infection. Nevertheless, swelling and vesicular degeneration of infected cells were a unique feature of this virus infection.

In the spinal cord, the viral antigen was mostly localized to neurons, and many neurons in both the anterior and posterior horns were strongly Ag-positive on days 7 and 10. On day 10 and thereafter, however, there were a number of Ag-positive cells in the white matter. They tended to locate near the surface of the cord or in the vicinity of the root entry zones. Most of the Ag-positive cells had a scanty cytoplasm and lined up in a row along myelinated fibers. They were most likely to be oligodendrocytes. No particular white matter lesion, however, was associated with the presence of these Ag-positive cells, and the implication of this finding remains to be elucidated. On the other hand, there were many small foci of vacuolar change in the white matter on day 21. These lesions were apparently formed by swollen axons, and the viral antigens were often localized to the degenerated axons. The presence of Ag-positive neurons in the dorsal root ganglion, although it was rare, suggested a centrifugal spread of the virus.

Although the diversity of pathogenesis of mouse hepatitis virus has been well recognized (4), much attention has been paid to the demyelinating activity of mouse hepatitis virus. The present experiment provided further evidence for the importance of neuronal degeneration in the development of vacuolar degeneration which sometimes mimicks the pathology of demyelination.

REFERENCES

1. N. Hirano, N. Goto, S. Makino and K. Fujiwara, Persistent infection with mouse hepatitis virus JHM strain in DBT cell culture, Adv. Exp. Med. Biol. 142:301 (1981)
2. N. Goto, M.Takaoka, N. Hirano, K. Takahashi and K. Fujiwara, Neuropathogenicity of a mutant of mouse hepatitis virus, JHM strain derived from persistently infecting DBT cells, Jpn. J. Vet. Sci. 46:755 (1984)
3. E. Lavi, P.S. Fishman, M.K. Highkin and S.R. Weiss, Limbic encephalitis after inhalation of a murine coronavirus, Lab. Invest. 58:31 (1988)
4. S.W. Barthold, D.S. Beck and A.L. Smith, Mouse hepatitis virus naso encephalopathy is dependent upon strain and host genotype. Arch. Virol. 91:247 (1986)

VACUOLAR ENCEPHALOMYELOPATHY IN MICE INDUCED BY INTRACEREBRAL INOCULATION WITH A CORONAVIRUS JHM-CC STRAIN

Tetsuro Tsukamoto*, Yuzo Iwasaki**, Norio Hirano***,
Satoru Haga***

*Department of Neurology, Fukushima Medical College, Fukushima,, Sendai, Japan
**Department of Neurological Sciences, Tohoku University School of Medicine
Sendai, Japan
***Department of Veterinary Microbiology, Iwate University, Morioka, Japan

INTRODUCTION

JHM-CC virus, a mutant strain of mouse hepatitis virus, was isolated by Hirano in 1980 from a DBT cell culture persistently infected with the neurovirulent strain, JHM[1]. This mutant strain is characterized by formation of smaller plaques on the DBT cells and by lower cell virulence than the original JHM[1]. Although several murine coronaviruses such as JHM are known to cause demyelinating encephalitis[2,4], we found that JHM-CC does not induce primary demyelination, but instead produces characteristic vacuolar degeneration in the brain and spinal cord. In this report we describe the clinical manifestations, neuropathological changes and viral antigen distribution in the central nervous system (CNS) of ICR mice infected intracerebrally with JHM-CC.

MATERIALS AND METHODS

A total of 107 four-week old ICR mice under periodical surveillance for antibody to MHV were inoculated intracerebrally with 0.02 ml of JHM-CC virus suspension (1x10^6 PFU). Twenty mice were maintained for two months after inoculation to observe any clinical manifestations.

For virus titration, 3 mice were sacrificed every day from 1 to 10 days after inoculation and on days 12 and 14. Individual 10% tissue homogenates (w/v) in MEM were prepared from the brain, spinal cord, liver and spleen. The infectivity of each tissue homogenate diluted in MEM was assayed by plaqueing in DBT cell culture as reported previously[5,6].

For histopathology and viral antigen detection, 3 mice were sacrificed and perfusion-fixed with a 10% buffered formalin solution on days 1,2,3,4,5,7,10,14,21,28,30, and 2,4, and 6 months after inoculation. Multiple 3 µm paraffin sections were prepared from the brain and spinal cord and were stained with hematoxylin-eosin and by the Kluver-Barrera and Bodian methods. For free-floating preparations, the formalin fixed tissues immersed in a PBS solution containing 20% sucrose and 0.1% dimethylsulfoxide, were rapidly frozen in liquid nitrogen and then cut into 40 µm thick sections with a cryostat. An immunohistochemical study was carried out on paraffin and free-floating sections by the avidin-biotin peroxidase complex (ABC) method using anti-JHM antibody raised in rabbits.

On days 3, 6 and 9 after inoculation, 3 mice each were fixed by perfusion with 4% paraformaldehyde and 0.5% glutaraldehyde in Millonig's phosphate buffer for electron microscopy. The tissues were postfixed with 1% OsO_4, dehydrated and embedded in epoxy resin. Ultrathin sections were stained with uranyl acetate and lead citrate and examined with a Hitachi H 600 electron microscope.

Coronaviruses and Their Diseases
Edited by D. Cavanagh and T.D.K. Brown
Plenum Press, New York, 1990

609

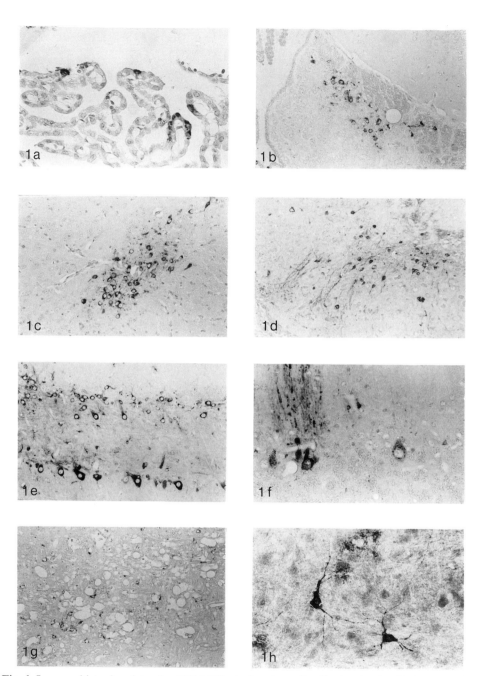

Fig. 1. Immunohistochemistry for JHM-CC viral antigen distribution in the CNS. a-g: 3 μm thick paraffin sections. h: 40 μm-thick floating sections. a. Choroidal plexus, one day post inoculation (p.i.). b. Habenular nucleus, 2 days p.i. c. Piriform cortex, 2 days p.i. d. Cingulate cortex, 3 days p.i. e. Olfactory bulb, 43 days p.i. f. Cerebellum, 4 days p.i. Purkinje cells and small cells in the molecular layer are positive. g. Brainstem, 7 days p.i. Vacuolar degeneration are progressing, whereas viral antigens are diminishing, h. Spinal cord neurons, 7 days p.i.

RESULTS

Close clinical observation of 20 mice showed all of them to be irritable and hypersensitive 5 to 7 days after inoculation. Two mice developed hind leg paresis on day 8 and 3 more on day 9. Four of 5 paralysed mice recovered from the disease after 15 days, whereas one mouse died of severe paresis on day 22. The other animals showed no symptoms.

Hindlimb paresis also developed 7 to 9 days after inoculation in about 20% of the mice designated for virus titration and for histopathology. A few severely paralysed animals died from difficulty in feeding. Even in the mice without clinical symptoms, the virus was constantly recovered from the brain and spinal cord during the first two weeks of the infection. The highest titer of the virus was recovered from the mice sacrificed on day 4 or 5 (10^6 PFU/0.2g). The titer declined gradually and became negative on day 14. Infectious virus was never recovered from the liver or spleen.

An immunohistochemical study revealed a spatial sequence for the progression of the viral infection in the CNS. On day 1, viral antigen positive cells were sporadically found in the ependyma, choroid plexus and corpus callosum (Fig.1a). On day 2, several neuronal cells in the habenular nucleus, piriform cortex and entorhinal cortex became positive for viral antigen (Fig.1b,c). By day 3, the infection had apparently spread to the cingulate cortex, accumbens nucleus, subiculum, caudate-putamen, thalamus, hypothalamus, substantia nigra, septal nucleus and even to the lower brain-stem (Fig.1d). On day 4, the viral antigens were

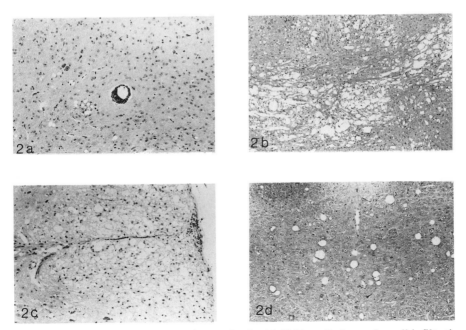

Fig. 2. Histopathology in paraffin sections stained with H-E. a. Perivascular cell infiltration in the pons, 28 days p.i. b. Marked vaculation in the pons with the paucity of inflammatory changes, 18 days p.i. c. Marked vacuolar changes in the spinal cord and subarachnoid inflammatory cell infiltration, 28 days p.i. d. Smaller vacuoles in the pons 2 months p.i. These possibly reflect an ongoing reparative process of vacuolation.

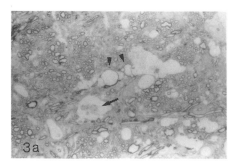

Fig. 3a. Vacuolar changes on day 9 p.i. One-μm plastic section of pons stained with toluidine blue. Myelin splitting (arrow heads) and axonal degeneration (arrow) are seen.

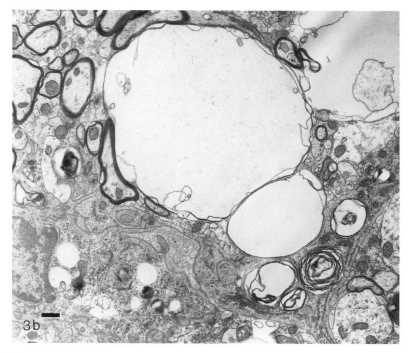

Fig. 3b. Ultrastructure of vacuolar changes on day 9 p.m. Myelin splitting and periaxonal edema. bar = 1μm.

demonstrable in the mitral cells and other neurons in the olfactory bulb, and occasionally in the Purkinje and granular cells of the cerebellum and spinal cord neurons (Fig.1e-g). The viral antigens were most strongly and widely expressed on day 5 when the antigens were almost exclusively localized to neurons and rarely to glial cells (Fig.1b). The viral antigens in the CNS gradually diminished and became undetectable by day 14.

Pathologically, inflammatory changes were rather inconspicuous. Mild mononuclear cell infiltration in the subarachnoid and perivascular spaces was noted on day 2 after inoculation. Between days 3 and 5, necrotic neurons were sporadically seen in the periaqueductal region,

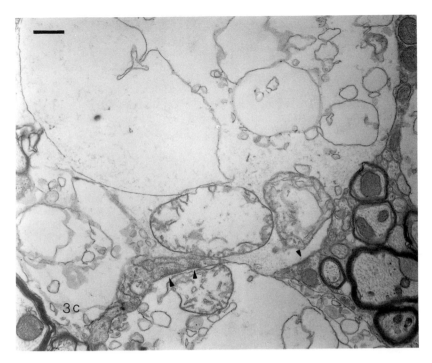

Fig. 3c. Ultrastructure of vacuolar changes in pons. Swollen axons containing bulging mitochondria and membrane-lined vacuoles. Synaptic vesicles are indicated by arrow heads. bar = 1μm.

pontine tegmentum and anterior horns of the spinal cord, often without inflammatory cell reaction. Mild ependymitis was evident in some mice. On day 7, severe neuronal degeneration developed in the olfactory bulb and lobe, and they often became totally necrotic. In other parts of the brain and spinal cord, however, such destructive changes were rare, and foci of microglial proliferation and perivascular mononuclear cell infiltration were sparsely distributed in the cerebral cortex and paraventricular tissues (Fig.2a). These inflammatory changes were most florid in the tissue examined on day 14.

In contrast to the relative paucity of inflammatory changes, the development of vacuolar or spongiform changes was impressive. Small foci of tissue vacuolation were first noted on day 4. These vacuolar changes progressed in size and number even after disappearance of the infectious virus and viral antigens from the CNS tissue and were most conspicuous in the mice sacrificed between days 14 and 28. Although numerous vacuoles of varying size were randomly distributed in the cingulate cortex, corpus callosum,basal ganglia, thalamus, internal capsule, midbrain and cerebellum, the brainstem and the spinal gray and white matter were most extensively involved (Fig.2b,c). Despite the presence of lymphocytes and some plasma cells in the subarachnoid space and thick perivascular cuffs around the parenchymal vessels, macrophages were almost completely absent at the sites of vacuolar degeneration. Following Kluver-Barrera and Bodian staining, the vacuolation did not appear to be related to either primary demylination or axonal swelling. After 2 months foci of vacuolar changes became smaller and decreased in number with the margins somewhat blurred and after 4 months they were no longer observed.

Electron microscopic observations disclosed that vacuolar degeneration was largely attributable to widening of the periaxonal spaces and intra-lamellar edema in the myelin sheath (Fig.3a,b). In addition, swollen axons with bulging mitochondria and membrane-lined vacuoles were occasionally seen (Fig.3c). There were, however, no evidence for primary demyelination. Viral particles were only rarely observed in neuronal cells.

DISCUSSION

In contrast to fulminant encephalitis induced by the parental strain of JHM, the intracerebral infection with JHM-CC virus[7,8], a mutant strain of mouse hepatitis virus (JHM), resulted only in mild hindlimb paresis in some mice or no symptoms in others. Irrespective of clinical manifestations, however, all mice developed histopathological lesions and viral antigens in the CNS. The most distinctive pathological findings were spongiform changes or severe vacuolization in the brain and spinal cord developing relatively delayed after early appearance of mild inflammatory cell infiltration in the subarachnoidal and perivascular spaces.

The progression of these vacuolar changes did not parallel chronologically the sequence of infectious virus levels and the intensity and extension of the viral antigens in the CNS, but these seemed anatomically to be related to the sites of viral replication. They increased in size and number where the viral antigens had been expressed immunohistochemically, even after disappearance of the infectious virus and viral antigens. It is worth noting, however, that vacuolar degeneration was no longer seen 4 months after inoculation. This could be suggestive of reversibility of the vacuolar changes. Furthermore, in the mice sacrificed 2 months after inoculation, vacuolar changes were less conspicuous than those in the mice sacrificed earlier. Smaller vacuoles with a somewhat obscure inner margin might reflect the ongoing reparative process of vacuolation.

Ultrastructural studies showed that these vacuolar changes were not primary demyelination, but were mostly attributable to periaxonal edema, intramyelinic splits and swollen axons containing degenerated mitochondria and membrane-lined vacuoles.

Similar spongiform or vacuolar changes have been found in some retrovirus infections[9-12]. Elucidation of the mechanism of vacuolar degeneration in this JHM-CC infection model could provide a better understanding of new types of neurological disorders associated with viral infections including vacuolar myelopathy in AIDS[11,12].

ACKNOWLEDGEMENT

This study was supported by a grant-in-aid for scientific research from the Ministry of Education, Science and Culture, Tokyo, Japan (61570381).

REFERENCES

1. N. Hirano, K. Fujiwara, S. Hino and M. Matumoto. Persistent infection with mouse hepatitis virus, JHM strain, in DBT cell culture. In: "Biochemistry and Biology of Coronaviruses", V. ter Meulen, S.Siddell and H. Wege eds., Plenum Publishing Corp., New York, 301-308 (1981).
2. L.P. Weiner. Pathogenesis of demyelination induced by a mouse hepatitis virus (JHM virus). Arch.Neurol. 28: 298-303 (1973).
3. S.A. Stohlman and L.P. Weiner. Chronic central nervous system demyelination in mice after JHM virus infection. Neurology (N.Y.) 31: 38-44 (1981).
4. R. Watanabe, H. Wege and V. ter Meulen. Comparative analysis of coronavirus JHM-induced demyelinating encephalomyelitis in Lewis and Brown Norway rats. Lab. Invest. 57: 375-384 (1987).
5. N. Hirano, K. Fujiwara, S.Hino and M. Matumoto. Replication and plaque formation of mouse hepatitis virus (MHV-2) in mouse cell line DBT culture. Arch. Gesamte Virusforsch.44: 298-302 (1978).
6. N. Hirano, T. Murakami, K.Fujiwara and M. Matumoto. Utility of mouse cell line for propagation and assay of mouse hepatitis virus. Jpn. J. Exp. Med.48: 71-75 (1978).
7. F.S. Cheever, J.B. Daniels, A.M. Pappenheimer and O.T. Bailey. A murine virus (JHM) causing disseminated encephalomyelitis with extensive destruction of myelin: I. Isolation and biological properties of the virus. J. Exp. Med. 90: 181-194 (1949).
8. N. Hirano, T.Murakami, F. Taguchi,K. Fujuwara and M.Matumoto. Comparison of mouse hepatitis virus strains for pathogenicity in weanling mice infected by various routes. Arch. Virol. 70: 69-73 (1981).

9. B.R. Brooks, J.R. Swarz and R.T. Johnson. Spongiform polioencephalomelopathy caused by a murine retrovirus. I. Pathogenesis of infection in newborn mice. Lab. Invest. 43: 480-486 (1980).

10. J.R. Swarz, B.R. Brooks and R.T. Johnson. Spongiform polioencephalomyelopathy caused by a murine retrovirus. II. Ultrastructural localization of virus replication and spongiform changes in the central nervous system. Neuropathol. Appl. Neurobiol. 7: 365-380 (1981).

11. C.K. Petito, B.A. Navia, E-S. Cho, B.D. Jordan, D.C. George and R.W. Price. Vacuolar myelopathy pathologically resembling subacute combined degeneration in patients with the acquired immunodeficiency syndrome. N. Engl. J. Med. 312: 874-879 (1985).

12. L.R. Sharer, L.G. Epstein, E-S. Cho and C.K. Petito. HTLV-III and vacuolar myelopathy. N. Engl. J. Med. 315: 62-63 (1986).

DIFFERENCE IN RESPONSE OF SUSCEPTIBLE MOUSE STRAINS TO A SMALL

PLAQUE MUTANT (JHM-CC) OF MOUSE CORONAVIRUS

Norio Hirano, Tetsuro Tsukamoto*, Satoshi Haga and Yuzo Iwasaki**

Department of Veterinary Microbiology, Iwate University, Morioka 020, Japan
Department of *Neurology, and**Neurological Science, Tohoku University
School of Medicine, Sendai 980, Japan

INTRODUCTION

The JHM-CC virus is a small plaque mutant isolated from the DBT cell culture persistently infected with JHM (1), the most neurotropic strain of mouse coronavirus (2). This JHM-CC virus had been shown to induce severe vacuolar degeneration in the brainstem and spinal cord of the infected ICR mice (1,3). Since the strain difference of mice in their susceptibility to various strains of mouse coronaviruses including parental JHM virus has been documented (4,5), we compared the kinetics of virus production and neuropathological changes after intracerebral inoculation of the JHM-CC virus in three strains of mice.

MATERIALS AND METHODS

Virus. Plaque-purified JHM-CC virus was propagated in DBT cells and infectivity was assayed by the plaque count method as reported previously (2).
Animal inoculation. Four-week-old male Balb/c, C3H and C57BL mice were obtained from a breeder colony, which has been serologically checked for the absence of mouse coronavirus infection. Mice were inoculated intracerebrally (i.c.) with 0.02 ml of virus material.
Infectivity of the brain and spinal cord. Ten percent tissue homogenates (w/v in Eagle's MEM) were prepared from the brain and spinal cord, and assayed for infectivity in DBT cell system as described previously (1).
Immunohistochemical study. Immunohistochemistry was carried out on paraffin sections by the avidin-biotin peroxidase complex (ABC) method using anti-JHM rabbit antibody (1:1000). For histopathological study, some of serial paraffin sections were stained with hematoxylin and eosin.

RESULTS

Thirty-one mice each of Balb/c, C3H and C57BL strains were inoculated i.c. with 1 x 10^6 PFU of JHM-CC virus, and were observed for the development of clinical signs for 14 days. All the mice became hypersensitive on day 4 to 6 post-inoculation. Among the three strains, C3H mice were most susceptible to the virus: half of them showed hind leg paresis and began to die on day 8. The Balb/c mice were most resistant and all survived for 14 days. Some of C57BL mice also showed hind leg paresis and died on day 10 and thereafter. The mortality of mice was about 50% (15/31) in C3H mice, 20% (6/31) in C57BL mice and 0% (0/31) in Balb/c mice. At autopsy, marked symmetrical dilatation of the entire ventricular system was the most conspicuous finding in the surviving mice of the C3H and C57BL strains.

Coronaviruses and Their Diseases
Edited by D. Cavanagh and T.D.K. Brown
Plenum Press, New York, 1990

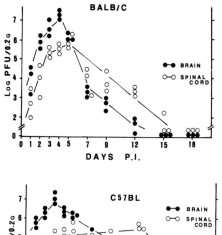

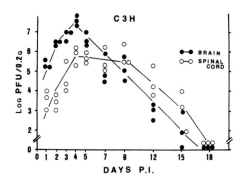

Fig. 1. Virus growth in the brain and spinal cord of Balb/c, C3H and C57BL mice after inoculation with 1×10^6 PFU of JHM-CC virus.

To correlate the kinetics of virus titer with histopathological changes in Balb/c, C3H and C57BL mice, 60 mice each of the above strains were inoculated with 1×10^6 PFU of the virus, and at various intervals, 2 mice each were sacrificed for immunohistochemical study and 3 mice each for virus assay of the brain and spinal cord. As shown in Fig.l, the virus infectivity of the brain reached a peak of 10^7 PFU/0.2g on day 3 to 4. The infectivity gradually declined afterwards and became undetectable on day 18 to 21. The titer of the spinal cord was 1 to 2 log units lower than that of the brain during first 5 days, and tended to be higher than that of the brain 7 days after inoculation. Among 3 strains, Balb/c mice showed a rapid decline of the infectivity titers, both of the brain and spinal cord, 4 to 5 days after inoculation, and the titers became undetectable by day 15. On the other hand the infectivity of the brain and spinal cord in C57BL mice was maintained at the detectable level of 10^3 PFU/0.2g even 15 days after inoculation. The virus growth in the brain and spinal cord of C3H mice was almost same to that of C57BL. The virus growth in the brain was parallel with the development of clinical signs as described above.

Using the ABC method, viral specific antigen was detected on day 3 in the olfactory bulb, cerebrum, brainstem, ependyma, choroid plexus and the aqueduct of Sylvius of the infected mice. Figure 2 shows viral antigens in the ependymal lining cells of the aqueduct of a C57BL mouse sacrificed on day 3. On day 5, virus antigen positive cells were also found in the cerebellum and spinal cord. In C57BL mice, the virus antigen was widely distributed in the CNS, and remained detectable in the cerebral cortex and brainstem even on day 15 when the antigen-positive cells were no longer detectable in the CNS of Balb/c and C3H mice. On day 3, a stenosis or occlusion of the aqueduct of Sylvius was suspected on the basis of histological examination of C57BL mice. On day 5, enlargement of the lateral ventricle was commonly seen in 3 mouse strains. The enlargement of the ventricles was accompanied by inflammatory cell infiltration and perivascular cuffings of lymphoid cells in the paraventricular tissue. By day 7, severe vacuolar changes developed in the brainstem of all the infected mice as described previously in ICR mice (1, 3). The hydrocephalic change was most remarkable in C57BL mice to compare with that in C3H and Balb/c mice. Figure 1 shows the hydrocephalus in C57BL mouse sacrificed on day 15.

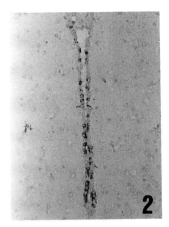
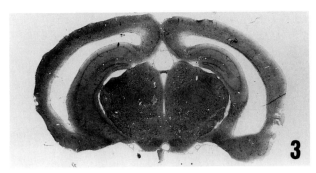

Fig. 2. Viral antigen in the aqueduct of C57BL mouse sacrificed on day 3.

Fig. 3. Hydrocephalus induced in C57BL mouse sacrificed on day 15.

DISCUSSION

In the present study, C3H mice were most susceptible to JHM-CC virus and Balb/c mice were most resistant. Strain difference in susceptibility to the virus was shown by mortality and virus growth in the CNS of each mouse strain. The mortality was considered to be dependent upon the virus growth in the CNS.

As neuropathological changes after virus inoculation, hydrocephalus due to enlargement of lateral ventricle and vacuolar degeneration in the brainstem and spinal cord were found in the infected mice. Viral specific antigen was demonstrated in the ependymal cells, choroid plexus and aqueduct as well as cerebral cortex and brainstem of the infected mice of 3 strains by the ABC method and a stenosis of the aqueduct was histopathologically suspected at early stage of the infection. Dilatation of the lateral ventricle and aqueduct were found on day 5. On day 7, vacuolar changes were produced in the brainstem and spinal cord and became severe with time, as previously reported on ICR mice (1,3). However, in ICR mice inoculated with the same dose of the virus, no hydrocephalic changes were observed. The highest titer in the brain of ICR mice was 10^6 PFU/0.2g, and was about 1 log unit lower than that of 3 strains examined in this study. The virus titer and persistence in the brain might play a role in inducing hydrocephalic changes. Hydrocephalus has been induced in experimental animals by a variety of virus infections (6). These experiments show that non-fatal infections with those viruses result in stenosis of the aqueduct leading to hydrocephalus. In the present study, viral growth in the ependyma and choroid plexus was suggested by the ABC method, and inflammatory cell infiltration was observed in the paraventricular tissue. The JHM-CC virus persisted in the CNS for 2 weeks. These findings suggest that hydrocephalic changes might be produced as a sequence to the stenosis of aqueduct by the virus. Further studies should be made to explain the early pathogenic events in C57BL mice after i.c. inoculation with JHM-CC virus.

REFERENCES

1. N. Hirano, N. Goto, S. Makino, and K. Fujiwara, Persistent infection with mouse hepatitis virus, JHM strain in DBT cell culture, Adv. Exp. Med. Biol. 142, 301-308 (1981).
2. N. Hirano, T. Murakami, F. Taguchi, K. Fujiwara, and M. Matumoto, Comparison of mouse hepatitis virus strains for pathogenicity in weanling mice infected by various routes, Arch. Virol. 70, 69-73 (1981).

3. N. Goto, M. Takaoka, N. Hirano, K. Takahashi, and K. Fujiwara, Neuropathogenicity of a mutant of mouse hepatitis virus, JHM strain derived from persistently infecting DBT cells, <u>Jpn. J. Vet. Sci.</u> 46, 755-760 (1984).

4. F. Taguchi, N. Hirano, Y. Kiuchi, and K. Fujiwara, Difference in response to mouse hepatitis virus among susceptible mouse strains. <u>Jpn. J. Microbiol.</u> 20, 293-302 (1979).

5. S. A. Stohlman, and J. A. Flelinger, Resistance to fatal central nevous system disease by mouse hepatitis virus strain JHM. I. Genetic analysis, <u>Immunogenetics</u> 6, 277-281 (1981).

6. R. T. Johnson, Hydrocephalus and viral infections, <u>Dev. Med. Child Neurol.</u> 17, 807-816 (1975).

Chapter 13

Neurological Consequences of Murine Hepatitis Virus Infection of Rats

BACKGROUND PAPER

ON THE ROLE OF THE IMMUNE RESPONSE IN THE COURSE OF CORONAVIRUS
JHM-INDUCED ENCEPHALOMYELITIDES IN MICE AND RATS

Rüdiger Dörries

Institut für Virologie und Immunbiologie der Üniversität
Versbacher Strasse 7
D-8700 Würzburg
Fed. Rep. Germany

Virus infections of the central nervous system (CNS) may result in the loss of myelin sheaths without axonal destruction. Severe neurological symptoms occur as a consequence of this phenomenon which is called primary demyelination. The sequence of events leading to primary demyelination during the course of viral infections of the CNS is only partially understood. Although it is well established that cytolytic infection of the oligodendroglia cell can cause primary demyelination, mononuclear infiltrates in subacute and chronic courses of the disease indicate that immunological events may take part in this process (reviewed by Johnson (l)). For several reasons, investigations into the dynamic interactions between virus infection of the CNS and the local immune response cannot be conducted in man. (1) Usually clinical specimens are restricted to cerebrospinal fluid which gives limited information about pathological events occuring in the brain parenchyma (2). It is not known at which time point of the preceeding systemic infection, the virus enters the brain and biopsies are taken too rarely and infrequently to understand the kinetics of the events (3). The general absence of genetic homogeneity in man complicates attempts to detect the influence of the immunogenetic background on the course of the disease. In contrast, intracerebral infections of rodents with the murine hepatitis virus JHM (MHV-4) are excellent models to study the relationships between virus-induced demyelination and the local immune response. Based on the work of Cheever (2), animal models of JHM virus-induced demyelinating encephalomyelitis have been developed in mice as well as in rats (3-5). In recent years striking similarities in the course of the infection in both rodents have been detected which might give the impression that these two models can substitute for each other. However, subtle but important differences do exist. Therefore, in the present review attempts are made to summarize and compare the knowledge about demyelinating encephalomyelitides in rats and mice, giving emphasis to the role of the local immune response in the brain.

In general, intracerebral infection of mice and rats may result in either an acute lethal panencephalitis or a subclinical infection (3-9). The acute disease is accompanied by paralytic symptoms and extensive damage in white as well as in grey matter of the brain. In subclinical infections small foci of chronic demyelination can be observed, but no involvement of grey matter is evident. The third type of disease, a subacute demyelinating encephalomyelitis with overt neurological symptoms is seen exclusively in rats (7-9). This subacute disease is characterized by a delayed onset and generally, reduced severity of the paralytic symptoms. Usually animals survive the clinical attack and histopathological changes are mostly confined to white matter with rare involvement of grey matter. Taken together, acute clinical disease is observed in rats and mice where the infection has spread from the periventricular white matter to large areas of the grey matter. In the rat, with decreasing grey matter involvement, clinical symptoms are less severe, although significant primary demyelination is seen. Asymptomatic

Coronaviruses and Their Diseases
Edited by D. Cavanagh and T.D.K. Brown
Plenum Press, New York, 1990

623

mice or rats have no grey matter destruction and primary demyelination can be detected up to several month of infection. However, the affected areas are very small.

A important factor that determines the outcome of the infection is the age of the animal (5,9,10). As a general rule, infection of suckling animals of all strains of mice and rats with mouse brain passaged wild type JHM will cause an acute fatal disease, whereas with increasing age, inoculation will result in a growing proportion of animals with clinically inapparent infection. Resistant inbred strains differ from susceptible ones in that they acquire disease resistance earlier in life and the proportion of animals without clinical symptoms can approach 100%. Moreover, at least in some inbred strains of susceptible rats, the transition from a fully susceptible to a more resistant stage is characterized by an increasing number of animals with a subacute demyelinating encephalitis. Clearly, factors acting in different inbred strains at different ages govern the susceptibility of mice and rats to clinically overt encephalomyelitis.

In both, rats and mice the age-dependent differentiation of the viral target cell is an endogenous factor which determines the course and the outcome of the infection (11-13). In mice, the role of the differentiating viral target cell was shown by *in vitro* examination of neurons from the resistant SJL strain. These cells are not permissive for JHM virus, whereas neurons of Balb/c mice support the replication of JHM easily (11). Moreover the yield of infectious virus obtained from SJL glial cell cultures is 50-100 fold lower than from glial cell cultures of Balb/c mice (12). *In situ* examination of infected brain from adult animals supported these findings, since viral antigen could not be detected in the grey matter of SJL mice, but was present in the grey matter of Balb/c animals (11). These data explain the resistant state of adult SJL mice to clinically overt neurological disease and the high rate of acute paralytic diseases observed in JHM-inoculated Balb/c mice. In rats of the strain Wistar Furth (WF) there is a correlation between onset of the resistant state and the rise of the enzyme CNPase in oligodendrocytes, which are the main target for JHM in the glial cell fraction of the brain (13). This enzyme is involved in the synthesis of myelin, a major component of oligodendrocytes.

The important role of the immune response during intracerebral infection with JHM was first recognized following immunosupressive treatment of rats and mice with cyclo-phosphamide or cyclosporin A (3,14,15). Wistar Furth (WF) rats, although highly susceptible to acute paralytic disease as suckling animals can be infected subclinically as adult animal. However, cyclophosphamide treatment after subclinical infection causes exacerbation of neurological symptoms (14). Wistar Lewis rats which acquire a resistant state to paralytic disease after a few days of life become very susceptible at the age of 35 days post partum (dpp) when immunosupressed by cyclosporin A (15). Adult swiss outbred mice usually reveal a considerable number of animals with clinically inapparent demyelinating encephalitis after infection with JHM virus. Immunosupression by cyclophosphamide prior to the infection causes a drift from inapparent demyelinating disease to acute lethal encephalomyelitis (3). In all immunosuppressed animals, involvement of grey matter is increased as compared to the untreated ones. This observation suggests that the immune response most likely interferes with the spread of the virus from the periventricular white matter to wide areas of the grey matter, which is a characteristic of the viral infection in mice and rats succumbing to acute encephalitis.

A virus-specific immune response is based on two effector mechanisms:
1. the synthesis of neutralizing antibodies and
2. the differentiation of cytotoxic T-lymphocytes which are able to kill virus-infected target cells.
Both axes of the response are dependent on the induction of helper T-lymphocytes providing help for differentiation of the contributing cells. Antibodies can prevent or delay neurological disease if passively given before infection. Suckling mice nursed by mothers preimmunized with JHM develop the subacute type of disease which is usually seen in weanling rats (16), and suckling rats protected by maternal antibodies develop a subacute disease instead of the fatal acute encephalomyelitis (17). In both cases, viral antigen is not eliminated from the brain, but is detected more often in the white- than in the grey matter. This suggests that virus-specific antibody selects for non-neurotropic variants, an assumption which is further strengthened by the fact that virus grown in the presence of neutralizing monoclonal antibodies with specificity for the S-protein is less neurotropic and preferentially infects glial cells (18-20). Such antibodies administered passively to susceptible mice protect the recipients from disease and

grey matter infection but do not prevent chronic demyelinating disease (21). High titres of neutralizing antibodies may favor the rise of escape mutants which preferentially infect glial cells leading to persistent infection and chronic demyelination. This idea is supported by findings that temperature sensitive mutants of JHM generated by chemical treatment of the wild type JHM strain reveal an altered cell tropism *in vivo* (22-24). In rats as well as in mice such ts-mutants are detected preferentially in glia and rarely infect neurons. This property corresponds to the fact that these viruses do not induce acute lethal encephalitis but rather a subacute- or clinically inapparent encephalomyelitis.

There is only limited data available on the function of the cellular immune response following JHM virus infection. Transfer experiments in mice with either T-cell clones or polyclonal T-cells into recipients which have been infected reveal the following picture (25-29). Nylon wool non-adherent CD4+ positive helper T-cells can protect syngeneic recipients from disease provided that they are specific for JHM and are compatible with class II antigens of the recipient. However, they do not eliminate the virus. This can only be achieved by transfer of a small nylon wool adherent T-cell fraction which consists of CD4+ helper and CD8+ cytotoxic T-cells into irradiated recipients. Depletion of the recepients of either CD4 cells or CD8 cells results in failure to eliminate the virus. This finding in combination with the fact, that only transfer into class I compatible recipients will result in clearance of the virus, clearly indicates that elimination of virus from the infected host is dependent on CD8 positive virus-specific T-cells, which probably require help from CD4+ T cells for sucessful action. Compared to these data, little is known in the rat about the function of individual T lymphocyte subsets. However it is clear, that either absence of a functional T-cell compartment as in athymic nu/nu rats (30) or immunosuppression by cyclosporin A results in prolonged susceptibility of animals to paralytic disease (15). Detailed functional data on individual lymphocyte subsets are lacking.

In summary, the local immune response of rats and mice infected intracerebrally with coronavirus JHM prevents disease and helps to overcome the infection of the CNS by clearing the virus from the body. However, many details about the local immunological effector mechanisms in the brains of these animals are still unknown. Two of the most important questions which remain to be answered are:

1. Does the action of cytotoxic T-lymphocytes contribute to primary demyelination *in vivo* and as a consequence, to the severity of the neurological symptoms?

2. Is the virus-specific antibody response generated within the CNS capable of selecting for variants of JHM which preferentially infect glial cells, thus driving the matter?

ACKNOWLEDGEMENTS

Dr. J. D. Sedgwick is gratefully acknowledged for giving editorial advice.

REFERENCES

1. R. T. Johnson, Chronic inflammatory and demyelinating diseases, In: "Viral infections of the Nervous System," R. T. Johnson, ed., Raven Press, New York, (1982).
2. F. S. Cheever, J. B. Daniels, A. M. Pappenheimer, and O. T. Bailey, A murine virus (JHM) causing disseminated encephalomyelitis with extensive destruction of myelin, J. Exp. Med. 90:181 (1949).
3. L. P. Weiner, Pathogenesis of demyelination induced by a mouse hepatitis virus, Arch. Neurol. 28:298 (1973)
4. K. Nagashima, H . Wege, R . Meyermann, and V . ter Meulen, Coronavirus-induced subacute demyelinating encephalomyelitis in rats. A morphological analysis, Acta Neuropathol 44: 63 (1978)
5. O. Sorensen, D. Perry, and S. Dales, In vivo and in vitro models of demyelinating diseases. III. JHM virus infection of rats. Arch. Neurol . 37: 478 (1980)
6. R. M. Herndon, D. E. Griffin, U. McCormick, and L. P. Weiner, Mouse hepatitis virus-induced recurrent demyelination, Arch. Neurol. 32: 32 (1975)
8. M. Koga, H. Wege, and V. ter Meulen, Sequence of murine coronavirus JHM-induced neuropathological changes in rats, Neuropathol. Appl . Neurobiol . 10 :173 (1984)

9. R. Watanabe, H. Wege, and V. ter Meulen, Comparative analysis of coronavirus JHM-induced demyelinating encephalomyelitis in Lewis and Brown Norway rats, Lab . Invest . 57: 375 (1987)

10. S. A . Stohlman, and L. P . Weiner, Chronic central nervous system demyelination in mice after JHM virus infection, Neurology 31:38 (1981)

11. R. L. Knobler, M. V. Haspel, and M. B. A. Oldstone, Mouse hepatitis virus type 4 (JHM strain) -induced fatal central nervous system disease. I. Genetic control and the murine neuron as the susceptible site of the disease, J. Exp . Med . 153: 832 (1981)

12. A. R. Collins, L. A. Tunison, and R. L. Knobler, Mouse hepatitis virus type 4 infection of primary glial cultures from genetically sysceptible and resistant mice, Infec . Immun. 40: 1192 (1983)

13. 5. Beushausen, and S. Dales, *In vivo* and *in vitro* models of demyelinating diseases. XI. Tropism and differentiation regulate the infectious process of coronaviruses in primary explants of the rat CNS, Virology 141: 89 (1985)

14. O. Sorensen, R. Dugre, D. Percy, and S. Dales, *In vivo* and *in vitro* models of demyelinating disease: Endogenous factors influencing demyelinating disease caused by mouse hepatitis virus in rats and mice, Infec. Immun. 37: 1248 (1982)

15. M. J. Zimmer, and S. Dales, *In vivo* and *In vitro* models of demyelinating diseases. XXIV. The infectious process in cyclosporin A-treated Wistar Lewis rats inoculated with JHM virus, Microb. Pathogen. 6: 7 (1989)

16. S. Perlman, R. Schelper, E. Bolger, and D. Ries, Late onset, symptomatic, demyelinating encephalomyelitis in mice infected with MHV-JHM in the presence of maternal antibody, Microb. Pathogen. 2: 185 (1987)

17. H. Wege, R. Watanabe, M. Koga and V. ter Meulen, Coronavirus JHM-induced demyelinating encephalomyelitis in rats: Influence of immunity on the course of disease, in: "Immunology of Nervous System Infections, Progress in Brain Research, Vol. 59," P. 0. Behan, V. ter Meulen, and F. Clifford Rose, eds., Elsevier Science Publishers, New York, (1983).

18. J. O. Fleming, M. D. Trousdale, J. Bradbury, S. A. Stohlman, and L.P. Weiner, Experimental demyelination induced by coronavirus JHM (MHV-4): molecular identification of a viral determinant of paralytic disease, Microb. Pathogen. 3: 9 (1987).

19. M. J. Buchmeier, R. G. Dalziel, and M. J. M. Koolen, Coronavirus-induced CNS disease: a model for virus-induced demyelination, J. Neuroimmunol. 20: 111 (1988)

20. H. Wege, J. Winter, P. Massa, R. Dörries, and V. ter Meulen, Coronavirus JHM-induced demyelinating disease: Specific domains on the E2-protein are associated with neurovirolence, in: "Coronaviruses. Advances in Experimental Medicine and Biology, Vol. 218," M. C. Lai, and S. A. Stohlman, eds., Plenum Publishing Corporation, New York, (1987).

21. M. J. Buchmeier, H. A. Lewicki, P. J. Talbot, and R. L. Knobler, Murine hepatitis virus-4 (strain JHM)-induced neurological disease is modulated *in vivo* by monoclonal antibody, Virology 132: 261 (1984).

22. M. V. Haspel, P. W. Lampert, and M. B. A. Oldstone, Temperature sensitive mutants of mouse hepatitis virus produce a high incidence of demyelination, Proc. Natl. Acad. Sci. USA 75: 4033 (1978)

23. R. L. Knobler, M. Dubois-Dalcq, M. V. Haspel, A. P. Claysmith, P. W. Lampert, and M. B. A. Oldstone, Selective localization of wild type and mutant mouse hepatitis virus (JHM strain) antigens in CNS tissue by fluorescence, light and electron microscopy, J. Neuroimmunol. 1: 81 (1981)

24. H. Wege, M. Koga, R. Watanabe, K. Nagashima, and V. ter Meulen, Neurovirulence of murine coronavirus JHM temperature-sensitive mutants in rats, Infec. Immun. 39: 1316 (1983)

25. J. G. Woodward, G. Matsushima, J. A. Frelinger, and S. A. Stohlman, Production and characterization of T cell clones specific for mouse hepatitis virus, strain JHM: *In vivo* and *in vitro* analysis, J. Immunol. 133: 1016 (1984).

26. S. A. Stohlman, G. K. Matsushima, N. Castell, and L. P. Weiner, *In vivo* effects of coronavirus-specific T cell clones: DTH inducer cells prevent a lethal infection, but do not inhibit virus replication, J. Immunol. 136: 3052 (1986).

27. S. A. Stohlman, M. A. Sussman, G. K. Matsushima, R. A. Shubin andS. S. Erlich, Delayed-type hypersensitivity response in the central nervous system during JHM virus infection requires viral specificity for protection, J. Neuroimmunol. 19: 255 (1988)

28. S. S. Erlich, G. K. Matsushima, and S. A. Stohlman, Studies on the mechanism of protection from acute viral encephalomyelitis by delayed-type hypersensitivity inducer T cell clones, J. Neurol. Sci. 90: 203 (1989).
29. M. A. Sussman, R. A. Shubin, S. Kyuwa, and S. A. Stohlman, T-cell-mediated clearance of mouse hepatitis virus strain JHM from the central nervous system, J. Virol. 63: 3051 (1989).
30. O. Sorensen, A. Saravani, and S. Dales, *In vivo* and *in vitro* models of demyelinating disease, XXIII: Infection by JHM virus of athymic rats, in: "Coronaviruses. Advances in Experimental Medicine and Biology, Vol. 218," M. C. Lai, and S. A. Stohlman, eds., Plenum Publishing Corporation, New York, (1987).

QUANTITATION, PHENOTYPIC CHARACTERIZATION AND IN SITU LOCALIZATION
OF LYMPHOID CELLS IN THE BRAIN PARENCHYMA OF RATS WITH DIFFERING
SUSCEPTIBILITY TO CORONAVIRUS JHM-INDUCED ENCEPHALOMYELITIS

Rüdiger Dörries, Stefan Schwender, Horst Imrich, Harry
Harms und Volker ter Meulen

Institut für Virologie und Immunbiologie der Universität
Versbacher Str. 7, 8700 Würzburg, Fed. Rep. Germany

INTRODUCTION

Intracerebral infection of rats with Coronavirus JHM may cause multiple neurological syndromes ranging from acute lethal encephalitis to
subclinical demyelination[1,2]. The outcome of the infection is determined
by both the type of virus used for inoculation as well as the genetic
background of the host animal[1,2,3,4]. Data accumulated from different
inbred strains of rats suggest that important host factors which influence the course of the disease include the maturation of viral target
cells[5] and the state of immunocompetence of the animal[6,7]. Although
virus-specific immunity in the cerebrospinal fluid of affected animals
has been examined repeatedly in the past[8,9,10], little information has
been collected about the dynamics of immune reactions taking place in
the brain parenchyma. However, these local immunological events are
almost certainly decisive for the clinical course of the infection.
Therefore, we attempted to analyse the kinetics of the lymphoid cell
infiltration following intracerebral inoculation of two rat strains with
coronvirus JHM. In order to detect relationships between neurological
symptomatology and local immune reactions in the brain tissue we selected two inbred strains which are known to behave differently after intracerebral infection. Whereas Lewis rats often develop a subacute demyelinating encephalomyelitis accompanied by severe paralytic signs of
disease, Brown Norway (BN) rats reveal no signs whatsoever, although
small foci of nodular demyelination can be detected in periventricular
areas of the brain[2].

MATERIAL AND METHODS

Preparation of virus

The virus we have used throughout all experiments is a derivative
of that we obtained from H. Wege[11]. In our laboratory it was passaged
once through mouse brain followed by a passage through sac(-) cells.
This virus was designated JHM (HS).

Inoculation of animals

Rats of the inbred strains, Lewis and BN (3 weeks old), were inoculated intracerebrally with 1000 plaque forming units (PFU) of JHM (HS) per animal in 40 µl of cell free tissue culture supernatant. For control purposes rats were inoculated with tissue culture medium from non-infected sac(-) cells. Inoculated animals were checked daily for signs of neurological disease.

Preparation of lymphocytes from rat brain

Animals were killed and perfused with PBS. Before removing the brain, cerebrospinal fluid was sampled from the cisterna magna. The brain and the spinal cord were minced through a steel sieve. The disso-ciated material was collected by low speed centrifugation and subjected to enzymatic digestion with collagenase and DNAse. Subsequently leuko-cytes were separated according to their density by a Percoll-step gra-dient.

Identification of lymphocyte subsets

Leukocytes isolated from the brain were stained by direct and in-direct immunofluorescence and analysed by flow cyto-fluorgraphy (FACS). Monoclonal antibodies (mabs) used for staining were OX1 (specific for rat leukocyte common antigen [L-CA]), OX33 (specific for a high molecu-lar weight L-CA present on B-cells), OX8 (specific for the CD8 molecule on cytotoxic T-cells), W3/25 (specific for the CD4 molecule on helper T-cells) and R73 (specific for the alpha/beta chains of the T-cell anti-gen receptor [TCR]). OX1, OX33, OX8 and W3/25 are commercially available antibodies, R73 was a gift from T. Hünig (Max-Planck Institut, Martins-ried, FRG).

Determination of antibody secreting cells

JHM-specific antibody secreting cells were determined by enzyme-linked immunospot (ELISPOT) assay as described by Sedgwick and Holt[12]. Leukocytes isolated from brain and resuspended in RPMI medium were plated on recangular plastic wells which had been coated with JHM virus. During an overnight incubation, antibodies secreted by JHM-specific plasma cells attached to the viral antigen coated to the bottom of the plate. These antibodies were detected by enzyme-labeled secondary anti-bodies and incubation in a substrate which is converted by the enzyme to a visible coloured spot. Each spot was counted as a single antibody secreting cell.

Titration of JHM specific antibodies

Heat-inactivated CSF samples were diluted in MEM and aliquots of 50 µl were incubated with 100 $TCID_{50}$ of JHM virus for one hour in a microtiter plate. Subsequently DBT cells were added to the wells and after 4 days the cultures were examined for cytopathogenic effects (CPE) after staining the cell monolayer with May-Grünwald stain. The neutrali-zation titer was considered as the highest dilution of CSF protecting more than 50% of the cell monolayer from CPE.

In situ localization of lymphocyte subsets and viral antigens

Serial frozen sections (7-8 µm thick) were cut from the cerebellum of an infected Lewis rat 23 days post infection (dpi). Each section was stained with a different mab to detect viral antigens as well as lym-phocyte subsets in situ. The following antigens were stained in sub-sequent sections: (1) viral nucleocapsid (mab #556 [gift of H. Wege from this institute]), (2) cytotoxic (CD8+) T-cells (mab OX8), (3) helper (CD4+) T-cells (mab W3/25), (4) B-cells (mab HIS 14 [gift of F. G. M.

Kroese, University of Groningen, The Netherlands]) and (5) macrophages (mab ED1 [gift of Ch. D. Dijkstra, Vrije Universiteit Amsterdam, The Netherlands]). Alkaline phosphatase labeled secondary antibody was used to localize primary mabs and incubation of the sections with fast red substrate resulted in a bright red precipitate. Digital pictures of the stained sections were taken by a video camera mounted on a microscope. With the aid of a computer program the red color of the precipitates could be changed in the picture to any desired color. Subsequently all pictures were merged into a single picture on the computer screen, resulting in a multi-colored topographical map of the examined area in the brain.

RESULTS

Clinical course of the infection

   Intracerebral inoculation of Lewis rats with JHM (HS) caused, in over 90% of the animals, a subacute demyelinating encephalomyelitis. Clinical signs of paralytic disease began at day 6 and were most severe 12 dpi. Thereafter animals started to recover and after 28 dpi no signs of an apparent neurological disease remained. In contrast, none of the BN rats inoculated with the same amount of the identical virus developed visible neurological symptoms.

Kinetics of lymphocyte infiltration into the CNS

   The dynamics of leukocyte populations in the brain parenchyma was analysed by killing one animal each day after infection up to 4 weeks pi and staining of the isolated leukocyte fraction with different mabs. FACS analysis of the cells confirmed that, in average more than 50 % carried the rat L-CA. Examination of B-lymphocytes within this leukocyte population (staining with either mab OX33 or polyclonal anti-rat IgG) revealed the following pattern: In both rat strains there was a sharp increase of B cells shortly before the onset of clinical symptoms in Lewis rats, followed by a drop in the B-cell count and a second smaller peak at the time when Lewis rats recovered from disease. CD4+ T-cells detected by the mab W3/25 were abundant in the brain of both rat strains. In Lewis rats their numbers peaked two times, first, just prior to the onset of overt disease at the time when B-cells reached their first maximum and a second time when these rats recovered. The course of the CD4+ T-cell infiltration in BN rats paralleled the influx of these cells into the brain of Lewis rats, but their number was slightly lower than in the latter strain. Striking differences between the rat strains were detectable in the numbers of CD8+ T-cells isolated from the CNS. FACS analysis after double labeling the cells with mabs OX8 and R73 revealed much higher numbers of cytotoxic T cells (CD8+, TCR α/β+) in the Lewis rats compared to BN rats. It is interesting to note that, in both rat strains an initial increase of these cells in the brain was noticeable. However, in BN rats, numbers dropped rapidly in the following weeks whereas in Lewis rats a second peak appeared at the same time that B-cells and CD4+ T-cells peaked and animals were reconvalescent.

Characterization of the humoral immune response in the CNS

   Using the ELISPOT assay we determined the number of JHM-specific antibody secreting plasma cells present in the CNS at different times after infection. Almost no antibody secreting plasma cells could be detected in the Lewis rats at the time of the initial peak of B-lymphocytes. However, during recovery from disease the number of JHM-specific antibody secretors reached its maximum. This was seen exactly at the time when numbers of B- and helper T-cells reached their second peak. BN rats showed more and earlier antibody secreting cells than the Lewis rat, although during the first increase of B-lymphocytes in the brain their numbers were almost as low as in Lewis rats. Since the amount (or possibly the affinity) of antibody which was secreted by the individual plasma cell was higher in BN rats than in Lewis, it was very likely that this would be reflected in the titer of virus-specific antibodies in the cerebrospinal fluid of individual animals. Using a microneutralization assay we determined the JHM-specific neutralization titers in CSF specimens. Animals from both rat strains revealed very low neutralizing titers at 6 dpi. In Lewis rats the titers increased slowly up to 3 weeks pi and dropped thereafter to almost non-detectable levels. The highest titers were detected shortly after the number of JHM-specific antibody secreting plasma cells was at a maximum in the CNS. At this time the animals had recovered almost completely from neurological disease signs. In contrast, neutralizing titers in BN rats increased quickly within the second week and reached much higher levels than in the Lewis rats. Maximal titers were seen roughly 2 days after JHM-specific plasma cells reached their maximum in the parenchyma. Subsequently a drop was noticeable but the titers remained significantly higher than in Lewis rats.

Arrangement of infiltrating cells in a demyelinated area of the CNS.

To establish a picture of the interaction of infiltrating cells with virus-infected cells at the site of demyelination we stained viral antigens and infiltrating leukocytes by immunohistochemistry in serial sections of a frozen cerebellum taken from a Lewis rat 23 dpi. Computer-aided image analysis of individual sections enabled the development of a multi-colored, single picture showing the topographical distribution of leukocytes and viral antigens within a demyelinated plaque close to the brain stem. CD8+ T-cells were detected in close proximity to viral antigen at the border of the demyelinated area. Macrophages occupied the virus-free center and CD4+ T-cells as well as a few B-cells were scattered in the suroundings of this plaque in the presence of viral antigen. All leukocyte populations could be identified in the perivascular cuff of an adjacent blood vessel. Double immunofluorescence studies in the same part of the brain revealed that oligodendrocytes were the major target of the virus and infected cells expressed major histocompatibility (MHC) class I antigens at high density.

DISCUSSION

In this paper we have attempted to summarize our present knowledge about the immunological events taking place in the CNS of Lewis- and BN rats after intracerebral infection with coronavirus JHM. In agreement with earlier reports this infection caused a subacute encephalomyelitis accompanied by transient paralysis in Lewis rats, whereas BN rats remained clinically healthy[2]. However, we also noticed distinct differences to data published previously. The number of Lewis rats which recovered from paralytic disease increased from 30%[2] to over 90% in our rats. Consequently the incidence of fatal encephalitides was lower than 10% in our animals, compared to 60%[2] as has been reported earlier. Moreover, no variation in the incubation time of the virus was evident. All of the paralytic Lewis rats revealed first signs of neurological symptoms between 4 to 6 dpi, whereas the onset of the classical subacute demyelinating encephalomyelitis has been reported to vary between 14 days and 8 months[13,14]. These differences most likely reflect the high degree of genetic variance of JHM virus, which makes comparison of data between different laboratories difficult, unless the same batch of virus is used. In recent years it has become clear, that multiple passages of

JHM virus through tissue culture results in a considerable loss of neuropathogenicity. Therefore, we prepared large amounts of a virus batch which was passaged only once through tissue culture after replication in the brain of suckling mice and used this virus throughout all experiments. This might explain the high reproducibilty of disease induction in our Lewis rats, which was a prerequisite for the kinetic analysis of the immunological events in the brain of these animals.

In the CNS of Lewis- as well as BN rats the numbers of B-lymphocytes revealed 2 maxima. The first peak was observed 1 or 2 days before onset of neurological symptoms in Lewis rats and the second peak shortly before Lewis rats started to recover from their disease. Previous examinations in this laboratory have shown that the permeability of the the blood brain barrier (BBB) is increased in diseased Lewis rats[9]. This could facilitate the transfer of leukocytes from blood vessels into the brain parenchyma and B-Lymphocytes would contribute to this infiltration. After sensitization of those cells which carry virus-specific immunoglobulin on their surface, differentiation into antibody secreting cells (ASC) could occur in the presence of helper T-cells. Our finding, that the numbers of helper T-cells in the brain of both rat strains followed exactly the alterations seen in the B-lymphocyte subset, is supportive of this hypothesis. As a result of these events the majority of ASC should be detectable in the second peak of lymphocytes and indeed in both rat strains, the number of ASC increased from almost non detectable levels in the first peak up to several thousand in the second peak.

A few days later, titers of neutralizing antibodies reached their maxiumum in cerebrospinal fluid specimens. Although in Lewis rats, titers remained significantly lower than in BN rats, they may have contributed to the recovery from neurological symptoms, because improvement of the Lewis rats started immediately after neutralizing antibodies had reached a certain level. Consistent with this is our observation that animals which died from acute encephalitis were antibody negative. Low titers of these antibodies as seen early in infection of Lewis rats and a slow rise in the subsequent days allows distribution of infectious virus in the CNS for a considerable period of time. Therefore, Lewis rats suffer frequently from wide spread infection of the CNS including the grey matter of the spinal cord, which undoubtly contributes to the severe paralytic disease. In contrast, the early rise of high neutralizing titers as seen in BN rats, may limit the spread of infectious virus into the grey matter and thus will prevent severe neurological symptomatology. As shown by Watanabe and coworkers[2], histopathological changes in BN rats indeed are confined to very small areas in the white matter close to the ventricles. However, these animals seemed to be infected persistently, because viral antigens were demonstrated in the brain up to 60 dpi[2]. As we have described earlier, the continous expression of viral antigens in these animals allows the maintenance of a vigorous synthesis of JHM-specific antibody response with restricted heterogeneity[10]. These data are in good agreement with our present observation, that even 4 weeks pi JHM-specific antibody titers were significantly higher in BN rats than in Lewis rats.

The persistent infection of BN rats probably is caused by the low numbers of cytotoxic T-lymphocytes recruited into the brain in the course of the infection. This is in sharp contrast to the Lewis rats. After a first increase of cytotoxic T-cells their numbers reached a much higher second peak at the time when these rats recovered from their clinical disease. At this time we cannot present functional data on these cells, however, we have good reason to believe that they act by killing JHM-infected oligodendrocytes. Computer-aided image analysis of serial sections of Lewis brain during convalescence, detected cytotoxic T-cells in close proximity to virus-infected cells and double immunofluorescence studies in the same area of the brain identified oligodendrocytes as the major target cell for the virus. In addition infected cells did express high levels of MHC class I antigens which is necessary for sucessful recognition of infected cells by CD8+ cytotoxic T-lymphocytes. Although these data do not directly prove a cytotoxic activity of T-cells in these animals, we believe that in convalescent Lewis rats, killing of JHM infected oligodendroglia cells is an important immunological effector mechanism. As a consequence, virus would be eliminated from the brain finally leading to recovery from the infection. However, it remains to be determined if, and to what extent, killing of infected oligodendrocytes contributes to the neurological symptomatology in these animals.

In summary, intracerebral infection of Lewis- and BN rats is a useful model to study the role of the local immune response during coronavirus-induced demyelinating encephalomyelitides. Our data suggest that both compartments of the immune system, the antibody response as well as the action of cytotoxic T cells, are required for a sucessful recovery from neurological disease. Lack of virus-specific antibodies will cause wide spread infection of the brain which may result in a fatal outcome and low numbers of cytotoxic T-cells will prevent efficient elimination of the virus from the brain leading to a persistent infection. At present, experiments are under way to functionallycharacterize cytotoxic T-cells from the brain of Lewis and BN rats.

REFERENCES

1. O. Sorensen, D. Perry, and S. Dales, In vivo and in vitro models of demyelinating diseases. III. JHM virus infection of rats. Arch. Neurol. 37:478 (1980)
2. R. Watanabe, H. Wege, and V. ter Meulen, Comparative analysis of coronavirus JHM-induced demyelinating encephalomyelitis in Lewis and Brown Norway rats, Lab. Invest. 57:375 (1987)
3. H. Wege, J. Winter, P. Massa, R. Dörries, and V. ter Meulen, Coronavirus JHM induced demyelinating disease: Specific domains on the E2-protein are associated with neurovirolence, in: "Coronaviruses. Advances in Experimental Medicine and Biology, Vol. 218," M. C. Lai, and S. A. Stohlman, eds., Plenum Publishing Corporation, New York, (1987).
4. H. Wege, M. Koga, R. Watanabe, K. Nagashima, and V. ter Meulen, Neurovirulence of murine coronavirus JHM temperature-sensitive mutants in rats, Infec. Immun. 39:1316 (1983).
5. S. Beushausen, and S. Dales, In vivo and in vitro models of demyelinating diseases. XI. Tropism and differentiation regulate the infectious process of coronaviruses in primary explants of the rat CNS, Virology 141:89 (1985)
6. M. J. Zimmer, and S. Dales, In vivo and in vitro models of demyelinating diseases. XXIV. The infectious process in cyclosporin A treated Wistar Lewis rats inoculated with JHM virus, Microb. Pathogen. 6:7 (1989)
7. H. Wege, R. Watanabe, M. Koga and V. ter Meulen, Coronavirus JHM-induced demyelinating encephalomyelitis in rats: Influence of immunity on the course of disease, in: "Immunology of Nervous System Infections, Progress in Brain Research, Vol. 59," P. O. Behan, V. ter Meulen, and F. Clifford Rose, eds., Elsevier Science Publishers, New York, (1983).

8. O. Sorensen, M. B. Coulter-Mackie, S. Puchalski, and S. Dales, _In vivo_ and _in vitro_ models of demyelinating disease. IX. Progression of JHM virus infection in the central nervous system of the rat during overt and asymptomatic phases, _Virology_ 137:347 (1984).

9. R. Dörries, R. Watanabe, H. Wege, and V. ter Meulen, Murine Coronavirus induced encephalomyelitides in rats: Analysis of immunoglobulins and virus-specific antibodies in serum and cerebrospinal fluid, _J. Neuroimmunol._ 12:131 (1986).

10. R. Dörries, R. Watanabe, H.Wege, and V. ter Meulen, Analysis of the intrathecal humoral immune response in Brown Norway (BN) rats, infected with the murine Coronavirus JHM, _J. Neuroimmunol._ 14:305 (1987).

11. K. Nagashima, H. Wege, R. Meyermann, and V. ter Meulen, Coronavirus induced subacute demyelinating encephalomyelitis in rats. A morphological analysis, _Acta Neuropathol._ 44:63 (1978)

12. J. D. Sedgwick and P. G. Holt, A solid-phase immunoenzymatic technique for the enumeration of specific antibody-secreting cells, _J. Immunol. Meth._ 57:301 (1983).

13. K. Nagashima, H. Wege, R. Meyermann, and V. ter Meulen, Demyelination by a long-term corona virus infection in rats, _Acta Neuropath._ 45:205 (1979)

14. M. Koga, H. Wege, and V. ter Meulen, Sequence of murine coronavirus JHM induced neuropathological changes in rats, _Neuropathol. Appl. Neurobiol._ 10:173 (1984)

CORONAVIRUS INDUCED DEMYELINATING ENCEPHALOMYELITIS IN RATS:

IMMUNOPATHOLOGICAL ASPECTS OF VIRAL PERSISTENCY

Helmut Wege, Jörn Winter, Heiner Körner, Egbert Flory[1],
Fritz Zimprich and Hans Lassmann[2]

Institute for Virology and Immunbiology, University
of Würzburg, Würzburg, West Germany[1]
Institute for Neurology, University of Vienna
Austria[2]

INTRODUCTION

Lesions of primary demyelination are a characteristic neuro-pathological finding for several important neurological diseases of humans and animals. Such diseases can be caused by virus infections like measles, herpes or distemper. In multiple sclerosis, a disease with unknown etiology, a viral agent could be a trigger factor[23]. Coronavirus infections of rodents are studied as interesting experimental models to investigate mechanisms of virus induced demyelination[19].

Lewis rats infected with the murine coronavirus JHM develop different forms of encephalomyelitis[11,12,21]. The host and viral factors which influence the outcome of infection had been described by several previous studies[9,16,17,22]. We have shown, that Lewis rats develop besides an antiviral immune response autoimmune reactions mediated by CD4+ T-cells against myelin basic protein[18]. However, as results from adoptive transfer experiments indicate, this autoimmune cellular response alone does not cause demyeli-nation. We demonstrated previously that antiviral antibodies can be produced locally within the CNS and are detectable within the cerebrospinal fluid of infected Lewis rats[3]. Results from experiments in other virus-host systems such as measles suggested, that the humoral immune response may not lead to the elimination of the virus, but result in an impaired expression of viral glycoproteins at least on the cell surface and promote the establishment of a persistent infection (immune modulation)[5]. Such events may be important for persistent virus infections of the central nervous system, because this compartment is relatively shielded from the peripheral immune system. On the other hand, later in the course of infection an immune response against virus may contribute to demyelination. We present here some evidence which suggest that the antiviral humoral immune response could play a pathogenetic role for primary demyelination and virus persistency after long incubation times.

Coronaviruses and Their Diseases
Edited by D. Cavanagh and T.D.K. Brown
Plenum Press. New York. 1990

637

RESULTS

Antiviral antibodies and virus infection in glia cell cultures

Primary glial cell cultures were established from brains of newborn Lewis rats[8,9]. The cultures consisted mainly of astrocytes, microglia and oligodentrocytes (e.g. 11 days post plating 48%, 24% and 12%). The cytopathogenicity of different JHM-virus variants is variable[9]. With the JHM-wt virus used in this study, infection leads to the destruction of the culture due to the formation of syncytia. Infectious virus is continuopusly released to the medium (Fig. 1 c). Only 6-10 % of the cells display viral antigen (Fig. 1 a). No significant difference was found in the number of cells positive for nucleocapsid and expressing spike protein on the cell surface. However, the outcome of infection was significantly changed if a mixture of monoclonal antibodies against S-protein was added five days post infection[20]. No visible cytopathology occured and no infectious virus was released to the medium after several days of treatment Fig. 1 d).The number of cells containing N-protein was higher than in untreated cultures. By contrast, relative to N-protein a significantly smaller number of cells displayed S-protein on the cell surface. The S- antigen appeared in a clustered and more polar distribution on the cell surface than in untreated cultures. Such cultures were passaged further in presence of anti- S antibodies. The passaged cultures consist predominantly of astrocytes. Infectious virus was reisolatable in form of a small plaque variant up to 60 days p.i., if the antibody treatment was terminated.

In similar experiments, the infected glia cultures were treated with single anti-S MAb's against defined epitopes. Most interesting was the observation, that some antibodies which do not neutralise infectious virus and are also not impairing cell fusion, suppress the release of infectious virus and promote the establishment of a chronic infection. These results are a first hint, that the antiviral humoral immune response could lead to immunomodulation and support the establishment of a chronic infection in brain tissue.

Neuropathological characterisation of different disease types

For the following study Lewis rats (4-6 weeks old) were infected by the intracerebral route with JHM virus passage designated MP2 SD. Animals at different stages of disease were bleeded after anesthesia and killed by perfusion with cold buffered formaldehyde. The tissue specimens were embedded in paraffin and processed for immunehistology[6]. Serial sections were stained for myelin, axons, different brain cell types, macrophages, T- and B cells, immuneglobulin, complement factor C9 and viral proteins. The disease types described in the following were strictly defined by neuropathological criteria.

Many rats developed an acute encephalomyelitis (**AE**) within 2 weeks p.i.and died rapidly. About 20-30 % of the rats appear to be healthy for several weeks, before neurological signs (ataxic gait, paresis, paralysis) occured. Animals which developed a late onset disease could be classified as either chronic panencephalomyelitis (**CPE**) or subacute demyelinating encephalomyelitis (**SDE**). In CPE,

lesions are localised in grey and white matter (Fig. 2). The
lesions are very necrotic, both neurons and glial cell harbor
virus antigen. In typical SDE animals however the lesions are
localised only in the white matter. Typical lesions of primary
demyelination are characterised by preservation of axons and
sparing of neurons (Fig. 2).

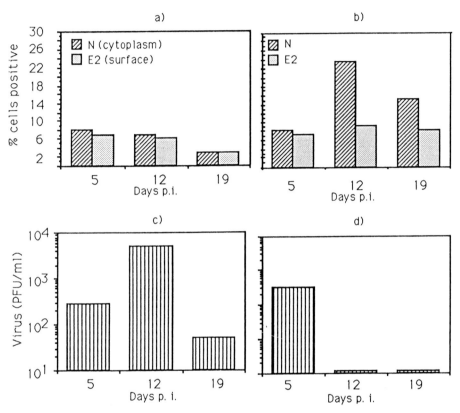

Fig. 1 Influence of anti- S Mab's on JHM infected glia cell
cultures. The infected cultures were maintained in parallel with
or without anti- S MAb's. At 5, 12 and 19 days p.i. the amount of
infectious virus was determined by plaque tests on L-cells. The
number of cells containing nucleocapsid protein was counted after
immunostaining with an anti- N MAb. Cells displaying spike protein
on the surface were quantitated with a mixture of anti- S MAb's.
Monolayers were disintegrated by trypsinisation and the cells
fixed on adhesion-slides. a) Amount of cells containing N protein
in the cytoplasm and S protein on the cell surface in JHM
infected cultures maintained without Anti- S MAb's. b) Amount of
virus proteins in cultures maintained in presence of anti- S
MAb's. c) Infectious virus released from cultures maintained
without anti- S MAb's (a). d) Infectious virus released from
cultures maintained with anti- S MAb's (b).

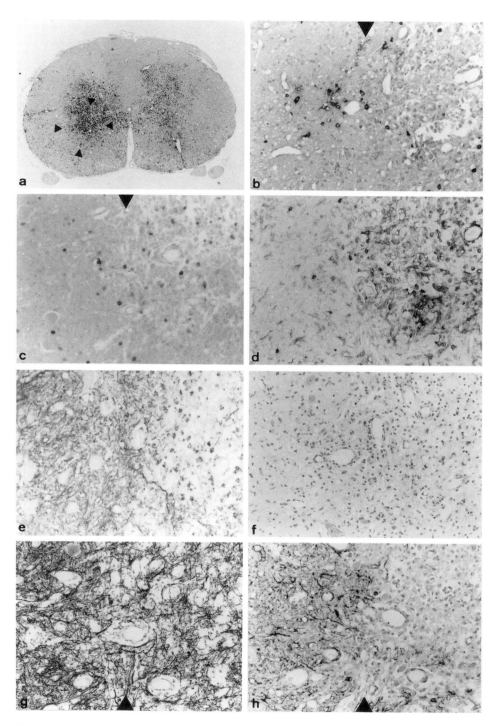

<u>Fig. 2</u> Chronic Panencephalitis (CPE). Rat with clinical signs 50 days p.i., dissection 2 days later. **a)** Symmetrical macrophage infiltrations in grey and white matter. Arrows show positions of pictures b-h (serial sections). ED 1, 23x **b)** Many viral antigen positive cells surround necrotic lesion. Rabbit anti JHM serum. 140x **c)** Pronounced T-cell infiltration. W3/13. 140x **d)** Ia antigen

on macrophages and dendritic (microglial) cells in the
surrounding.Ox6. 140x **e)** Demyelination, degraded myelin in
macrophages. Anti-MBP MAb. 140x **f)** Perivascular infiltration.
Hematoxilin-eosin, 140x **g)** Reduced axonal density, loss of nerve
cells. Bielschovsky silver impregnation. 140x **h)** Loss of
astrocytes, gliosis in surrounding tissue. GFAP. 140x

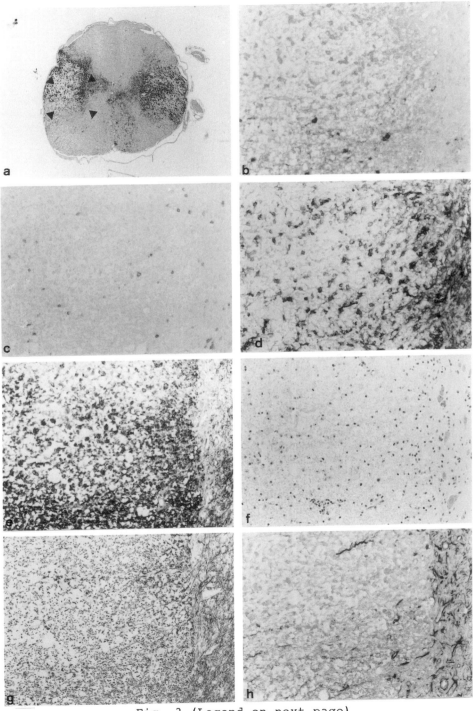

Fig. 3 (Legend on next page)

Type and quantitative composition of inflammatory infiltrates

Quantitative evaluations including statistical analysis were performed by counting cells positive for the marker in question from several lesions and from at least six animals for each disease type In all cases, macrophages and T-cells dominate within the lesion. About 3.5-5 times more macrophages were counted than T-cells (about 500 cells/mm^2). With regard to macrophages and T-cells, no essential differences were found between CPE and SDE. By contrast, in SDE 3x more plasma cells (about 55 cells/mm^2) were counted than in CPE. Moreover, a pronounced immuneglobulins staining was a typical finding for SDE- lesions. In addition to that, within the lesions complement factor C9 was detectable by immunehistology.

Distribution of viral nucleocapsid and spike protein in vivo

In parallel to the quantitative evaluation of cellular infiltrates, the number of cells positive for virus proteins and viral RNA were determined by immune histology and in situ hybridisation. Independent of the stage and kind of disease, identical numbers cells were found positive for either viral antigen or RNA. The amount of cells containing nucleocapsid and spike protein was quantitiated by immunostaining with monoclonal antibodies. Between AE and CPE, no essential difference was found between the relative proportions of cells positive for nucleocapsid and spike protein. If the number of cells positive for N-protein is set to 100%, about 45-60% of cells are positive for S-protein.Such a difference has to be expected, because the amount of N-protein exceeds that of S-protein. An interesting shift in the relative proportions was found for SDE. In these animals, the proportion of cells positive for S-protein was only 15-25 % of the values obtained for N-protein.

SUMMARY AND DISCUSSION

It was shown, that antibodies against the spike protein promoted the establishment of a chronic infection in primary glial cultures. By neuropathological criteria, three different types of disease were defined (AE, CPE and SDE). The relative amount of viral nucleocapsid and spike protein was quantitated in different types of demyelinating lesions. In rats, where primary demyelination was restricted to the white matter (SDE), a

---

Fig. 3 Subacute Demyelinating Encephalomyelitis (SDE). The rat was dissected 96 days p.i., 11 days after onset of disease. a) Symmetrical macrophage infiltration in the lateral white matter. Arrows show positions of pictures b-h (serial sections) ED1, 23x b) Viral antigen in the surrounding white matter. Rabbit- anti JHM serum, 140x c) Distinct T-cell infiltration in and around the lesion. W3/13. 140x d) Ia expression in regions of ongoing demyelination, rim of the lesion. Ox6. 140x e) Complete loss of myelin, degradation products in macrophages. Anti-MBP MAb, 140x f) Perivascular cuffing, cellular infiltration, small edema. Hematoxilin-eosin, 140x g) Axons within the lesion are well preserved. Bielschovsky silver impregnation, 140x h) Loss of astrocytes in the lesion, surrounded by marked gliosis. GFAP. 140x

significantly lower amount of cells was found to contain spike protein than nucleocapsid. Furthermore, in SDE lesions a higher amount of plasma cells than in AE and CPE was counted. Within demyelinated areas, immunoglobulins and the complement component C9 were detected in addition to intensive infiltrates of macrophages and T-cells.

Several observations indicate, that virus persistency could be promoted by the immune response, if infectious virus is not eliminated during the acute phase of disease. Treatment of JHM virus infected mice with monoclonal antibodies against S-protein modulated the disease from an acute fatal infection to a disease with more pronounced demyelination[1]. Furthermore, mice wich were infected in presence of maternal antibodies against JHM virus developed a late onset demyelinating disease[13]. At the present stage not much is known on the molecular mechanisms of coronavirus persistency in the brain tissue. By combining in situ hybridisation and immune histology, we could not obtain evidence for the existence of cells containing only viral RNA without expression of viral structural proteins. For measles virus, immune modulation results not only in a reduced surface expression of viral glycoproteins but also in a reduced transcription and translation rate of viral proteins[5]. Due to the coronavirus gene organisation (positive strandedness, nested set structure) a detailed analysis on presence of genome, expression of various mRNA species and viral proteins in brain tissue was not yet possible. It is conceivable, that the interaction between antibody induced modulation of S-protein expression on the cell surface and selection for variants with antigenic changes of the S-protein interact during establishment of persistency. It is known, that variants which escape neutralisation are less neurovirulent and reveal molecular changes of the S-protein[2,4,22]. In addition, the role of antibodies against other viral structural proteins (M, N and HE) should be further evaluated by in vivo. Furthermore, independently of immunity a selective replication of variants occurs in rat neural cells during the acute stage of infection[10,16].

The predominant mechanism of demyelination may differ depending on the virus-host system and time cinetics in individual animals. In acute disease the cytolytic destruction of oligodendroglia by virus infection, activated macrophages and the T-cell response may be the major mechanism (see Dörries et al., this vol.). Our data suggest that in SDE antibody mediated cytotoxicity against infected cells could lead to virus induced primary demyelination. This does not disclose the possibility, that a combination of a cellular autoimmune response and antiviral immunity lead to demyelination. It had been shown, that in chronic relapsing allergic encephalomyelitis the intensity and type of demyelination can be influenced by the combination of encephalitogenic T-cells and demyelinating antibodies[6]. The pathogenesis of SDE may start with an early phase of sensitation against virus- and neuroantigens during the acute phase. Besides antigen presentation by perivascular macrophages and microglia, astrocytes could provide an additional amplification loop for activation of T-cells[7,10] (see Mößner et al., this vol.). The early cellular immune response could help to survive the acute stage of disease without complete virus clearance[14] (Dörries et al. this vol.). During the incubation time, a smoldering chronic infection may be favoured by the local humoral immune response. As a consequence of a disturbance of the blood- brain barrier or if viral variants emerge, a SDE or CPE with pronounced inflammatory

demyelination and clinical symptoms could be incuced. The
neuropathological differences between CPE and SPE may be related
to the specific cellular tropism of variant viruses for neuronal
cells.

ACKNOWLEDGEMENTS

    We thank Hanna Wege for excellent technical assistance. The
work was supported by the Deutsche Forschungsgemeinschaft and
Hertie Stiftung.

REFERENCES

1. Buchmeier, M.J., Lewicki, H.A., Talbot, P.J., Knobler, R.L.
    Murine hepatitis virus-4 (strain JHM)-induced neurologic
    disease is modulated in vivo by monoclonal antibody. Virol.
    132, 261-270 (1984).
2. Dalziel, R.G., Lampert, P.W., Talbot, P.J., Buchmeier, M.J.
    Site-Specific alteration of murine hepatitis virus type 4
    peplomer glycoprotein E2 results in reduced neurovirulence. J.
    Virol. 59, 463-471 (1986).
3. Dörries, R., Watanabe, R., Wege, H., ter Meulen, V. Murine
    coronavirus induced encephalomyelitides in rats: Analysis of
    immunoglobulins and virus-specific antibodies in serum and
    cerebrospinal fluid. J. Neuroimmunol. 12, 131-142 (1986).
4. Fleming, J.O., Trousdale, M.D., Bradbury, J., Stohlman, S.A.,
    Weiner, L.P. Experimental demyelination induced by coronavirus
    JHM (MHV-4): Molecular identification of a viral determinant of
    paralytic disease. Microbial Pathogenesis 3, 9-20 (1987).
5. Fujinami, R.S, Oldstone, M.B.A. Antibody initiates virus
    persistence: Immune modulation and measles virus infection. In:
    Notkins, A.L. and Oldstone, M.B.A. (ed). Concepts in viral
    path. Springer Verlag 1986
6. Lassmann, H., Brunner, C., Bradl, M., Linington, C.
    Experimental allergic encephalomyelitis: the balance between
    encephalitogenic T lymphocytes and demyelinating antibodies
    determines size and structure of demyelinated lesions. Acta
    Neuropathol.(Berl.) 75, 566-576 (1988)
7. Massa, P.T., Dörries, R., ter Meulen, V. Viral Particles induce
    Ia Antigen Expression on Astrocytes. Nature 320, 543-546
    (1986).
8. Massa, P.T., Wege, H., ter Meulen, V. Analysis of murine
    hepatitis virus (JHM strain) tropism toward Lewis rat glial
    cells in vitro: type I astrocytes and brain macrophages
    (microglia) are the primary glial cell targets. 55, 318-327
    (1986).
9. Massa, P.T., Wege, H., ter Meulen, V. Growth pattern of various
    JHM coronavirus isolates in primary rat glial cell cultures
    correlates with differing neurotropism in vivo. Virus Res. 9,
    133-144 (1988).
10. Morris, V.L., Tieszer, C., Mackinnon, J., Percy, D.
    Characterization of coronavirus JHM variants isolated from
    Wistar Furth rats with a viral-induced demyelinating disease.
    Virology 169, 127-136 (1989)
11. Nagashima, K., Wege, H., Meyermann, R., ter Meulen, V.
    Coronavirus induced subacute demyelinating encephalomyelitis in
    rats. A morphological analysis. Acta Neuropath. 44, 63-70
    (1978).

12. Nagashima, K., Wege, H., Meyermann, R., ter Meulen, V. Demyelinating encephalomyelitis induced by a long-term corona virus infection in rats. Acta Neuropath. 45, 205-213 (1979).

13. Perlman, S., Schelper, R., Bolger, E., Ries, S. Late onset, symptomatic, demyelinating encephalomyelitis in mice infected with MHV-JHM in the presence of maternal antibody. Microbial Pathogen. 2, 185-194 (1987).

14. Stohlman, S.A., Matsushima, G.K., Casteel, N., Weiner, L.P. In vivo effects of coronavirus-specific T cell clones: DTH inducer cells prevent a lethal infection but do not inhibit virus replication. J. Immunol. 136, 8, 3052-3056 (1986).

15. Suzumura, A., Lavi, E., Weiss, S.R., Silberberg, D.H. Coronavirus infection induces H-2 antigen expression on oligodendrocytes and astrocytes. Science 232, 991-993 (1986).

16. Taguchi, F., Siddell, S.G., Wege, H., ter Meulen, V. Characterization of a variant virus selected in rat brain after infection by murine coronavirus MHV-JHM. J. Virol. 54, 429-435 (1985).

17. Watanabe, R., Wege, H., ter Meulen, V. Comparative analysis of coronavirus JHM induced demyelinating encephalomyelitis in Lewis and Brown-Norway rats. Lab. Invest. 57, 375-384 (1987).

18. Watanabe, R., Wege, H., ter Meulen, V. Adoptive transfer of EAE-like lesions by BMP stimulated lymphocytes from rats with coronavirus-induced demyelinating encephalomyelitis. Nature 305, 150-153 (1983).

19. Wege, H., Dörries, R., Massa, P., Watanabe, R. Autoimmunity and immune pathological aspects of virus disease. In:"Perspectives on autoimmunity" I.R. Cohen (ed.). CRC Press, Inc. Boca Raton, Florida (1988).

20. Wege, H., Dörries, R., Wege, H. Hybridoma antibodies to the murine coronavirus JHM: Characterisation of Epitopes on the Peplomer protein (E2). J. gen. Virol. 65, 1931-1942 (1984).

21. Wege, H., Watanabe, R., ter Meulen, V. Relapsing subacute demyelinating encephalomyelitis in rats in the course of coronavirus JHM infection. J. Neuroimmunol. 6, 325-336 (1984).

22. Wege, H., Winter, J., Meyermann, R. the Peplomer protein E2 of coronavirus JHM as a determinant of neurovirulence: Definition of critical epitopes by variant-analysis. J. gen. Virol. 69, 87-98 (1988).

23. Wisniewski, H.M., Schuller-Levis, G.B., Mehta, P.D., Madrid,.E., Lassmann, H. Pathogenetic aspects of multiple sclerosis and experimental models of inflammatory demyelination. Concepts Immunopathol. 2, 128-150 (1985).

ASTROCYTES AS ANTIGEN PRESENTING CELLS FOR PRIMARY AND SECONDARY
T CELL RESPONSES: EFFECT OF ASTROCYTE INFECTION BY MURINE
HEPATITIS VIRUS

Rainald Mößner, Jonathon Sedgwick*, Egbert Flory,
Heiner Körner, Helmut Wege and Volker ter Meulen

Institute for Virology and Immunobiology, University
of Würzburg, Würzburg, West Germany
*Correspondence

ABSTRACT

CD4$^+$ T cell lines specific for murine hepatitis virus (MHV)-
JHM or myelin basic protein (MBP) proliferated when cultured
together with MHC class I and II positive syngeneic rat
astrocytes and either inactivated virus or MBP as antigen. The
magnitude of the T cell proliferative response was comparable to
that seen when thymocytes were used as a source of antigen presenting cells (APC).

In contrast, MHC class I and II positive astrocytes were unable to significantly stimulate the proliferation of highly
purified populations of naive CD4$^+$ and CD8$^+$ T cells in an allogeneic mixed lymphocyte reaction (MLR). Both T cell populations
proliferated when mixed with allogeneic lymph node cells.
Infection of the astrocytes with a variant of MHV-JHM (PI-AS22D)
did not alter this cells incapacity to stimulate the naive CD4$^+$
and CD8$^+$ T cells to proliferate.

INTRODUCTION

Intracerebral (i.c.) inoculation of young adult rats with
the coronavirus, MHV-JHM, can induce either an acute, fatal
encephalitis or a delayed-onset subacute demyelinating
encephalomyelitis[1]. Susceptibility is rat strain dependent and
may potentially be influenced at many levels including
differences in the anti-viral immune response seen in different
rat strains[1-3] or the capacity of virus to stimulate MHC
expression on glial cells in susceptible strains[4], which may
initiate or perpetuate an encephalomyelitis. With regard to the
latter possibility, it is now well established that astrocytes
may act as APC for secondary T cell responses (i.e. in the
restimulation of T cell lines and clones). However, if astrocytes
were to participate in the initiation of a T cell response and
subsequent induction of encephalitis, for example following viral
infection <u>in vivo</u>, then these cells should, in principle, be
effective stimulators of a primary immune response.

Coronaviruses and Their Diseases
Edited by D. Cavanagh and T.D.K. Brown
Plenum Press, New York, 1990

However, relatively few cell types appear capable of acting as primary APC at least for CD4[+] T cell responses, the most potent of these being the dendritic cell[5] but such cells are not normally found in the central nervous system (CNS).

In these experiments we assessed the capacity of astrocytes to act as APC in primary and secondary T cell responses and present preliminary data from experiments which examined whether virus infection may have any effect on astrocyte function in this context.

METHODS

Primary Astrocyte Cultures

Primary astrocyte cultures from newborn Brown Norway (BN, RT1[n]) or Lewis (Lew, RT1[l]) rats were prepared essentially as described previously[6] and maintained in 50ml or 260 ml tissue culture flasks (Falcon). The cells were characterized using a range of monoclonal antibodies (MAbs) and a combination of immunoflourescence microscopy and flow cyto-fluorography (FACScan). MAbs used were mGalC (labels galactocerebroside, an oligodendrocyte marker)[7], MRC OX1 and MRC OX30 (both label the leucocyte common antigen (L-CA), found on cells of bone marrow origin), MRC OX42, a putative marker for microglia, MRC OX18 (anti-rat MHC Class I), and MRC OX6 (anti-rat MHC Class II). Glial fibrillary acidic protein (GFAP) was detected using a rabbit polyclonal antibody (DAKO). See refs. 8,9 for cross reference details of MAbs used.

Virus Preparation

MHV-JHM was adapted to a persistent infection of Sac(-) cells to generate JHM-PI[10]. This virus stock was then subjected to one passage on a rat mixed glial culture and two passages over purified rat astrocyte cultures then expanded by one passage over DBT cells. The resultant virus is designated JHM-PIAS22D.

Virus Infection and interferon gamma (IFN γ) pre-treatment

Astrocyte cultures were inoculated with virus at an MOI of approximately 1, for 1 hour at 37°C. Excess virus was then removed by washing and replaced by normal growth media. The level of infection 2-3 days later was determined by immunoflourescence microscopy using the mouse MAb #556 (anti-Nucleocapsid (60K) protein)[11].
For IFN γ treatment, astrocytes were pulsed daily for 3 days with a final concentration of 20 U/ml rat recombinant IFN γ.

T Cell Isolation

T cell lines. Standard procedures[12] were used to produce stable CD4[+] T cell lines specific for either MBP (designated 266/87B) or MHV-JHM (designated 146/88A). The MBP line was from a Lew rat inoculated s.c. with MBP in FCA while the virus-specific line was derived from an i.c. infected Lew rat.

Purification of T cell subsets. Pooled cervical and mesenteric lymph nodes from naive Lewis rats were depleted of various subpopulations by incubating the cells with the appropriate cocktail of monoclonal antibodies followed by a rosetting procedure using sheep erythrocytes coated with rabbit-anti-mouse Ig and the labelled cell population removed by a brief centrifugation step[13]. CD4+ T cells were depleted of all other cells expressing CD8 (MRC OX8), MHC Class II (MRC OX6) and surface Ig (B cells; MRC OX12). CD8+ T cells were depleted of cells expressing CD4 (MRC OX35 and W3/25), MHC class II and surface Ig and subjected to a second purification step using magnetic beads[14]. See refs. (8,9,15) for cross reference details of monoclonal antibodies used.

RESULTS

Astrocyte Characterization

Normal (untreated) astrocytes were 90-95 % pure as determined by staining for GFAP. Few cells were positive for the leukocyte common antigen (L-CA) found on cells of bone marrow origin and we could not detect cells positive either for the MAb MRC OX42, a putative marker for microglia or GalC an oligodendrocyte marker.

Most cells (> 95%) were MHC Class I positive, but only expressed MHC Class II after treatment with IFN γ. Significant expression of MHC Class II was seen on about 40 % of Lew and about 20 % of BN astrocytes. IFN γ also upregulated the expression of MHC Class I. The majority of cells were infected after 3 days as indicated by the presence of intracellular Nucleocapsid protein. Infection with this particular variant did not induce MHC Class II and inconsistently upregulated the expression of MHC Class I.

Astrocytes as APC for Secondary T Cell Responses.

Resting CD4+ T cell lines were cultured together with either syngeneic thymocytes or astrocytes plus or minus specific antigen (Fig. 1). Addition of thymocytes, the usual source of APC for rat T cell lines, resulted in a high specific proliferation of both T cell lines. IFN γ pre-treated astrocytes induced a comparable degree of T cell line proliferation while addition of normal (not IFN γ treated) astrocytes also resulted in specific T cell proliferation but the magnitude was less, at least at the time point shown here.

Astrocytes as Stimulators of Primary T Cell Responses

The MLR was employed to examine the capacity of astrocytes to stimulate primary T cell responses. Responding cells were CD4+ and CD8+ T cells isolated from the lymph nodes of naive Lew rats. Purities of around 99 % (as assessed by FACScan analysis) were obtained in all experiments.

Varying numbers of these cells were mixed with a constant number of stimulator cells which were either irradiated lymph node cells from Lew or BN rats (Fig. 2, A and B) or astrocytes from these two rat strains (Fig. 2, C and D).

When mixed with lymph node stimulators, both the CD4+ and CD8+ T cells responded to the allogeneic stimulus (BN). The proliferative response of CD4+ T cells was about twenty times greater than the CD8+ T cell response. Addition of the anti-CD4 MAb, W3/25, significantly blocked only the CD4+ T cell response (Fig. 2, A and B).
Astrocytes were also tested for their ability to stimulate CD4+ and CD8+ T cells in the MLR. Astrocytes were either untreated, pre-treated with IFNγ or inoculated with JHM-PI-AS22D for 1 hour prior to addition of responder T cells (Fig. 2, C and D). In all cases, the curves were relatively flat indicating that a dose dependent uptake of ^{3}H-thymidine by the responder T cells had not occurred. Astrocytes were not irradiated in these experiments (see Discussion) and some proliferation by these cells may account for the background counts recorded.

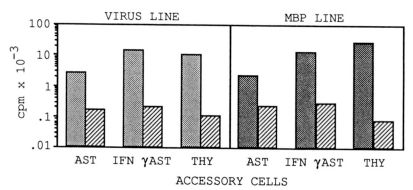

Fig 1. Astrocytes are good accessory cells for secondary T cell responses. 2×10^4 resting cells of each T cell line were cultured in the presence of irradiated (2000 R γ) syngeneic accessory cells together with specific antigen (shaded bars; 10µg/ml UV inactivated JHMV or 20µg/ml MBP) or no antigen (hatched bars). Accessory cells were 2×10^4 normal (AST) or IFN pre-treated astrocytes (IFN γ AST) or 10^6 thymocytes. Assay time was 48 hours inclusive of an 18 hour pulse with 3H-Thymidine. Shown are means of triplicate cultures.

DISCUSSION

The data presented here confirm that astrocytes may function as accessory cells for secondary T lymphocyte responses and, in these experiments, were shown to induce proliferation of T cell lines specific for both viral and self (MBP) antigens as effectively as thymocyte APC. Prior induction of MHC class II on these astrocytes by IFN γ pre-treatment enhanced their capacity to stimulate these CD4+ T cell lines above that seen when untreated astrocytes were used. The observation made here and elsewhere[16]

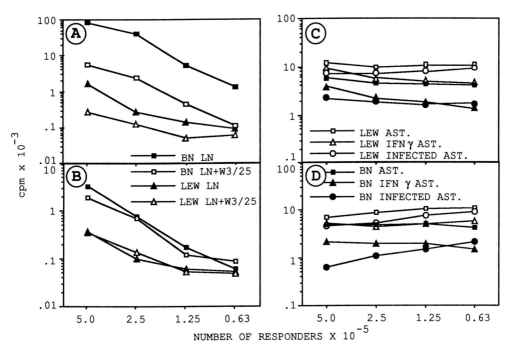

Fig. 2. Comparison of Astrocytes (AST) and lymph node (LN) cells as stimulators of the primary MLR. Responder cells were purified CD4 (A and C) and CD8 (B and D) positive T cells from Lew rats at the indicated number per well. Stimulators were either irradiated LN cells (5×10^5 per well) or non-irradiated AST (2×10^4 per well) which were untreated, IFN γ pre-treated, or infected with JHM-PI-AS22D. 5μg/ml W3/25 MAb (anti-rat CD4) was added to some of the wells. Assay time was 78 hours inclusive of an 18 hour 3H-Thymidine pulse.

that non-IFN γ pre-treated, ostensibly MHC Class II- negative astrocyte may also act as APC for T cell lines (Fig. 1) probably indicates that low-level induction of MHC Class II on the astrocytes occurs as a consequence of some IFN γ release (and possibly other cytokines) from the added T cells resulting in further T cell stimulation as the level of MHC class II on the astrocytes increases during culture.

Irradiated lymph node cells were effective stimulators of the primary allogeneic MLR. Both Lew CD4+ and CD8+ T cells proliferated in response to stimulation by BN lymph node cells although the level of CD8+ T cell proliferation was low. The magnitude of CD8+ T cell proliferation in the MLR is generally much lower than the CD4+ T cell response[17] and appears to be dependent on the responder strain used[18]. Anti-CD4 MAb did not block the proliferation of the CD8+ T cell population demonstrating that the response was indeed due to autonomous CD8+ T cell proliferation.

In preliminary experiments we attempted to infect astrocytes for two to three days prior to irradiation and establishment of the MLR but this resulted in rapid, presumably virus-mediated, destruction of the astrocytes during the 3 day course of the MLR. Thus, infection of non-irradiated astrocytes just prior to establishment of the MLR was necessary and, without irradiation, some uptake of tritiated thymidine occurred as evidenced by the high background counts.

When naive Lew CD4+ and CD8+ T cells were added to these non-irradiated syngeneic or allogeneic astrocytes there was no apparent responder cell proliferation above the 2000-10,000 cpm background contributed by the astrocytes themselves (Fig. 2C and D). Thus, one may conclude that allogeneic astrocytes whether untreated (i.e. expressing only MHC Class I), IFN γ pretreated (expressing increased levels of MHC Class I and also MHC Class II) or virus infected, do not stimulate naive T cells to proliferate.

Certainly this is clear for the CD4+ T cell response, which when positive, is normally at least 1 log above background, but the low magnitude of the CD8 T cell response (Fig. 2, B) means that a positive response to astrocyte stimulators may be disguised by the high background and experiments are underway to remedy this problem. It is unclear why the allogeneic (BN) astrocyte stimulators always incorporated less label than the Lew astrocytes and it could simply be related to a slightly different proliferative potential of the astrocytes from these two strains. A second possibility is that the growth of BN astrocytes was affected by the presence of the LEW T cells (i.e. that cytotoxic T cells were generated) and that this occurred in the absence of significant T cell proliferation.

Infection of astrocytes by this coronavirus did not alter the cells incapacity to stimulate T cells in the MLR. We considered it possible that such infection may enhance the stimulator capacity of astrocytes as, for example, astrocytes infected with this virus secrete IL-6 (data not shown) which appears to be an important co-factor in the induction of T cell responses following mitogenic or allogeneic stimulus[19,20]. However, no induction of MHC Class II occurred with this virus variant as it appears to do with others[4] so a CD4[+] T cell response was unlikely but also, no CD8[+] T cell proliferation was observed and certainly the astrocytes were highly MHC Class I positive. The limitations to the detection of CD8[+] T cell proliferation discussed above must be considered, but clearly, CD8[+] T cell proliferation was not very significant (if it in fact occurred at all) and virus infection of the astrocytes did not change this.

The principle conclusion to be drawn from these studies is that astrocytes are probably not functional stimulators of primary immune responses. Certainly, this is the case for CD4[+] T cell responses but it is less clear for CD8[+] T cells. Furthermore, infection of astrocytes by a virus which has the potential to induce the cell to secrete factors important in the initiation of T cell responses does not seem to change this situation. Other coronavirus-JHM isolates (or indeed other viruses) may be different in this regard.

In contrast, the same astrocytes are potent presenting cells for secondary T cell responses so we would envisage that once a T cell response is initiated peripherally (to self or viral antigen), astrocytes may then, if a pre-activated T cell is encountered in the CNS, re-stimulate the cell. Thus, astrocytes may play only a secondary role in enhancing or perpetuating, rather than initiating, immunopathological responses in the CNS.

ACKNOWLEDGEMENTS

We would like to thank Hanna Wege and Hanne Weinand for excellent technical assistance and Helga Kriesinger for typing the manuscript. This study was supported by Deutsche Forschungs-gemeinschaft and the Herti Foundation.

REFERENCES

1. R. Watanabe, H. Wege, and V. ter Meulen, Comparative analysis of coronavirus JHM-induced demyelinating encephalomyelitis in Lewis and Brown Norway rats, Lab. Invest. 57:375 (1987).
2. R. Dörries, R. Watanabe, H. Wege, and V. ter Meulen, Murine coronavirus-induced encephalomyelitides in rats: Analysis of immunoglobulins and virus-specific antibodies in serum and cerebrospinal fluid, J. Neuroimmunol. 12:131 (1986).
3. R. Dörries, R. Watanabe, H. Wege, and V. ter Meulen, Analysis of intrathecal humoral immune response in Brown Norway (BN) rats, infected with the murine coronavirus JHM, J.Neuroimmunol. 14:305 (1987).
4. P.T. Massa, R. Brinkmann, and V. ter Meulen, Inducibility of Ia antigen on astrocytes by murine coronavirus JHM is rat strain dependent, J. Exp. Med. 166:259 (1987)
5. R.M. Steinman, B. Gutchinov, M.D. Witmer, and N.C. Nussenzweig, Dendritic cells are the principal stimulators of the primary mixed leukocyte reaction in mice, J. Exp. Med. 157:613 (1983).

6. P.T. Massa, V. ter Meulen, and A. Fontana, Hyperinducibility of Ia antigen on astrocytes correlates with strain-specific susceptibility to experimental autoimmune encephalomyelitis, Proc. Natl. Acad. Sci. USA. 84:4219 (1987).

7. B. Ranscht, P.A. Clapshaw, J. Price, M. Noble, and W. Seifert, Development of oligodendrocytes and Schwann cells studied with a monoclonal antibody against galactocerebroside, Proc. Natl. Acad. Sci. USA. 79:2709 (1982).

8. J. Sedgwick, S. Brostoff and D. Mason, Experimental allergic encephalomyelitis in the absence of a classical delayed-type hypersensitivity reaction. Severe paralytic disease correlates with the presence of interleukin 2 receptor-positive cells infiltrating the central nervous system, J. Exp. Med. 165:1058 (1987).

9. D.J. Paterson, J.R. Green, W.A. Jefferies, M. Puklavec, and A.F. Williams, The MRC OX44 antigen marks a functionally relevant subset among rat thymocytes, J. Exp. Med. 165:1 (1987).

10. H.N. Baybutt, H. Wege, M.J. Carter, and V. ter Meulen, Adaption of coronavirus JHM to persistent infection of murine Sac(-) cells, J. gen. Virol. 65:915 (1984).

11. H. Wege, J. Winter, P. Massa, R. Dörries, and V. ter Meulen, Coronavirus JHM-induced demyelinating disease: Specific domains on the E2-protein are associated with neurovirulence, in: "Coronaviruses", M.M.C. Lai and S.A. Stohlman, ed., Plenum Publishing Corporation, New York (1987).

12. J.D. Sedgwick, I.A.M. MacPhee, and M. Puklavec, Isolation of encephalitogenic CD4+ T cell clones in the rat. Cloning methodology and interferon-γ secretion, J. Immunol. Methods, 121:185 (1989).

13. D.W. Mason, W.J. Penhale, and J.D. Sedgwick, Preparation of lymphocyte subpopulations, in: "Lymphocytes, a practical approach", G.G.B. Klaus, ed., IRL Press, Oxford (1987).

14. S. Funderud, K. Nustad, T. Lea, F. Vartdal, G. Gaudernack, P. Stenstad, and J. Ugelstad, Fractionation of lymphocytes by immunomagnetic beads, in: "Lymphocytes, a practical approach", G.G.B. Klaus, ed., IRL Press, Oxford (1987).

15. S.V. Hunt, and M.H. Fowler, A repopulation assay for B and T lymphocyte stem cells employing radiation chimaeras, Cell Tissue Kinet. 14:445 (1981).

16. A. Fontana, W. Fierz, and H. Wekerle, Astrocytes present myelin basic protein to encephalitogenic T-cell lines, Nature 307:273 (1984).

17. D.W. Mason and S.J. Simmonds, The autonomy of CD8+ T cells in vitro and in vivo, Immunology, 65:249 (1988).

18. J. Sprent and M. Schaefer, Antigen-presenting cells for unprimed T cells, Immunol. Today, 10:17 (1989).

19. C. Uyttenhove, P.G. Coulie, and J. Van Snick, T cell growth and differentiation induced by interleukin-HP1/IL-6, the murine hybridoma/plasmacytoma growth factor, J. Exp. Med. 167:1417 (1988).

20. D. McKenzie, Alloantigen presentation by B cells. Requirement for IL-1 and IL-6, J. Immunol. 141:2907 (1988).

EPIGENETIC FACTORS INFLUENCING THE MORPHOGENESIS OF
PRIMARY NEURAL CELL CULTURES AND THE CONCOMITANT EFFECTS
ON ESTABLISHING JHMV INFECTIONS

J. M. M. Pasick and S. Dales

Department of Microbiology and Immunology
University of Western Ontario
London, Ontario, Canada, N6A 5C1

INTRODUCTION

The murine coronavirus, JHM, produces a spectrum of
disease in the postnatal rat ranging from an acute
encephalomyelitis to a delayed onset disease
clinicopathologically characterized by limb paresis
progressing to paralysis, with associated foci of
demyelination within white matter tracts of the
rhombencephalon and spinal cord. The type of disease
predominating in intracerebrally inoculated rat pups was
found by previous work in our laboratory to be a function
of the following host determinants: strain of animal
challenged, age at which the animal was inoculated and the
host's immunologic status (1,2,3). Other parameters such
as the phenotype of the virion's major envelope
glycoprotein, E2 (4,5,6) and the length of the latent
period or time elapsing between inoculation and
development of disease (1), are examples of other
determinants involved in the pathogenic outcome of virus
challenge in vivo.

Because of the complexity and dynamic interactions
occurring among virus, host and environment, in vivo
models by their nature make fundamental studies of basic
pathogenic mechanisms such as cell tropism and virus-cell
interactions difficult. For this reason, our laboratory
has adopted a simplified in vitro system using primary
dissociated neural cells explanted from neonatal cerebral
hemispheres for the purpose of studying fundamental virus-
cell interactions. This approach has proved particularly
fruitful in establishing the tropism of JHMV for rat
oligodendrocytes, and in providing a model which partially
explains the mechanism by which animals acquire resistance
to disease when inoculated with virus after weaning. This
latter aspect of virus-host interaction was based on the
observed restriction of virus replication in
oligodendrocyte targets induced to differentiate by the
experimental elevation of intracellular cAMP levels (7,8).

The present study extends the utility of this in vitro paradigm focusing on epigenetic factors influencing the survival and proliferation of primary neural cell populations, the influence this has on histotypic cellular organization of cultures and the concomitant consequences these have on the ability to establish persistent JHMV infections. Numerous studies have recently begun to address the developmental effects of specific hormones and growth factors on defined stages of glial precursors belonging to the oligodendrocyte lineage (9,10,11,12,13),as well as cells that have committed to become oligodendrocytes (14,15,16,17,18,19,20). Furthermore many of these same substances are also being examined for their potential neuronotrophic effects (21,22,23). A study of this nature is only possible when the composition of the extracellular environment is completely defined, thus necessitating the elimination of serum from the culture medium due to its unknown composition as well as the potential for variation to occur from batch to batch.

RESULTS AND DISCUSSION

(a) Comparison of the Morphological Appearance of Primary Dissociated Cerebral Hemisphere Cultures Grown in Either Serum Containing or Chemically Defined Medium. Primary cerebral hemisphere cultures were prepared as described previously (7) from neonatal rat pups less than 12 hours old (P0) and seeded onto poly-L-lysine treated polystyrene culture vessels in basal minimum essential medium supplemented with 10% fetal bovine serum (BME_{10}). The initial seeding density varied from .1 to .15 cerebral hemispheres per square centimeter of culture surface. At three days in vitro (DIV) and postnatal day 3 (P3), the culture medium was changed and cultures either maintained in BME_{10}, or switched to BME supplemented with 1% fetal bovine serum (BME_1), or to a serum free chemically defined medium first described by Bottenstein (19). Briefly, this latter medium, O1, consists of Dulbecco's modified Eagle's medium (DMEM) supplemented with 1.2 g of $NaHCO_3$/l, 15mM Hepes (pH 7.3), 5ug bovine insulin/ml, 50ug human transferrin/ml, 30 nM sodium selenite, and 10 ng d-biotin/ml. In the initial experiments tri-iodothyronine (T3) was also added to O1 at a concentration of 30 nM. This additional supplement was included because of the well documented effects this hormone is known to have on postnatal CNS development in the rat, particularly myelination (24,25,26,27).

The morphological differences observed between primary cultures grown either in the presence of serum or in chemically defined medium were substantial and are illustrated in figure 1. Generally speaking, cultures under either situation possessed a similar phenotypic appearance when viewed with phase contrast microscopy until 6-7 DIV. At this time cultures grown in the presence of 10% FBS began to take on a typical stratified appearance in which phase light, glial fibrillary acidic protein positive (GFAP+), epithelioid astrocytes proliferated to form a basal layer over which an upper layer of evenly spaced, phase dark, process bearing, galactosyl cerebroside positive (GC+) oligodendrocytes were located (Fig. 1a). By contrast, at 6-7 DIV, primary dissociated cerebral explant cultures grown in O1 since 3 DIV did not exhibit a notable proliferation of an epithelioid, astrocytic sub-layer but rather, most of the cells were of relatively high phase density, were heterogenous with respect to morphology, and produced a highly extensive network of processes (Fig. 1b).Many of these basal, process bearing cells were labelled positively with the monoclonal antibody A2B5 which recognizes a surface tetraganglioside, and is both a weak marker for neurons and a high avidity marker for O2-A progenitor cells of the oligodendrocytic-type 2 astrocytic lineage (28,29). Overlying this basal layer was a cell type with a relatively small cell soma which was organized into clusters and chains that covered the culture surface. Early in culture these cells are labelled positively with A2B5 and later become GC+. The marked differences in morphogenesis between the two culture conditions were a consistent finding and it is interesting to note that in a previous report dealing with primary murine cerebellar cultures, the removal of neurons from culture was associated with a change of astrocytes from star-shaped to epithelioid in morphology and also accompanied by concomitant astrocyte proliferation (30).

Electron microscopic studies of primary neural cultures grown under the two environmental conditions described above complement the observations noted in phase contrast images. Cultures grown in BME_{10} are relatively simple in terms of cells types present and their organization. These cultures consisted of a basal layer of cells comprised of flat, intermediate filament containing astrocytes over which lie rounded oligodendrocytes. Cells cultured in O1 were more heterogenous in ultrastructural appearance and possessed a more complex organization. Many areas of these cultures bore processes which on cross-section contained regularly arranged arrays of microtubules and mitochondria characteristics of both dendrites and axons (Fig. 2a,b).

(b) <u>Comparison of the Ability of JHMV to Establish Persistent Infections in Primary Neural Cultures Grown in the Presence and Absence of Serum.</u> The initial experiments sought to determine if the presence of T3, a hormone putatively involved in postnatal myelination, could influence the ability of JHMV to establish persistent infections in primary dissociated cerebral hemisphere cultures derived from Wistar Furth neonates. Cultures grown under no serum, low serum, or high serum conditions in the presence or absence of T3 or the cAMP analogue N6,O2'-dibutyryladenosine 3':5'-cyclic monophosphate (dbcAMP) were infected at P10 with JHMV at a m.o.i. of 1. At regular intervals post inoculation, dilutions of the culture supernatants were assayed for virus titre on monolayers of L-2 murine fibroblasts. A representative example of one such experiment is illustrated in figure 3. As can be seen, a marked difference was observed in both the magnitude of virus production and the length of time

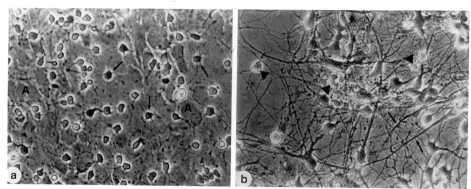

Fig. 1. a. Selected area from brain explant cultured in vitro for 10 days in the presence of BME_{10} nutrient medium. A = astrocytic cell type; arrows point towards oligodendrocytic cell type. Mag. x 1,600.

b. Selected area from a brain explant cultured in vitro for 10 days in the presence of defined 01 nutrient medium. Arrows point towards extensive processes emanating from cells with neuronal morphology. Arrowheads identify adherent cells of the GC+ type (oligodendrocytes). Mag. x 1,600.

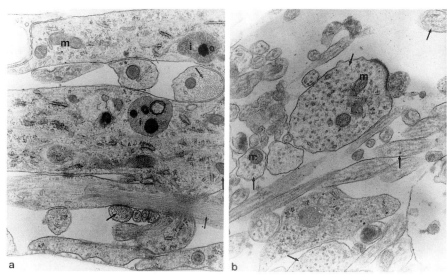

Fig. 2.   a. Selected area of a culture like
             that in 1a, preserved in situ for
             electron microscopy. Arrows point
             towards prominent bundles of
             intermediate filaments of the type
             associated with GFAP+ astrocytes.
             Stratification of cell layers is
             evident. m = mitochondrion, i =
             inclusion of indeterminate type. x
             32,000.

          b. Selected area of a culture like
             that in figure 1b, preserved in
             situ for electron microscopy.
             Arrows point towards processes
             containing numerous microtubules,
             evident in longitudinal and cross
             sections. Note absence of bundles
             of intermediate filaments,
             prominent in 2a. m =
             mitochondrion. x 41,000.

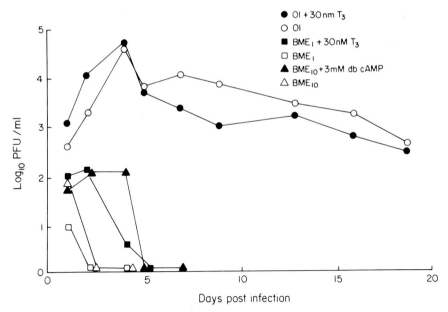

Fig. 3. JHMV replication was assayed on dissociated
cerebral hemisphere cultures derived
from PO Wistar Furth (WF) rats.
Cultures were either grown continuously
in BME_{10} or switched to BME_1 or nutrient
medium 01 with or without T3 at 3 DIV.
Cultures receiving dbcAMP were treated
48 hrs. prior to and 48 hrs., after JHMV
infection. All cultures were infected
at 10 DIV and all points represent the
mean titre of duplicate cultures.

which the cultures were persistently infected in serum
free versus low or high serum conditions. In our
experience T3 did not appear to influence the character of
virus production in cultures grown under chemically
defined conditions and thus the role it plays in the
differentiation of cells of the oligodendrocyte lineage,
and the effect this has on JHMV replication at this stage
remains ambiguous.

These results did prompt us, however, to question the
influence that pre-exposure to varying concentrations of
dbcAMP would have on the ability of JHMV to establish
persistent infections in primary cultures grown under
chemically defined conditions. The results of one such
experiment are illustrated in figure 4. Instead of
inhibition of virus replication as was previously reported
in oligodendrocyte enriched cultures (7,8), either no
inhibition or varying degrees of enhancement of virus
replication were observed. This result led us to consider

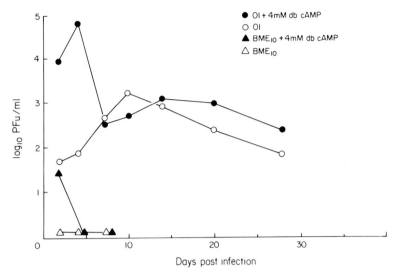

Fig. 4. JHMV replication was assayed on dissociated cerebral hemisphere cultures derived from PO WF rats. Cultures were either grown continuously in BME_{10} or switched to defined nutrient medium O1 at 3 DIV. Cultures receiving dbcAMP were treated for 48 hrs. prior to and 72 hrs. after being infected with JHMV at an m.o.i. of 1. All cultures were infected at 10 DIV, and all points represent the mean titre of duplicate cultures.

the possibilities that either oligodendrocytes were arrested at a stage in their differentiation process which was refractive to the viral inhibitory effects of experimental elevation of intracellular cAMP levels or that another cell type was responsible for replicating the virus. The former explanation seemed unlikely because of a number of reports (12,13,14,15,16,17,18,20) which indicated that precursor cells of the oligodendrocyte lineage and cells committed to become oligodendrocytes can undergo normal or accelerated differentiation in chemically defined media similar in composition to the one used in our experiments. To help distinguish between these two possibilities, it was decided to assess the direct effects of medium O1 both in the presence and absence of dbcAMP on cultures enriched for oligodendrocytes with respect to their ability to support a JHMV infection.

(c) <u>Comparison of Enriched Cultures of Oligodendrocytes in Serum containing and Chemically Defined Conditions to Support JHMV Infection.</u> Oligodendrocytes were released from primary mixed cultures grown in BME_{10} at 7 DIV as previously described (7). Briefly, mixed cultures in 75 cm$_2$ Corning flat bottom flasks were replenished with 10 ml of fresh medium. The flasks were then sealed and placed on a rotary shaker and agitated for 120 minutes at 300 rpm. This method selectively releases oligodendrocytes from mixed culture on the basis of their less adherent nature. The cells in suspension were pelleted by centrifugation, resuspended and plated onto a 24 well plate (Nunc) at a density of 5 x 10^5 cells per well. Half of the released oligodendrocytes were continued in BME$_{10}$, and the remainder were seeded onto wells previously coated with FBS and propagated in defined medium O1. At 24 hours after seeding (8 DIV), one half of cultures grown in BME$_{10}$ and O1 were exposed to 5 mM dbcAMP. Exposure to dbcAMP continued for a total of 48 hours prior to inoculating cultures with 1 m.o.i. of JHMV (11 DIV) and for an additional 24 hours post inoculation. Culture supernatants were removed at 24 hour intervals from cultures of each treatment and virus titre determined by inoculating serial dilutions onto L-2 cell monolayers.

Consistent with previous experiments in this laboratory, shaken oligodendrocyte cultures grown in BME$_{10}$ were able to replicate JHMV efficiently over several days, whereas prior exposure to dbcAMP under these culture conditions inhibited virus replication (Fig 5). Oligodendrocytes cultured in O1 either in the absence or presence of dbcAMP however, were unable to replicate virus. This result is consistent with the observations that oligodendrocytes are capable of differentiating in defined medium in the absence of other cell types, and suggests the possibility that this cell type is not responsible for replicating the virus under mixed culture conditions. A possible explanation for the apparent inability of oligodendrocytes in mixed culture conditions grown in BME$_{10}$ to establish persistent infections may involve cell density as has already shown to play a role in establishing infections in enriched cultures (7). A second possibility is that some mode of heterotypic intercellular interaction either in the form of a soluble factor released by astrocytes, or the direct physical contact with astrocytes may somehow suppress virus replication in oligodendrocytes derived from mixed cultures.

The complementary experiment to the one just described involved assessing the ability of the tightly adherent, residual cells remaining after releasing oligodendrocytes from mixed culture to replicate JHMV under the identical conditions assayed for enriched oligodendrocyte cultures. For this purpose, primary cerebral hemisphere cultures derived from P0 Wistar Furth rats were grown either continuously in BME$_{10}$ or switched to nutrient medium O1 after 3 DIV. At 7 DIV, loosely adherent cells in both culture conditions were removed by shaking. The cells remaining in cultures, grown continuously in BME10 from the time of explantation, were very homogeneous in appearance and consisted almost entirely of astrocytes with epithelioid morphology. By contrast, the residual cells in cultures grown in nutrient medium O1 were heterogenous in appearance and were characterized by cells possessing various sized cell soma from which irradiated a complex network of processes. Many of these cells possessed processes with a definite polarity typical of neurites.

Residual cells in BME_{10} were either exposed to 5 mM dbcAMP or were left as unexposed controls. Residual cells cultured in O1 were also treated in a similar manner. After 72 hours of exposure to dbcAMP and 10 DIV, all cultures were inoculated with JHMV at a m.o.i. of 1. Dilutions of culture supernatant were assayed on L-2 cell monolayers for virus titre at 24 hour intervals. The results of one such experiment are summarized in Table 1.

REPLICATION OF JHMV IN SHAKEN WISTAR FURTH CEREBRAL CULTURES ENRICHED FOR OLIGODENDROCYTES

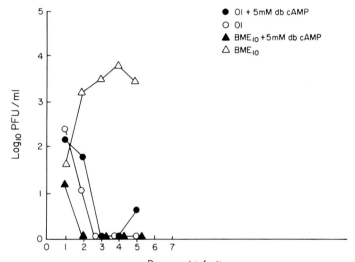

Fig. 5. Oligodendrocytes were mechanically released from primary culture grown in BME_{10} at 7 DIV as described in the text. Secondary culture of enriched oligodendrocytes were then established at a density of $2 \times 10^5/cm^2$ in either BME_{10} or defined nutrient medium O1. One half of the cultures were exposed to dbcAMP 48 hrs. prior to and 24 hrs. after infecting with JHMV at an m.o.i. of 1. All cultures were infected at 11 DIV, and all points represent the mean titre of triplicate cultures.

This demonstrates that the population of tightly adherent cells grown in nutrient medium O1 are different with respect to both morphology and ability to replicate virus when compared with the residual cells grown in BME_{10}.

Based on the data we have acquired to date, it appears that serum free conditions favour the survival of a cell type which we tentatively believe to be neuronal. The current data also leads us to speculate that this presumed neuronal cell type may not respond to the experimental elevation of intracellular cAMP levels in the same way that oligodendrocytes do with respect to JHMV replication. Experiments conducted on murine C1300 neuroblastomas have shown that pretreatment with dbcAMP enhances instead of inhibits virus production over that of untreated controls, a result which is consistent with the hypothesis that elevation of intracellular cAMP levels within neurons does not inhibit JHMV replication. This may have important implications with respect to spread of virus in the CNS, the cell type it may persist in after weaning, as well as the type of disease it is capable of producing as a function of the age of the host in vivo. Studies are presently under way to characterize the ability of cultures enriched in primary neurons as well as cultures of other rodent neuroblastomas to replicate JHMV after exposure to dbcAMP. We are particularly interested in the biochemical effects this has on the production of the free regulatory subunit, RI, of the cAMP-dependent protein kinases in primary neurons and cell lines of neuronal origin as compared with that observed in oligodendrocytes (8). Results from such studies may provide valuable lessons on the neurobiological determinants involved in establishing a persistent viral infection within the CNS.

JHMV Replication in Cultures
of Tightly Adherent Cells.

TREATMENT OF CULTURES	DAYS POST INFECTION			
	1	2	3	4
01 + 5mm dbcAMP	10	200	98	110
01	10	190	71	22
BME_{10} + 5mm dbcAMP	5.0	2.7	1.2	1.3
BME_{10}	6.8	.75	.05	0

Note: All titres expressed as 10^2 PFU/ml.
       All cultures infected at an M.O.1. of 1

ACKNOWLEDGEMENTS

We acknowledge the technical assistance of Sharon Wilton in the preparation of electron micrographs. This study was supported by the Multiple Sclerosis Society and Medical Research Council of Canada. J.M.M.P. is a recipient of a Multiple Sclerosis Society Postdoctoral Fellowship.

REFERENCES

1. O. Sorensen, D. Percy, and S. Dales, In vivo and in vitro models of demyelinating diseases III. JHM virus infections of rats, <u>Archives of Neurol.</u> 37:478-484 (1980).

2. O. Soresen, R. Dugre, D. Percy, and S. Dales, In vivo and in vitro models of demylinating disease: Endogenous factors, influencing demyelinating disease caused by mouse hepatitis virus in rats and mice, <u>Infect. and Immun.</u> 37:1248-1260 (1982).

3. M. J. Zimmer, and S. Dales, In vivo and in vitro models of demyelinating diseases XXIV. The infectious process in cyclosporin A treated wistar lewis rats inoculated with JHMV virus, <u>Microbial Path.</u> 6:7-16 (1989).

4. H. Wege, J. Winter, and R. Meyermann, The peplomer protein E2 of coronavirus JHMV as a determinant of neurovirulence: Definition of critical epitopes by variant analysis, <u>J. Gen. Virol.</u> 69:87-98 (1988).

5. M. J. Buchmeier, R. G. Dalziel, and M. J. M. Koolen, Coronavirus-induced CNS disease: a model for virus-induced demyelination, <u>J. Neuroimmunol.</u> 20:111-116 (1988).

6. V. L. Morris, C. Tieszer, J, Mackinnon, and D. Percy, Characterization of coronavirus JHM variants isolated from wistar furth rats with a viral-induced demyelinating disease, <u>Virology</u> 169:127--136 (1989).

7. S. Beushausen, and S. Dales, In vivo and in vitro models of demyelinating disease XI. Tropism and differentiation regulate the infectious process of coronaviruses in primary explants of the rat CNS, <u>Virology.</u> 141:89-101 (1985).

8. S. Beushausen, S. Narindrasorasak, B. D. Sanwal, and S. Dales, In vivo and vitro models of demyelinating disease: Activation of the adenylate cyclase system influences JHM virus expression in explanted rat oligodendrocytes, <u>J. Virol.</u> 61:3795-3803 (1987).

9. W. D. Richardson, N. Pringle, M. J. Mosley, B. Westermark, and M. Dubois-Dalcy, A role for platelet-derived growth factor in normal gliogenesis in the central nervous system, <u>Cell.</u> 53:309-319 (1988).

10. M. Noble, K. Murray, P. Stroobant, M. D. Waterfield, and P. Riddle, Platelet-derived growth factor promotes division and mobility and inhibits premature differentiation of the oligodendrocyte/type 2 astrocyte progenitor cell, <u>Nature.</u> 333:560-562 (1988).

11. M. C. Roff, L. E. Lillien, W. D. Richardson, J. F. Burne, and M. D. Noble, Platelet-derived growth factor from astroytes drives the clock that times oligodendrocyte development in culture, <u>Nature.</u> 333:562-565 (1988).

12. T. Bahar, F. A. McMorris, E. A. Novotny, J. L. Barker, and M. Dubois-Daley, Growth and differentiation properties of O-2A progenitors purified from rat cerebral hemispheres, <u>J. Neurosci Res.</u> 21:168-180 (1988).

13. F. A. McMorris and M. Dubois-Dalcy, Insulin-like growth factor promotes cell proliferation and oligodendrogial commitment it rat glial pronitor cells developing in vitro, <u>J. Neurosci. Res.</u> 21:168-180 (1988).

14. F. A. McMorris, T. M. Smith, S. DeSalvo, and R. Furlanetto, Insulin-like growth factor I/somatomedin C: A potent inducer of oligodendrocyte development, <u>Proc. Natl. Acad. Sci. USA</u> 83:822-826 (1986).

15. R. H. M. van der Pal, J. W. Koper, L. M. G. van Golde, and M. Lopes-Cardozo, Effects of insulin-like growth factor (IGF-I) on oligodendrocyte-enriched glial cultures, <u>J. Neurosci. Res.</u> 19:483-490 (1988).

16. P. A. Eccleston, and D. H. Silberberg, The differentiation of oligodendrocytes in a serum-free hormone-supplemented medium, <u>Develop. Brain Res.</u> 16:1-9 (1984).

17. R. P. Saneto, and J. DeVellis, Characterization of cultured rat oligodendrocytes proliferating in a serum-free, chemically defined medium, <u>Proc. Natl. Acad. Sci. U.S.A.</u> 82:3509-3513 (1985).

18. J. W. Koper, M. Lopes-Cardozo, H. J. Romijn, and L. M. G. Van Golde, Culture of rat cerebral oligodendrocytes in a serum-free, chemically defined medium, <u>J. Neurosci. Methods.</u> 10:157-169 (1984).

19. J. E. Bottenstein, Growth requirements in vitro of oligodendrocyte cell lines and neonatal rat brain oligodendrocytes, <u>Pro. Natl. Acad. Sci. U.S.A.</u> 83:1955-1959 (1986).

20. A. L. Gard and S. E. Pfeiffer, Oligodendrocyte progenitors isolated directly from developing telencephalon at a specific phenotypic stage: myelinogenic potential in a defined environment, <u>Development</u> 106:119-132 (1989).

21. J. E. Bottenstein, and G. H. Sato, Growth of a rat neuroblastmoma cell line in serum-free supplemented medium, <u>Proc. Natl. Acad. Sci. U.S.A.</u> 76:514-517 (1979).

22. R. Garza, J. H. Dussault, and J. Puymirat, Influence of triiodothyronine (L-T3) on the morphological and biochemical development of fetal brain acetycholinesterase-positive neurons cultured in a chemically defined medium, <u>Develop. Brain Res.</u> 43:287-297 (1988).

23. A. J. Patel, M. Hayashi, and A. Hunt, Role of thyroid hormone and nerve growth factor in the development of choline acetyltransferase and other cell-specific marker enzymes in the basal forebrain of the rat, <u>J. Neurochem.</u> 50:803-811 (1988).

24. A. Rami, A Rabie, and A. J. Patel, Thyroid hormone and development of the rat hippocampus: Cell acquisition in the dentate gyrus, Neuroscience 19:1207-1216 (1986).
25. A. Rami, A. J. Patel, and A. Ralsie, Thyroid hormond and development of the rat hippocampus: Morphological alterations in gramule and pyramidal cells, Neuroscience 19:1217-1226 (1986).
26. J. W. Koper, R. C. Hoeben, F. M. H. Hachstenback, L. M. G. Van Golde, and M, Lopes-Cardozo, Effects of triiodothyromine on the synthesis of sulfolipids by oligodendroyte-enriched glial cultures, Biochim. et Biophys. Acta 887:321-334 (1986).
27. F. Courtin, F. Chantoux, and J. Franeon, Thyroid hormone metabolism by glial cells in primary culture, Mol. Cell. Endocrin. 48:167-178 (1986).
28. G. S. Eisenbarth, F. S. Walsh, and M. Nirenberg, Monoclonal antibody to a plasma membrane antigen of neurons, Proc. Natl. Acad. Sci. U. S. A. 76:4913-4917 (1979).
29. M. C. Raff, R. H. Miller, M. Noble, A glial progenitor cell that develops in vitro into an astrocyte or an oligodendrocyte depending on culture medium, Nature 303:390-396 (1983).
30. I. Nagata, G. Keilhauer, and M. Schachner, Neuronal influence on antigenic marker profile, cell shape and proliferation of cultured astrocytes obtained by microdisection of distinct layers from the postnatal mouse cerebellum, Develop. Brain Res. 24: 217-232 (1986).

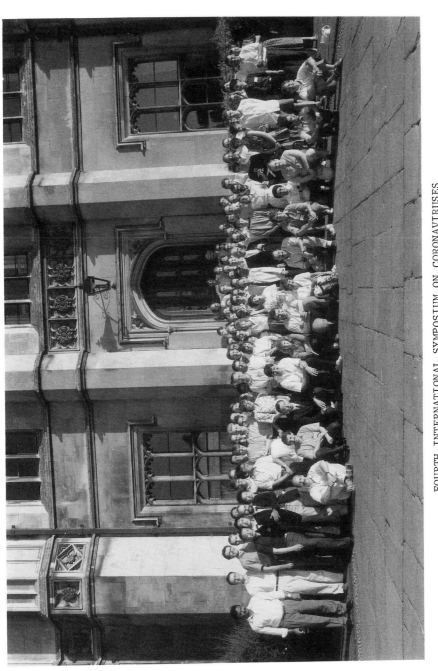

FOURTH INTERNATIONAL SYMPOSIUM ON CORONAVIRUSES
July 16–21, 1989, Cambridge, United Kingdom

A59 virus, see Murine hepatitis virus, A59 strain
Antibody (see also Monoclonal antibody
  Fc binding to S protein, 51
  to HE protein, 103, 173
  IgA in milk after PRCV, 421
  PRCV - maternal antibody, 429
  to MHV non-structural proteins, 291
Antibody neutralization
  anti-HE protein antibodies, 103, 173, 457
  anti-S protein antibodies, 143, 151, 159, 173, 181, 211, 457
  neutralizing IgA in milk, 421
Astrocytes (see also Glial cells)
  as antigen presenting cells, 647
  MHC antigens after MHV4 infection, 579
Avian infectious bronchitis virus see infectious bronchitis virus

Baculovirus expression
  of M protein of TGEV, 223
  of N protein of TGEV, 223
  of S protein of MHV-JHM, 211
  of S protein of TGEV, 223
Berne virus, 307
Bovine coronavirus (BCV)
  detection in clinical specimens, 467
  genome organisation, 81, 103
  HE protein, 81, 95, 103, 173
  monoclonal antibodies, 457, 461
  relationship with TCV, 457
  sequence comparison with MHV, 81
  variation among isolates, 461

Canine coronavirus (CCV)
  CCV infection in cats, 475
  monoclonal antibodies, 159
Cardiomyopathy, 511

Cell-mediated immunity in MHV infection
  astrocytes as antigen presenting cells, 647
  lymphoid cells in brain parenchyma, 629
  MHV clearance, 557, 573
  reviews, 555, 623
Central nervous system diseases
    (see also demyelination)
    (see also encephalomyelitis)
  astrocytes as antigen presenting cells, 647
  epigenetic factors and neural cell cultures, 655
  expression of MHC antigens, 557, 579, 593
  immune response and CNS disease, 557, 565, 573, 629, 637
  response of different mouse strains to JHM-CC, 617
  primary dissociated neural cell cultures, 655
  reviews, 555, 623
  T cell-mediated clearance of MHV-JHM in mice, 557, 573
  vacuolar degeneration and JHM-CC, 601
  vacuolar encephalomyelopathy and JHM-CC, 609

Defective-interfering particles, leader RNA switching, 341
Demyelination (see also Central nervous system disease)
  abrogation of by immunosuppression, 565
  immunopathogenesis induced by MHV-4, 565
  late onset in suckling mice, 573
  reviews, 555, 623

E.coli, expression in,
  of IBV N protein, 189

E.coli, expression in (continued)
of IBV S protein, 181
of MHV non-structural proteins, 291, 317
of MHV-A59 S protein, 181
of TGEV S protein polypeptides, 151, 159, 181
E1 protein, see Membrane protein (M)
E2 protein, see Spike protein (S)
Encephalomyelitis (see also Central nervous system diseases)
encephalomyelopathy and JHM-CC, 601, 609, 617
lymphoid cells in brain parenchyma, of Lewis and BN rats, 629
review, 623
types of encephalopathy, 637
Endoglycosidase H, 9
Epitopes
linear neutralizing epitopes, 181
of TGEV S protein fragments, 151, 159
on S protein, 139
of BCV, 173
of FIPV, 181
of IBV, 143, 181
of MHV-A59, 181
of PRVC, 435
of TGEV, 151, 159, 181
on M protein, 139
on HE protein, 139
of BCV, 173
on N protein, T cell epitopes, 181
on proteolytic fragments, 151, 159
review, 139
role of glycosylation, 143
Evolution
deletions in genome, 385
influenza C virus and corona-virus relationships, 2 1 , 81, 103
organ tropism, 379, 385, 395, 403, 411
recombination, 341
review, 367
TGEV and PRCV, 159, 419, 421, 435, 441
torovirus and coronavirus relationships, 307
Expression see Baculovirus expression,
see E.coli, expression in,
see Vaccinia virus expression

Feline enteric coronavirus (FECV)
monoclonal antibodies, 159
Feline infectious peritonitis virus (FIPV)
attenuated ts vaccine variant, 481
biosynthesis of S protein, 9
candidate vaccine variant, 481
early death syndrome, 217, 475
expression of S protein, 9, 217
CCV role in feline infectious peritonitis, 475
monoclonal antibodies, 159
Fusion
FIPV recombinant S protein, 9
IBV in Vero cells, 33
MHV-A59 recombinant S protein, 9
MHV-JHM recombinant S protein, 21
pH, 33
variation among MHV isolates, 411

Genes, see RNA
Genome organisation
BCV, 81, 103
TGEV, 357
Glial cells (see also Astrocytes, and Oligodendrocytes)
increase in mRNAs for MHC antigens, 593

H-2, see Major histocompatibility complex
Hemagglutinating encephalomyelitis virus (HEV)
HE protein purification, 109
monoclonal antibodies, 159
Hemagglutinin-esterase protein (HE)
acetylesterase activity, 5, 21, 103, 109
action on erythrocytes, 109
antibody inhibition of esterase, 103
cell surface location, 95
epitopes, 139
expression with vaccinia virus, 21
membrane orientation, 95
nomenclature, 1
of TCV, 449
purification, 109
review, 5, 91
sequence, BCV, 81, 95, 103
structure, 5, 81
Hemagglutination
inhibition by anti-HE antibody, 103, 449

Hemadsorption
    by cells expressing HE protein,
        21
Human coronavirus OC43
    replication in human colon cells
        and mouse intestine, 497
Human coronavirus 229E
    growth curve, 73
    virion polypeptides, 73
    monoclonal antibodies, 159
Humoral Immunity see Antibody,
        see Monoclonal antibody,
        see Antibody neutralization
Hygromycin B, 67

Immunopathology
    FIPV and S protein, 217
    in MHV persistency, 637
    role in demyelination, 565
Infectious bronchitis virus (IBV)
    ammonium chloride, 33
    neutralising   monoclonal
        antibodies, 143
    organ tropism, 379
    polymerase, 275
    recombination, 369
    ribosomal   frameshift   signals,
        269
    susceptibility of chicken lines,
        491
    syncytium-induction, 33
    T-cell epitopes of N protein,
        189
    T-cell hybridomas, 189
    variation, 369, 373, 379
Influenza C virus
    cell receptors, 115
    relationship with coronaviruses,
        21, 81, 103
In situ hybridization
    coronavirus RNA in human CNS
        tissue, 505
    of MHC H-2 class RNA probes with
        MHV A59 infected brain
        cells, 593
    MHV-JHM route to CNS, 573

JHM, see Murine hepatitis virus,
        JHM strain

Leader RNA
    leader RNA switching, 341
    leader-primed transcription, 327
    structure and binding to N, 247

Major   histocompatibility   complex
        (MHC)

Major   histocompatibility   complex
        (MHC) (continued)
    modulation   of   MHC   antigens
        following MHV infection,
        557, 579, 593
Membrane protein (M)
    epitopes, 139
    expression, 121, 127
    function, 5, 91
    intracellular   transport,   121,
        127
    nomenclature, 1
    of HCV-229E, 73
    of TCV, 449
    review, 5, 91
    structure, 1, 73
MHV-S
    N protein sequence, 239
Monoclonal   antibody   (see   also
        Neutralization   resistant
        variants)
    purification of S protein, 205
    to non-structural proteins, 317
    to S protein
        of BCV, 173
        of IBV, 143, 181
        of MHV-A59, 181, 265
        of MHV-JHM, 211, 385
        of TGEV, 151, 159, 181
        of TCV, 449, 457
    to HE protein
        of BCV, 103, 173
        of TCV, 449, 457
    to M protein of TCV, 449
    to N protein of TCV, 449, 457
Monoclonal   antibody-resistant
        mutants, see neutraliza-
        tion-resistant variants
Murine hepatitis virus-3 (MHV-3)
    B and T lymphotropisms, 543
    N protein sequence, 239
    organ tropism of variants, 403
    protective   effect   of
        prostaglandin E, 533
Murine   hepatitis   virus-4   (MHV-4)
        see   Murine   hepatitis
        virus-JHM strain
Murine hepatitis virus, A59 strain
    cell receptor, 37, 45
    fusion, 9, 59
    in mouse fibroblast mutants, 59
    leader RNA secondary structure,
        247
    M protein, 127
    membrane   permeability   alter-
        ations, 67
    non-structural   proteins,   283,
        291

Murine hepatitis virus, A59 strain
      (continued)
   N protein sequence, 239
   polymerase, 291
   species specificity, 37, 45
   protection by S protein, 205
Murine hepatitis virus, JHM strain
   defective-interfering RNA, 341
   deletions in S protein, 385,
      395, 411
   dephosphorylation of N protein,
      255, 261
   Fc binding by S protein, 51
   fusion, 21, 411
   HE protein expression, 21
   hemadsorption, 21
   JHM-CC variant, 601, 609, 617
   N protein sequence, 239
   non-structural proteins, 317
   polymerase, 283
   retinopathy in mice, 519
Multiple sclerosis
   presence of coronavirus RNA, 505

Neuroattenuated MHV variants
   deletions in S protein, 385,
      395, 411
   non-fatal disease and JHM-CC,
      601, 609, 617
Neutralization-resistant variants
      (see also Antibody
      neutralization)
   of TGEV, 151, 159
   of MHV, 385, 395, 403
Non-structural proteins
   BCV, 81
   IBV, 275, 307
   MHV, 283, 291, 307, 317
   TGEV, 301, 357
Nucleocapsid protein (N)
   binding to leader RNA, 247
   dephosphorylation, 255
   distribution in CNS tissue, 637
   nomenclature, 1
   of HCV-229E
   of TCV, 449
   review, 235
   structure and function, 235, 239

Oligodendrocytes (see also Glial
      cells)
   MHV-JHM infection, 565, 655
   MHV,JHM replication inhibition,
      261

Organ tropism
   IBV, 379
   MHV, 385, 395, 403

Oligodendrocytes (continued)
   MHV3 in B and T lymphocytes, 543
   PRCV, 419, 429

Peplomer see Spike protein (S)
Peptides (see also Antibody,
      see also Antibody neutraliz-
      ation
   of IBV S protein, 181
   of MHV-A59 S protein, 181
   of TGEV S protein, 151, 159, 181
Persistent infection
   differential role of humoral and
      cell-mediated immunity,
      573
   of MHV in primary neural
      cultures, 657
   immunopathological aspects in
      rats, 637
   MHV-A59, 59, 67
Phosphoprotein phosphatase, 255,
      261
Polymerase, RNA
   autoproteolytic activity, 283
   comparison with toroviruses, 307
   polypeptides of, 275, 283, 307
   ribosomal frameshift signal,
      269, 307
   sequence data, 283, 301, 307
Polymerase chain reaction, 467
Porcine epidemic diarrhoea virus
      (PEDV)
   monoclonal antibodies, 159
Porcine respiratory coronavirus
      (PRCV)
   differentiation from TGEV, 159,
      435, 441
   milk IgA antibodies, 421
   mRNAs, 441
   monoclonal antibody analysis,
      159, 435
   organ tropism, 429
   proteins, 441
   review, 419
   role of maternal antibody, 429
Porcine transmissible gastro-
      enteritis virus, see
      Transmissible gastro-
      enteritis virus
Probes, labelling systems, 467
Prostaglandin E, 533
Protective immune responses
   induced by S protein, 205

Rabbit coronavirus (RbCV)
   rabbit dilated cardiomyopathy,
      511

Receptors, cell
  on erythrocytes, 109, 115
  for MHV-A59, 37, 45
  resialylation of erythrocytes,
    115
Recombinant vaccines
  review, 201
  see also Baculovirus expression
  see also E.coli, expression in
  see also Peptides
  see also Vaccinia virus
    expression
  review, 201
Recombination
  evidence for in IBV, 369
  leader RNA switching, 341
Reproductive disorders in rats, 525
Resistance, genetic
  cell receptors, 37, 45
  differential recovery from IBV,
    491
  mouse fibroblast mutants, 59
Retinopathy, 519
Ribosomal frameshifting, 269
RNA (see also Sequence, RNA)
  gene nomenclature, 1
  mRNA nomenclature, 1

Sequence, protein
  BCV HE protein, 81, 95, 103
  MHV S protein, 395
  protease domain of gene 1, 283
  TGEV neutralization resistant
    variants, 151, 159
  TGEV S protein, 223, 301
Sequence, RNA
  3′ end of IBV genome, 373
  BCV HE protein, 95
  MHV S protein, 395
  protease domain of gene 1, 283
  TGEV S protein, 301
Sequence similarity
  of S protein of MHV variants,
    395
  of Massachusetts variants of
    IBV, 369
  HE protein and influenza C virus
    HEF protein, 21, 81, 103
Sialodacryoadenitis virus, 525
Spike protein (S)
  attachment to cells, 5, 37, 45
  BCV S characteristics, 81
  binding to Fc of immunoglobulin,
    51
  biosynthesis, 9
  deletions, 385, 395, 411, 441
  distribution in CNS tissue, 637

Spike protein (S) (continued)
  epitopes, 139, 143, 151, 159,
    385, 395, 435
  expression with baculovirus, 211
  expression with vaccinia virus,
    9, 21
  fusion, see Fusion
  hemadsorption, 21
  induction of protection, 205
  intracellular transport, 9
  nomenclature, 1
  of TCV, 449
  oligomerization, 9
  purification by monoclonal
    antibody, 205
  review, 5
  structure, 5, 9, 73, 84, 223,
    301, 385, 395
Susceptibility, see Resistance,
    genetic
Syncytia, see Fusion

T-cell (see also Cell-mediated
    immunity)
  T-cell hybridomas, 189
Temperature-sensitive (ts) mutants
  genetic map of ts mutants of
    MHV-A59, 349
  N gene of MHV-A59, 239
  of FIPV, for vaccine, 481
Tissue tropism, see Organ tropism
Toroviruses, 307
Transcription
  review, 327
  subgenomic minus strand RNA, 335
  subgenomic replicons, 335
Transmissible gastroenteritis virus
    (TGEV)
  antigenic sites on S protein,
    151, 159
  expression of M protein, 121,
    223
  expression of N protein, 223
  expression of S protein, 223
  genome organisation, 357
  polymerase, 301
  subgenomic minus strand RNA, 335
Tunicamycin, 449
Turkey coronavirus TCV
  monoclonal antibodies, 449, 457
  protease treatment, 449
  relationship with BCV, 457
  virion proteins, 449

Uncoating, virus (see also Fusion)
  IBV, 33
  MHV, 411

Vaccines (see also Recombinant
        vaccines)
  candidate vaccine for FIPV, 481
Vaccinia virus expression
    of FIPV S protein, 9, 217
    of IBV S protein, 9
    of MHV-A59 M protein, 127
    of MHV-A59 S protein, 9
    of MHV-JHM HE protein, 21
    of MHV-JHM S protein, 21
    of TGEV M protein, 121, 223
    of TGEV N protein, 223
    of TGEV S protein, 223

Variants of viruses (see also
        Neutralization-resistant
        variants)
  HCV OC43, 497
  IBV, 369, 373, 379,
  MHV N protein, 239
  PRCV, 159, 435
  TGEV, 159, 301